Neural Network Design

Martin T. Hagan
Oklahoma State University

Howard B. Demuth
University of Idaho

Mark Beale
MHB, Inc.

PWS Publishing Company

I(T)P

An International Thomson Publishing Company

Boston • Albany • Bonn • Cincinnati • Detroit • London • Madrid • Melbourne
Mexico City • New York • Paris • San Francisco • Singapore • Tokyo • Toronto • Washington

PWS PUBLISHING COMPANY

20 Park Plaza, Boston, MA 02116-4324

MTH
To Janet, Thomas, Daniel, Mom and Dad
HBD
To Hal, Katherine, Kimberly, and Mary
MHB
To Teri, Mom and Dad

I(T)P™
International Thomson Publishing
The trademark ITP is used under license

For more information, contact:

PWS Publishing Co.
20 Park Plaza
Boston, MA 02116

International Thomson Publishing Europe
Berkshire House I68-I73
High Holborn
London WC1V 7AA
England

Thomas Nelson Australia
102 Dodds Street
South Melbourne, 3205
Victoria, Australia

Nelson Canada
1120 Birchmount Road
Scarborough, Ontario
Canada M1K 5G4

International Thomson Editores
Campos Eliseos 385, Piso 7
Col. Polanco
11560 Mexico D.F., Mexico

International Thomson Publishing GmbH
Konigswinterer Strasse 418
53227 Bonn, Germany

International Thomson Publishing Asia
221 Henderson Road
#05-10 Henderson Building
Singapore 0315

International Thomson Publishing Japan
Hirakawacho Kyowa Building, 31
2-2-1 Hirakawacho
Chiyoda-ku, Tokyo 102
Japan

Acquisitions Editor: Bill Barter
Assistant Editor: Ken Morton
Editorial Assistant: Monica Bond
Production Editor and Cover Design: Pamela Rockwell
Cover Art: Vanessa Pineiro
Manufacturing Coordinator: Ellen Glisker
Marketing Manager: Nathan Wilbur
Cover Printer: Coral Graphic Services, Inc.
Text Printer and Binder: Quebecor/Hawkins

Library of Congress Cataloging-in-Publication Data
Hagan, Martin T.
   Neural network design / Martin T. Hagan, Howard B. Demuth, Mark Beale.
      p.   cm.
   Includes bibliographical references and index.
      ISBN 0-534-94332-2 (hard cover)
      1. Neural networks (Computer science)   I. Demuth, Howard B.
   II. Beale, Mark H.   III. Title.
   QA76.87.H34 1995
   006.3--dc20   95-43658
                                                                        CIP

Printed and bound in the United States of America.

96 97 98 99 -- 10 9 8 7 6 5 4 3 2 1

Contents

Preface

An Illustrative Example

Perceptron Learning Rule

Signal and Weight Vector Spaces

Linear Transformations for Neural Networks

Supervised Hebbian Learning

Performance Surfaces and Optimum Points

Performance Optimization

9

Widrow-Hoff Learning

10

Backpropagation

Variations on Backpropagation

17 Stability

18 Hopfield Network

Epilogue

Appendices

Bibliography

Notation

Software

Index

Preface

This book gives an introduction to basic neural network architectures and learning rules. Emphasis is placed on the mathematical analysis of these networks, on methods of training them and on their application to practical engineering problems in such areas as pattern recognition, signal processing and control systems.

Every effort has been made to present material in a clear and consistent manner so that it can be read and applied with ease. We have included many solved problems to illustrate each topic of discussion.

Since this is a book on the design of neural networks, our choice of topics was guided by two principles. First, we wanted to present the most useful and practical neural network architectures, learning rules and training techniques. Second, we wanted the book to be complete in itself and to flow easily from one chapter to the next. For this reason, various introductory materials and chapters on applied mathematics are included just before they are needed for a particular subject. In summary, we have chosen some topics because of their practical importance in the application of neural networks, and other topics because of their importance in explaining how neural networks operate.

We have omitted many topics that might have been included. We have not, for instance, made this book a catalog or compendium of all known neural network architectures and learning rules, but have instead concentrated on the fundamental concepts. Second, we have not discussed neural network implementation technologies, such as VLSI, optical devices and parallel computers. Finally, we do not present the biological and psychological foundations of neural networks in any depth. These are all important topics, but we hope that we have done the reader a service by focusing on those topics that we consider to be most useful in the design of neural networks and by treating those topics in some depth.

This book has been organized for a one-semester introductory course in neural networks at the senior or first-year graduate level. (It is also suitable for short courses, self-study and reference.) The reader is expected to have some background in linear algebra, probability and differential equations.

Each chapter of the book is divided into the following sections: Objectives, Theory and Examples, Summary of Results, Solved Problems, Epilogue,

Further Reading and Exercises. The *Theory and Examples* section comprises the main body of each chapter. It includes the development of fundamental ideas as well as worked examples (indicated by the icon shown here in the left margin). The *Summary of Results* section provides a convenient listing of important equations and concepts and facilitates the use of the book as an industrial reference. About a third of each chapter is devoted to the *Solved Problems* section, which provides detailed examples for all key concepts.

The following figure illustrates the dependencies among the chapters.

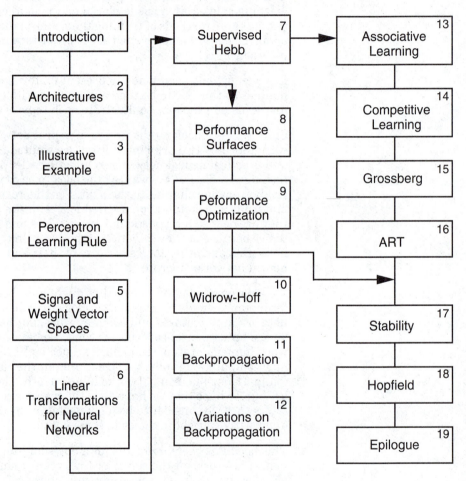

Chapters 1 through 6 cover basic concepts that are required for all of the remaining chapters. Chapter 1 is an introduction to the text, with a brief historical background and some basic biology. Chapter 2 describes the basic neural network architectures. The notation that is introduced in this chapter is used throughout the book. In Chapter 3 we present a simple pattern recognition problem and show how it can be solved using three different types of neural networks. These three networks are representative of the types of networks that are presented in the remainder of the text. In addition, the pattern recognition problem presented here provides a common thread of experience throughout the book.

Much of the focus of this book will be on methods for training neural networks to perform various tasks. In Chapter 4 we introduce learning algorithms and present the first practical algorithm: the perceptron learning rule. The perceptron network has fundamental limitations, but it is important for historical reasons and is also a useful tool for introducing key concepts that will be applied to more powerful networks in later chapters.

One of the main objectives of this book is to explain how neural networks operate. For this reason we will weave together neural network topics with important introductory material. For example, linear algebra, which is the core of the mathematics required for understanding neural networks, is reviewed in Chapters 5 and 6. The concepts discussed in these chapters will be used extensively throughout the remainder of the book.

Chapters 7 and 13–16 describe networks and learning rules that are heavily inspired by biology and psychology. They fall into two categories: associative networks and competitive networks. Chapters 7 and 13 introduce basic concepts, while Chapters 14–16 describe more advanced networks.

Chapters 8–12 develop a class of learning called performance learning, in which a network is trained to optimize its performance. Chapters 8 and 9 introduce the basic concepts of performance learning. Chapters 10–12 apply these concepts to feedforward neural networks of increasing power and complexity.

Chapters 17 and 18 discuss recurrent networks. These networks, which have feedback connections, are dynamical systems. Chapter 17 investigates the stability of these systems. Chapter 18 presents the Hopfield network, which has been one of the most influential recurrent networks.

In Chapter 19 we summarize the networks presented in this book and discuss their relationships to other networks that we do not cover. We also point the reader to other sources for further study. If you want to know "Where do I go from here?" look to Chapter 19.

Software

MATLAB is not essential for using this book. The computer exercises can be performed with any available programming language, and the *Neural Network Design Demonstrations*, while helpful, are not critical to understanding the material covered in this book.

However, we have made use of the MATLAB software package to supplement the textbook. This software is widely available and, because of its matrix/vector notation and graphics, is a convenient environment in which to experiment with neural networks. We use MATLAB in two different ways. First, we have included a number of exercises for the reader to perform in MATLAB. Many of the important features of neural networks become apparent only for large-scale problems, which are computationally intensive and not feasible for hand calculations. With MATLAB, neural network algorithms can be quickly implemented, and large-scale problems can be tested conveniently. These MATLAB exercises are identified by the icon shown here to the left. (If MATLAB is not available, any other programming language can be used to perform the exercises.)

The second way in which we use MATLAB is through the *Neural Network Design Demonstrations*, which are on a disk included with this book. These interactive demonstrations illustrate important concepts in each chapter. After the software has been loaded into the MATLAB directory on your computer, it can be invoked by typing **nnd** at the MATLAB prompt. All demonstrations are easily accessible from a master menu. The icon shown here to the left identifies references to these demonstrations in the text.

The demonstrations require MATLAB version 4.0 or later, or the student edition of MATLAB version 4.0. In addition, a few of the demonstrations require The MathWorks' *Neural Network Toolbox* version 1.0 or later. See Appendix C for specific information on using the demonstration software.

Acknowledgments

We are deeply indebted to the reviewers who have given freely of their time to read all or parts of the drafts of this book and to test various versions of the software. In particular we are most grateful to Professor John Andreae, University of Canterbury; Dan Foresee, AT&T; Dr. Carl Latino, Oklahoma State University; Jack Hagan, MCI; Dr. Gerry Andeen, SRI; and Joan Miller and Margie Jenks, University of Idaho. We also had constructive inputs from our graduate students in ECEN 5713 at Oklahoma State University and ENEL 621 at the University of Canterbury who read early drafts, tested the software and provided helpful suggestions for improving the book. We are also grateful to the anonymous reviewers who provided several useful recommendations.

We wish to thank Dr. Peter Gough for inviting us to join the staff in the Electrical and Electronic Engineering Department at the University of Canterbury, Christchurch, New Zealand. Thanks also to Mike Surety for his computer help and to the departmental staff for their assistance. A sabbatical from Oklahoma State University and a year's leave from the University of Idaho gave us the time to write this book. Thanks to Texas Instruments, and in particular Bill Harland, for their support of our neural network research. Thanks to The Mathworks for permission to use material from the *Neural Network Toolbox*.

We are grateful to Joan Pilgram for her encouragement and business advice, and to Mrs. Bernice Hewitt, Christchurch, for her good spirit and hospitality.

Finally, we wish to express our appreciation to the staff at PWS Publishing Company, especially Bill Barter, Pam Rockwell, Amy Mayfield, Ken Morton and Nathan Wilbur. Thanks to Vanessa Pineiro for the lovely cover art.

1 Introduction

Objectives

As you read these words you are using a complex biological neural network. You have a highly interconnected set of some 10^{11} neurons to facilitate your reading, breathing, motion and thinking. Each of your biological neurons, a rich assembly of tissue and chemistry, has the complexity, if not the speed, of a microprocessor. Some of your neural structure was with you at birth. Other parts have been established by experience.

Scientists have only just begun to understand how biological neural networks operate. It is generally understood that all biological neural functions, including memory, are stored in the neurons and in the connections between them. Learning is viewed as the establishment of new connections between neurons or the modification of existing connections. This leads to the following question: Although we have only a rudimentary understanding of biological neural networks, is it possible to construct a small set of simple artificial "neurons" and perhaps train them to serve a useful function? The answer is "yes." This book, then, is about *artificial* neural networks.

The neurons that we consider here are not biological. They are extremely simple abstractions of biological neurons, realized as elements in a program or perhaps as circuits made of silicon. Networks of these artificial neurons do not have a fraction of the power of the human brain, but they can be trained to perform useful functions. This book is about such neurons, the networks that contain them and their training.

History

The history of artificial neural networks is filled with colorful, creative individuals from many different fields, many of whom struggled for decades to develop concepts that we now take for granted. This history has been documented by various authors. One particularly interesting book is *Neurocomputing: Foundations of Research* by John Anderson and Edward Rosenfeld. They have collected and edited a set of some 43 papers of special historical interest. Each paper is preceded by an introduction that puts the paper in historical perspective.

Histories of some of the main neural network contributors are included at the beginning of various chapters throughout this text and will not be repeated here. However, it seems appropriate to give a brief overview, a sample of the major developments.

At least two ingredients are necessary for the advancement of a technology: concept and implementation. First, one must have a concept, a way of thinking about a topic, some view of it that gives a clarity not there before. This may involve a simple idea, or it may be more specific and include a mathematical description. To illustrate this point, consider the history of the heart. It was thought to be, at various times, the center of the soul or a source of heat. In the 17th century medical practitioners finally began to view the heart as a pump, and they designed experiments to study its pumping action. These experiments revolutionized our view of the circulatory system. Without the pump concept, an understanding of the heart was out of grasp.

Concepts and their accompanying mathematics are not sufficient for a technology to mature unless there is some way to implement the system. For instance, the mathematics necessary for the reconstruction of images from computer-aided tomography (CAT) scans was known many years before the availability of high-speed computers and efficient algorithms finally made it practical to implement a useful CAT system.

The history of neural networks has progressed through both conceptual innovations and implementation developments. These advancements, however, seem to have occurred in fits and starts rather than by steady evolution.

Some of the background work for the field of neural networks occurred in the late 19th and early 20th centuries. This consisted primarily of interdisciplinary work in physics, psychology and neurophysiology by such scientists as Hermann von Helmholtz, Ernst Mach and Ivan Pavlov. This early work emphasized general theories of learning, vision, conditioning, etc., and did not include specific mathematical models of neuron operation.

The modern view of neural networks began in the 1940s with the work of Warren McCulloch and Walter Pitts [McPi43], who showed that networks of artificial neurons could, in principle, compute any arithmetic or logical function. Their work is often acknowledged as the origin of the neural network field.

McCulloch and Pitts were followed by Donald Hebb [Hebb49], who proposed that classical conditioning (as discovered by Pavlov) is present because of the properties of individual neurons. He proposed a mechanism for learning in biological neurons (see Chapter 7).

The first practical application of artificial neural networks came in the late 1950s, with the invention of the perceptron network and associated learning rule by Frank Rosenblatt [Rose58]. Rosenblatt and his colleagues built a perceptron network and demonstrated its ability to perform pattern recognition. This early success generated a great deal of interest in neural network research. Unfortunately, it was later shown that the basic perceptron network could solve only a limited class of problems. (See Chapter 4 for more on Rosenblatt and the perceptron learning rule.)

At about the same time, Bernard Widrow and Ted Hoff [WiHo60] introduced a new learning algorithm and used it to train adaptive linear neural networks, which were similar in structure and capability to Rosenblatt's perceptron. The Widrow-Hoff learning rule is still in use today. (See Chapter 10 for more on Widrow-Hoff learning.)

Unfortunately, both Rosenblatt's and Widrow's networks suffered from the same inherent limitations, which were widely publicized in a book by Marvin Minsky and Seymour Papert [MiPa69]. Rosenblatt and Widrow were aware of these limitations and proposed new networks that would overcome them. However, they were not able to successfully modify their learning algorithms to train the more complex networks.

Many people, influenced by Minsky and Papert, believed that further research on neural networks was a dead end. This, combined with the fact that there were no powerful digital computers on which to experiment, caused many researchers to leave the field. For a decade neural network research was largely suspended.

Some important work, however, did continue during the 1970s. In 1972 Teuvo Kohonen [Koho72] and James Anderson [Ande72] independently and separately developed new neural networks that could act as memories. (See Chapters 13 and 14 for more on Kohonen networks.) Stephen Grossberg [Gros76] was also very active during this period in the investigation of self-organizing networks. (See Chapters 15 and 16.)

Interest in neural networks had faltered during the late 1960s because of the lack of new ideas and powerful computers with which to experiment. During the 1980s both of these impediments were overcome, and research in neural networks increased dramatically. New personal computers and workstations, which rapidly grew in capability, became widely available. In addition, important new concepts were introduced.

Two new concepts were most responsible for the rebirth of neural networks. The first was the use of statistical mechanics to explain the operation of a certain class of recurrent network, which could be used as an associative memory. This was described in a seminal paper by physicist John Hopfield [Hopf82]. (Chapters 17 and 18 discuss these Hopfield networks.)

The second key development of the 1980s was the backpropagation algorithm for training multilayer perceptron networks, which was discovered independently by several different researchers. The most influential publication of the backpropagation algorithm was by David Rumelhart and James McClelland [RuMc86]. This algorithm was the answer to the criticisms Minsky and Papert had made in the 1960s. (See Chapters 11 and 12 for a development of the backpropagation algorithm.)

These new developments reinvigorated the field of neural networks. In the last ten years, thousands of papers have been written, and neural networks have found many applications. The field is buzzing with new theoretical and practical work. As noted below, it is not clear where all of this will lead us.

The brief historical account given above is not intended to identify all of the major contributors, but is simply to give the reader some feel for how knowledge in the neural network field has progressed. As one might note, the progress has not always been "slow but sure." There have been periods of dramatic progress and periods when relatively little has been accomplished.

Many of the advances in neural networks have had to do with new concepts, such as innovative architectures and training rules. Just as important has been the availability of powerful new computers on which to test these new concepts.

Well, so much for the history of neural networks to this date. The real question is, "What will happen in the next ten to twenty years?" Will neural networks take a permanent place as a mathematical/engineering tool, or will they fade away as have so many promising technologies? At present, the answer seems to be that neural networks will not only have their day but will have a permanent place, not as a solution to every problem, but as a tool to be used in appropriate situations. In addition, remember that we still know very little about how the brain works. The most important advances in neural networks almost certainly lie in the future.

Although it is difficult to predict the future success of neural networks, the large number and wide variety of applications of this new technology are very encouraging. The next section describes some of these applications.

Applications

A recent newspaper article described the use of neural networks in literature research by Aston University. It stated that "the network can be taught to recognize individual writing styles, and the researchers used it to compare works attributed to Shakespeare and his contemporaries." A popular science television program recently documented the use of neural networks by an Italian research institute to test the purity of olive oil. These examples are indicative of the broad range of applications that can be found for neural networks. The applications are expanding because neural networks are good at solving problems, not just in engineering, science and mathematics, but in medicine, business, finance and literature as well. Their application to a wide variety of problems in many fields makes them very attractive. Also, faster computers and faster algorithms have made it possible to use neural networks to solve complex industrial problems that formerly required too much computation.

The following note and Table of Neural Network Applications are reproduced here from the *Neural Network Toolbox* for MATLAB with the permission of the MathWorks, Inc.

The 1988 DARPA Neural Network Study [DARP88] lists various neural network applications, beginning with the adaptive channel equalizer in about 1984. This device, which is an outstanding commercial success, is a single-neuron network used in long distance telephone systems to stabilize voice signals. The DARPA report goes on to list other commercial applications, including a small word recognizer, a process monitor, a sonar classifier and a risk analysis system.

Neural networks have been applied in many fields since the DARPA report was written. A list of some applications mentioned in the literature follows.

Aerospace

High performance aircraft autopilots, flight path simulations, aircraft control systems, autopilot enhancements, aircraft component simulations, aircraft component fault detectors

Automotive

Automobile automatic guidance systems, warranty activity analyzers

Banking

Check and other document readers, credit application evaluators

Defense

Weapon steering, target tracking, object discrimination, facial recognition, new kinds of sensors, sonar, radar and image signal processing including data compression, feature extraction and noise suppression, signal/image identification

Electronics

Code sequence prediction, integrated circuit chip layout, process control, chip failure analysis, machine vision, voice synthesis, nonlinear modeling

Entertainment

Animation, special effects, market forecasting

Financial

Real estate appraisal, loan advisor, mortgage screening, corporate bond rating, credit line use analysis, portfolio trading program, corporate financial analysis, currency price prediction

Insurance

Policy application evaluation, product optimization

Manufacturing

Manufacturing process control, product design and analysis, process and machine diagnosis, real-time particle identification, visual quality inspection systems, beer testing, welding quality analysis, paper quality prediction, computer chip quality analysis, analysis of grinding operations, chemical product design analysis, machine maintenance analysis, project bidding, planning and management, dynamic modeling of chemical process systems

Medical

Breast cancer cell analysis, EEG and ECG analysis, prosthesis design, optimization of transplant times, hospital expense reduction, hospital quality improvement, emergency room test advisement

Oil and Gas

Exploration

Robotics

Trajectory control, forklift robot, manipulator controllers, vision systems

Speech

Speech recognition, speech compression, vowel classification, text to speech synthesis

Securities

Market analysis, automatic bond rating, stock trading advisory systems

Telecommunications

Image and data compression, automated information services, real-time translation of spoken language, customer payment processing systems

Transportation

Truck brake diagnosis systems, vehicle scheduling, routing systems

Conclusion

The number of neural network applications, the money that has been invested in neural network software and hardware, and the depth and breadth of interest in these devices have been growing rapidly.

Biological Inspiration

The artificial neural networks discussed in this text are only remotely related to their biological counterparts. In this section we will briefly describe those characteristics of brain function that have inspired the development of artificial neural networks.

The brain consists of a large number (approximately 10^{11}) of highly connected elements (approximately 10^4 connections per element) called neurons. For our purposes these neurons have three principal components: the dendrites, the cell body and the axon. The dendrites are tree-like receptive networks of nerve fibers that carry electrical signals into the cell body. The cell body effectively sums and thresholds these incoming signals. The axon is a single long fiber that carries the signal from the cell body out to other neurons. The point of contact between an axon of one cell and a dendrite of another cell is called a synapse. It is the arrangement of neurons and the strengths of the individual synapses, determined by a complex chemical process, that establishes the function of the neural network. Figure 1.1 is a simplified schematic diagram of two biological neurons.

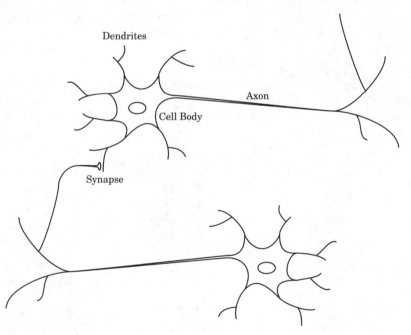

Figure 1.1 Schematic Drawing of Biological Neurons

Some of the neural structure is defined at birth. Other parts are developed through learning, as new connections are made and others waste away. This development is most noticeable in the early stages of life. For example, it has been shown that if a young cat is denied use of one eye during a critical window of time, it will never develop normal vision in that eye.

Neural structures continue to change throughout life. These later changes tend to consist mainly of strengthening or weakening of synaptic junctions. For instance, it is believed that new memories are formed by modification of these synaptic strengths. Thus, the process of learning a new friend's face consists of altering various synapses.

Artificial neural networks do not approach the complexity of the brain. There are, however, two key similarities between biological and artificial neural networks. First, the building blocks of both networks are simple computational devices (although artificial neurons are much simpler than biological neurons) that are highly interconnected. Second, the connections between neurons determine the function of the network. The primary objective of this book will be to determine the appropriate connections to solve particular problems.

It is worth noting that even though biological neurons are very slow when compared to electrical circuits (10^{-3} s compared to 10^{-9} s), the brain is able to perform many tasks much faster than any conventional computer. This is in part because of the massively parallel structure of biological neural networks; all of the neurons are operating at the same time. Artificial neural networks share this parallel structure. Even though most artificial neural networks are currently implemented on conventional digital computers, their parallel structure makes them ideally suited to implementation using VLSI, optical devices and parallel processors.

In the following chapter we will introduce our basic artificial neuron and will explain how we can combine such neurons to form networks. This will provide a background for Chapter 3, where we take our first look at neural networks in action.

Further Reading

[Ande72]   J. A. Anderson, "A simple neural network generating an interactive memory," *Mathematical Biosciences*, vol. 14, pp. 197–220, 1972.

Anderson proposed a "linear associator" model for associative memory. The model was trained, using a generalization of the Hebb postulate, to learn an association between input and output vectors. The physiological plausibility of the network was emphasized. Kohonen published a closely related paper at the same time [Koho72], although the two researchers were working independently.

[AnRo88]   J. A. Anderson and E. Rosenfeld, *Neurocomputing: Foundations of Research*, Cambridge, MA: MIT Press, 1989.

Neurocomputing is a fundamental reference book. It contains over forty of the most important neurocomputing writings. Each paper is accompanied by an introduction that summarizes its results and gives a perspective on the position of the paper in the history of the field.

[DARP88]   *DARPA Neural Network Study*, Lexington, MA: MIT Lincoln Laboratory, 1988.

This study is a compendium of knowledge of neural networks as they were known to 1988. It presents the theoretical foundations of neural networks and discusses their current applications. It contains sections on associative memories, recurrent networks, vision, speech recognition, and robotics. Finally, it discusses simulation tools and implementation technology.

[Gros76]   S. Grossberg, "Adaptive pattern classification and universal recoding: I. Parallel development and coding of neural feature detectors," *Biological Cybernetics*, Vol. 23, pp. 121–134, 1976.

Grossberg describes a self-organizing neural network based on the visual system. The network, which consists of short-term and long-term memory mechanisms, is a continuous-time competitive network. It forms a basis for the adaptive resonance theory (ART) networks.

1

[Gros80]   S. Grossberg, "How does the brain build a cognitive code?" *Psychological Review*, Vol. 88, pp. 375–407, 1980.

Grossberg's 1980 paper proposes neural structures and mechanisms that can explain many physiological behaviors including spatial frequency adaptation, binocular rivalry, etc. His systems perform error correction by themselves, without outside help.

[Hebb 49]   D. O. Hebb, *The Organization of Behavior*. New York: Wiley, 1949.

The main premise of this seminal book is that behavior can be explained by the action of neurons. In it, Hebb proposed one of the first learning laws, which postulated a mechanism for learning at the cellular level.

Hebb proposes that classical conditioning in biology is present because of the properties of individual neurons.

[Hopf82]   J. J. Hopfield, "Neural networks and physical systems with emergent collective computational abilities," *Proceedings of the National Academy of Sciences*, Vol. 79, pp. 2554–2558, 1982.

Hopfield describes a content-addressable neural network. He also presents a clear picture of how his neural network operates, and of what it can do.

[Koho72]   T. Kohonen, "Correlation matrix memories," *IEEE Transactions on Computers*, vol. 21, pp. 353–359, 1972.

Kohonen proposed a correlation matrix model for associative memory. The model was trained, using the outer product rule (also known as the Hebb rule), to learn an association between input and output vectors. The mathematical structure of the network was emphasized. Anderson published a closely related paper at the same time [Ande72], although the two researchers were working independently.

[McPi43]   W. McCulloch and W. Pitts, "A logical calculus of the ideas immanent in nervous activity," *Bulletin of Mathematical Biophysics.*, Vol. 5, pp. 115–133, 1943.

This article introduces the first mathematical model of a neuron, in which a weighted sum of input signals is compared to a threshold to determine whether or not the neuron fires. This was the first attempt to describe what the brain does, based on computing elements known at the time. It shows that simple neural networks can compute any arithmetic or logical function.

[MiPa69]   M. Minsky and S. Papert, *Perceptrons*, Cambridge, MA: MIT Press, 1969.

A landmark book that contains the first rigorous study devoted to determining what a perceptron network is capable of learning. A formal treatment of the perceptron was needed both to explain the perceptron's limitations and to indicate directions for overcoming them. Unfortunately, the book pessimistically predicted that the limitations of perceptrons indicated that the field of neural networks was a dead end. Although this was not true it temporarily cooled research and funding for research for several years.

[Rose58]   F. Rosenblatt, "The perceptron: A probabilistic model for information storage and organization in the brain," *Psychological Review*, Vol. 65, pp. 386–408, 1958.

Rosenblatt presents the first practical artificial neural network — the perceptron.

[RuMc86]   D. E. Rumelhart and J. L. McClelland, eds., *Parallel Distributed Processing: Explorations in the Microstructure of Cognition*, Vol. 1, Cambridge, MA: MIT Press, 1986.

One of the two key influences in the resurgence of interest in the neural network field during the 1980s. Among other topics, it presents the backpropagation algorithm for training multilayer networks.

[WiHo60]   B. Widrow and M. E. Hoff, "Adaptive switching circuits,"*1960 IRE WESCON Convention Record*, New York: IRE Part 4, pp. 96–104, 1960.

This seminal paper describes an adaptive perceptron-like network that can learn quickly and accurately. The authors assume that the system has inputs and a desired output classification for each input, and that the system can calculate the error between the actual and desired output. The weights are adjusted, using a gradient descent method, so as to minimize the mean square error. (Least Mean Square error or LMS algorithm.)

This paper is reprinted in [AnRo88].

2 Neuron Model and Network Architectures

Objectives

In Chapter 1 we presented a simplified description of biological neurons and neural networks. Now we will introduce our simplified mathematical model of the neuron and will explain how these artificial neurons can be interconnected to form a variety of network architectures. We will also illustrate the basic operation of these networks through some simple examples. The concepts and notation introduced in this chapter will be used throughout this book.

This chapter does not cover all of the architectures that will be used in this book, but it does present the basic building blocks. More complex architectures will be introduced and discussed as they are needed in later chapters. Even so, a lot of detail is presented here. Please note that it is not necessary for the reader to memorize all of the material in this chapter on a first reading. Instead, treat it as a sample to get you started and a resource to which you can return.

Theory and Examples

Notation

Neural networks are so new that standard mathematical notation and architectural representations for them have not yet been firmly established. In addition, papers and books on neural networks have come from many diverse fields, including engineering, physics, psychology and mathematics, and many authors tend to use vocabulary peculiar to their specialty. As a result, many books and papers in this field are difficult to read, and concepts are made to seem more complex than they actually are. This is a shame, as it has prevented the spread of important new ideas. It has also led to more than one "reinvention of the wheel."

In this book we have tried to use standard notation where possible, to be clear and to keep matters simple without sacrificing rigor. In particular, we have tried to define practical conventions and use them consistently.

Figures, mathematical equations and text discussing both figures and mathematical equations will use the following notation:

Scalars — small *italic* letters: *a,b,c*

Vectors — small **bold** nonitalic letters: **a,b,c**

Matrices — capital **BOLD** nonitalic letters: **A,B,C**

Additional notation concerning the network architectures will be introduced as you read this chapter. A complete list of the notation that we use throughout the book is given in Appendix B, so you can look there if you have a question.

Neuron Model

Single-Input Neuron

Weight
Bias
Net Input
Transfer Function

A single-input neuron is shown in Figure 2.1. The scalar input p is multiplied by the scalar *weight* w to form wp, one of the terms that is sent to the summer. The other input, 1, is multiplied by a *bias* b and then passed to the summer. The summer output n, often referred to as the *net input*, goes into a *transfer function* f, which produces the scalar neuron output a. (Some authors use the term "activation function" rather than *transfer function* and "offset" rather than *bias*.)

If we relate this simple model back to the biological neuron that we discussed in Chapter 1, the weight w corresponds to the strength of a synapse, the cell body is represented by the summation and the transfer function, and the neuron output a represents the signal on the axon.

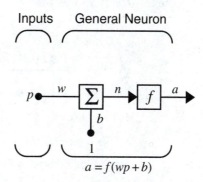

Figure 2.1 Single-Input Neuron

The neuron output is calculated as

$$a = f(wp + b) .$$

If, for instance, $w = 3$, $p = 2$ and $b = -1.5$, then

$$a = f(3(2) - 1.5) = f(4.5)$$

The actual output depends on the particular transfer function that is chosen. We will discuss transfer functions in the next section.

The bias is much like a weight, except that it has a constant input of 1. However, if you do not want to have a bias in a particular neuron, it can be omitted. We will see examples of this in Chapters 3, 7 and 14.

Note that w and b are both *adjustable* scalar parameters of the neuron. Typically the transfer function is chosen by the designer and then the parameters w and b will be adjusted by some learning rule so that the neuron input/output relationship meets some specific goal (see Chapter 4 for an introduction to learning rules). As described in the following section, we have different transfer functions for different purposes.

Transfer Functions

The transfer function in Figure 2.1 may be a linear or a nonlinear function of n. A particular transfer function is chosen to satisfy some specification of the problem that the neuron is attempting to solve.

A variety of transfer functions have been included in this book. Three of the most commonly used functions are discussed below.

Hard Limit
Transfer Function

The *hard limit transfer function*, shown on the left side of Figure 2.2, sets the output of the neuron to 0 if the function argument is less than 0, or 1 if its argument is greater than or equal to 0. We will use this function to create neurons that classify inputs into two distinct categories. It will be used extensively in Chapter 4.

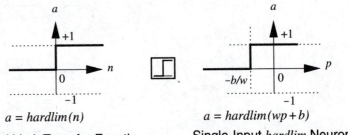

$$a = hardlim(n)$$

Hard Limit Transfer Function

$$a = hardlim(wp + b)$$

Single-Input *hardlim* Neuron

Figure 2.2 Hard Limit Transfer Function

The graph on the right side of Figure 2.2 illustrates the input/output characteristic of a single-input neuron that uses a hard limit transfer function. Here we can see the effect of the weight and the bias. Note that an icon for the hard limit transfer function is shown between the two figures. Such icons will replace the general f in network diagrams to show the particular transfer function that is being used.

Linear Transfer Function

The output of a *linear transfer function* is equal to its input:

$$a = n, \tag{2.1}$$

as illustrated in Figure 2.3.

Neurons with this transfer function are used in the ADALINE networks, which are discussed in Chapter 10.

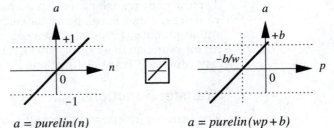

$$a = purelin(n)$$

Linear Transfer Function

$$a = purelin(wp + b)$$

Single-Input *purelin* Neuron

Figure 2.3 Linear Transfer Function

The output (a) versus input (p) characteristic of a single-input linear neuron with a bias is shown on the right of Figure 2.3.

Log-Sigmoid Transfer Function

The *log-sigmoid transfer function* is shown in Figure 2.4.

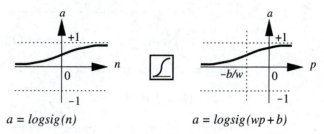

$$a = logsig(n)$$

Log-Sigmoid Transfer Function

$$a = logsig(wp + b)$$

Single-Input *logsig* Neuron

Figure 2.4 Log-Sigmoid Transfer Function

This transfer function takes the input (which may have any value between plus and minus infinity) and squashes the output into the range 0 to 1, according to the expression:

$$a = \frac{1}{1 + e^{-n}}.$$

$$(2.2)$$

The log-sigmoid transfer function is commonly used in multilayer networks that are trained using the backpropagation algorithm, in part because this function is differentiable (see Chapter 11).

Most of the transfer functions used in this book are summarized in Table 2.1. Of course, you can define other transfer functions in addition to those shown in Table 2.1 if you wish.

To experiment with a single-input neuron, use the Neural Network Design Demonstration One-Input Neuron **nnd2n1**.

Name	Input/Output Relation	Icon	MATLAB Function
Hard Limit	$a = 0 \quad n < 0$ $a = 1 \quad n \geq 0$		hardlim
Symmetrical Hard Limit	$a = -1 \quad n < 0$ $a = +1 \quad n \geq 0$		hardlims
Linear	$a = n$		purelin
Saturating Linear	$a = 0 \quad n < 0$ $a = n \quad 0 \leq n \leq 1$ $a = 1 \quad n > 1$		satlin
Symmetric Saturating Linear	$a = -1 \quad n < -1$ $a = n \quad -1 \leq n \leq 1$ $a = 1 \quad n > 1$		satlins
Log-Sigmoid	$a = \dfrac{1}{1 + e^{-n}}$		logsig
Hyperbolic Tangent Sigmoid	$a = \dfrac{e^n - e^{-n}}{e^n + e^{-n}}$		tansig
Positive Linear	$a = 0 \quad n < 0$ $a = n \quad 0 \leq n$		poslin
Competitive	$a = 1 \quad$ neuron with max n $a = 0 \quad$ all other neurons	C	compet

Table 2.1 Transfer Functions

Multiple-Input Neuron

Typically, a neuron has more than one input. A neuron with R inputs is shown in Figure 2.5. The individual inputs $p_1, p_2, ..., p_R$ are each weighted **Weight Matrix** by corresponding elements $w_{1,1}, w_{1,2}, ..., w_{1,R}$ of the *weight matrix* **W**.

Inputs   Multiple-Input Neuron

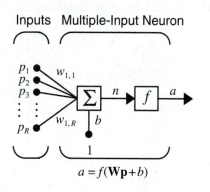

$$a = f(\mathbf{W}p + b)$$

Figure 2.5 Multiple-Input Neuron

The neuron has a bias b, which is summed with the weighted inputs to form the net input n:

$$n = w_{1,1}p_1 + w_{1,2}p_2 + \cdots + w_{1,R}p_R + b \,. \tag{2.3}$$

This expression can be written in matrix form:

$$n = \mathbf{W}p + b \,, \tag{2.4}$$

where the matrix **W** for the single neuron case has only one row.

Now the neuron output can be written as

$$a = f(\mathbf{W}p + b) \,. \tag{2.5}$$

Fortunately, neural networks can often be described with matrices. This kind of matrix expression will be used throughout the book. Don't be concerned if you are rusty with matrix and vector operations. We will review these topics in Chapters 5 and 6, and we will provide many examples and solved problems that will spell out the procedures.

Weight Indices   We have adopted a particular convention in assigning the indices of the elements of the weight matrix. The first index indicates the particular neuron destination for that weight. The second index indicates the source of the signal fed to the neuron. Thus, the indices in $w_{1,2}$ say that this weight represents the connection *to* the first (and only) neuron *from* the second source. Of course, this convention is more useful if there is more than one neuron, as will be the case later in this chapter.

We would like to draw networks with several neurons, each having several inputs. Further, we would like to have more than one layer of neurons. You can imagine how complex such a network might appear if all the lines were drawn. It would take a lot of ink, could hardly be read, and the mass of detail might obscure the main features. Thus, we will use an *abbreviated notation*. A multiple-input neuron using this notation is shown in Figure 2.6.

Abbreviated Notation

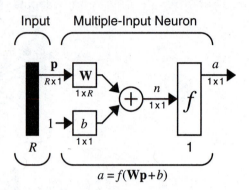

$$a = f(\mathbf{W}\mathbf{p}+b)$$

Figure 2.6 Neuron with R Inputs, Abbreviated Notation

As shown in Figure 2.6, the input vector **p** is represented by the solid vertical bar at the left. The dimensions of **p** are displayed below the variable as $R \times 1$, indicating that the input is a single vector of R elements. These inputs go to the weight matrix **W**, which has R columns but only one row in this single neuron case. A constant 1 enters the neuron as an input and is multiplied by a scalar bias b. The net input to the transfer function f is n, which is the sum of the bias b and the product **Wp**. The neuron's output a is a scalar in this case. If we had more than one neuron, the network output would be a vector.

The dimensions of the variables in these abbreviated notation figures will always be included, so that you can tell immediately if we are talking about a scalar, a vector or a matrix. You will not have to guess the kind of variable or its dimensions.

Note that the number of inputs to a network is set by the external specifications of the problem. If, for instance, you want to design a neural network that is to predict kite-flying conditions and the inputs are air temperature, wind velocity and humidity, then there would be three inputs to the network.

*To experiment with a two-input neuron, use the Neural Network Design Demonstration Two-Input Neuron (**nnd2n2**).*

Network Architectures

Commonly one neuron, even with many inputs, may not be sufficient. We might need five or ten, operating in parallel, in what we will call a "layer." This concept of a layer is discussed below.

A Layer of Neurons

Layer   A single-*layer* network of S neurons is shown in Figure 2.7. Note that each of the R inputs is connected to each of the neurons and that the weight matrix now has S rows.

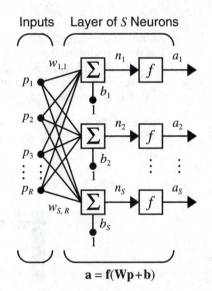

$$a = f(Wp+b)$$

Figure 2.7 Layer of S Neurons

The layer includes the weight matrix, the summers, the bias vector $\mathbf{b}$, the transfer function boxes and the output vector $\mathbf{a}$. Some authors refer to the inputs as another layer, but we will not do that here.

Each element of the input vector $\mathbf{p}$ is connected to each neuron through the weight matrix $\mathbf{W}$. Each neuron has a bias b_i, a summer, a transfer function f and an output a_i. Taken together, the outputs form the output vector $\mathbf{a}$.

It is common for the number of inputs to a layer to be different from the number of neurons (i.e., $R \neq S$).

You might ask if all the neurons in a layer must have the same transfer function. The answer is no; you can define a single (composite) layer of neurons having different transfer functions by combining two of the networks shown above in parallel. Both networks would have the same inputs, and each network would create some of the outputs.

The input vector elements enter the network through the weight matrix **W**:

$$\mathbf{W} = \begin{bmatrix} w_{1,1} & w_{1,2} & \cdots & w_{1,R} \\ w_{2,1} & w_{2,2} & \cdots & w_{2,R} \\ \vdots & \vdots & & \vdots \\ w_{S,1} & w_{S,2} & \cdots & w_{S,R} \end{bmatrix}. \tag{2.6}$$

As noted previously, the row indices of the elements of matrix **W** indicate the destination neuron associated with that weight, while the column indices indicate the source of the input for that weight. Thus, the indices in $w_{3,2}$ say that this weight represents the connection *to* the third neuron *from* the second source.

Fortunately, the S-neuron, R-input, one-layer network also can be drawn in abbreviated notation, as shown in Figure 2.8.

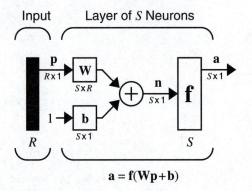

$$\mathbf{a} = \mathbf{f}(\mathbf{Wp} + \mathbf{b})$$

Figure 2.8 Layer of S Neurons, Abbreviated Notation

Here again, the symbols below the variables tell you that for this layer, **p** is a vector of length R, **W** is an $S \times R$ matrix, and **a** and **b** are vectors of length S. As defined previously, the layer includes the weight matrix, the summation and multiplication operations, the bias vector **b**, the transfer function boxes and the output vector.

Multiple Layers of Neurons

Now consider a network with several layers. Each layer has its own weight matrix **W**, its own bias vector **b**, a net input vector **n** and an output vector **a**. We need to introduce some additional notation to distinguish between these layers. We will use superscripts to identify the layers. Specifically, we

2

Layer Superscript   append the number of the layer as a *superscript* to the names for each of these variables. Thus, the weight matrix for the first layer is written as $\mathbf{W}^1$, and the weight matrix for the second layer is written as $\mathbf{W}^2$. This notation is used in the three-layer network shown in Figure 2.9.

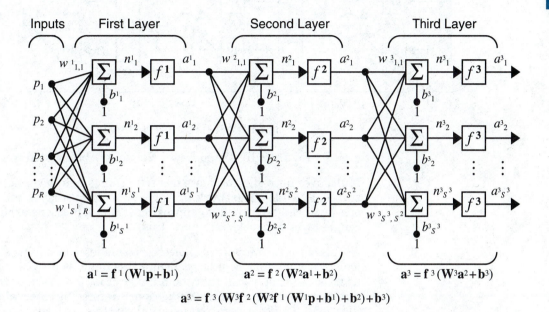

$$\mathbf{a}^1 = \mathbf{f}^1(\mathbf{W}^1\mathbf{p}+\mathbf{b}^1) \qquad \mathbf{a}^2 = \mathbf{f}^2(\mathbf{W}^2\mathbf{a}^1+\mathbf{b}^2) \qquad \mathbf{a}^3 = \mathbf{f}^3(\mathbf{W}^3\mathbf{a}^2+\mathbf{b}^3)$$

$$\mathbf{a}^3 = \mathbf{f}^3(\mathbf{W}^3\mathbf{f}^2(\mathbf{W}^2\mathbf{f}^1(\mathbf{W}^1\mathbf{p}+\mathbf{b}^1)+\mathbf{b}^2)+\mathbf{b}^3)$$

Figure 2.9 Three-Layer Network

As shown, there are R inputs, S^1 neurons in the first layer, S^2 neurons in the second layer, etc. As noted, different layers can have different numbers of neurons.

The outputs of layers one and two are the inputs for layers two and three. Thus layer 2 can be viewed as a one-layer network with $R = S^1$ inputs, $S = S^2$ neurons, and an $S^1 \times S^2$ weight matrix $\mathbf{W}^2$. The input to layer 2 is $\mathbf{a}^1$, and the output is $\mathbf{a}^2$.

Output Layer   A layer whose output is the network output is called an *output layer*. The
Hidden Layers   other layers are called *hidden layers*. The network shown above has an output layer (layer 3) and two hidden layers (layers 1 and 2).

The same three-layer network discussed previously also can be drawn using our abbreviated notation, as shown in Figure 2.10.

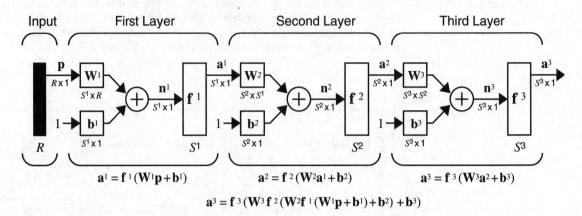

$$\mathbf{a}^1 = \mathbf{f}^{\,1}(\mathbf{W}^1\mathbf{p}+\mathbf{b}^1) \qquad \mathbf{a}^2 = \mathbf{f}^{\,2}(\mathbf{W}^2\mathbf{a}^1+\mathbf{b}^2) \qquad \mathbf{a}^3 = \mathbf{f}^{\,3}(\mathbf{W}^3\mathbf{a}^2+\mathbf{b}^3)$$

$$\mathbf{a}^3 = \mathbf{f}^{\,3}(\mathbf{W}^3\mathbf{f}^{\,2}(\mathbf{W}^2\mathbf{f}^{\,1}(\mathbf{W}^1\mathbf{p}+\mathbf{b}^1)+\mathbf{b}^2)+\mathbf{b}^3)$$

Figure 2.10 Three-Layer Network, Abbreviated Notation

Multilayer networks are more powerful than single-layer networks. For instance, a two-layer network having a sigmoid first layer and a linear second layer can be trained to approximate most functions arbitrarily well. Single-layer networks cannot do this.

At this point the number of choices to be made in specifying a network may look overwhelming, so let us consider this topic. The problem is not as bad as it looks. First, recall that the number of inputs to the network and the number of outputs from the network are defined by external problem specifications. So if there are four external variables to be used as inputs, there are four inputs to the network. Similarly, if there are to be seven outputs from the network, there must be seven neurons in the output layer. Finally, the desired characteristics of the output signal also help to select the transfer function for the output layer. If an output is to be either –1 or 1, then a symmetrical hard limit transfer function should be used. Thus, the architecture of a single-layer network is almost completely determined by problem specifications, including the specific number of inputs and outputs and the particular output signal characteristic.

Now, what if we have more than two layers? Here the external problem does not tell you directly the number of neurons required in the hidden layers. In fact, there are few problems for which one can predict the optimal number of neurons needed in a hidden layer. This problem is an active area of research. We will develop some feeling on this matter as we proceed to Chapter 11, Backpropagation.

As for the number of layers, most practical neural networks have just two or three layers. Four or more layers are used rarely.

We should say something about the use of biases. One can choose neurons with or without biases. The bias gives the network an extra variable, and so you might expect that networks with biases would be more powerful than those without, and that is true. Note, for instance, that a neuron without a bias will always have a net input n of zero when the network inputs **p** are zero. This may not be desirable and can be avoided by the use of a bias. The effect of the bias is discussed more fully in Chapters 3, 4 and 5.

In later chapters we will omit a bias in some examples or demonstrations. In some cases this is done simply to reduce the number of network parameters. With just two variables, we can plot system convergence in a two-dimensional plane. Three or more variables are difficult to display.

Recurrent Networks

Delay   Before we discuss recurrent networks, we need to introduce some simple building blocks. The first is the *delay* block, which is illustrated in Figure 2.11.

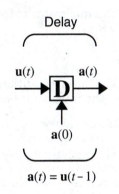

$$\mathbf{a}(t) = \mathbf{u}(t-1)$$

Figure 2.11 Delay Block

The delay output $\mathbf{a}(t)$ is computed from its input $\mathbf{u}(t)$ according to

$$\mathbf{a}(t) \;=\; \mathbf{u}(t-1)\,. \tag{2.7}$$

Thus the output is the input delayed by one time step. (This assumes that time is updated in discrete steps and takes on only integer values.) Eq. (2.7) requires that the output be initialized at time $t = 0$. This initial condition is indicated in Figure 2.11 by the arrow coming into the bottom of the delay block.

Integrator   Another related building block, which we will use for the continuous-time recurrent networks in Chapters 15–18, is the *integrator*, which is shown in Figure 2.12.

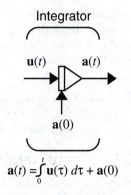

$$\mathbf{a}(t) = \int_0^t \mathbf{u}(\tau)\, d\tau + \mathbf{a}(0)$$

Figure 2.12 Integrator Block

The integrator output $\mathbf{a}(t)$ is computed from its input $\mathbf{u}(t)$ according to

$$\mathbf{a}(t) \;=\; \int_0^t \mathbf{u}(\tau)\, d\tau + \mathbf{a}(0)\,. \tag{2.8}$$

The initial condition $\mathbf{a}(0)$ is indicated by the arrow coming into the bottom of the integrator block.

Recurrent Network We are now ready to introduce recurrent networks. A *recurrent network* is a network with feedback; some of its outputs are connected to its inputs. This is quite different from the networks that we have studied thus far, which were strictly feedforward with no backward connections. One type of discrete-time recurrent network is shown in Figure 2.13.

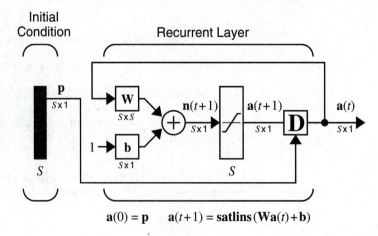

$$\mathbf{a}(0) = \mathbf{p} \qquad \mathbf{a}(t+1) = \mathbf{satlins}\,(\mathbf{Wa}(t) + \mathbf{b})$$

Figure 2.13 Recurrent Network

In this particular network the vector **p** supplies the initial conditions (i.e., **a**(0) = **p**). Then future outputs of the network are computed from previous outputs:

$$\mathbf{a}(1) = satlins(\mathbf{W}\mathbf{a}(0) + \mathbf{b}) , \mathbf{a}(2) = satlins(\mathbf{W}\mathbf{a}(1) + \mathbf{b}) , \ldots$$

2

Recurrent networks are potentially more powerful than feedforward networks and can exhibit temporal behavior. These types of networks are discussed in Chapters 3 and 15–18.

Summary of Results

Single-Input Neuron

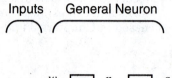

$$a = f(wp + b)$$

Multiple-Input Neuron

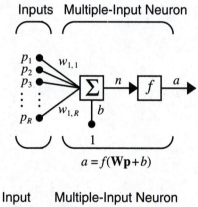

$$a = f(\mathbf{W}\mathbf{p} + b)$$

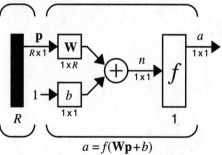

$$a = f(\mathbf{W}\mathbf{p} + b)$$

Transfer Functions

Name	Input/Output Relation	Icon	MATLAB Function
Hard Limit	$a = 0 \quad n < 0$ $a = 1 \quad n \geq 0$		hardlim
Symmetrical Hard Limit	$a = -1 \quad n < 0$ $a = +1 \quad n \geq 0$		hardlims
Linear	$a = n$		purelin
Saturating Linear	$a = 0 \quad n < 0$ $a = n \quad 0 \leq n \leq 1$ $a = 1 \quad n > 1$		satlin
Symmetric Saturating Linear	$a = -1 \quad n < -1$ $a = n \quad -1 \leq n \leq 1$ $a = 1 \quad n > 1$		satlins
Log-Sigmoid	$a = \dfrac{1}{1 + e^{-n}}$		logsig
Hyperbolic Tangent Sigmoid	$a = \dfrac{e^{n} - e^{-n}}{e^{n} + e^{-n}}$		tansig
Positive Linear	$a = 0 \quad n < 0$ $a = n \quad 0 \leq n$		poslin
Competitive	$a = 1 \quad$ neuron with max n $a = 0 \quad$ all other neurons	C	compet

Layer of Neurons

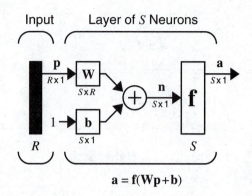

$$\mathbf{a} = \mathbf{f}(\mathbf{Wp}+\mathbf{b})$$

Three Layers of Neurons

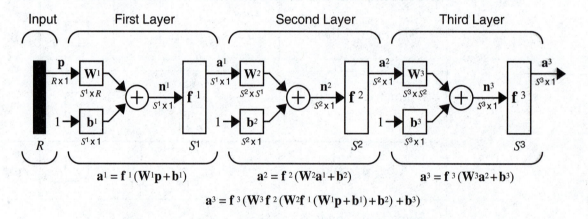

$$\mathbf{a}^1 = \mathbf{f}^1(\mathbf{W}^1\mathbf{p}+\mathbf{b}^1) \qquad \mathbf{a}^2 = \mathbf{f}^2(\mathbf{W}^2\mathbf{a}^1+\mathbf{b}^2) \qquad \mathbf{a}^3 = \mathbf{f}^3(\mathbf{W}^3\mathbf{a}^2+\mathbf{b}^3)$$

$$\mathbf{a}^3 = \mathbf{f}^3(\mathbf{W}^3\mathbf{f}^2(\mathbf{W}^2\mathbf{f}^1(\mathbf{W}^1\mathbf{p}+\mathbf{b}^1)+\mathbf{b}^2)+\mathbf{b}^3)$$

Delay

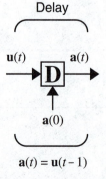

$$\mathbf{a}(t) = \mathbf{u}(t-1)$$

Integrator

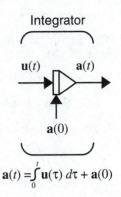

Integrator

$$\mathbf{a}(t) = \int_0^t \mathbf{u}(\tau)\, d\tau + \mathbf{a}(0)$$

Recurrent Network

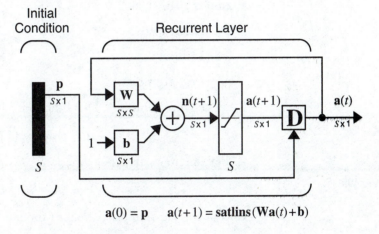

$$\mathbf{a}(0) = \mathbf{p} \qquad \mathbf{a}(t+1) = \mathbf{satlins}\,(\mathbf{W}\mathbf{a}(t) + \mathbf{b})$$

How to Pick an Architecture

Problem specifications help define the network in the following ways:

1. Number of network inputs = number of problem inputs

2. Number of neurons in output layer = number of problem outputs

3. Output layer transfer function choice at least partly determined by problem specification of the outputs

Solved Problems

P2.1 **The input to a single-input neuron is 2.0, its weight is 2.3 and its bias is –3.**

   i. What is the net input to the transfer function?

   ii. What is the neuron output?

i. The net input is given by:

$$n = wp + b = (2.3)(2) + (-3) = 1.6$$

ii. The output cannot be determined because the transfer function is not specified.

P2.2 **What is the output of the neuron of P2.1 if it has the following transfer functions?**

   i. Hard limit

   ii. Linear

   iii. Log-sigmoid

i. For the hard limit transfer function:

$$a = hardlim(1.6) = 1.0$$

ii. For the linear transfer function:

$$a = purelin(1.6) = 1.6$$

iii. For the log-sigmoid transfer function:

$$a = logsig(1.6) = \frac{1}{1 + e^{-1.6}} = 0.8320$$

Verify this result using MATLAB and the function **logsig**, which is in the MININNET directory (see Appendix B).

P2.3 **Given a two-input neuron with the following parameters:** $b = 1.2$, $\mathbf{W} = \begin{bmatrix} 3 & 2 \end{bmatrix}$ **and** $\mathbf{p} = \begin{bmatrix} -5 & 6 \end{bmatrix}^T$, **calculate the neuron output for the following transfer functions:**

   i. A symmetrical hard limit transfer function

   ii. A saturating linear transfer function

iii. A hyperbolic tangent sigmoid (tansig) transfer function

First calculate the net input n :

$$n = \mathbf{Wp} + b = \begin{bmatrix} 3 & 2 \end{bmatrix} \begin{bmatrix} -5 \\ 6 \end{bmatrix} + (1.2) = -1.8 .$$

Now find the outputs for each of the transfer functions.

i. $a = hardlims\,(-1.8) = -1$

ii. $a = satlin\,(-1.8) = 0$

iii. $a = tansig\,(-1.8) = -0.9468$

P2.4 **A single-layer neural network is to have six inputs and two outputs. The outputs are to be limited to and continuous over the range 0 to 1. What can you tell about the network architecture? Specifically:**

　　i. **How many neurons are required?**

　　ii. **What are the dimensions of the weight matrix?**

　　iii. **What kind of transfer functions could be used?**

　　iv. **Is a bias required?**

The problem specifications allow you to say the following about the network.

i. Two neurons, one for each output, are required.

ii. The weight matrix has two rows corresponding to the two neurons and six columns corresponding to the six inputs. (The product $\mathbf{Wp}$ is a two-element vector.)

iii. Of the transfer functions we have discussed, the *logsig* transfer function would be most appropriate.

iv. Not enough information is given to determine if a bias is required.

Epilogue

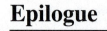

This chapter has introduced a simple artificial neuron and has illustrated how different neural networks can be created by connecting groups of neurons in various ways. One of the main objectives of this chapter has been to introduce our basic notation. As the networks are discussed in more detail in later chapters, you may wish to return to Chapter 2 to refresh your memory of the appropriate notation.

This chapter was not meant to be a complete presentation of the networks we have discussed here. That will be done in the chapters that follow. We will begin in Chapter 3, which will present a simple example that uses some of the networks described in this chapter, and will give you an opportunity to see these networks in action. The networks demonstrated in Chapter 3 are representative of the types of networks that are covered in the remainder of this text.

Exercises

E2.1 The input to a single input neuron is 2.0, its weight is 1.3 and its bias is 3.0. What possible kinds of transfer function, from Table 2.1, could this neuron have, if its output is:

    i. 1.6

    ii. 1.0

    iii. 0.9963

    iv. –1.0

E2.2 Consider a single-input neuron with a bias. We would like the output to be –1 for inputs less than 3 and +1 for inputs greater than or equal to 3.

    i. What kind of a transfer function is required?

    ii. What bias would you suggest? Is your bias in any way related to the input weight? If yes, how?

    iii. Summarize your network by naming the transfer function and stating the bias and the weight. Draw a diagram of the network. Verify the network performance using MATLAB.

```
» 2 + 2
ans =
    4
```

E2.3 Given a two-input neuron with the following weight matrix and input vector: $\mathbf{W} = \begin{bmatrix} 3 & 2 \end{bmatrix}$ and $\mathbf{p} = \begin{bmatrix} -5 & 7 \end{bmatrix}^T$, we would like to have an output of 0.5. Do you suppose that there is a combination of bias and transfer function that might allow this?

    i. Is there a transfer function from Table 2.1 that will do the job if the bias is zero?

    ii. Is there a bias that will do the job if the linear transfer function is used? If yes, what is it?

    iii. Is there a bias that will do the job if a log-sigmoid transfer function is used? Again, if yes, what is it?

    iv. Is there a bias that will do the job if a symmetrical hard limit transfer function is used? Again, if yes, what is it?

E2.4 A two-layer neural network is to have four inputs and six outputs. The range of the outputs is to be continuous between 0 and 1. What can you tell about the network architecture? Specifically:

i. How many neurons are required in each layer?

   ii. What are the dimensions of the first-layer and second-layer weight matrices?

  iii. What kinds of transfer functions can be used in each layer?

   iv. Are biases required in either layer?

3 An Illustrative Example

Objectives

Think of this chapter as a preview of coming attractions. We will take a simple pattern recognition problem and show how it can be solved using three different neural network architectures. It will be an opportunity to see how the architectures described in the previous chapter can be used to solve a practical (although extremely oversimplified) problem. Do not expect to completely understand these three networks after reading this chapter. We present them simply to give you a taste of what can be done with neural networks, and to demonstrate that there are many different types of networks that can be used to solve a given problem.

The three networks presented in this chapter are representative of the types of networks discussed in the remaining chapters: feedforward networks (represented here by the perceptron), competitive networks (represented here by the Hamming network) and recurrent associative memory networks (represented here by the Hopfield network).

Theory and Examples

Problem Statement

A produce dealer has a warehouse that stores a variety of fruits and vegetables. When fruit is brought to the warehouse, various types of fruit may be mixed together. The dealer wants a machine that will sort the fruit according to type. There is a conveyer belt on which the fruit is loaded. This conveyer passes through a set of sensors, which measure three properties of the fruit: *shape*, *texture* and *weight*. These sensors are somewhat primitive. The shape sensor will output a 1 if the fruit is approximately round and a –1 if it is more elliptical. The texture sensor will output a 1 if the surface of the fruit is smooth and a –1 if it is rough. The weight sensor will output a 1 if the fruit is more than one pound and a –1 if it is less than one pound.

The three sensor outputs will then be input to a neural network. The purpose of the network is to decide which kind of fruit is on the conveyor, so that the fruit can be directed to the correct storage bin. To make the problem even simpler, let's assume that there are only two kinds of fruit on the conveyor: apples and oranges.

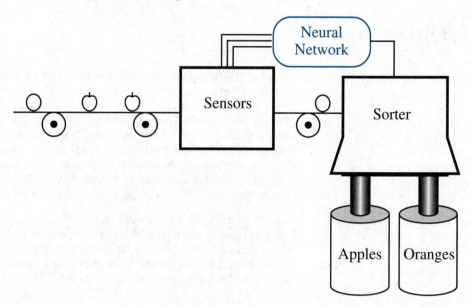

As each fruit passes through the sensors it can be represented by a three-dimensional vector. The first element of the vector will represent shape, the second element will represent texture and the third element will represent weight:

$$\mathbf{p} = \begin{bmatrix} shape \\ texture \\ weight \end{bmatrix}. \tag{3.1}$$

Therefore, a prototype orange would be represented by

$$\mathbf{p}_1 = \begin{bmatrix} 1 \\ -1 \\ -1 \end{bmatrix}, \tag{3.2}$$

and a prototype apple would be represented by

$$\mathbf{p}_2 = \begin{bmatrix} 1 \\ 1 \\ -1 \end{bmatrix}. \tag{3.3}$$

The neural network will receive one three-dimensional input vector for each fruit on the conveyer and must make a decision as to whether the fruit is an *orange* ($\mathbf{p}_1$) or an *apple* ($\mathbf{p}_2$).

Now that we have defined this simple (trivial?) pattern recognition problem, let's look briefly at three different neural networks that could be used to solve it. The simplicity of our problem will facilitate our understanding of the operation of the networks.

Perceptron

The first network we will discuss is the perceptron. Figure 3.1 illustrates a single-layer perceptron with a symmetric hard limit transfer function *hardlims*.

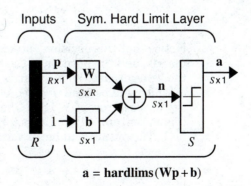

$$a = \mathbf{hardlims}(\mathbf{Wp} + \mathbf{b})$$

Figure 3.1 Single-Layer Perceptron

Two-Input Case

Before we use the perceptron to solve the orange and apple recognition problem (which will require a three-input perceptron, i.e., $R = 3$), it is useful to investigate the capabilities of a two-input/single-neuron perceptron ($R = 2$), which can be easily analyzed graphically. The two-input perceptron is shown in Figure 3.2.

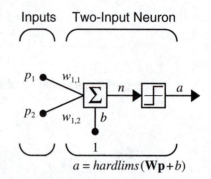

Figure 3.2 Two-Input/Single-Neuron Perceptron

Single-neuron perceptrons can classify input vectors into two categories. For example, for a two-input perceptron, if $w_{1,1} = -1$ and $w_{1,2} = 1$ then

$$a = hardlims\,(n) = hardlims\,\left(\begin{bmatrix} -1 & 1 \end{bmatrix}\mathbf{p} + b\right).\qquad(3.4)$$

Therefore, if the inner product of the weight matrix (a single row vector in this case) with the input vector is greater than or equal to $-b$, the output will be 1. If the inner product of the weight vector and the input is less than $-b$, the output will be -1. This divides the input space into two parts. Figure 3.3 illustrates this for the case where $b = -1$. The blue line in the figure represents all points for which the net input n is equal to 0:

$$n = \begin{bmatrix} -1 & 1 \end{bmatrix}\mathbf{p} - 1 = 0.\qquad(3.5)$$

Notice that this decision boundary will always be orthogonal to the weight matrix, and the position of the boundary can be shifted by changing b. (In the general case, $\mathbf{W}$ is a matrix consisting of a number of row vectors, each of which will be used in an equation like Eq. (3.5). There will be one boundary for each row of $\mathbf{W}$. See Chapter 4 for more on this topic.) The shaded region contains all input vectors for which the output of the network will be 1. The output will be -1 for all other input vectors.

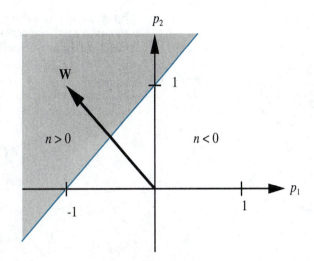

Figure 3.3 Perceptron Decision Boundary

The key property of the single-neuron perceptron, therefore, is that it can separate input vectors into two categories. The decision boundary between the categories is determined by the equation

$$\mathbf{W}\mathbf{p} + b = 0.\tag{3.6}$$

Because the boundary must be linear, the single-layer perceptron can only be used to recognize patterns that are linearly separable (can be separated by a linear boundary). These concepts will be discussed in more detail in Chapter 4.

Pattern Recognition Example

Now consider the apple and orange pattern recognition problem. Because there are only two categories, we can use a single-neuron perceptron. The vector inputs are three-dimensional ($R = 3$), therefore the perceptron equation will be

$$a = hardlims\left(\begin{bmatrix} w_{1,1} & w_{1,2} & w_{1,3} \end{bmatrix}\begin{bmatrix} p_1 \\ p_2 \\ p_3 \end{bmatrix} + b\right).\tag{3.7}$$

We want to choose the bias b and the elements of the weight matrix so that the perceptron will be able to distinguish between apples and oranges. For example, we may want the output of the perceptron to be 1 when an apple is input and -1 when an orange is input. Using the concept illustrated in Figure 3.3, let's find a linear boundary that can separate oranges and apples. The two prototype vectors (recall Eq. (3.2) and Eq. (3.3)) are shown in Figure 3.4. From this figure we can see that the linear boundary that divides these two vectors symmetrically is the p_1, p_3 plane.

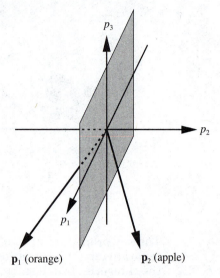

$\mathbf{p}_1$ (orange) $\mathbf{p}_2$ (apple)

Figure 3.4   Prototype Vectors

The p_1, p_3 plane, which will be our decision boundary, can be described by the equation

$$p_2 = 0 ,$$
(3.8)

or

$$\begin{bmatrix} 0 & 1 & 0 \end{bmatrix} \begin{bmatrix} p_1 \\ p_2 \\ p_3 \end{bmatrix} + 0 = 0 .$$
(3.9)

Therefore the weight matrix and bias will be

$$\mathbf{W} = \begin{bmatrix} 0 & 1 & 0 \end{bmatrix}, \, b = 0 .$$
(3.10)

The weight matrix is orthogonal to the decision boundary and points toward the region that contains the prototype pattern $\mathbf{p}_2$ (*apple*) for which we want the perceptron to produce an output of 1. The bias is 0 because the decision boundary passes through the origin.

Now let's test the operation of our perceptron pattern classifier. It classifies perfect apples and oranges correctly since

Orange:

$$a = hardlims\left(\begin{bmatrix} 0 & 1 & 0 \end{bmatrix}\begin{bmatrix} 1 \\ -1 \\ -1 \end{bmatrix} + 0\right) = -1 \ (orange)\,, \qquad (3.11)$$

Apple:

$$a = hardlims\left(\begin{bmatrix} 0 & 1 & 0 \end{bmatrix}\begin{bmatrix} 1 \\ 1 \\ -1 \end{bmatrix} + 0\right) = 1 \ (apple)\,. \qquad (3.12)$$

But what happens if we put a not-so-perfect orange into the classifier? Let's say that an orange with an elliptical shape is passed through the sensors. The input vector would then be

$$\mathbf{p} = \begin{bmatrix} -1 \\ -1 \\ -1 \end{bmatrix}\,. \qquad (3.13)$$

The response of the network would be

$$a = hardlims\left(\begin{bmatrix} 0 & 1 & 0 \end{bmatrix}\begin{bmatrix} -1 \\ -1 \\ -1 \end{bmatrix} + 0\right) = -1 \ (orange)\,. \qquad (3.14)$$

In fact, any input vector that is closer to the orange prototype vector than to the apple prototype vector (in Euclidean distance) will be classified as an orange (and vice versa).

 To experiment with the perceptron network and the apple/orange classification problem, use the Neural Network Design Demonstration Perceptron Classification (**nnd3pc**).

This example has demonstrated some of the features of the perceptron network, but by no means have we exhausted our investigation of perceptrons. This network, and variations on it, will be examined in Chapters 4 through 12. Let's consider some of these future topics.

In the apple/orange example we were able to design a network graphically, by choosing a decision boundary that clearly separated the patterns. What about practical problems, with high dimensional input spaces? In Chapters 4, 7, 10 and 11 we will introduce learning algorithms that can be used to train networks to solve complex problems by using a set of examples of proper network behavior.

The key characteristic of the single-layer perceptron is that it creates linear decision boundaries to separate categories of input vector. What if we have categories that cannot be separated by linear boundaries? This question will be addressed in Chapter 11, where we will introduce the multilayer perceptron. The multilayer networks are able to solve classification problems of arbitrary complexity.

Hamming Network

The next network we will consider is the Hamming network [Lipp87]. It was designed explicitly to solve binary pattern recognition problems (where each element of the input vector has only two possible values — in our example 1 or –1). This is an interesting network, because it uses both feedforward and recurrent (feedback) layers, which were both described in Chapter 2. Figure 3.5 shows the standard Hamming network. Note that the number of neurons in the first layer is the same as the number of neurons in the second layer.

The objective of the Hamming network is to decide which prototype vector is closest to the input vector. This decision is indicated by the output of the recurrent layer. There is one neuron in the recurrent layer for each prototype pattern. When the recurrent layer converges, there will be only one neuron with nonzero output. This neuron indicates the prototype pattern that is closest to the input vector. Now let's investigate the two layers of the Hamming network in detail.

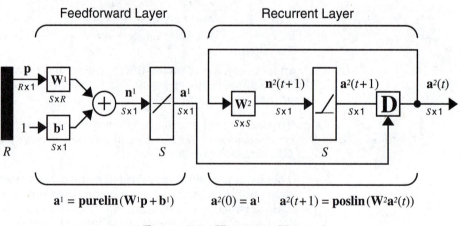

$$\mathbf{a}^1 = \mathbf{purelin}(\mathbf{W}^1\mathbf{p} + \mathbf{b}^1) \qquad \mathbf{a}^2(0) = \mathbf{a}^1 \qquad \mathbf{a}^2(t+1) = \mathbf{poslin}(\mathbf{W}^2\mathbf{a}^2(t))$$

Figure 3.5   Hamming Network

Feedforward Layer

The feedforward layer performs a correlation, or inner product, between each of the prototype patterns and the input pattern (as we will see in Eq. (3.17)). In order for the feedforward layer to perform this correlation, the rows of the weight matrix in the feedforward layer, represented by the connection matrix $\mathbf{W}^1$, are set to the prototype patterns. For our apple and orange example this would mean

$$\mathbf{W}^1 = \begin{bmatrix} \mathbf{p}_1^T \\ \mathbf{p}_2^T \end{bmatrix} = \begin{bmatrix} 1 & -1 & -1 \\ 1 & 1 & -1 \end{bmatrix}. \tag{3.15}$$

The feedforward layer uses a linear transfer function, and each element of the bias vector is equal to R, where R is the number of elements in the input vector. For our example the bias vector would be

$$\mathbf{b}^1 = \begin{bmatrix} 3 \\ 3 \end{bmatrix}. \tag{3.16}$$

With these choices for the weight matrix and bias vector, the output of the feedforward layer is

$$\mathbf{a}^1 = \mathbf{W}^1 \mathbf{p} + \mathbf{b}^1 = \begin{bmatrix} \mathbf{p}_1^T \\ \mathbf{p}_2^T \end{bmatrix} \mathbf{p} + \begin{bmatrix} 3 \\ 3 \end{bmatrix} = \begin{bmatrix} \mathbf{p}_1^T \mathbf{p} + 3 \\ \mathbf{p}_2^T \mathbf{p} + 3 \end{bmatrix}. \tag{3.17}$$

Note that the outputs of the feedforward layer are equal to the inner products of each prototype pattern with the input, plus R. For two vectors of equal length (norm), their inner product will be largest when the vectors point in the same direction, and will be smallest when they point in opposite directions. (We will discuss this concept in more depth in Chapters 5, 8 and 9.) By adding R to the inner product we guarantee that the outputs of the feedforward layer can never be negative. This is required for proper operation of the recurrent layer.

This network is called the Hamming network because the neuron in the feedforward layer with the largest output will correspond to the prototype pattern that is closest in Hamming distance to the input pattern. (The Hamming distance between two vectors is equal to the number of elements that are different. It is defined only for binary vectors.) We leave it to the reader to show that the outputs of the feedforward layer are equal to $2R$ minus twice the Hamming distances from the prototype patterns to the input pattern.

Recurrent Layer

The recurrent layer of the Hamming network is what is known as a "competitive" layer. The neurons in this layer are initialized with the outputs of the feedforward layer, which indicate the correlation between the prototype patterns and the input vector. Then the neurons compete with each other to determine a winner. After the competition, only one neuron will have a nonzero output. The winning neuron indicates which category of input was presented to the network (for our example the two categories are *apples* and *oranges*). The equations that describe the competition are:

$$\mathbf{a}^2(0) = \mathbf{a}^1 \quad \text{(Initial Condition)}, \tag{3.18}$$

and

$$\mathbf{a}^2(t+1) = \mathbf{poslin}(\mathbf{W}^2\mathbf{a}^2(t)). \tag{3.19}$$

(Don't forget that the superscripts here indicate the layer number, not a power of 2.) The *poslin* transfer function is linear for positive values and zero for negative values. The weight matrix $\mathbf{W}^2$ has the form

$$\mathbf{W}^2 = \begin{bmatrix} 1 & -\varepsilon \\ -\varepsilon & 1 \end{bmatrix}, \tag{3.20}$$

where ε is some number less than $1/(S-1)$, and S is the number of neurons in the recurrent layer. (Can you show why ε must be less than $1/(S-1)$?)

An iteration of the recurrent layer proceeds as follows:

$$\mathbf{a}^2(t+1) = \mathbf{poslin}\left(\begin{bmatrix} 1 & -\varepsilon \\ -\varepsilon & 1 \end{bmatrix}\mathbf{a}^2(t)\right) = \mathbf{poslin}\left(\begin{bmatrix} a_1^2(t) - \varepsilon a_2^2(t) \\ a_2^2(t) - \varepsilon a_1^2(t) \end{bmatrix}\right). \tag{3.21}$$

Each element is reduced by the same fraction of the other. The larger element will be reduced by less, and the smaller element will be reduced by more, therefore the difference between large and small will be increased. The effect of the recurrent layer is to zero out all neuron outputs, except the one with the largest initial value (which corresponds to the prototype pattern that is closest in Hamming distance to the input).

To illustrate the operation of the Hamming network, consider again the oblong orange that we used to test the perceptron:

$$\mathbf{p} = \begin{bmatrix} -1 \\ -1 \\ -1 \end{bmatrix}. \tag{3.22}$$

The output of the feedforward layer will be

$$a^1 = \begin{bmatrix} 1 & -1 & -1 \\ 1 & 1 & -1 \end{bmatrix} \begin{bmatrix} -1 \\ -1 \\ -1 \end{bmatrix} + \begin{bmatrix} 3 \\ 3 \end{bmatrix} = \begin{bmatrix} (1+3) \\ (-1+3) \end{bmatrix} = \begin{bmatrix} 4 \\ 2 \end{bmatrix}, \tag{3.23}$$

which will then become the initial condition for the recurrent layer.

The weight matrix for the recurrent layer will be given by Eq. (3.20) with $\varepsilon = 1/2$ (any number less than 1 would work). The first iteration of the recurrent layer produces

$$\mathbf{a}^2(1) = \mathbf{poslin}(\mathbf{W}^2\mathbf{a}^2(0)) = \begin{cases} \mathbf{poslin}\left(\begin{bmatrix} 1 & -0.5 \\ -0.5 & 1 \end{bmatrix} \begin{bmatrix} 4 \\ 2 \end{bmatrix} \right) \\ \mathbf{poslin}\left(\begin{bmatrix} 3 \\ 0 \end{bmatrix} \right) = \begin{bmatrix} 3 \\ 0 \end{bmatrix} \end{cases}. \tag{3.24}$$

The second iteration produces

$$\mathbf{a}^2(2) = \mathbf{poslin}(\mathbf{W}^2\mathbf{a}^2(1)) = \begin{cases} \mathbf{poslin}\left(\begin{bmatrix} 1 & -0.5 \\ -0.5 & 1 \end{bmatrix} \begin{bmatrix} 3 \\ 0 \end{bmatrix} \right) \\ \mathbf{poslin}\left(\begin{bmatrix} 3 \\ -1.5 \end{bmatrix} \right) = \begin{bmatrix} 3 \\ 0 \end{bmatrix} \end{cases}. \tag{3.25}$$

Since the outputs of successive iterations produce the same result, the network has converged. Prototype pattern number one, the *orange*, is chosen as the correct match, since neuron number one has the only nonzero output. (Recall that the first element of $\mathbf{a}^1$ was $(\mathbf{p}_1^T\mathbf{p} + 3)$.) This is the correct choice, since the Hamming distance from the *orange* prototype to the input pattern is 1, and the Hamming distance from the *apple* prototype to the input pattern is 2.

To experiment with the Hamming network and the apple/orange classification problem, use the Neural Network Design Demonstration Hamming Classification (nnd3hamc).

There are a number of networks whose operation is based on the same principles as the Hamming network; that is, where an inner product operation (feedforward layer) is followed by a competitive dynamic layer. These competitive networks will be discussed in Chapters 13 through 16. They are *self-organizing* networks, which can learn to adjust their prototype vectors based on the inputs that have been presented.

Hopfield Network

The final network we will discuss in this brief preview is the Hopfield network. This is a recurrent network that is similar in some respects to the recurrent layer of the Hamming network, but which can effectively perform the operations of both layers of the Hamming network. A diagram of the Hopfield network is shown in Figure 3.6. (This figure is actually a slight variation of the standard Hopfield network. We use this variation because it is somewhat simpler to describe and yet demonstrates the basic concepts.)

The neurons in this network are initialized with the input vector, then the network iterates until the output converges. When the network is operating correctly, the resulting output should be one of the prototype vectors. Therefore, whereas in the Hamming network the nonzero neuron indicates which prototype pattern is chosen, the Hopfield network actually produces the selected prototype pattern at its output.

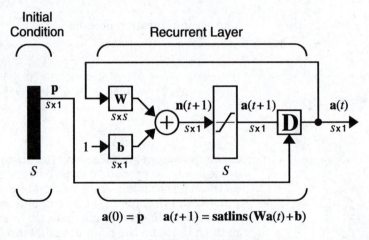

$$\mathbf{a}(0) = \mathbf{p} \qquad \mathbf{a}(t+1) = \mathbf{satlins}(\mathbf{Wa}(t) + \mathbf{b})$$

Figure 3.6   Hopfield Network

The equations that describe the network operation are

$$\mathbf{a}(0) = \mathbf{p} \tag{3.26}$$

and

$$\mathbf{a}(t+1) = \mathbf{satlins}(\mathbf{Wa}(t) + \mathbf{b}), \tag{3.27}$$

where *satlins* is the transfer function that is linear in the range $[-1, 1]$ and saturates at 1 for inputs greater than 1 and at -1 for inputs less than -1.

The design of the weight matrix and the bias vector for the Hopfield network is a more complex procedure than it is for the Hamming network, where the weights in the feedforward layer are the prototype patterns. Hopfield design procedures will be discussed in detail in Chapter 18.

To illustrate the operation of the network, we have determined a weight matrix and a bias vector that can solve our orange and apple pattern recognition problem. They are given in Eq. (3.28).

$$\mathbf{W} = \begin{bmatrix} 0.2 & 0 & 0 \\ 0 & 1.2 & 0 \\ 0 & 0 & 0.2 \end{bmatrix}, \mathbf{b} = \begin{bmatrix} 0.9 \\ 0 \\ -0.9 \end{bmatrix} \tag{3.28}$$

Although the procedure for computing the weights and biases for the Hopfield network is beyond the scope of this chapter, we can say a few things about why the parameters in Eq. (3.28) work for the apple and orange example.

We want the network output to converge to either the orange pattern, $\mathbf{p}_1$, or the apple pattern, $\mathbf{p}_2$. In both patterns, the first element is 1, and the third element is -1. The difference between the patterns occurs in the second element. Therefore, no matter what pattern is input to the network, we want the first element of the output pattern to converge to 1, the third element to converge to -1, and the second element to go to either 1 or -1, whichever is closer to the second element of the input vector.

The equations of operation of the Hopfield network, using the parameters given in Eq. (3.28), are

$$a_1(t+1) = satlins(0.2a_1(t) + 0.9)$$

$$a_2(t+1) = satlins(1.2a_2(t))$$

$$a_3(t+1) = satlins(0.2a_3(t) - 0.9) \tag{3.29}$$

Regardless of the initial values, $a_i(0)$, the first element will be increased until it saturates at 1, and the third element will be decreased until it saturates at -1. The second element is multiplied by a number larger than 1. Therefore, if it is initially negative, it will eventually saturate at -1; if it is initially positive it will saturate at 1.

(It should be noted that this is not the only ($\mathbf{W}$, $\mathbf{b}$) pair that could be used. You might want to try some others. See if you can discover what makes these work.)

Let's again take our oblong orange to test the Hopfield network. The outputs of the Hopfield network for the first three iterations would be

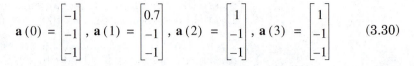

$$\mathbf{a}(0) = \begin{bmatrix} -1 \\ -1 \\ -1 \end{bmatrix}, \ \mathbf{a}(1) = \begin{bmatrix} 0.7 \\ -1 \\ -1 \end{bmatrix}, \ \mathbf{a}(2) = \begin{bmatrix} 1 \\ -1 \\ -1 \end{bmatrix}, \ \mathbf{a}(3) = \begin{bmatrix} 1 \\ -1 \\ -1 \end{bmatrix} \qquad (3.30)$$

The network has converged to the *orange* pattern, as did both the Hamming network and the perceptron, although each network operated in a different way. The perceptron had a single output, which could take on values of –1 (*orange*) or 1 (*apple*). In the Hamming network the single nonzero neuron indicated which prototype pattern had the closest match. If the first neuron was nonzero, that indicated *orange*, and if the second neuron was nonzero, that indicated *apple*. In the Hopfield network the prototype pattern itself appears at the output of the network.

To experiment with the Hopfield network and the apple / orange classification problem, use the Neural Network Design Demonstration Hopfield Classification (**nnd3hopc**).

As with the other networks demonstrated in this chapter, do not expect to feel completely comfortable with the Hopfield network at this point. There are a number of questions that we have not discussed. For example, "How do we know that the network will eventually converge?" It is possible for recurrent networks to oscillate or to have chaotic behavior. In addition, we have not discussed general procedures for designing the weight matrix and the bias vector. These topics will be discussed in detail in Chapters 17 and 18.

Epilogue

The three networks that we have introduced in this chapter demonstrate many of the characteristics that are found in the architectures which are discussed throughout this book.

Feedforward networks, of which the perceptron is one example, are presented in Chapters 4, 7, 11 and 12. In these networks, the output is computed directly from the input in one pass; no feedback is involved. Feedforward networks are used for pattern recognition, as in the apple and orange example, and also for function approximation (see Chapter 11). Function approximation applications are found in such areas as adaptive filtering (see Chapter 10) and automatic control.

Competitive networks, represented here by the Hamming network, are characterized by two properties. First, they compute some measure of distance between stored prototype patterns and the input pattern. Second, they perform a competition to determine which neuron represents the prototype pattern closest to the input. In the competitive networks that are discussed in Chapters 14–16, the prototype patterns are adjusted as new inputs are applied to the network. These adaptive networks learn to cluster the inputs into different categories.

Recurrent networks, like the Hopfield network, were originally inspired by statistical mechanics. They have been used as associative memories, in which stored data is recalled by association with input data, rather than by an address. They have also been used to solve a variety of optimization problems. We will discuss these recurrent networks in Chapters 17 and 18.

We hope this chapter has piqued your curiosity about the capabilities of neural networks and has raised some questions. A few of the questions we will answer in later chapters are:

1. How do we determine the weight matrix and bias for perceptron networks with many inputs, where it is impossible to visualize the decision boundary? (Chapters 4 and 10)

2. If the categories to be recognized are not linearly separable, can we extend the standard perceptron to solve the problem? (Chapters 11 and 12)

3. Can we learn the weights and biases of the Hamming network when we don't know the prototype patterns? (Chapters 14–16)

4. How do we determine the weight matrix and bias vector for the Hopfield network? (Chapter 18)

5. How do we know that the Hopfield network will eventually converge? (Chapters 17 and 18)

Exercise

E3.1 In this chapter we have designed three different neural networks to distinguish between apples and oranges, based on three sensor measurements (shape, texture and weight). Suppose that we want to distinguish between bananas and pineapples:

$$\mathbf{p}_1 = \begin{bmatrix} -1 \\ 1 \\ -1 \end{bmatrix} \text{ (Banana)}$$

$$\mathbf{p}_2 = \begin{bmatrix} -1 \\ -1 \\ 1 \end{bmatrix} \text{ (Pineapple)}$$

   i. Design a perceptron to recognize these patterns.

   ii. Design a Hamming network to recognize these patterns.

   iii. Design a Hopfield network to recognize these patterns.

   iv. Test the operation of your networks by applying several different input patterns. Discuss the advantages and disadvantages of each network.

4 Perceptron Learning Rule

4

Objectives

One of the questions we raised in Chapter 3 was: "How do we determine the weight matrix and bias for perceptron networks with many inputs, where it is impossible to visualize the decision boundaries?" In this chapter we will describe an algorithm for *training* perceptron networks, so that they can *learn* to solve classification problems. We will begin by explaining what a learning rule is and will then develop the perceptron learning rule. We will conclude by discussing the advantages and limitations of the single-layer perceptron network. This discussion will lead us into future chapters.

Theory and Examples

In 1943, Warren McCulloch and Walter Pitts introduced one of the first artificial neurons [McPi43]. The main feature of their neuron model is that a weighted sum of input signals is compared to a threshold to determine the neuron output. When the sum is greater than or equal to the threshold, the output is 1. When the sum is less than the threshold, the output is 0. They went on to show that networks of these neurons could, in principle, compute any arithmetic or logical function. Unlike biological networks, the parameters of their networks had to be designed, as no training method was available. However, the perceived connection between biology and digital computers generated a great deal of interest.

In the late 1950s, Frank Rosenblatt and several other researchers developed a class of neural networks called perceptrons. The neurons in these networks were similar to those of McCulloch and Pitts. Rosenblatt's key contribution was the introduction of a learning rule for training perceptron networks to solve pattern recognition problems [Rose58]. He proved that his learning rule will always converge to the correct network weights, if weights exist that solve the problem. Learning was simple and automatic. Examples of proper behavior were presented to the network, which learned from its mistakes. The perceptron could even learn when initialized with random values for its weights and biases.

Unfortunately, the perceptron network is inherently limited. These limitations were widely publicized in the book *Perceptrons* [MiPa69] by Marvin Minsky and Seymour Papert. They demonstrated that the perceptron networks were incapable of implementing certain elementary functions. It was not until the 1980s that these limitations were overcome with improved (multilayer) perceptron networks and associated learning rules. We will discuss these improvements in Chapters 11 and 12.

Today the perceptron is still viewed as an important network. It remains a fast and reliable network for the class of problems that it can solve. In addition, an understanding of the operations of the perceptron provides a good basis for understanding more complex networks. Thus, the perceptron network, and its associated learning rule, are well worth discussion here.

In the remainder of this chapter we will define what we mean by a learning rule, explain the perceptron network and learning rule, and discuss the limitations of the perceptron network.

Learning Rules

Learning Rule   As we begin our discussion of the perceptron learning rule, we want to discuss learning rules in general. By *learning rule* we mean a procedure for modifying the weights and biases of a network. (This procedure may also be referred to as a training algorithm.) The purpose of the learning rule is to train the network to perform some task. There are many types of neural network learning rules. They fall into three broad categories: supervised learning, unsupervised learning and reinforcement (or graded) learning.

Supervised Learning
Training Set

In *supervised learning*, the learning rule is provided with a set of examples (the *training set*) of proper network behavior:

$$\{\mathbf{p}_1, \mathbf{t}_1\}, \{\mathbf{p}_2, \mathbf{t}_2\}, \dots, \{\mathbf{p}_Q, \mathbf{t}_Q\}, \tag{4.1}$$

Target

where $\mathbf{p}_q$ is an input to the network and $\mathbf{t}_q$ is the corresponding correct (*target*) output. As the inputs are applied to the network, the network outputs are compared to the targets. The learning rule is then used to adjust the weights and biases of the network in order to move the network outputs closer to the targets. The perceptron learning rule falls in this supervised learning category. We will also investigate supervised learning algorithms in Chapters 7–12.

Reinforcement Learning

Reinforcement learning is similar to supervised learning, except that, instead of being provided with the correct output for each network input, the algorithm is only given a grade. The grade (or score) is a measure of the network performance over some sequence of inputs. This type of learning is currently much less common than supervised learning. It appears to be most suited to control system applications (see [BaSu83], [WhSo92]).

Unsupervised Learning

In *unsupervised learning*, the weights and biases are modified in response to network inputs only. There are no target outputs available. At first glance this might seem to be impractical. How can you train a network if you don't know what it is supposed to do? Most of these algorithms perform some kind of clustering operation. They learn to categorize the input patterns into a finite number of classes. This is especially useful in such applications as vector quantization. We will see in Chapters 13–16 that there are a number of unsupervised learning algorithms.

Perceptron Architecture

Before we present the perceptron learning rule, let's expand our investigation of the perceptron network, which we began in Chapter 3. The general perceptron network is shown in Figure 4.1.

The output of the network is given by

$$\mathbf{a} = \mathbf{hardlim}(\mathbf{Wp} + \mathbf{b}). \tag{4.2}$$

(Note that in Chapter 3 we used the *hardlims* transfer function, instead of *hardlim*. This does not affect the capabilities of the network. See Exercise E4.6.)

4

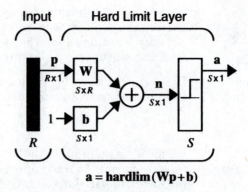

$$a = \text{hardlim}(\mathbf{W}\mathbf{p}+\mathbf{b})$$

Figure 4.1 Perceptron Network

It will be useful in our development of the perceptron learning rule to be able to conveniently reference individual elements of the network output. Let's see how this can be done. First, consider the network weight matrix:

$$\mathbf{W} = \begin{bmatrix} w_{1,1} & w_{1,2} & \cdots & w_{1,R} \\ w_{2,1} & w_{2,2} & \cdots & w_{2,R} \\ \vdots & \vdots & & \vdots \\ w_{S,1} & w_{S,2} & \cdots & w_{S,R} \end{bmatrix}. \tag{4.3}$$

We will define a vector composed of the elements of the ith row of $\mathbf{W}$:

$$_i\mathbf{w} = \begin{bmatrix} w_{i,1} \\ w_{i,2} \\ \vdots \\ w_{i,R} \end{bmatrix}. \tag{4.4}$$

Now we can partition the weight matrix:

$$\mathbf{W} = \begin{bmatrix} _1\mathbf{w}^T \\ _2\mathbf{w}^T \\ \vdots \\ _S\mathbf{w}^T \end{bmatrix}. \tag{4.5}$$

This allows us to write the ith element of the network output vector as

$$a_i = hardlim(n_i) = hardlim(_iw^Tp + b_i) . \qquad (4.6)$$

$a = hardlim(n)$

Recall that the *hardlim* transfer function (shown at left) is defined as:

$$a = hardlim(n) = \begin{cases} 1 & if \ n \geq 0 \\ 0 & otherwise. \end{cases} \qquad (4.7)$$

$n = \mathbf{Wp} + b$

Therefore, if the inner product of the ith row of the weight matrix with the input vector is greater than or equal to $-b_i$, the output will be 1, otherwise the output will be 0. *Thus each neuron in the network divides the input space into two regions.* It is useful to investigate the boundaries between these regions. We will begin with the simple case of a single-neuron perceptron with two inputs.

Single-Neuron Perceptron

Let's consider a two-input perceptron with one neuron, as shown in Figure 4.2.

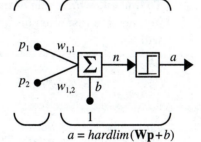

Figure 4.2 Two-Input/Single-Output Perceptron

The output of this network is determined by

$$a = hardlim(n) = hardlim(\mathbf{Wp} + b)$$
$$= hardlim(_1w^Tp + b) = hardlim(w_{1,1}p_1 + w_{1,2}p_2 + b) \qquad (4.8)$$

Decision Boundary   The *decision boundary* is determined by the input vectors for which the net input n is zero:

$$n = _1w^Tp + b = w_{1,1}p_1 + w_{1,2}p_2 + b = 0. \qquad (4.9)$$

To make the example more concrete, let's assign the following values for the weights and bias:

$$w_{1,1} = 1, \; w_{1,2} = 1, \; b = -1.$$ (4.10)

The decision boundary is then

$$n = {}_1\mathbf{w}^T\mathbf{p} + b = w_{1,1}p_1 + w_{1,2}p_2 + b = p_1 + p_2 - 1 = 0.$$ (4.11)

This defines a line in the input space. On one side of the line the network output will be 0; on the line and on the other side of the line the output will be 1. To draw the line, we can find the points where it intersects the p_1 and p_2 axes. To find the p_2 intercept set $p_1 = 0$:

$$p_2 = -\frac{b}{w_{1,2}} = -\frac{-1}{1} = 1 \quad \text{if } p_1 = 0.$$ (4.12)

To find the p_1 intercept, set $p_2 = 0$:

$$p_1 = -\frac{b}{w_{1,1}} = -\frac{-1}{1} = 1 \quad \text{if } p_2 = 0.$$ (4.13)

The resulting decision boundary is illustrated in Figure 4.3.

To find out which side of the boundary corresponds to an output of 1, we just need to test one point. For the input $\mathbf{p} = \begin{bmatrix} 2 & 0 \end{bmatrix}^T$, the network output will be

$$a = hardlim\left({}_1\mathbf{w}^T\mathbf{p} + b\right) = hardlim\left(\begin{bmatrix} 1 & 1 \end{bmatrix}\begin{bmatrix} 2 \\ 0 \end{bmatrix} - 1\right) = 1.$$ (4.14)

Therefore, the network output will be 1 for the region above and to the right of the decision boundary. This region is indicated by the shaded area in Figure 4.3.

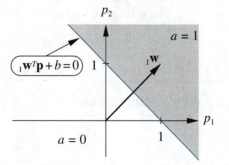

Figure 4.3 Decision Boundary for Two-Input Perceptron

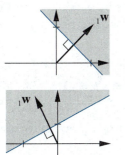

We can also find the decision boundary graphically. The first step is to note that the boundary is always orthogonal to $_1\mathbf{w}$, as illustrated in the adjacent figures. The boundary is defined by

$$_1\mathbf{w}^T\mathbf{p} + b = 0.\qquad(4.15)$$

For all points on the boundary, the inner product of the input vector with the weight vector is the same. This implies that these input vectors will all have the same projection onto the weight vector, so they must lie on a line orthogonal to the weight vector. (These concepts will be covered in more detail in Chapter 5.) In addition, any vector in the shaded region of Figure 4.3 will have an inner product greater than $-b$, and vectors in the unshaded region will have inner products less than $-b$. Therefore the weight vector $_1\mathbf{w}$ will always point toward the region where the neuron output is 1.

After we have selected a weight vector with the correct angular orientation, the bias value can be computed by selecting a point on the boundary and satisfying Eq. (4.15).

Let's apply some of these concepts to the design of a perceptron network to implement a simple logic function: the AND gate. The input/target pairs for the AND gate are

$$\left\{\mathbf{p}_1 = \begin{bmatrix}0\\0\end{bmatrix}, t_1 = 0\right\}\ \left\{\mathbf{p}_2 = \begin{bmatrix}0\\1\end{bmatrix}, t_2 = 0\right\}\ \left\{\mathbf{p}_3 = \begin{bmatrix}1\\0\end{bmatrix}, t_3 = 0\right\}\ \left\{\mathbf{p}_4 = \begin{bmatrix}1\\1\end{bmatrix}, t_4 = 1\right\}.$$

The figure to the left illustrates the problem graphically. It displays the input space, with each input vector labeled according to its target. The dark circles ● indicate that the target is 1, and the light circles ○ indicate that the target is 0.

The first step of the design is to select a decision boundary. We want to have a line that separates the dark circles and the light circles. There are an infinite number of solutions to this problem. It seems reasonable to choose the line that falls "halfway" between the two categories of inputs, as shown in the adjacent figure.

Next we want to choose a weight vector that is orthogonal to the decision boundary. The weight vector can be any length, so there are infinite possibilities. One choice is

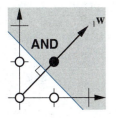

$$_1\mathbf{w} = \begin{bmatrix}2\\2\end{bmatrix},\qquad(4.16)$$

as displayed in the figure to the left.

Finally, we need to find the bias, b. We can do this by picking a point on the decision boundary and satisfying Eq. (4.15). If we use $\mathbf{p} = \begin{bmatrix} 1.5 & 0 \end{bmatrix}^T$ we find

$$_1\mathbf{w}^T\mathbf{p} + b = \begin{bmatrix} 2 & 2 \end{bmatrix}\begin{bmatrix} 1.5 \\ 0 \end{bmatrix} + b = 3 + b = 0 \quad \Rightarrow \quad b = -3. \tag{4.17}$$

We can now test the network on one of the input/target pairs. If we apply $\mathbf{p}_2$ to the network, the output will be

$$a = hardlim\,(_1\mathbf{w}^T\mathbf{p}_2 + b) = hardlim\left(\begin{bmatrix} 2 & 2 \end{bmatrix}\begin{bmatrix} 0 \\ 1 \end{bmatrix} - 3\right) \tag{4.18}$$

$$a = hardlim\,(-1) = 0,$$

which is equal to the target output t_2. Verify for yourself that all inputs are correctly classified.

To experiment with decision boundaries, use the Neural Network Design Demonstration Decision Boundaries *(nnd4db).*

Multiple-Neuron Perceptron

Note that for perceptrons with multiple neurons, as in Figure 4.1, there will be one decision boundary for each neuron. The decision boundary for neuron i will be defined by

$$_i\mathbf{w}^T\mathbf{p} + b_i = 0. \tag{4.19}$$

A single-neuron perceptron can classify input vectors into two categories, since its output can be either 0 or 1. A multiple-neuron perceptron can classify inputs into many categories. Each category is represented by a different output vector. Since each element of the output vector can be either 0 or 1, there are a total of 2^S possible categories, where S is the number of neurons.

Perceptron Learning Rule

Now that we have examined the performance of perceptron networks, we are in a position to introduce the perceptron learning rule. This learning rule is an example of supervised training, in which the learning rule is provided with a set of examples of proper network behavior:

$$\{\mathbf{p}_1, \mathbf{t}_1\}, \{\mathbf{p}_2, \mathbf{t}_2\}, \dots, \{\mathbf{p}_Q, \mathbf{t}_Q\}, \tag{4.20}$$

where $\mathbf{p}_q$ is an input to the network and $\mathbf{t}_q$ is the corresponding target output. As each input is applied to the network, the network output is compared to the target. The learning rule then adjusts the weights and biases of the network in order to move the network output closer to the target.

Test Problem

In our presentation of the perceptron learning rule we will begin with a simple test problem and will experiment with possible rules to develop some intuition about how the rule should work. The input/target pairs for our test problem are

$$\left\{ \mathbf{p}_1 = \begin{bmatrix} 1 \\ 2 \end{bmatrix}, t_1 = 1 \right\} \left\{ \mathbf{p}_2 = \begin{bmatrix} -1 \\ 2 \end{bmatrix}, t_2 = 0 \right\} \left\{ \mathbf{p}_3 = \begin{bmatrix} 0 \\ -1 \end{bmatrix}, t_3 = 0 \right\}.$$

The problem is displayed graphically in the adjacent figure, where the two input vectors whose target is 0 are represented with a light circle $\bigcirc$, and the vector whose target is 1 is represented with a dark circle $\bullet$. This is a very simple problem, and we could almost obtain a solution by inspection. This simplicity will help us gain some intuitive understanding of the basic concepts of the perceptron learning rule.

The network for this problem should have two-inputs and one output. To simplify our development of the learning rule, we will begin with a network without a bias. The network will then have just two parameters, $w_{1,1}$ and $w_{1,2}$, as shown in Figure 4.4.

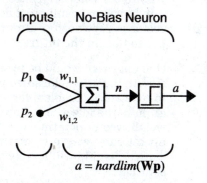

Figure 4.4 Test Problem Network

By removing the bias we are left with a network whose decision boundary must pass through the origin. We need to be sure that this network is still able to solve the test problem. There must be an allowable decision boundary that can separate the vectors $\mathbf{p}_2$ and $\mathbf{p}_3$ from the vector $\mathbf{p}_1$. The figure to the left illustrates that there are indeed an infinite number of such boundaries.

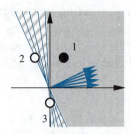

The adjacent figure shows the weight vectors that correspond to the allowable decision boundaries. (Recall that the weight vector is orthogonal to the decision boundary.) We would like a learning rule that will find a weight vector that points in one of these directions. Remember that the length of the weight vector does not matter; only its direction is important.

Constructing Learning Rules

Training begins by assigning some initial values for the network parameters. In this case we are training a two-input/single-output network without a bias, so we only have to initialize its two weights. Here we set the elements of the weight vector, $_1\mathbf{w}$, to the following randomly generated values:

$$_1\mathbf{w}^T = \begin{bmatrix} 1.0 & -0.8 \end{bmatrix}. \tag{4.21}$$

We will now begin presenting the input vectors to the network. We begin with $\mathbf{p}_1$:

$$a = hardlim\,(_1\mathbf{w}^T\mathbf{p}_1) = hardlim\left(\begin{bmatrix} 1.0 & -0.8 \end{bmatrix}\begin{bmatrix} 1 \\ 2 \end{bmatrix}\right) \tag{4.22}$$

$$a = hardlim\,(-0.6) = 0.$$

The network has not returned the correct value. The network output is 0, while the target response, t_1, is 1.

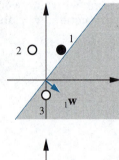

We can see what happened by looking at the adjacent diagram. The initial weight vector results in a decision boundary that incorrectly classifies the vector $\mathbf{p}_1$. We need to alter the weight vector so that it points more toward $\mathbf{p}_1$, so that in the future it has a better chance of classifying it correctly.

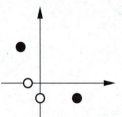

One approach would be to set $_1\mathbf{w}$ equal to $\mathbf{p}_1$. This is simple and would ensure that $\mathbf{p}_1$ was classified properly in the future. Unfortunately, it is easy to construct a problem for which this rule cannot find a solution. The diagram to the lower left shows a problem that cannot be solved with the weight vector pointing directly at either of the two class 1 vectors. If we apply the rule $_1\mathbf{w} = \mathbf{p}$ every time one of these vectors is misclassified, the network's weights will simply oscillate back and forth and will never find a solution.

Another possibility would be to add $\mathbf{p}_1$ to $_1\mathbf{w}$. Adding $\mathbf{p}_1$ to $_1\mathbf{w}$ would make $_1\mathbf{w}$ point more in the direction of $\mathbf{p}_1$. Repeated presentations of $\mathbf{p}_1$ would cause the direction of $_1\mathbf{w}$ to asymptotically approach the direction of $\mathbf{p}_1$. This rule can be stated:

$$\text{If } t = 1 \text{ and } a = 0, \text{ then } _1\mathbf{w}^{new} = _1\mathbf{w}^{old} + \mathbf{p}. \tag{4.23}$$

Applying this rule to our test problem results in new values for ${}_1\mathbf{w}$:

$$
{}_1\mathbf{w}^{new} = {}_1\mathbf{w}^{old} + \mathbf{p}_1 = \begin{bmatrix} 1.0 \\ -0.8 \end{bmatrix} + \begin{bmatrix} 1 \\ 2 \end{bmatrix} = \begin{bmatrix} 2.0 \\ 1.2 \end{bmatrix}. \tag{4.24}
$$

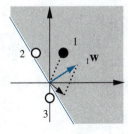

This operation is illustrated in the adjacent figure.

We now move on to the next input vector and will continue making changes to the weights and cycling through the inputs until they are all classified correctly.

The next input vector is $\mathbf{p}_2$. When it is presented to the network we find:

$$
a = hardlim\left({}_1\mathbf{w}^T\mathbf{p}_2\right) = hardlim\left(\begin{bmatrix} 2.0 & 1.2 \end{bmatrix} \begin{bmatrix} -1 \\ 2 \end{bmatrix} \right) \tag{4.25}
$$

$$
= hardlim\,(0.4) = 1 .
$$

The target t_2 associated with $\mathbf{p}_2$ is 0 and the output a is 1. A class 0 vector was misclassified as a 1.

Since we would now like to move the weight vector ${}_1\mathbf{w}$ away from the input, we can simply change the addition in Eq. (4.23) to subtraction:

$$
\text{If } t = 0 \text{ and } a = 1, \text{ then } {}_1\mathbf{w}^{new} = {}_1\mathbf{w}^{old} - \mathbf{p} . \tag{4.26}
$$

If we apply this to the test problem we find:

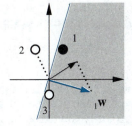

$$
{}_1\mathbf{w}^{new} = {}_1\mathbf{w}^{old} - \mathbf{p}_2 = \begin{bmatrix} 2.0 \\ 1.2 \end{bmatrix} - \begin{bmatrix} -1 \\ 2 \end{bmatrix} = \begin{bmatrix} 3.0 \\ -0.8 \end{bmatrix}, \tag{4.27}
$$

which is illustrated in the adjacent figure.

Now we present the third vector $\mathbf{p}_3$:

$$
a = hardlim\left({}_1\mathbf{w}^T\mathbf{p}_3\right) = hardlim\left(\begin{bmatrix} 3.0 & -0.8 \end{bmatrix} \begin{bmatrix} 0 \\ -1 \end{bmatrix} \right) \tag{4.28}
$$

$$
= hardlim\,(0.8) = 1 .
$$

The current ${}_1\mathbf{w}$ results in a decision boundary that misclassifies $\mathbf{p}_3$. This is a situation for which we already have a rule, so ${}_1\mathbf{w}$ will be updated again, according to Eq. (4.26):

$$
{}_1\mathbf{w}^{new} = {}_1\mathbf{w}^{old} - \mathbf{p}_3 = \begin{bmatrix} 3.0 \\ -0.8 \end{bmatrix} - \begin{bmatrix} 0 \\ -1 \end{bmatrix} = \begin{bmatrix} 3.0 \\ 0.2 \end{bmatrix}. \tag{4.29}
$$

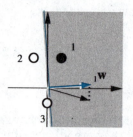

The diagram to the left shows that the perceptron has finally learned to classify the three vectors properly. If we present any of the input vectors to the neuron, it will output the correct class for that input vector.

This brings us to our third and final rule: if it works, don't fix it.

$$\text{If } t = a, \text{ then } {}_1\mathbf{w}^{new} = {}_1\mathbf{w}^{old}. \tag{4.30}$$

Here are the three rules, which cover all possible combinations of output and target values:

$$\text{If } t = 1 \text{ and } a = 0, \text{ then } {}_1\mathbf{w}^{new} = {}_1\mathbf{w}^{old} + \mathbf{p}.$$
$$\text{If } t = 0 \text{ and } a = 1, \text{ then } {}_1\mathbf{w}^{new} = {}_1\mathbf{w}^{old} - \mathbf{p}. \tag{4.31}$$
$$\text{If } t = a, \text{ then } {}_1\mathbf{w}^{new} = {}_1\mathbf{w}^{old}.$$

Unified Learning Rule

The three rules in Eq. (4.31) can be rewritten as a single expression. First we will define a new variable, the perceptron error e:

$$e = t - a. \tag{4.32}$$

We can now rewrite the three rules of Eq. (4.31) as:

$$\text{If } e = 1, \text{ then } {}_1\mathbf{w}^{new} = {}_1\mathbf{w}^{old} + \mathbf{p}.$$
$$\text{If } e = -1, \text{ then } {}_1\mathbf{w}^{new} = {}_1\mathbf{w}^{old} - \mathbf{p}. \tag{4.33}$$
$$\text{If } e = 0, \text{ then } {}_1\mathbf{w}^{new} = {}_1\mathbf{w}^{old}.$$

Looking carefully at the first two rules in Eq. (4.33) we can see that the sign of $\mathbf{p}$ is the same as the sign on the error, e. Furthermore, the absence of $\mathbf{p}$ in the third rule corresponds to an e of 0. Thus, we can unify the three rules into a single expression:

$$_1\mathbf{w}^{new} = {}_1\mathbf{w}^{old} + e\mathbf{p} = {}_1\mathbf{w}^{old} + (t - a)\mathbf{p}. \tag{4.34}$$

This rule can be extended to train the bias by noting that a bias is simply a weight whose input is always 1. We can thus replace the input $\mathbf{p}$ in Eq. (4.34) with the input to the bias, which is 1. The result is the perceptron rule for a bias:

$$b^{new} = b^{old} + e. \tag{4.35}$$

Training Multiple-Neuron Perceptrons

The perceptron rule, as given by Eq. (4.34) and Eq. (4.35), updates the weight vector of a single neuron perceptron. We can generalize this rule for the multiple-neuron perceptron of Figure 4.1 as follows. To update the ith row of the weight matrix use:

$$_i\mathbf{w}^{new} = {}_i\mathbf{w}^{old} + e_i\mathbf{p}. \tag{4.36}$$

To update the ith element of the bias vector use:

$$b_i^{\,new} = b_i^{\,old} + e_i. \tag{4.37}$$

Perceptron Rule The *perceptron rule* can be written conveniently in matrix notation:

$$\mathbf{W}^{new} = \mathbf{W}^{old} + \mathbf{e}\mathbf{p}^T, \tag{4.38}$$

and

$$\mathbf{b}^{new} = \mathbf{b}^{old} + \mathbf{e}. \tag{4.39}$$

To test the perceptron learning rule, consider again the apple/orange recognition problem of Chapter 3. The input/output prototype vectors will be

$$\left\{ \mathbf{p}_1 = \begin{bmatrix} 1 \\ -1 \\ -1 \end{bmatrix}, t_1 = \begin{bmatrix} 0 \end{bmatrix} \right\} \qquad \left\{ \mathbf{p}_2 = \begin{bmatrix} 1 \\ 1 \\ -1 \end{bmatrix}, t_2 = \begin{bmatrix} 1 \end{bmatrix} \right\}. \tag{4.40}$$

(Note that we are using 0 as the target output for the orange pattern, $\mathbf{p}_1$, instead of –1, as was used in Chapter 3. This is because we are using the *hardlim* transfer function, instead of *hardlims*.)

Typically the weights and biases are initialized to small random numbers. Suppose that here we start with the initial weight matrix and bias:

$$\mathbf{W} = \begin{bmatrix} 0.5 & -1 & -0.5 \end{bmatrix}, b = 0.5. \tag{4.41}$$

The first step is to apply the first input vector, $\mathbf{p}_1$, to the network:

$$a = hardlim(\mathbf{W}\mathbf{p}_1 + b) = hardlim\left(\begin{bmatrix} 0.5 & -1 & -0.5 \end{bmatrix} \begin{bmatrix} 1 \\ -1 \\ -1 \end{bmatrix} + 0.5 \right) \tag{4.42}$$

$$= hardlim(2.5) = 1$$

Then we calculate the error:

$$e = t_1 - a = 0 - 1 = -1.$$ (4.43)

The weight update is

$$\mathbf{W}^{new} = \mathbf{W}^{old} + e\mathbf{p}^T = \begin{bmatrix} 0.5 & -1 & -0.5 \end{bmatrix} + (-1)\begin{bmatrix} 1 & -1 & -1 \end{bmatrix}$$ (4.44)
$$= \begin{bmatrix} -0.5 & 0 & 0.5 \end{bmatrix}.$$

The bias update is

$$b^{new} = b^{old} + e = 0.5 + (-1) = -0.5.$$ (4.45)

This completes the first iteration.

The second iteration of the perceptron rule is:

$$a = hardlim\,(\mathbf{W}\mathbf{p}_2 + b) = hardlim\,(\begin{bmatrix} -0.5 & 0 & 0.5 \end{bmatrix}\begin{bmatrix} 1 \\ 1 \\ -1 \end{bmatrix} + (-0.5))$$ (4.46)

$$= hardlim\,(-0.5) = 0$$

$$e = t_2 - a = 1 - 0 = 1$$ (4.47)

$$\mathbf{W}^{new} = \mathbf{W}^{old} + e\mathbf{p}^T = \begin{bmatrix} -0.5 & 0 & 0.5 \end{bmatrix} + 1\begin{bmatrix} 1 & 1 & -1 \end{bmatrix} = \begin{bmatrix} 0.5 & 1 & -0.5 \end{bmatrix}$$ (4.48)

$$b^{new} = b^{old} + e = -0.5 + 1 = 0.5$$ (4.49)

The third iteration begins again with the first input vector:

$$a = hardlim\,(\mathbf{W}\mathbf{p}_1 + b) = hardlim\,(\begin{bmatrix} 0.5 & 1 & -0.5 \end{bmatrix}\begin{bmatrix} 1 \\ -1 \\ -1 \end{bmatrix} + 0.5)$$ (4.50)

$$= hardlim\,(0.5) = 1$$

$$e = t_1 - a = 0 - 1 = -1$$ (4.51)

$$\mathbf{W}^{new} = \mathbf{W}^{old} + e\mathbf{p}^T = \begin{bmatrix} 0.5 & 1 & -0.5 \end{bmatrix} + (-1)\begin{bmatrix} 1 & -1 & -1 \end{bmatrix}$$ (4.52)
$$= \begin{bmatrix} -0.5 & 2 & 0.5 \end{bmatrix}$$

$$b^{new} = b^{old} + e = 0.5 + (-1) = -0.5 \,. \tag{4.53}$$

If you continue with the iterations you will find that both input vectors will now be correctly classified. The algorithm has converged to a solution. Note that the final decision boundary is not the same as the one we developed in Chapter 3, although both boundaries correctly classify the two input vectors.

To experiment with the perceptron learning rule, use the Neural Network Design Demonstration Perceptron Rule (**nnd4pr**).

Proof of Convergence

Although the perceptron learning rule is simple, it is quite powerful. In fact, it can be shown that the rule will always converge to weights that accomplish the desired classification (assuming that such weights exist). In this section we will present a proof of convergence for the perceptron learning rule for the single-neuron perceptron shown in Figure 4.5.

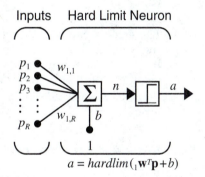

Figure 4.5 Single-Neuron Perceptron

The output of this perceptron is obtained from

$$a = hardlim\,(_1\mathbf{w}^T\mathbf{p} + b) \,. \tag{4.54}$$

The network is provided with the following examples of proper network behavior:

$$\{\mathbf{p}_1, t_1\}, \{\mathbf{p}_2, t_2\}, ..., \{\mathbf{p}_Q, t_Q\} \,. \tag{4.55}$$

where each target output, t_q, is either 0 or 1.

Notation

To conveniently present the proof we will first introduce some new notation. We will combine the weight matrix and the bias into a single vector:

$$\mathbf{x} = \begin{bmatrix} {}_1\mathbf{w} \\ b \end{bmatrix}. \tag{4.56}$$

We will also augment the input vectors with a 1, corresponding to the bias input:

$$\mathbf{z}_q = \begin{bmatrix} \mathbf{p}_q \\ 1 \end{bmatrix}. \tag{4.57}$$

Now we can express the net input to the neuron as follows:

$$n = {}_1\mathbf{w}^T\mathbf{p} + b = \mathbf{x}^T\mathbf{z}. \tag{4.58}$$

The perceptron learning rule for a single-neuron perceptron (Eq. (4.34) and Eq. (4.35)) can now be written

$$\mathbf{x}^{new} = \mathbf{x}^{old} + e\mathbf{z}. \tag{4.59}$$

The error e can be either 1, -1 or 0. If $e = 0$, then no change is made to the weights. If $e = 1$, then the input vector is added to the weight vector. If $e = -1$, then the negative of the input vector is added to the weight vector. If we count only those iterations for which the weight vector is changed, the learning rule becomes

$$\mathbf{x}(k) = \mathbf{x}(k-1) + \mathbf{z}'(k-1), \tag{4.60}$$

where $\mathbf{z}'(k-1)$ is the appropriate member of the set

$$\{\mathbf{z}_1, \mathbf{z}_2, ..., \mathbf{z}_Q, -\mathbf{z}_1, -\mathbf{z}_2, ..., -\mathbf{z}_Q\}. \tag{4.61}$$

We will assume that a weight vector exists that can correctly categorize all Q input vectors. This solution will be denoted $\mathbf{x}^*$. For this weight vector we will assume that

$$\mathbf{x}^{*T}\mathbf{z}_q > \delta > 0 \text{ if } t_q = 1, \tag{4.62}$$

and

$$\mathbf{x}^{*T}\mathbf{z}_q < -\delta < 0 \text{ if } t_q = 0. \tag{4.63}$$

Proof

We are now ready to begin the proof of the perceptron convergence theorem. The objective of the proof is to find upper and lower bounds on the length of the weight vector at each stage of the algorithm.

Assume that the algorithm is initialized with the zero weight vector: $\mathbf{x}(0) = \mathbf{0}$. (This does not affect the generality of our argument.) Then, after k iterations (changes to the weight vector), we find from Eq. (4.60):

$$\mathbf{x}(k) = \mathbf{z}'(0) + \mathbf{z}'(1) + \cdots + \mathbf{z}'(k-1) . \qquad (4.64)$$

If we take the inner product of the solution weight vector with the weight vector at iteration k we obtain

$$\mathbf{x}^{*T}\mathbf{x}(k) = \mathbf{x}^{*T}\mathbf{z}'(0) + \mathbf{x}^{*T}\mathbf{z}'(1) + \cdots + \mathbf{x}^{*T}\mathbf{z}'(k-1) . \qquad (4.65)$$

From Eq. (4.61)–Eq. (4.63) we can show that

$$\mathbf{x}^{*T}\mathbf{z}'(i) > \delta . \qquad (4.66)$$

Therefore

$$\mathbf{x}^{*T}\mathbf{x}(k) > k\delta . \qquad (4.67)$$

From the Cauchy-Schwartz inequality (see [Brog91])

$$\left(\mathbf{x}^{*T}\mathbf{x}(k)\right)^2 \leq \|\mathbf{x}^*\|^2 \|\mathbf{x}(k)\|^2 , \qquad (4.68)$$

where

$$\|\mathbf{x}\|^2 = \mathbf{x}^T\mathbf{x} . \qquad (4.69)$$

If we combine Eq. (4.67) and Eq. (4.68) we can put a lower bound on the squared length of the weight vector at iteration k:

$$\|\mathbf{x}(k)\|^2 \geq \frac{\left(\mathbf{x}^{*T}\mathbf{x}(k)\right)^2}{\|\mathbf{x}^*\|^2} > \frac{(k\delta)^2}{\|\mathbf{x}^*\|^2} . \qquad (4.70)$$

Next we want to find an upper bound for the length of the weight vector. We begin by finding the change in the length at iteration k:

$$\begin{aligned}
\|\mathbf{x}(k)\|^2 &= \mathbf{x}^T(k)\mathbf{x}(k) \\
&= [\mathbf{x}(k-1) + \mathbf{z}'(k-1)]^T[\mathbf{x}(k-1) + \mathbf{z}'(k-1)] \\
&= \mathbf{x}^T(k-1)\mathbf{x}(k-1) + 2\mathbf{x}^T(k-1)\mathbf{z}'(k-1) \\
&\quad + \mathbf{z}'^T(k-1)\mathbf{z}'(k-1)
\end{aligned} \qquad (4.71)$$

Note that

$$\mathbf{x}^T(k-1)\,\mathbf{z'}(k-1) \leq 0 \,, \tag{4.72}$$

since the weights would not be updated unless the previous input vector had been misclassified. Now Eq. (4.71) can be simplified to

$$\|\mathbf{x}(k)\|^2 \leq \|\mathbf{x}(k-1)\|^2 + \|\mathbf{z'}(k-1)\|^2 \,. \tag{4.73}$$

We can repeat this process for $\|\mathbf{x}(k-1)\|^2$, $\|\mathbf{x}(k-2)\|^2$, etc., to obtain

$$\|\mathbf{x}(k)\|^2 \leq \|\mathbf{z'}(0)\|^2 + \cdots + \|\mathbf{z'}(k-1)\|^2 \,. \tag{4.74}$$

If $\Pi = max\{\|\mathbf{z'}(i)\|^2\}$, this upper bound can be simplified to

$$\|\mathbf{x}(k)\|^2 \leq k\Pi \,. \tag{4.75}$$

We now have an upper bound (Eq. (4.75)) and a lower bound (Eq. (4.70)) on the squared length of the weight vector at iteration k. If we combine the two inequalities we find

$$k\Pi \geq \|\mathbf{x}(k)\|^2 > \frac{(k\delta)^2}{\|\mathbf{x*}\|^2} \text{ or } k < \frac{\Pi\|\mathbf{x*}\|^2}{\delta^2} \,. \tag{4.76}$$

Because k has an upper bound, this means that the weights will only be changed a finite number of times. Therefore, the perceptron learning rule will converge in a finite number of iterations.

The maximum number of iterations (changes to the weight vector) is inversely related to the square of δ. This parameter is a measure of how close the solution decision boundary is to the input patterns. This means that if the input classes are difficult to separate (are close to the decision boundary) it will take many iterations for the algorithm to converge.

Note that there are only three key assumptions required for the proof:

1. A solution to the problem exists, so that Eq. (4.66) is satisfied.

2. The weights are only updated when the input vector is misclassified, therefore Eq. (4.72) is satisfied.

3. An upper bound, Π, exists for the length of the input vectors.

Because of the generality of the proof, there are many variations of the perceptron learning rule that can also be shown to converge. (See Exercise E4.9.)

Limitations

The perceptron learning rule is guaranteed to converge to a solution in a finite number of steps, so long as a solution exists. This brings us to an important question. What problems can a perceptron solve? Recall that a single-neuron perceptron is able to divide the input space into two regions. The boundary between the regions is defined by the equation

$$_1\mathbf{w}^T\mathbf{p} + b = 0.$$ (4.77)

This is a linear boundary (hyperplane). The perceptron can be used to classify input vectors that can be separated by a linear boundary. We call such vectors *linearly separable*. The logical AND gate example on page 4-7 illustrates a two-dimensional example of a linearly separable problem. The apple/orange recognition problem of Chapter 3 was a three-dimensional example.

Linear Separability

Unfortunately, many problems are not linearly separable. The classic example is the XOR gate. The input/target pairs for the XOR gate are

$$\left\{ \mathbf{p}_1 = \begin{bmatrix} 0 \\ 0 \end{bmatrix}, t_1 = 0 \right\} \left\{ \mathbf{p}_2 = \begin{bmatrix} 0 \\ 1 \end{bmatrix}, t_2 = 1 \right\} \left\{ \mathbf{p}_3 = \begin{bmatrix} 1 \\ 0 \end{bmatrix}, t_3 = 1 \right\} \left\{ \mathbf{p}_4 = \begin{bmatrix} 1 \\ 1 \end{bmatrix}, t_4 = 0 \right\}.$$

This problem is illustrated graphically on the left side of Figure 4.6, which also shows two other linearly inseparable problems. Try drawing a straight line between the vectors with targets of 1 and those with targets of 0 in any of the diagrams of Figure 4.6.

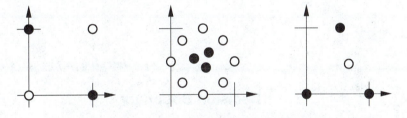

Figure 4.6 Linearly Inseparable Problems

It was the inability of the basic perceptron to solve such simple problems that led, in part, to a reduction in interest in neural network research during the 1970s. Rosenblatt had investigated more complex networks, which he felt would overcome the limitations of the basic perceptron, but he was never able to effectively extend the perceptron rule to such networks. In Chapter 11 we will introduce multilayer perceptrons, which can solve arbitrary classification problems, and will describe the backpropagation algorithm, which can be used to train them.

Summary of Results

Perceptron Architecture

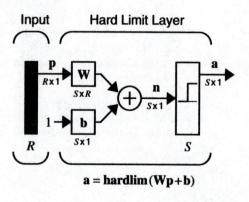

$$a = \mathbf{hardlim}(\mathbf{Wp+b})$$

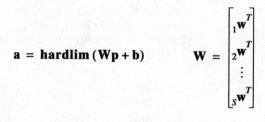

$$\mathbf{a} = \mathbf{hardlim}\,(\mathbf{Wp} + \mathbf{b}) \qquad \mathbf{W} = \begin{bmatrix} {}_1\mathbf{w}^T \\ {}_2\mathbf{w}^T \\ \vdots \\ {}_S\mathbf{w}^T \end{bmatrix}$$

$$a_i = hardlim\,(n_i) = hardlim\,({}_i\mathbf{w}^T\mathbf{p} + b_i)$$

Decision Boundary

$${}_i\mathbf{w}^T\mathbf{p} + b_i = 0.$$

The decision boundary is always orthogonal to the weight vector.

Single-layer perceptrons can only classify linearly separable vectors.

Perceptron Learning Rule

$$\mathbf{W}^{new} = \mathbf{W}^{old} + \mathbf{ep}^T$$

$$\mathbf{b}^{new} = \mathbf{b}^{old} + \mathbf{e}$$

where $\mathbf{e} = \mathbf{t} - \mathbf{a}$.

Solved Problems

P4.1 **Solve the three simple classification problems shown in Figure P4.1 by drawing a decision boundary. Find weight and bias values that result in single-neuron perceptrons with the chosen decision boundaries.**

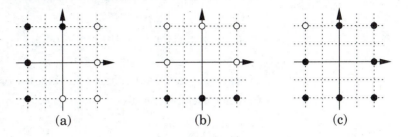

Figure P4.1   Simple Classification Problems

First we draw a line between each set of dark and light data points.

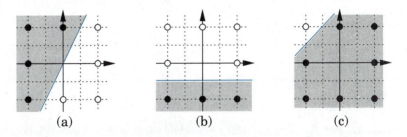

The next step is to find the weights and biases. The weight vectors must be orthogonal to the decision boundaries, and pointing in the direction of points to be classified as 1 (the dark points). The weight vectors can have any length we like.

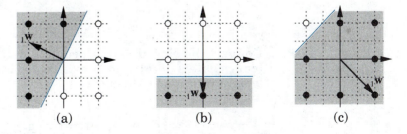

Here is one set of choices for the weight vectors:

$$\text{(a) } {}_1\mathbf{w}^T = \begin{bmatrix} -2 & 1 \end{bmatrix}, \quad \text{(b) } {}_1\mathbf{w}^T = \begin{bmatrix} 0 & -2 \end{bmatrix}, \quad \text{(c) } {}_1\mathbf{w}^T = \begin{bmatrix} 2 & -2 \end{bmatrix}.$$

Now we find the bias values for each perceptron by picking a point on the decision boundary and satisfying Eq. (4.15).

$$_1\mathbf{w}^T \mathbf{p} + b = 0$$
$$b = -_1\mathbf{w}^T \mathbf{p}$$

This gives us the following three biases:

(a) $b = -\begin{bmatrix} -2 & 1 \end{bmatrix} \begin{bmatrix} 0 \\ 0 \end{bmatrix} = 0$, (b) $b = -\begin{bmatrix} 0 & -2 \end{bmatrix} \begin{bmatrix} 0 \\ -1 \end{bmatrix} = -2$, (c) $b = -\begin{bmatrix} 2 & -2 \end{bmatrix} \begin{bmatrix} -2 \\ 1 \end{bmatrix} = 4$

We can now check our solution against the original points. Here we test the first network on the input vector $\mathbf{p} = \begin{bmatrix} -2 & 2 \end{bmatrix}^T$.

$$a = hardlim\left(_1\mathbf{w}^T \mathbf{p} + b\right)$$

$$= hardlim\left(\begin{bmatrix} -2 & 1 \end{bmatrix} \begin{bmatrix} -2 \\ 2 \end{bmatrix} + 0\right)$$

$$= hardlim\,(6)$$

$$= 1$$

We can use MATLAB to automate the testing process and to try new points. Here the first network is used to classify a point that was not in the original problem.

```
» 2 + 2
ans =
     4
```

```
w=[-2 1]; b = 0;
a = hardlim(w*[1;1]+b)
a =
         0
```

P4.2 **Convert the classification problem defined below into an equivalent problem definition consisting of inequalities constraining weight and bias values.**

$$\left\{ \mathbf{p}_1 = \begin{bmatrix} 0 \\ 2 \end{bmatrix}, t_1 = 1 \right\} \left\{ \mathbf{p}_2 = \begin{bmatrix} 1 \\ 0 \end{bmatrix}, t_2 = 1 \right\} \left\{ \mathbf{p}_3 = \begin{bmatrix} 0 \\ -2 \end{bmatrix}, t_3 = 0 \right\} \left\{ \mathbf{p}_4 = \begin{bmatrix} 2 \\ 0 \end{bmatrix}, t_4 = 0 \right\}$$

Each target t_i indicates whether or not the net input in response to $\mathbf{p}_i$ must be less than 0, or greater than or equal to 0. For example, since t_1 is 1, we know that the net input corresponding to $\mathbf{p}_1$ must be greater than or equal to 0. Thus we get the following inequality:

$$\mathbf{W}\mathbf{p}_1 + b \geq 0$$
$$0w_{1,1} + 2w_{1,2} + b \geq 0$$
$$2w_{1,2} + b \geq 0.$$

Applying the same procedure to the input/target pairs for $\{\mathbf{p}_2, t_2\}$, $\{\mathbf{p}_3, t_3\}$ and $\{\mathbf{p}_4, t_4\}$ results in the following set of inequalities.

$$2w_{1,2} + b \geq 0 \quad (i)$$
$$w_{1,1} + b \geq 0 \quad (ii)$$
$$-2w_{1,2} + b < 0 \quad (iii)$$
$$2w_{1,1} + b < 0 \quad (iv)$$

Solving a set of inequalities is more difficult than solving a set of equalities. One added complexity is that there are often an infinite number of solutions (just as there are often an infinite number of linear decision boundaries that can solve a linearly separable classification problem).

However, because of the simplicity of this problem, we can solve it by graphing the solution spaces defined by the inequalities. Note that $w_{1,1}$ only appears in inequalities (ii) and (iv), and $w_{1,2}$ only appears in inequalities (i) and (iii). We can plot each pair of inequalities with two graphs.

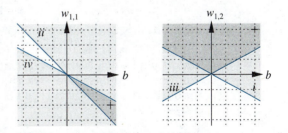

Any weight and bias values that fall in both dark gray regions will solve the classification problem.

Here is one such solution:

$$\mathbf{W} = \begin{bmatrix} -2 & 3 \end{bmatrix} \qquad b = 3.$$

P4.3 **We have a classification problem with four classes of input vector. The four classes are**

$$\text{class 1: } \left\{ \mathbf{p}_1 = \begin{bmatrix} 1 \\ 1 \end{bmatrix}, \mathbf{p}_2 = \begin{bmatrix} 1 \\ 2 \end{bmatrix} \right\}, \text{ class 2: } \left\{ \mathbf{p}_3 = \begin{bmatrix} 2 \\ -1 \end{bmatrix}, \mathbf{p}_4 = \begin{bmatrix} 2 \\ 0 \end{bmatrix} \right\},$$

$$\text{class 3: } \left\{ \mathbf{p}_5 = \begin{bmatrix} -1 \\ 2 \end{bmatrix}, \mathbf{p}_6 = \begin{bmatrix} -2 \\ 1 \end{bmatrix} \right\}, \text{ class 4: } \left\{ \mathbf{p}_7 = \begin{bmatrix} -1 \\ -1 \end{bmatrix}, \mathbf{p}_8 = \begin{bmatrix} -2 \\ -2 \end{bmatrix} \right\}.$$

Design a perceptron network to solve this problem.

To solve a problem with four classes of input vector we will need a perceptron with at least two neurons, since an S-neuron perceptron can categorize 2^S classes. The two-neuron perceptron is shown in Figure P4.2.

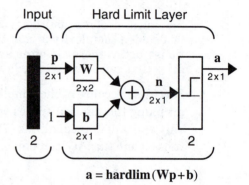

$$\mathbf{a} = \mathbf{hardlim}(\mathbf{Wp} + \mathbf{b})$$

Figure P4.2 Two-Neuron Perceptron

Let's begin by displaying the input vectors, as in Figure P4.3. The light circles ○ indicate class 1 vectors, the light squares □ indicate class 2 vectors, the dark circles ● indicate class 3 vectors, and the dark squares ■ indicate class 4 vectors.

A two-neuron perceptron creates two decision boundaries. Therefore, to divide the input space into the four categories, we need to have one decision boundary divide the four classes into two sets of two. The remaining boundary must then isolate each class. Two such boundaries are illustrated in Figure P4.4. We now know that our patterns are linearly separable.

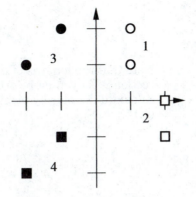

Figure P4.3 Input Vectors for Problem P4.3

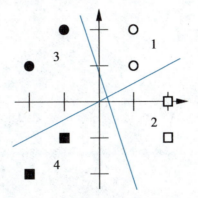

Figure P4.4 Tentative Decision Boundaries for Problem P4.3

The weight vectors should be orthogonal to the decision boundaries and should point toward the regions where the neuron outputs are 1. The next step is to decide which side of each boundary should produce a 1. One choice is illustrated in Figure P4.5, where the shaded areas represent outputs of 1. The darkest shading indicates that both neuron outputs are 1. Note that this solution corresponds to target values of

$$\text{class 1: } \left\{ \mathbf{t}_1 = \begin{bmatrix} 0 \\ 0 \end{bmatrix}, \mathbf{t}_2 = \begin{bmatrix} 0 \\ 0 \end{bmatrix} \right\}, \text{ class 2: } \left\{ \mathbf{t}_3 = \begin{bmatrix} 0 \\ 1 \end{bmatrix}, \mathbf{t}_4 = \begin{bmatrix} 0 \\ 1 \end{bmatrix} \right\},$$

$$\text{class 3: } \left\{ \mathbf{t}_5 = \begin{bmatrix} 1 \\ 0 \end{bmatrix}, \mathbf{t}_6 = \begin{bmatrix} 1 \\ 0 \end{bmatrix} \right\}, \text{ class 4: } \left\{ \mathbf{t}_7 = \begin{bmatrix} 1 \\ 1 \end{bmatrix}, \mathbf{t}_8 = \begin{bmatrix} 1 \\ 1 \end{bmatrix} \right\}.$$

We can now select the weight vectors:

$$_1\mathbf{w} = \begin{bmatrix} -3 \\ -1 \end{bmatrix} \text{ and } _2\mathbf{w} = \begin{bmatrix} 1 \\ -2 \end{bmatrix}.$$

Note that the lengths of the weight vectors is not important, only their directions. They must be orthogonal to the decision boundaries. Now we can calculate the bias by picking a point on a boundary and satisfying Eq. (4.15):

$$b_1 = -_1\mathbf{w}^T\mathbf{p} = -\begin{bmatrix} -3 & -1 \end{bmatrix}\begin{bmatrix} 0 \\ 1 \end{bmatrix} = 1,$$

$$b_2 = -_2\mathbf{w}^T\mathbf{p} = -\begin{bmatrix} 1 & -2 \end{bmatrix}\begin{bmatrix} 0 \\ 0 \end{bmatrix} = 0.$$

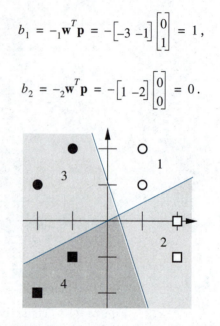

Figure P4.5 Decision Regions for Problem P4.3

In matrix form we have

$$\mathbf{W} = \begin{bmatrix} _1\mathbf{w}^T \\ _2\mathbf{w}^T \end{bmatrix} = \begin{bmatrix} -3 & -1 \\ 1 & -2 \end{bmatrix} \text{ and } \mathbf{b} = \begin{bmatrix} 1 \\ 0 \end{bmatrix},$$

which completes our design.

P4.4 **Solve the following classification problem with the perceptron rule. Apply each input vector in order, for as many repetitions as it takes to ensure that the problem is solved. Draw a graph of the problem only after you have found a solution.**

$$\left\{ \mathbf{p}_1 = \begin{bmatrix} 2 \\ 2 \end{bmatrix}, t_1 = 0 \right\} \left\{ \mathbf{p}_2 = \begin{bmatrix} 1 \\ -2 \end{bmatrix}, t_2 = 1 \right\} \left\{ \mathbf{p}_3 = \begin{bmatrix} -2 \\ 2 \end{bmatrix}, t_3 = 0 \right\} \left\{ \mathbf{p}_4 = \begin{bmatrix} -1 \\ 1 \end{bmatrix}, t_4 = 1 \right\}$$

Use the initial weights and bias:

$$\mathbf{W}(0) = \begin{bmatrix} 0 & 0 \end{bmatrix} \qquad b(0) = 0 .$$

We start by calculating the perceptron's output a for the first input vector $\mathbf{p}_1$, using the initial weights and bias.

$$a = hardlim(\mathbf{W}(0)\mathbf{p}_1 + b(0))$$

$$= hardlim\left(\begin{bmatrix} 0 & 0 \end{bmatrix} \begin{bmatrix} 2 \\ 2 \end{bmatrix} + 0 \right) = hardlim(0) = 1$$

The output a does not equal the target value t_1, so we use the perceptron rule to find new weights and biases based on the error.

$$e = t_1 - a = 0 - 1 = -1$$

$$\mathbf{W}(1) = \mathbf{W}(0) + e\mathbf{p}_1^T = \begin{bmatrix} 0 & 0 \end{bmatrix} + (-1) \begin{bmatrix} 2 & 2 \end{bmatrix} = \begin{bmatrix} -2 & -2 \end{bmatrix}$$

$$b(1) = b(0) + e = 0 + (-1) = -1$$

We now apply the second input vector $\mathbf{p}_2$, using the updated weights and bias.

$$a = hardlim(\mathbf{W}(1)\mathbf{p}_2 + b(1))$$

$$= hardlim\left(\begin{bmatrix} -2 & -2 \end{bmatrix} \begin{bmatrix} 1 \\ -2 \end{bmatrix} - 1 \right) = hardlim(1) = 1$$

This time the output a is equal to the target t_2. Application of the perceptron rule will not result in any changes.

$$\mathbf{W}(2) = \mathbf{W}(1)$$

$$b(2) = b(1)$$

We now apply the third input vector.

$$a = hardlim\,(\mathbf{W}\,(2)\,\mathbf{p}_3 + b\,(2)\,)$$

$$= hardlim\left(\begin{bmatrix} -2 & -2 \end{bmatrix}\begin{bmatrix} -2 \\ 2 \end{bmatrix} - 1\right) = hardlim\,(-1)\ =\ 0$$

The output in response to input vector $\mathbf{p}_3$ is equal to the target t_3, so there will be no changes.

$$\mathbf{W}\,(3)\ =\ \mathbf{W}\,(2)$$
$$b\,(3)\ =\ b\,(2)$$

We now move on to the last input vector $\mathbf{p}_4$.

$$a = hardlim\,(\mathbf{W}\,(3)\,\mathbf{p}_4 + b\,(3)\,)$$

$$= hardlim\left(\begin{bmatrix} -2 & -2 \end{bmatrix}\begin{bmatrix} -1 \\ 1 \end{bmatrix} - 1\right) = hardlim\,(-1)\ =\ 0$$

This time the output a does not equal the appropriate target t_4. The perceptron rule will result in a new set of values for $\mathbf{W}$ and b.

$$e = t_4 - a = 1 - 0 = 1$$
$$\mathbf{W}\,(4)\ =\ \mathbf{W}\,(3) + e\mathbf{p}_4^T\ =\ \begin{bmatrix} -2 & -2 \end{bmatrix} + (1)\begin{bmatrix} -1 & 1 \end{bmatrix}\ =\ \begin{bmatrix} -3 & -1 \end{bmatrix}$$
$$b\,(4)\ =\ b\,(3) + e\ =\ -1 + 1\ =\ 0$$

We now must check the first vector $\mathbf{p}_1$ again. This time the output a is equal to the associated target t_1.

$$a\ =\ hardlim\,(\mathbf{W}\,(4)\,\mathbf{p}_1 + b\,(4)\,)$$

$$= hardlim\left(\begin{bmatrix} -3 & -1 \end{bmatrix}\begin{bmatrix} 2 \\ 2 \end{bmatrix} + 0\right) = hardlim\,(-8)\ =\ 0$$

Therefore there are no changes.

$$\mathbf{W}\,(5)\ =\ \mathbf{W}\,(4)$$
$$b\,(5)\ =\ b\,(4)$$

The second presentation of $\mathbf{p}_2$ results in an error and therefore a new set of weight and bias values.

$$a = hardlim\left(\mathbf{W}(5)\,\mathbf{p}_2 + b(5)\right)$$

$$= hardlim\left(\begin{bmatrix} -3 & -1 \end{bmatrix}\begin{bmatrix} 1 \\ -2 \end{bmatrix} + 0\right) = hardlim(-1) = 0$$

Here are those new values:

$$e = t_2 - a = 1 - 0 = 1$$
$$\mathbf{W}(6) = \mathbf{W}(5) + e\mathbf{p}_2^T = \begin{bmatrix} -3 & -1 \end{bmatrix} + (1)\begin{bmatrix} 1 & -2 \end{bmatrix} = \begin{bmatrix} -2 & -3 \end{bmatrix}$$
$$b(6) = b(5) + e = 0 + 1 = 1.$$

Cycling through each input vector once more results in no errors.

$$a = hardlim(\mathbf{W}(6)\,\mathbf{p}_3 + b(6)) = hardlim\left(\begin{bmatrix} -2 & -3 \end{bmatrix}\begin{bmatrix} -2 \\ 2 \end{bmatrix} + 1\right) = 0 = t_3$$

$$a = hardlim(\mathbf{W}(6)\,\mathbf{p}_4 + b(6)) = hardlim\left(\begin{bmatrix} -2 & -3 \end{bmatrix}\begin{bmatrix} -1 \\ 1 \end{bmatrix} + 1\right) = 1 = t_4$$

$$a = hardlim(\mathbf{W}(6)\,\mathbf{p}_1 + b(6)) = hardlim\left(\begin{bmatrix} -2 & -3 \end{bmatrix}\begin{bmatrix} 2 \\ 2 \end{bmatrix} + 1\right) = 0 = t_1$$

$$a = hardlim(\mathbf{W}(6)\,\mathbf{p}_2 + b(6)) = hardlim\left(\begin{bmatrix} -2 & -3 \end{bmatrix}\begin{bmatrix} 1 \\ -2 \end{bmatrix} + 1\right) = 1 = t_2$$

Therefore the algorithm has converged. The final solution is:

$$\mathbf{W} = \begin{bmatrix} -2 & -3 \end{bmatrix} \qquad b = 1.$$

Now we can graph the training data and the decision boundary of the solution. The decision boundary is given by

$$n = \mathbf{W}\mathbf{p} + b = w_{1,1}p_1 + w_{1,2}p_2 + b = -2p_1 - 3p_2 + 1 = 0.$$

To find the p_2 intercept of the decision boundary, set $p_1 = 0$:

$$p_2 = -\frac{b}{w_{1,2}} = -\frac{1}{-3} = \frac{1}{3} \quad \text{if } p_1 = 0.$$

To find the p_1 intercept, set $p_2 = 0$:

$$p_1 = -\frac{b}{w_{1,1}} = -\frac{1}{-2} = \frac{1}{2} \quad \text{if } p_2 = 0.$$

The resulting decision boundary is illustrated in Figure P4.6.

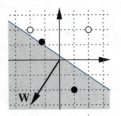

Figure P4.6 Decision Boundary for Problem P4.4

Note that the decision boundary falls across one of the training vectors. This is acceptable, given the problem definition, since the hard limit function returns 1 when given an input of 0, and the target for the vector in question is indeed 1.

P4.5 **Consider again the four-class decision problem that we introduced in Problem P4.3. Train a perceptron network to solve this problem using the perceptron learning rule.**

If we use the same target vectors that we introduced in Problem P4.3, the training set will be:

$$\left\{ \mathbf{p}_1 = \begin{bmatrix} 1 \\ 1 \end{bmatrix}, \mathbf{t}_1 = \begin{bmatrix} 0 \\ 0 \end{bmatrix} \right\} \left\{ \mathbf{p}_2 = \begin{bmatrix} 1 \\ 2 \end{bmatrix}, \mathbf{t}_2 = \begin{bmatrix} 0 \\ 0 \end{bmatrix} \right\} \left\{ \mathbf{p}_3 = \begin{bmatrix} 2 \\ -1 \end{bmatrix}, \mathbf{t}_3 = \begin{bmatrix} 0 \\ 1 \end{bmatrix} \right\}$$

$$\left\{ \mathbf{p}_4 = \begin{bmatrix} 2 \\ 0 \end{bmatrix}, \mathbf{t}_4 = \begin{bmatrix} 0 \\ 1 \end{bmatrix} \right\} \left\{ \mathbf{p}_5 = \begin{bmatrix} -1 \\ 2 \end{bmatrix}, \mathbf{t}_5 = \begin{bmatrix} 1 \\ 0 \end{bmatrix} \right\} \left\{ \mathbf{p}_6 = \begin{bmatrix} -2 \\ 1 \end{bmatrix}, \mathbf{t}_6 = \begin{bmatrix} 1 \\ 0 \end{bmatrix} \right\}$$

$$\left\{ \mathbf{p}_7 = \begin{bmatrix} -1 \\ -1 \end{bmatrix}, \mathbf{t}_7 = \begin{bmatrix} 1 \\ 1 \end{bmatrix} \right\} \left\{ \mathbf{p}_8 = \begin{bmatrix} -2 \\ -2 \end{bmatrix}, \mathbf{t}_8 = \begin{bmatrix} 1 \\ 1 \end{bmatrix} \right\} .$$

Let's begin the algorithm with the following initial weights and biases:

$$\mathbf{W}(0) = \begin{bmatrix} 1 & 0 \\ 0 & 1 \end{bmatrix}, \mathbf{b}(0) = \begin{bmatrix} 1 \\ 1 \end{bmatrix} .$$

The first iteration is

$$\mathbf{a} = hardlim \left(\mathbf{W}(0) \mathbf{p}_1 + \mathbf{b}(0) \right) = hardlim \left(\begin{bmatrix} 1 & 0 \\ 0 & 1 \end{bmatrix} \begin{bmatrix} 1 \\ 1 \end{bmatrix} + \begin{bmatrix} 1 \\ 1 \end{bmatrix} \right) = \begin{bmatrix} 1 \\ 1 \end{bmatrix},$$

$$\mathbf{e} = \mathbf{t}_1 - \mathbf{a} = \begin{bmatrix} 0 \\ 0 \end{bmatrix} - \begin{bmatrix} 1 \\ 1 \end{bmatrix} = \begin{bmatrix} -1 \\ -1 \end{bmatrix},$$

$$\mathbf{W}(1) = \mathbf{W}(0) + \mathbf{e}\mathbf{p}_1^T = \begin{bmatrix} 1 & 0 \\ 0 & 1 \end{bmatrix} + \begin{bmatrix} -1 \\ -1 \end{bmatrix} \begin{bmatrix} 1 & 1 \end{bmatrix} = \begin{bmatrix} 0 & -1 \\ -1 & 0 \end{bmatrix},$$

$$\mathbf{b}(1) = \mathbf{b}(0) + \mathbf{e} = \begin{bmatrix} 1 \\ 1 \end{bmatrix} + \begin{bmatrix} -1 \\ -1 \end{bmatrix} = \begin{bmatrix} 0 \\ 0 \end{bmatrix}.$$

The second iteration is

$$\mathbf{a} = hardlim\,(\mathbf{W}(1)\mathbf{p}_2 + \mathbf{b}(1)) = hardlim\,(\begin{bmatrix} 0 & -1 \\ -1 & 0 \end{bmatrix} \begin{bmatrix} 1 \\ 2 \end{bmatrix} + \begin{bmatrix} 0 \\ 0 \end{bmatrix}) = \begin{bmatrix} 0 \\ 0 \end{bmatrix},$$

$$\mathbf{e} = \mathbf{t}_2 - \mathbf{a} = \begin{bmatrix} 0 \\ 0 \end{bmatrix} - \begin{bmatrix} 0 \\ 0 \end{bmatrix} = \begin{bmatrix} 0 \\ 0 \end{bmatrix},$$

$$\mathbf{W}(2) = \mathbf{W}(1) + \mathbf{e}\mathbf{p}_2^T = \begin{bmatrix} 0 & -1 \\ -1 & 0 \end{bmatrix} + \begin{bmatrix} 0 \\ 0 \end{bmatrix} \begin{bmatrix} 1 & 2 \end{bmatrix} = \begin{bmatrix} 0 & -1 \\ -1 & 0 \end{bmatrix},$$

$$\mathbf{b}(2) = \mathbf{b}(1) + \mathbf{e} = \begin{bmatrix} 0 \\ 0 \end{bmatrix} + \begin{bmatrix} 0 \\ 0 \end{bmatrix} = \begin{bmatrix} 0 \\ 0 \end{bmatrix}.$$

The third iteration is

$$\mathbf{a} = hardlim\,(\mathbf{W}(2)\mathbf{p}_3 + \mathbf{b}(2)) = hardlim\,(\begin{bmatrix} 0 & -1 \\ -1 & 0 \end{bmatrix} \begin{bmatrix} 2 \\ -1 \end{bmatrix} + \begin{bmatrix} 0 \\ 0 \end{bmatrix}) = \begin{bmatrix} 1 \\ 0 \end{bmatrix},$$

$$\mathbf{e} = \mathbf{t}_3 - \mathbf{a} = \begin{bmatrix} 0 \\ 1 \end{bmatrix} - \begin{bmatrix} 1 \\ 0 \end{bmatrix} = \begin{bmatrix} -1 \\ 1 \end{bmatrix},$$

$$\mathbf{W}(3) = \mathbf{W}(2) + \mathbf{e}\mathbf{p}_3^T = \begin{bmatrix} 0 & -1 \\ -1 & 0 \end{bmatrix} + \begin{bmatrix} -1 \\ 1 \end{bmatrix} \begin{bmatrix} 2 & -1 \end{bmatrix} = \begin{bmatrix} -2 & 0 \\ 1 & -1 \end{bmatrix},$$

4

$$\mathbf{b}(3) = \mathbf{b}(2) + \mathbf{e} = \begin{bmatrix} 0 \\ 0 \end{bmatrix} + \begin{bmatrix} -1 \\ 1 \end{bmatrix} = \begin{bmatrix} -1 \\ 1 \end{bmatrix}.$$

Iterations four through eight produce no changes in the weights.

$$\mathbf{W}(8) = \mathbf{W}(7) = \mathbf{W}(6) = \mathbf{W}(5) = \mathbf{W}(4) = \mathbf{W}(3)$$

$$\mathbf{b}(8) = \mathbf{b}(7) = \mathbf{b}(6) = \mathbf{b}(5) = \mathbf{b}(4) = \mathbf{b}(3)$$

The ninth iteration produces

$$\mathbf{a} = hardlim \,(\mathbf{W}(8)\,\mathbf{p}_1 + \mathbf{b}(8)) = hardlim \,(\begin{bmatrix} -2 & 0 \\ 1 & -1 \end{bmatrix}\begin{bmatrix} 1 \\ 1 \end{bmatrix} + \begin{bmatrix} -1 \\ 1 \end{bmatrix}) = \begin{bmatrix} 0 \\ 1 \end{bmatrix},$$

$$\mathbf{e} = \mathbf{t}_1 - \mathbf{a} = \begin{bmatrix} 0 \\ 0 \end{bmatrix} - \begin{bmatrix} 0 \\ 1 \end{bmatrix} = \begin{bmatrix} 0 \\ -1 \end{bmatrix},$$

$$\mathbf{W}(9) = \mathbf{W}(8) + \mathbf{e}\mathbf{p}_1^T = \begin{bmatrix} -2 & 0 \\ 1 & -1 \end{bmatrix} + \begin{bmatrix} 0 \\ -1 \end{bmatrix}\begin{bmatrix} 1 & 1 \end{bmatrix} = \begin{bmatrix} -2 & 0 \\ 0 & -2 \end{bmatrix},$$

$$\mathbf{b}(9) = \mathbf{b}(8) + \mathbf{e} = \begin{bmatrix} -1 \\ 1 \end{bmatrix} + \begin{bmatrix} 0 \\ -1 \end{bmatrix} = \begin{bmatrix} -1 \\ 0 \end{bmatrix}.$$

At this point the algorithm has converged, since all input patterns will be correctly classified. The final decision boundaries are displayed in Figure P4.7. Compare this result with the network we designed in Problem P4.3.

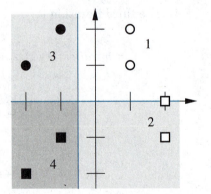

Figure P4.7 Final Decision Boundaries for Problem P4.5

Epilogue

In this chapter we have introduced our first learning rule — the perceptron learning rule. It is a type of learning called *supervised learning*, in which the learning rule is provided with a set of examples of proper network behavior. As each input is applied to the network, the learning rule adjusts the network parameters so that the network output will move closer to the target.

The perceptron learning rule is very simple, but it is also quite powerful. We have shown that the rule will always converge to a correct solution, if such a solution exists. The weakness of the perceptron network lies not with the learning rule, but with the structure of the network. The standard perceptron is only able to classify vectors that are linearly separable. We will see in Chapter 11 that the perceptron architecture can be generalized to mutlilayer perceptrons, which can solve arbitrary classification problems. The backpropagation learning rule, which is introduced in Chapter 11, can be used to train these networks.

In Chapters 3 and 4 we have used many concepts from the field of linear algebra, such as inner product, projection, distance (norm), etc. We will find in later chapters that a good foundation in linear algebra is essential to our understanding of all neural networks. In Chapters 5 and 6 we will review some of the key concepts from linear algebra that will be most important in our study of neural networks. Our objective will be to obtain a fundamental understanding of how neural networks work.

4

Further Reading

[BaSu83]   A. Barto, R. Sutton and C. Anderson, "Neuron-like adaptive elements can solve difficult learning control problems," *IEEE Transactions on Systems, Man and Cybernetics*, Vol. 13, No. 5, pp. 834–846, 1983.

A classic paper in which a reinforcement learning algorithm is used to train a neural network to balance an inverted pendulum.

[Brog91]   W. L. Brogan, *Modern Control Theory*, 3rd Ed., Englewood Cliffs, NJ: Prentice-Hall, 1991.

A well-written book on the subject of linear systems. The first half of the book is devoted to linear algebra. It also has good sections on the solution of linear differential equations and the stability of linear and nonlinear systems. It has many worked problems.

[McPi43]   W. McCulloch and W. Pitts, "A logical calculus of the ideas immanent in nervous activity," *Bulletin of Mathematical Biophysics*, Vol. 5, pp. 115–133, 1943.

This article introduces the first mathematical model of a neuron, in which a weighted sum of input signals is compared to a threshold to determine whether or not the neuron fires.

[MiPa69]   M. Minsky and S. Papert, *Perceptrons*, Cambridge, MA: MIT Press, 1969.

A landmark book that contains the first rigorous study devoted to determining what a perceptron network is capable of learning. A formal treatment of the perceptron was needed both to explain the perceptron's limitations and to indicate directions for overcoming them. Unfortunately, the book pessimistically predicted that the limitations of perceptrons indicated that the field of neural networks was a dead end. Although this was not true, it temporarily cooled research and funding for research for several years.

[Rose58]   F. Rosenblatt, "The perceptron: A probabilistic model for information storage and organization in the brain," *Psychological Review*, Vol. 65, pp. 386–408, 1958.

This paper presents the first practical artificial neural network — the perceptron.

[Rose61]   F. Rosenblatt, *Principles of Neurodynamics*, Washington DC: Spartan Press, 1961.

One of the first books on neurocomputing.

[WhSo92]   D. White and D. Sofge (Eds.), *Handbook of Intelligent Control*, New York: Van Nostrand Reinhold, 1992.

Collection of articles describing current research and applications of neural networks and fuzzy logic to control systems.

4

Exercises

E4.1 Consider the classification problem defined below:

$$\left\{ \mathbf{p}_1 = \begin{bmatrix} -1 \\ 1 \end{bmatrix}, t_1 = 1 \right\} \left\{ \mathbf{p}_2 = \begin{bmatrix} 0 \\ 0 \end{bmatrix}, t_2 = 1 \right\} \left\{ \mathbf{p}_3 = \begin{bmatrix} 1 \\ -1 \end{bmatrix}, t_3 = 1 \right\} \left\{ \mathbf{p}_4 = \begin{bmatrix} 1 \\ 0 \end{bmatrix}, t_4 = 0 \right\}$$

$$\left\{ \mathbf{p}_5 = \begin{bmatrix} 0 \\ 1 \end{bmatrix}, t_5 = 0 \right\}.$$

  i. Draw a diagram of the single-neuron perceptron you would use to solve this problem. How many inputs are required?

  ii. Draw a graph of the data points, labeled according to their targets. Is this problem solvable with the network you defined in part (i)? Why or why not?

E4.2 Consider the classification problem defined below.

$$\left\{ \mathbf{p}_1 = \begin{bmatrix} -1 \\ 1 \end{bmatrix}, t_1 = 1 \right\} \left\{ \mathbf{p}_2 = \begin{bmatrix} -1 \\ -1 \end{bmatrix}, t_2 = 1 \right\} \left\{ \mathbf{p}_3 = \begin{bmatrix} 0 \\ 0 \end{bmatrix}, t_3 = 0 \right\} \left\{ \mathbf{p}_4 = \begin{bmatrix} 1 \\ 0 \end{bmatrix}, t_4 = 0 \right\}.$$

  i. Design a single-neuron perceptron to solve this problem. Design the network graphically, by choosing weight vectors that are orthogonal to the decision boundaries.

  ii. Test your solution with all four input vectors.

  iii. Classify the following input vectors with your solution. You can either perform the calculations manually or with MATLAB.

$$\mathbf{p}_5 = \begin{bmatrix} -2 \\ 0 \end{bmatrix} \qquad \mathbf{p}_6 = \begin{bmatrix} 1 \\ 1 \end{bmatrix} \qquad \mathbf{p}_7 = \begin{bmatrix} 0 \\ 1 \end{bmatrix} \qquad \mathbf{p}_8 = \begin{bmatrix} -1 \\ -2 \end{bmatrix}$$

  iv. Which of the vectors in part (iii) will always be classified the same way, regardless of the solution values for $\mathbf{W}$ and b? Which may vary depending on the solution? Why?

E4.3 Solve the classification problem in Exercise E4.2 by solving inequalities (as in Problem P4.2), and repeat parts (ii) and (iii) with the new solution. (The solution is more difficult than Problem P4.2, since you can't isolate the weights and biases in a pairwise manner.)

E4.4 Solve the classification problem in Exercise E4.2 by applying the perceptron rule to the following initial parameters, and repeat parts (ii) and (iii) with the new solution.

$$\mathbf{W}(0) = \begin{bmatrix} 0 & 0 \end{bmatrix} \qquad b(0) = 0$$

E4.5 Prove mathematically (not graphically) that the following problem is unsolvable for a two-input/single-neuron perceptron.

$$\left\{ \mathbf{p}_1 = \begin{bmatrix} -1 \\ 1 \end{bmatrix}, t_1 = 1 \right\} \left\{ \mathbf{p}_2 = \begin{bmatrix} -1 \\ -1 \end{bmatrix}, t_2 = 0 \right\} \left\{ \mathbf{p}_3 = \begin{bmatrix} 1 \\ -1 \end{bmatrix}, t_3 = 1 \right\} \left\{ \mathbf{p}_4 = \begin{bmatrix} 1 \\ 1 \end{bmatrix}, t_4 = 0 \right\}$$

(Hint: start by rewriting the input/target requirements as inequalities that constrain the weight and bias values.)

E4.6 The symmetric hard limit function is sometimes used in perceptron networks, instead of the hard limit function. Target values are then taken from the set [-1, 1] instead of [0, 1].

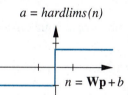

$a = hardlims(n)$

$n = \mathbf{W}\mathbf{p} + b$

   i. Write a simple expression that maps numbers in the ordered set [0, 1] into the ordered set [-1, 1]. Write the expression that performs the inverse mapping.

   ii. Consider two single-neuron perceptrons with the same weight and bias values. The first network uses the hard limit function ([0, 1] values), and the second network uses the symmetric hard limit function. If the two networks are given the same input $\mathbf{p}$, and updated with the perceptron learning rule, will their weights continue to have the same value?

   iii. If the changes to the weights of the two neurons are different, how do they differ? Why?

   iv. Given initial weight and bias values for a standard hard limit perceptron, create a method for initializing a symmetric hard limit perceptron so that the two neurons will always respond identically when trained on identical data.

E4.7 The vectors in the ordered set defined below were obtained by measuring the weight and ear lengths of toy rabbits and bears in the Fuzzy Wuzzy Animal Factory. The target values indicate whether the respective input vector was taken from a rabbit (0) or a bear (1). The first element of the input vector is the weight of the toy, and the second element is the ear length.

$$\left\{ \mathbf{p}_1 = \begin{bmatrix} 1 \\ 4 \end{bmatrix}, t_1 = 0 \right\} \left\{ \mathbf{p}_2 = \begin{bmatrix} 1 \\ 5 \end{bmatrix}, t_2 = 0 \right\} \left\{ \mathbf{p}_3 = \begin{bmatrix} 2 \\ 4 \end{bmatrix}, t_3 = 0 \right\} \left\{ \mathbf{p}_4 = \begin{bmatrix} 2 \\ 5 \end{bmatrix}, t_4 = 0 \right\}$$

$$\left\{ \mathbf{p}_5 = \begin{bmatrix} 3 \\ 1 \end{bmatrix}, t_5 = 1 \right\} \left\{ \mathbf{p}_6 = \begin{bmatrix} 3 \\ 2 \end{bmatrix}, t_6 = 1 \right\} \left\{ \mathbf{p}_7 = \begin{bmatrix} 4 \\ 1 \end{bmatrix}, t_7 = 1 \right\} \left\{ \mathbf{p}_8 = \begin{bmatrix} 4 \\ 2 \end{bmatrix}, t_8 = 1 \right\}$$

   i. Use MATLAB to initialize and train a network to solve this "practical" problem.

   ii. Use MATLAB to test the resulting weight and bias values against the input vectors.

   iii. Alter the input vectors to ensure that the decision boundary of any solution will not intersect one of the original input vectors (i.e., to ensure only robust solutions are found). Then retrain the network.

E4.8 Consider again the four-category classification problem described in Problems P4.3 and P4.5. Suppose that we change the input vector $\mathbf{p}_3$ to

$$\mathbf{p}_3 = \begin{bmatrix} 2 \\ 2 \end{bmatrix}.$$

   i. Is the problem still linearly separable? Demonstrate your answer graphically.

   ii. Use MATLAB and to initialize and train a network to solve this problem. Explain your results.

   iii. If $\mathbf{p}_3$ is changed to

$$\mathbf{p}_3 = \begin{bmatrix} 2 \\ 1.5 \end{bmatrix}$$

   is the problem linearly separable?

   iv. With the $\mathbf{p}_3$ from (iii), use MATLAB to initialize and train a network to solve this problem. Explain your results.

E4.9 One variation of the perceptron learning rule is

$$\mathbf{W}^{new} = \mathbf{W}^{old} + \alpha \mathbf{e}\mathbf{p}^T$$

$$\mathbf{b}^{new} = \mathbf{b}^{old} + \alpha \mathbf{e}$$

where α is called the learning rate. Prove convergence of this algorithm. Does the proof require a limit on the learning rate? Explain.

5 Signal and Weight Vector Spaces

5

Objectives

It is clear from Chapters 3 and 4 that it is very useful to think of the inputs and outputs of a neural network, and the rows of a weight matrix, as vectors. In this chapter we want to examine these vector spaces in detail and to review those properties of vector spaces that are most helpful when analyzing neural networks. We will begin with general definitions and then apply these definitions to specific neural network problems. The concepts that are discussed in this chapter and in Chapter 6 will be used extensively throughout the remaining chapters of this book. They are critical to our understanding of why neural networks work.

Theory and Examples

Linear algebra is the core of the mathematics required for understanding neural networks. In Chapters 3 and 4 we saw the utility of representing the inputs and outputs of neural networks as vectors. In addition, we saw that it is often useful to think of the rows of a weight matrix as vectors in the same vector space as the input vectors.

Recall from Chapter 3 that in the Hamming network the rows of the weight matrix of the feedforward layer were equal to the prototype vectors. In fact, the purpose of the feedforward layer was to calculate the inner products between the prototype vectors and the input vector.

In the single neuron perceptron network we noted that the decision boundary was always orthogonal to the weight matrix (a row vector).

In this chapter we want to review the basic concepts of vector spaces (e.g., inner products, orthogonality) in the context of neural networks. We will begin with a general definition of vector spaces. Then we will present the basic properties of vectors that are most useful for neural network applications.

One comment about notation before we begin. All of the vectors we have discussed so far have been ordered n-tuples (columns) of real numbers and are represented by bold small letters, e.g.,

$$\mathbf{x} = \begin{bmatrix} x_1 & x_2 & \dots & x_n \end{bmatrix}^T. \tag{5.1}$$

These are vectors in $\Re^n$, the standard n-dimensional Euclidean space. In this chapter we will also be talking about more general vector spaces than $\Re^n$. These more general vectors will be represented with a script typeface, as in χ. We will show in this chapter how these general vectors can often be represented by columns of numbers.

Linear Vector Spaces

What do we mean by a vector space? We will begin with a very general definition. While this definition may seem abstract, we will provide many concrete examples. By using a general definition we can solve a larger class of problems, and we can impart a deeper understanding of the concepts.

Vector Space   **Definition.** A linear *vector space*, X, is a set of elements (vectors) defined over a scalar field, F, that satisfies the following conditions:

1.   An operation called vector addition is defined such that if $\chi \in X$ (χ is an element of X) and $y \in X$, then $\chi + y \in X$.

2. $x + y = y + x$.

3. $(x + y) + z = x + (y + z)$.

4. There is a unique vector $0 \in X$, called the zero vector, such that $x + 0 = x$ for all $x \in X$.

5. For each vector $x \in X$ there is a unique vector in X, to be called $-x$, such that $x + (-x) = 0$.

6. An operation, called multiplication, is defined such that for all scalars $a \in F$, and all vectors $x \in X$, $ax \in X$.

7. For any $x \in X$, $1x = x$ (for scalar 1).

8. For any two scalars $a \in F$ and $b \in F$, and any $x \in X$, $a(bx) = (ab)x$.

9. $(a + b)x = ax + bx$.

10. $a(x + y) = ax + ay$.

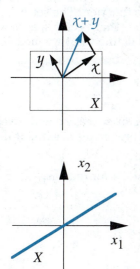

To illustrate these conditions, let's investigate a few sample sets and determine whether or not they are vector spaces. First consider the standard two-dimensional Euclidean space, $\Re^2$, shown in the upper left figure. This is clearly a vector space, and all ten conditions are satisfied for the standard definitions of vector addition and scalar multiplication.

What about subsets of $\Re^2$? What subsets of $\Re^2$ are also vector spaces (subspaces)? Consider the boxed area (X) in the center left figure. Does it satisfy all ten conditions? No. Clearly even condition 1 is not satisfied. The vectors x and y shown in the figure are in X, but $x + y$ is not. From this example it is clear that no bounded sets can be vector spaces.

Are there any subsets of $\Re^2$ that are vector spaces? Consider the line (X) shown in the bottom left figure. (Assume that the line extends to infinity in both directions.) Is this line a vector space? We leave it to you to show that indeed all ten conditions are satisfied. Will any such infinite line satisfy the ten conditions? Well, any line that passes through the origin will work. If it does not pass through the origin then condition 4, for instance, would not be satisfied.

In addition to the standard Euclidean spaces, there are other sets that also satisfy the ten conditions of a vector space. Consider, for example, the set P^2 of all polynomials of degree less than or equal to 2. Two members of this set would be

$$\chi = 2 + t + 4t^2$$

$$y = 1 + 5t . \tag{5.2}$$

If you are used to thinking of vectors only as columns of numbers, these may seem to be strange vectors indeed. However, recall that to be a vector space, a set need only satisfy the ten conditions we presented. Are these conditions satisfied for the set P^2? If we add two polynomials of degree less than or equal to 2, the result will also be a polynomial of degree less than or equal to 2. Therefore condition 1 is satisfied. We can also multiply a polynomial by a scalar without changing the order of the polynomial. Therefore condition 6 is satisfied. It is not difficult to show that all ten conditions are satisfied, showing that P^2 is a vector space.

Consider the set $C_{[0, 1]}$ of all continuous functions defined on the interval $[0, 1]$. Two members of this set would be

$$\chi = \sin (t)$$

$$y = e^{-2t} . \tag{5.3}$$

Another member of the set is shown in the figure to the left.

The sum of two continuous functions is also a continuous function, and a scalar times a continuous function is a continuous function. The set $C_{[0, 1]}$ is also a vector space. This set is different than the other vector spaces we have discussed; it is infinite dimensional. We will define what we mean by dimension later in this chapter.

Linear Independence

Now that we have defined what we mean by a vector space, we will investigate some of the properties of vectors. The first properties are linear dependence and linear independence.

Consider n vectors $\{\chi_1, \chi_2, \dots, \chi_n\}$. If there exist n scalars $a_1, a_2, \dots, a_n$, at least one of which is nonzero, such that

$$a_1\chi_1 + a_2\chi_2 + \cdots + a_n\chi_n = 0, \tag{5.4}$$

then the $\{\chi_i\}$ are linearly dependent.

Linear Independence   The converse statement would be: If $a_1\chi_1 + a_2\chi_2 + \cdots + a_n\chi_n = 0$ implies that each $a_i = 0$, then $\{\chi_i\}$ is a set of *linearly independent* vectors.

Note that these definitions are equivalent to saying that if a set of vectors is independent then no vector in the set can be written as a linear combination of the other vectors.

As an example of independence, consider the pattern recognition problem of Chapter 3. The two prototype patterns (*orange* and *apple*) were given by:

$$\mathbf{p}_1 = \begin{bmatrix} 1 \\ -1 \\ -1 \end{bmatrix}, \mathbf{p}_2 = \begin{bmatrix} 1 \\ 1 \\ -1 \end{bmatrix}. \tag{5.5}$$

Let $a_1\mathbf{p}_1 + a_2\mathbf{p}_2 = 0$, then

$$\begin{bmatrix} a_1 + a_2 \\ -a_1 + a_2 \\ -a_1 + (-a_2) \end{bmatrix} = \begin{bmatrix} 0 \\ 0 \\ 0 \end{bmatrix}, \tag{5.6}$$

but this can only be true if $a_1 = a_2 = 0$. Therefore $\mathbf{p}_1$ and $\mathbf{p}_2$ are linearly independent.

Consider vectors from the space P^2 of polynomials of degree less than or equal to 2. Three vectors from this space would be

$$\chi_1 = 1 + t + t^2, \chi_2 = 2 + 2t + t^2, \chi_3 = 1 + t. \tag{5.7}$$

Note that if we let $a_1 = 1$, $a_2 = -1$ and $a_3 = 1$, then

$$a_1\chi_1 + a_2\chi_2 + a_n\chi_n = 0. \tag{5.8}$$

Therefore these three vectors are linearly dependent.

Spanning a Space

Next we want to define what we mean by the dimension (size) of a vector space. To do so we must first define the concept of a spanning set.

Let X be a linear vector space and let $\{u_1, u_2, \dots, u_m\}$ be a subset of general vectors in X. This subset spans X if and only if for every vector $\chi \in X$ there exist scalars $x_1, x_2, \dots, x_n$ such that $\chi = x_1u_1 + x_2u_2 + \cdots + x_mu_m$. In other words, a subset spans a space if every vector in the space can be written as a linear combination of the vectors in the subset.

The dimension of a vector space is determined by the minimum number of vectors it takes to span the space. This leads to the definition of a basis set. Basis Set A *basis set* for X is a set of linearly independent vectors that spans X. Any basis set contains the minimum number of vectors required to span the

5

space. The dimension of X is therefore equal to the number of elements in the basis set. Any vector space can have many basis sets, but each one must contain the same number of elements. (See [Stra80] for a proof of this fact.)

Take, for example, the linear vector space P^2. One possible basis for this space is

$$u_1 = 1 , u_2 = t , u_3 = t^2 . \tag{5.9}$$

Clearly any polynomial of degree two or less can be created by taking a linear combination of these three vectors. Note, however, that *any* three independent vectors from P^2 would form a basis for this space. One such alternate basis is:

$$u_1 = 1 , u_2 = 1 + t , u_3 = 1 + t + t^2 . \tag{5.10}$$

Inner Product

From our brief encounter with neural networks in Chapters 3 and 4, it is clear that the inner product is fundamental to the operation of many neural networks. Here we will introduce a general definition for inner products and then give several examples.

Inner Product   Any scalar function of x and y can be defined as an *inner product*, (x,y), provided that the following properties are satisfied:

1. $(x,y) = (y,x)$.

2. $(x,ay_1 + by_2) = a(x,y_1) + b(x,y_2)$.

3. $(x,x) \geq 0$, where equality holds if and only if x is the zero vector.

The standard inner product for vectors in R^n is

$$\mathbf{x}^T\mathbf{y} = x_1 y_1 + x_2 y_2 + \cdots + x_n y_n , \tag{5.11}$$

but this is not the only possible inner product. Consider again the set $C_{[0,1]}$ of all continuous functions defined on the interval [0, 1]. Show that the following scalar function is an inner product (see Problem P5.6).

$$(x,y) = \int_0^1 x(t) y(t) \, dt \tag{5.12}$$

Norm

The next operation we need to define is the norm, which is based on the concept of vector length.

Norm A scalar function $\|x\|$ is called a *norm* if it satisfies the following properties:

1. $\|x\| \geq 0$.
2. $\|x\| = 0$ if and only if $x = 0$.
3. $\|ax\| = |a|\|x\|$ for scalar a.
4. $\|x + y\| \leq \|x\| + \|y\|$.

There are many functions that would satisfy these conditions. One common norm is based on the inner product:

$$\|x\| = (x,x)^{1/2}. \tag{5.13}$$

For Euclidean spaces, $\Re^n$, this yields the norm with which we are most familiar:

$$\|\mathbf{x}\| = (\mathbf{x}^T\mathbf{x})^{1/2} = \sqrt{x_1^2 + x_2^2 + \cdots + x_n^2}. \tag{5.14}$$

In neural network applications it is often useful to normalize the input vectors. This means that $\|\mathbf{p}_i\| = 1$ for each input vector.

Angle Using the norm and the inner product we can generalize the concept of angle for vector spaces of dimension greater than two. The *angle* θ between two vectors x and y is defined by

$$\cos\theta = \frac{(x,y)}{\|x\|\|y\|}. \tag{5.15}$$

Orthogonality

Now that we have defined the inner product operation, we can introduce the important concept of orthogonality.

Orthogonality Two vectors $x, y \in X$ are said to be *orthogonal* if $(x,y) = 0$.

Orthogonality is an important concept in neural networks. We will see in Chapter 7 that when the prototype vectors of a pattern recognition problem are orthogonal and normalized, a linear associator neural network can be trained, using the Hebb rule, to achieve perfect recognition.

In addition to orthogonal vectors, we can also have orthogonal spaces. A vector $x \in X$ is orthogonal to a subspace X_1 if x is orthogonal to every vec-

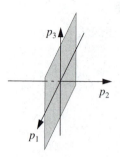

tor in X_1. This is typically represented as $\chi \perp X_1$. A subspace X_1 is orthogonal to a subspace X_2 if every vector in X_1 is orthogonal to every vector in X_2. This is represented by $X_1 \perp X_2$.

The figure to the left illustrates the two orthogonal spaces that were used in the perceptron example of Chapter 3. (See Figure 3.4.) The p_1, p_3 plane is a subspace of $\Re^3$, which is orthogonal to the p_2 axis (which is another subspace of $\Re^3$). The p_1, p_3 plane was the decision boundary of a perceptron network. In Solved Problem P5.1 we will show that the perceptron decision boundary will be a vector space whenever the bias value is zero.

Gram-Schmidt Orthogonalization

There is a relationship between orthogonality and independence. It is possible to convert a set of independent vectors into a set of orthogonal vectors that spans the same vector space. The standard procedure to accomplish this is called Gram-Schmidt orthogonalization.

Assume that we have n independent vectors $y_1, y_2, \ldots, y_n$. From these vectors we want to obtain n orthogonal vectors $v_1, v_2, \ldots, v_n$. The first orthogonal vector is chosen to be the first independent vector:

$$v_1 = y_1. \tag{5.16}$$

To obtain the second orthogonal vector we use y_2, but subtract off the portion of y_2 that is in the direction of v_1. This leads to the equation

$$v_2 = y_2 - av_1, \tag{5.17}$$

where a is chosen so that v_2 is orthogonal to v_1. This requires that

$$(v_1, v_2) = (v_1, y_2 - av_1) = (v_1, y_2) - a(v_1, v_1) = 0, \tag{5.18}$$

or

$$a = \frac{(v_1, y_2)}{(v_1, v_1)}. \tag{5.19}$$

Therefore to find the component of y_2 in the direction of v_1, av_1, we need to find the inner product between the two vectors. We call av_1 the *projection* of y_2 on the vector v_1.

Projection

If we continue this process, the kth step will be

$$v_k = y_k - \sum_{i=1}^{k-1} \frac{(v_i, y_k)}{(v_i, v_i)} v_i. \tag{5.20}$$

To illustrate this process, we consider the following independent vectors in $\mathfrak{R}^2$:

$$\mathbf{y}_1 = \begin{bmatrix} 2 \\ 1 \end{bmatrix}, \mathbf{y}_2 = \begin{bmatrix} 1 \\ 2 \end{bmatrix}. \tag{5.21}$$

The first orthogonal vector would be

$$\mathbf{v}_1 = \mathbf{y}_1 = \begin{bmatrix} 2 \\ 1 \end{bmatrix}. \tag{5.22}$$

The second orthogonal vector is calculated as follows:

$$\mathbf{v}_2 = \mathbf{y}_2 - \frac{\mathbf{v}_1^T \mathbf{y}_2}{\mathbf{v}_1^T \mathbf{v}_1}\mathbf{v}_1 = \begin{bmatrix} 1 \\ 2 \end{bmatrix} - \frac{\begin{bmatrix} 2 & 1 \end{bmatrix}\begin{bmatrix} 1 \\ 2 \end{bmatrix}}{\begin{bmatrix} 2 & 1 \end{bmatrix}\begin{bmatrix} 2 \\ 1 \end{bmatrix}}\begin{bmatrix} 2 \\ 1 \end{bmatrix} = \begin{bmatrix} 1 \\ 2 \end{bmatrix} - \begin{bmatrix} 1.6 \\ 0.8 \end{bmatrix} = \begin{bmatrix} -0.6 \\ 1.2 \end{bmatrix}. \tag{5.23}$$

See Figure 5.1 for a graphical representation of this process.

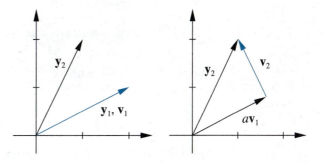

Figure 5.1 Gram-Schmidt Orthogonalization Example

Orthonormal We could convert $\mathbf{v}_1$ and $\mathbf{v}_2$ to a set of *orthonormal* (orthogonal and normalized) vectors by dividing each vector by its norm.

To experiment with this orthogonalization process, use the Neural Network Design Demonstration Gram-Schmidt (**nnd5gs**).

Vector Expansions

Note that we have been using a script font (χ) to represent general vectors and bold type ($\mathbf{x}$) to represent vectors in $\mathfrak{R}^n$, which can be written as columns of numbers. In this section we will show that general vectors in finite dimensional vector spaces can also be written as columns of numbers and therefore are in some ways equivalent to vectors in $\Re^n$.

Vector Expansion

If a vector space X has a basis set $\{v_1, v_2, \ldots, v_n\}$, then any $\chi \in X$ has a unique *vector expansion*:

$$\chi = \sum_{i=1}^{n} x_i v_i = x_1 v_1 + x_2 v_2 + \cdots + x_n v_n.$$ (5.24)

Therefore any vector in a finite dimensional vector space can be represented by a column of numbers:

$$\mathbf{x} = \begin{bmatrix} x_1 & x_2 & \ldots & x_n \end{bmatrix}^T.$$ (5.25)

This $\mathbf{x}$ is a representation of the general vector χ. Of course in order to interpret the meaning of $\mathbf{x}$ we need to know the basis set. If the basis set changes, $\mathbf{x}$ will change, even though it still represents the same general vector χ. We will discuss this in more detail in the next subsection.

If the vectors in the basis set are orthogonal $((v_i, v_j) = 0, i \neq j)$ it is very easy to compute the coefficients in the expansion. We simply take the inner product of v_j with both sides of Eq. (5.24):

$$(v_j, \chi) = (v_j, \sum_{i=1}^{n} x_i v_i) = \sum_{i=1}^{n} x_i (v_j, v_i) = x_j (v_j, v_j).$$ (5.26)

Therefore the coefficients of the expansion are given by

$$x_j = \frac{(v_j, \chi)}{(v_j, v_j)}.$$ (5.27)

When the vectors in the basis set are not orthogonal, the computation of the coefficients in the vector expansion is more complex. This case is covered in the following subsection.

Reciprocal Basis Vectors

If a vector expansion is required and the basis set is not orthogonal, the reciprocal basis vectors are introduced. These are defined by the following equations:

$$(r_i, v_j) = 0 \qquad i \neq j$$

$$= 1 \qquad i = j,$$ (5.28)

Reciprocal Basis Vectors where the basis vectors are $\{v_1, v_2, \ldots, v_n\}$ and the *reciprocal basis vectors* are $\{r_1, r_2, \ldots, r_n\}$.

If the vectors have been represented by columns of numbers (through vector expansion), and the standard inner product is used

$$(r_i, v_j) = \mathbf{r}_i^T \mathbf{v}_j, \qquad (5.29)$$

then Eq. (5.28) can be represented in matrix form as

$$\mathbf{R}^T \mathbf{B} = \mathbf{I}, \qquad (5.30)$$

where

$$\mathbf{B} = \begin{bmatrix} \mathbf{v}_1 & \mathbf{v}_2 & \cdots & \mathbf{v}_n \end{bmatrix}, \qquad (5.31)$$

$$\mathbf{R} = \begin{bmatrix} \mathbf{r}_1 & \mathbf{r}_2 & \cdots & \mathbf{r}_n \end{bmatrix}. \qquad (5.32)$$

Therefore $\mathbf{R}$ can be found from

$$\mathbf{R}^T = \mathbf{B}^{-1}, \qquad (5.33)$$

and the reciprocal basis vectors can be obtained from the columns of $\mathbf{R}$.

Now consider again the vector expansion

$$\chi = x_1 v_1 + x_2 v_2 + \cdots + x_n v_n. \qquad (5.34)$$

Taking the inner product of r_1 with both sides of Eq. (5.34) we obtain

$$(r_1, \chi) = x_1(r_1, v_1) + x_2(r_1, v_2) + \cdots + x_n(r_1, v_n). \qquad (5.35)$$

By definition

$$(r_1, v_2) = (r_1, v_3) = \cdots = (r_1, v_n) = 0$$

$$(r_1, v_1) = 1. \qquad (5.36)$$

Therefore the first coefficient of the expansion is

$$x_1 = (r_1, \chi), \qquad (5.37)$$

and in general

$$x_j = (r_j, \chi). \qquad (5.38)$$

As an example, consider the two basis vectors

$$\mathbf{v}_1^s = \begin{bmatrix} 2 \\ 1 \end{bmatrix}, \ \mathbf{v}_2^s = \begin{bmatrix} 1 \\ 2 \end{bmatrix}. \tag{5.39}$$

Suppose that we want to expand the vector

$$\mathbf{x}^s = \begin{bmatrix} 0 \\ 3 \\ 2 \end{bmatrix} \tag{5.40}$$

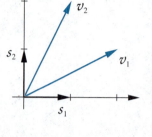

in terms of the two basis vectors. (We are using the superscript s to indicate that these columns of numbers represent expansions of the vectors in terms of the standard basis in $\Re^2$. The elements of the standard basis are indicated in the adjacent figure as the vectors s_1 and s_2. We need to use this explicit notation in this example because we will be expanding the vectors in terms of two different basis sets.)

The first step in the vector expansion is to find the reciprocal basis vectors.

$$\mathbf{R}^T = \begin{bmatrix} 2 & 1 \\ 1 & 2 \end{bmatrix}^{-1} = \begin{bmatrix} \dfrac{2}{3} & -\dfrac{1}{3} \\ -\dfrac{1}{3} & \dfrac{2}{3} \end{bmatrix} \quad \mathbf{r}_1 = \begin{bmatrix} \dfrac{2}{3} \\ -\dfrac{1}{3} \end{bmatrix} \quad \mathbf{r}_2 = \begin{bmatrix} -\dfrac{1}{3} \\ \dfrac{2}{3} \end{bmatrix}. \tag{5.41}$$

Now we can find the coefficients in the expansion.

$$x_1^v = \mathbf{r}_1^T \mathbf{x}^s = \begin{bmatrix} \dfrac{2}{3} & -\dfrac{1}{3} \end{bmatrix} \begin{bmatrix} 0 \\ 3 \\ 2 \end{bmatrix} = -\dfrac{1}{2}$$

$$x_2^v = \mathbf{r}_2^T \mathbf{x}^s = \begin{bmatrix} -\dfrac{1}{3} & \dfrac{2}{3} \end{bmatrix} \begin{bmatrix} 0 \\ 3 \\ 2 \end{bmatrix} = 1 \tag{5.42}$$

or, in matrix form,

$$\mathbf{x}^v = \mathbf{R}^T \mathbf{x}^s = \mathbf{B}^{-1} \mathbf{x}^s = \begin{bmatrix} \dfrac{2}{3} & -\dfrac{1}{3} \\ -\dfrac{1}{3} & \dfrac{2}{3} \end{bmatrix} \begin{bmatrix} 0 \\ 3 \\ 2 \end{bmatrix} = \begin{bmatrix} -\dfrac{1}{2} \\ 1 \end{bmatrix}. \tag{5.43}$$

So that

$$\chi = -\frac{1}{2}v_1 + 1v_2,$$

(5.44)

as indicated in Figure 5.2.

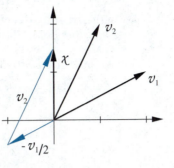

Figure 5.2 Vector Expansion

Note that we now have two different vector expansions for χ, represented by $\mathbf{x}^s$ and $\mathbf{x}^v$. In other words,

$$\chi = 0s_1 + \frac{3}{2}s_2 = -\frac{1}{2}v_1 + 1v_2.$$

(5.45)

When we represent a general vector as a column of numbers we need to know what basis set was used for the expansion. In this text, unless otherwise stated, assume the standard basis set was used.

Eq. (5.43) shows the relationship between the two different representations of χ, $\mathbf{x}^v = \mathbf{B}^{-1}\mathbf{x}^s$. This operation, called a change of basis, will become very important in later chapters for the performance analysis of certain neural networks.

 *To experiment with the vector expansion process, use the Neural Network Design Demonstration Reciprocal Basis (**nnd5rb**).*

Summary of Results

Linear Vector Spaces

Definition. A linear vector space, X, is a set of elements (vectors) defined over a scalar field, F, that satisfies the following conditions:

1. An operation called vector addition is defined such that if $\chi \in X$ and $y \in X$, then $\chi + y \in X$.

2. $\chi + y = y + \chi$.

3. $(\chi + y) + z = \chi + (y + z)$.

4. There is a unique vector $0 \in X$, called the zero vector, such that $\chi + 0 = \chi$ for all $\chi \in X$.

5. For each vector $\chi \in X$ there is a unique vector in X, to be called $-\chi$, such that $\chi + (-\chi) = 0$.

6. An operation, called multiplication, is defined such that for all scalars $a \in F$, and all vectors $\chi \in X$, $a\chi \in X$.

7. For any $\chi \in X$, $1\chi = \chi$ (for scalar 1).

8. For any two scalars $a \in F$ and $b \in F$, and any $\chi \in X$, $a(b\chi) = (ab)\chi$.

9. $(a + b)\chi = a\chi + b\chi$.

10. $a(\chi + y) = a\chi + ay$.

Linear Independence

Consider n vectors $\{\chi_1, \chi_2, \dots, \chi_n\}$. If there exist n scalars $a_1, a_2, \dots, a_n$, at least one of which is nonzero, such that

$$a_1\chi_1 + a_2\chi_2 + \cdots + a_n\chi_n = 0,$$

then the $\{\chi_i\}$ are linearly dependent.

Spanning a Space

Let X be a linear vector space and let $\{u_1, u_2, \ldots, u_m\}$ be a subset of vectors in X. This subset spans X if and only if for every vector $\chi \in X$ there exist scalars $x_1, x_2, \ldots, x_n$ such that $\chi = x_1 u_1 + x_2 u_2 + \cdots + x_m u_m$.

Inner Product

Any scalar function of χ and y can be defined as an inner product, (χ,y), provided that the following properties are satisfied.

1. $(\chi,y) = (y,\chi)$.

2. $(\chi, ay_1 + by_2) = a(\chi,y_1) + b(\chi,y_2)$.

3. $(\chi,\chi) \geq 0$, where equality holds if and only if χ is the zero vector.

Norm

A scalar function $\|\chi\|$ is called a norm if it satisfies the following properties:

1. $\|\chi\| \geq 0$.

2. $\|\chi\| = 0$ if and only if $\chi = 0$.

3. $\|a\chi\| = |a|\|\chi\|$ for scalar a.

4. $\|\chi + y\| \leq \|\chi\| + \|y\|$.

Angle

The angle θ between two vectors χ and y is defined by

$$\cos\theta = \frac{(\chi,y)}{\|\chi\|\|y\|}.$$

Orthogonality

Two vectors $\chi, y \in X$ are said to be orthogonal if $(\chi,y) = 0$.

Gram-Schmidt Orthogonalization

Assume that we have n independent vectors $y_1, y_2, \ldots, y_n$. From these vectors we will obtain n orthogonal vectors $v_1, v_2, \ldots, v_n$.

$$v_1 = y_1$$

$$v_k = y_k - \sum_{i=1}^{k-1} \frac{(v_i,y_k)}{(v_i,v_i)} v_i,$$

where

$$\frac{(v_i, y_k)}{(v_i, v_i)} v_i$$

is the projection of y_k on v_i.

Vector Expansions

$$x = \sum_{i=1}^{n} x_i v_i = x_1 v_1 + x_2 v_2 + \cdots + x_n v_n.$$

For orthogonal vectors,

$$x_j = \frac{(v_j, x)}{(v_j, v_j)}$$

Reciprocal Basis Vectors

$$(r_i, v_j) = 0 \qquad i \neq j$$

$$= 1 \qquad i = j$$

$$x_j = (r_j, x).$$

To compute the reciprocal basis vectors:

$$\mathbf{B} = \left[\mathbf{v}_1 \; \mathbf{v}_2 \; \cdots \; \mathbf{v}_n \right],$$

$$\mathbf{R} = \left[\mathbf{r}_1 \; \mathbf{r}_2 \; \cdots \; \mathbf{r}_n \right],$$

$$\mathbf{R}^T = \mathbf{B}^{-1}.$$

In matrix form:

$$\mathbf{x}^v = \mathbf{B}^{-1} \mathbf{x}^s.$$

Solved Problems

P5.1 **Consider the single-neuron perceptron network shown in Figure P5.1. Recall from Chapter 3 (see Eq. (3.6)) that the decision boundary for this network is given by $\mathbf{W}\mathbf{p} + b = 0$. Show that the decision boundary is a vector space if $b = 0$.**

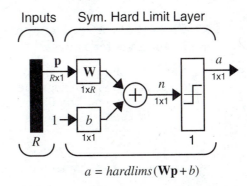

$$a = hardlims(\mathbf{W}\mathbf{p} + b)$$

Figure P5.1 Single-Neuron Perceptron

To be a vector space the boundary must satisfy the ten conditions given at the beginning of this chapter. Condition 1 requires that when we add two vectors together the sum remains in the vector space. Let $\mathbf{p}_1$ and $\mathbf{p}_2$ be two vectors on the decision boundary. To be on the boundary they must satisfy

$$\mathbf{W}\mathbf{p}_1 = 0 \qquad \mathbf{W}\mathbf{p}_2 = 0.$$

If we add these two equations together we find

$$\mathbf{W}(\mathbf{p}_1 + \mathbf{p}_2) = 0.$$

Therefore the sum is also on the decision boundary.

Conditions 2 and 3 are clearly satisfied. Condition 4 requires that the zero vector be on the boundary. Since $\mathbf{W}\mathbf{0} = 0$, the zero vector is on the decision boundary. Condition 5 implies that if $\mathbf{p}$ is on the boundary, then $-\mathbf{p}$ must also be on the boundary. If $\mathbf{p}$ is on the boundary, then

$$\mathbf{W}\mathbf{p} = 0.$$

If we multiply both sides of this equation by -1 we find

$$\mathbf{W}(-\mathbf{p}) = 0.$$

Therefore condition 5 is satisfied.

Condition 6 will be satisfied if for any **p** on the boundary $a\mathbf{p}$ is also on the boundary. This can be shown in the same way as condition 5. Just multiply both sides of the equation by a instead of by 1.

$$\mathbf{W}(a\mathbf{p}) = 0$$

Conditions 7 through 10 are clearly satisfied. Therefore the perceptron decision boundary is a vector space.

P5.2 **Show that the set Y of nonnegative ($f(t) \geq 0$) continuous functions is not a vector space.**

This set violates several of the conditions required of a vector space. For example, there are no negative vectors, so condition 5 cannot be satisfied. Also, consider condition 6. The function $f(t) = |t|$ is a member of Y. Let $a = -2$. Then

$$af(2) = -2|2| = -4 < 0.$$

Therefore $af(t)$ is not a member of Y, and condition 6 is not satisfied.

P5.3 **Which of the following sets of vectors are independent? Find the dimension of the vector space spanned by each set.**

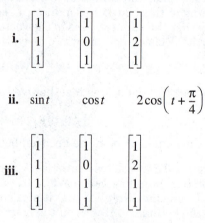

i. $\begin{bmatrix} 1 \\ 1 \\ 1 \end{bmatrix} \quad \begin{bmatrix} 1 \\ 0 \\ 1 \end{bmatrix} \quad \begin{bmatrix} 1 \\ 2 \\ 1 \end{bmatrix}$

ii. $\sin t \qquad \cos t \qquad 2\cos\left(t + \frac{\pi}{4}\right)$

iii. $\begin{bmatrix} 1 \\ 1 \\ 1 \\ 1 \end{bmatrix} \quad \begin{bmatrix} 1 \\ 0 \\ 1 \\ 1 \end{bmatrix} \quad \begin{bmatrix} 1 \\ 2 \\ 1 \\ 1 \end{bmatrix}$

i. We can solve this problem several ways. First, let's assume that the vectors are dependent. Then we can write

$$a_1 \begin{bmatrix} 1 \\ 1 \\ 1 \end{bmatrix} + a_2 \begin{bmatrix} 1 \\ 0 \\ 1 \end{bmatrix} + a_3 \begin{bmatrix} 1 \\ 2 \\ 1 \end{bmatrix} = \begin{bmatrix} 0 \\ 0 \\ 0 \end{bmatrix}.$$

If we can solve for the coefficients and they are not all zero, then the vectors are dependent. By inspection we can see that if we let $a_1 = 2$, $a_2 = -1$ and $a_3 = -1$, then the equation is satisfied. Therefore the vectors are dependent.

Another approach, when we have n vectors in $\Re^n$, is to write the above equation in matrix form:

$$\begin{bmatrix} 1 & 1 & 1 \\ 1 & 0 & 2 \\ 1 & 1 & 1 \end{bmatrix} \begin{bmatrix} a_1 \\ a_2 \\ a_3 \end{bmatrix} = \begin{bmatrix} 0 \\ 0 \\ 0 \end{bmatrix}$$

If the matrix in this equation has an inverse, then the solution will require that all coefficients be zero; therefore the vectors are independent. If the matrix is singular (has no inverse), then a nonzero set of coefficients will work, and the vectors are dependent. The test, then, is to create a matrix using the vectors as columns. If the determinant of the matrix is zero (singular matrix), then the vectors are dependent; otherwise they are independent. Using the Laplace expansion [Brog91] on the first column, the determinant of this matrix is

$$\begin{vmatrix} 1 & 1 & 1 \\ 1 & 0 & 2 \\ 1 & 1 & 1 \end{vmatrix} = 1 \begin{vmatrix} 0 & 2 \\ 1 & 1 \end{vmatrix} + (-1) \begin{vmatrix} 1 & 1 \\ 1 & 1 \end{vmatrix} + 1 \begin{vmatrix} 1 & 1 \\ 0 & 2 \end{vmatrix} = -2 + 0 + 2 = 0$$

Therefore the vectors are dependent.

The dimension of the space spanned by the vectors is two, since any two of the vectors can be shown to be independent.

ii. By using some trigonometric identities we can write

$$\cos\left(t + \frac{\pi}{4}\right) = \frac{-1}{\sqrt{2}} \sin t + \frac{1}{\sqrt{2}} \cos t .$$

Therefore the vectors are dependent. The dimension of the space spanned by the vectors is two, since no linear combination of $\sin t$ and $\cos t$ is identically zero.

iii. This is similar to part (i), except that the number of vectors is less than the size of the vector space they are drawn from (three vectors in $\Re^4$). In this case the matrix made up of the vectors will not be square, so we will not be able to compute a determinant. However, we can use something called the Gramian [Brog91]. It is the determinant of a matrix whose i,j element is the inner product of vector i and vector j. The vectors are dependent if and only if the Gramian is zero.

For our problem the Gramian would be

$$G = \begin{vmatrix} (\mathbf{x}_1,\mathbf{x}_1) & (\mathbf{x}_1,\mathbf{x}_2) & (\mathbf{x}_1,\mathbf{x}_3) \\ (\mathbf{x}_2,\mathbf{x}_1) & (\mathbf{x}_2,\mathbf{x}_2) & (\mathbf{x}_2,\mathbf{x}_3) \\ (\mathbf{x}_3,\mathbf{x}_1) & (\mathbf{x}_3,\mathbf{x}_2) & (\mathbf{x}_3,\mathbf{x}_3) \end{vmatrix},$$

where

$$\mathbf{x}_1 = \begin{bmatrix} 1 \\ 1 \\ 1 \\ 1 \end{bmatrix} \qquad \mathbf{x}_2 = \begin{bmatrix} 1 \\ 0 \\ 1 \\ 1 \end{bmatrix} \qquad \mathbf{x}_3 = \begin{bmatrix} 1 \\ 2 \\ 1 \\ 1 \end{bmatrix}.$$

Therefore

$$G = \begin{vmatrix} 4 & 3 & 5 \\ 3 & 3 & 3 \\ 5 & 3 & 7 \end{vmatrix} = 4 \begin{vmatrix} 3 & 3 \\ 3 & 7 \end{vmatrix} + (-3) \begin{vmatrix} 3 & 5 \\ 3 & 7 \end{vmatrix} + 5 \begin{vmatrix} 3 & 5 \\ 3 & 3 \end{vmatrix} = 48 - 18 - 30 = 0.$$

We can also show that these vectors are dependent by noting

$$2\begin{bmatrix} 1 \\ 1 \\ 1 \\ 1 \end{bmatrix} - 1\begin{bmatrix} 1 \\ 0 \\ 1 \\ 1 \end{bmatrix} - 1\begin{bmatrix} 1 \\ 2 \\ 1 \\ 1 \end{bmatrix} = \begin{bmatrix} 0 \\ 0 \\ 0 \\ 0 \end{bmatrix}.$$

The dimension of the space must therefore be less than 3. We can show that $\mathbf{x}_1$ and $\mathbf{x}_2$ are independent, since

$$G = \begin{vmatrix} 4 & 3 \\ 3 & 3 \end{vmatrix} = 4 \neq 0.$$

Therefore the dimension of the space is 2.

P5.4 **Recall from Chapters 3 and 4 that one-layer perceptrons can only be used to recognize patterns that are linearly separable (can be separated by a linear boundary — see Figure 3.3). If two patterns are linearly separable, are they always linearly independent?**

No, these are two unrelated concepts. Take the following simple example. Consider the two input perceptron shown in Figure P5.2.

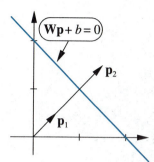

Suppose that we want to separate the two vectors

$$\mathbf{p}_1 = \begin{bmatrix} 0.5 \\ 0.5 \end{bmatrix} \qquad \mathbf{p}_2 = \begin{bmatrix} 1.5 \\ 1.5 \end{bmatrix} .$$

If we choose the weights and offsets to be $w_{11} = 1$, $w_{12} = 1$ and $b = -2$, then the decision boundary ($\mathbf{Wp} + b = 0$) is shown in the figure to the left. Clearly these two vectors are linearly separable. However, they are not linearly independent since $\mathbf{p}_2 = 3\mathbf{p}_1$.

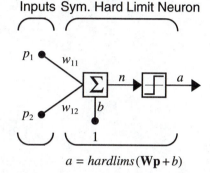

$$a = hardlims(\mathbf{Wp} + b)$$

Figure P5.2 Two-Input Perceptron

P5.5 **Using the following basis vectors, find an orthogonal set using Gram-Schmidt orthogonalization.**

$$\mathbf{y}_1 = \begin{bmatrix} 1 \\ 1 \\ 1 \end{bmatrix} \qquad \mathbf{y}_2 = \begin{bmatrix} 1 \\ 0 \\ 0 \end{bmatrix} \qquad \mathbf{y}_3 = \begin{bmatrix} 0 \\ 1 \\ 0 \end{bmatrix}$$

Step 1.

$$\mathbf{v}_1 = \mathbf{y}_1 = \begin{bmatrix} 1 \\ 1 \\ 1 \end{bmatrix}$$

Step 2.

$$\mathbf{v}_2 = \mathbf{y}_2 - \frac{\mathbf{v}_1^T \mathbf{y}_2}{\mathbf{v}_1^T \mathbf{v}_1} \mathbf{v}_1 = \begin{bmatrix} 1 \\ 0 \\ 0 \end{bmatrix} - \frac{\begin{bmatrix} 1 & 1 & 1 \end{bmatrix} \begin{bmatrix} 1 \\ 0 \\ 0 \end{bmatrix}}{\begin{bmatrix} 1 & 1 & 1 \end{bmatrix} \begin{bmatrix} 1 \\ 1 \\ 1 \end{bmatrix}} \begin{bmatrix} 1 \\ 1 \\ 1 \end{bmatrix} = \begin{bmatrix} 1 \\ 0 \\ 0 \end{bmatrix} - \begin{bmatrix} 1/3 \\ 1/3 \\ 1/3 \end{bmatrix} = \begin{bmatrix} 2/3 \\ -1/3 \\ -1/3 \end{bmatrix}$$

Step 3.

$$\mathbf{v}_3 = \mathbf{y}_3 - \frac{\mathbf{v}_1^T \mathbf{y}_3}{\mathbf{v}_1^T \mathbf{v}_1} \mathbf{v}_1 - \frac{\mathbf{v}_2^T \mathbf{y}_3}{\mathbf{v}_2^T \mathbf{v}_2} \mathbf{v}_2$$

$$\mathbf{v}_3 = \begin{bmatrix} 0 \\ 1 \\ 0 \end{bmatrix} - \frac{\begin{bmatrix} 1 & 1 & 1 \end{bmatrix} \begin{bmatrix} 0 \\ 1 \\ 0 \end{bmatrix}}{\begin{bmatrix} 1 & 1 & 1 \end{bmatrix} \begin{bmatrix} 1 \\ 1 \\ 1 \end{bmatrix}} \begin{bmatrix} 1 \\ 1 \\ 1 \end{bmatrix} - \frac{\begin{bmatrix} 2/3 & -1/3 & -1/3 \end{bmatrix} \begin{bmatrix} 0 \\ 1 \\ 0 \end{bmatrix}}{\begin{bmatrix} 2/3 & -1/3 & -1/3 \end{bmatrix} \begin{bmatrix} 2/3 \\ -1/3 \\ -1/3 \end{bmatrix}} \begin{bmatrix} 2/3 \\ -1/3 \\ -1/3 \end{bmatrix}$$

$$\mathbf{v}_3 = \begin{bmatrix} 0 \\ 1 \\ 0 \end{bmatrix} - \begin{bmatrix} 1/3 \\ 1/3 \\ 1/3 \end{bmatrix} - \begin{bmatrix} -1/3 \\ 1/6 \\ 1/6 \end{bmatrix} = \begin{bmatrix} 0 \\ 1/2 \\ -1/2 \end{bmatrix}$$

P5.6 **Consider the vector space of all polynomials defined on the interval [-1, 1]. Show that** $(\chi , y) = \int_{-1}^{1} \chi(t) y(t)\, dt$ **is a valid inner product.**

An inner product must satisfy the following properties.

1. $(\chi , y) = (y , \chi)$

$$(\chi , y) = \int_{-1}^{1} \chi(t) y(t)\, dt = \int_{-1}^{1} y(t) \chi(t)\, dt = (y , \chi)$$

2. $(\chi , a y_1 + b y_2) = a(\chi , y_1) + b(\chi , y_2)$

$$(\chi, ay_1 + by_2) = \int_{-1}^{1} \chi(t) \, (ay_1(t) + by_2(t)) \, dt = a \int_{-1}^{1} \chi(t) y_1(t) \, dt + b \int_{-1}^{1} \chi(t) y_2(t) \, dt$$

$$= a(\chi, y_1) + b(\chi, y_2)$$

3. $(\chi, \chi) \geq 0$, where equality holds if and only if χ is the zero vector.

$$(\chi, \chi) = \int_{-1}^{1} \chi(t) \chi t \, dt = \int_{-1}^{1} \chi^2(t) \, dt \geq 0$$

Equality holds here only if $\chi(t) = 0$ for $-1 \leq t \leq 1$, which is the zero vector.

P5.7 **Two vectors from the vector space described in the previous problem (polynomials defined on the interval [-1, 1]) are $1 + t$ and $1 - t$. Find an orthogonal set of vectors based on these two vectors.**

Step 1.

$$v_1 = y_1 = 1 + t$$

Step 2.

$$v_2 = y_2 - \frac{(v_1, y_2)}{(v_1, v_1)} v_1$$

where

$$(v_1, y_2) = \int_{-1}^{1} (1 + t)(1 - t) \, dt = \left(t - \frac{t^3}{3} \right) \Bigg|_{-1}^{1} = \left(\frac{2}{3} \right) - \left(-\frac{2}{3} \right) = \frac{4}{3}$$

$$(v_1, v_1) = \int_{-1}^{1} (1 + t)^2 \, dt = \frac{(1 + t)^3}{3} \Bigg|_{-1}^{1} = \left(\frac{8}{3} \right) - (0) = \frac{8}{3}.$$

Therefore

$$v_2 = (1 - t) - \frac{4/3}{8/3}(1 + t) = \frac{1}{2} - \frac{3}{2}t.$$

P5.8 Expand $x = \begin{bmatrix} 6 & 9 & 9 \end{bmatrix}^T$ **in terms of the following basis set.**

$$v_1 = \begin{bmatrix} 1 \\ 1 \\ 1 \end{bmatrix} \qquad v_2 = \begin{bmatrix} 1 \\ 2 \\ 3 \end{bmatrix} \qquad v_3 = \begin{bmatrix} 1 \\ 3 \\ 2 \end{bmatrix}$$

The first step is to calculate the reciprocal basis vectors.

$$B = \begin{bmatrix} 1 & 1 & 1 \\ 1 & 2 & 3 \\ 1 & 3 & 2 \end{bmatrix} \qquad B^{-1} = \begin{bmatrix} \dfrac{5}{3} & -\dfrac{1}{3} & -\dfrac{1}{3} \\ -\dfrac{1}{3} & -\dfrac{1}{3} & \dfrac{2}{3} \\ -\dfrac{1}{3} & \dfrac{2}{3} & -\dfrac{1}{3} \end{bmatrix}$$

Therefore taking the rows of B^{-1},

$$r_1 = \begin{bmatrix} 5/3 \\ -1/3 \\ -1/3 \end{bmatrix} \qquad r_2 = \begin{bmatrix} -1/3 \\ -1/3 \\ 2/3 \end{bmatrix} \qquad r_3 = \begin{bmatrix} -1/3 \\ 2/3 \\ -1/3 \end{bmatrix}.$$

The coefficients in the expansion are calculated

$$x_1^v = r_1^T x = \begin{bmatrix} \dfrac{5}{3} & \dfrac{-1}{3} & \dfrac{-1}{3} \end{bmatrix} \begin{bmatrix} 6 \\ 9 \\ 9 \end{bmatrix} = 4$$

$$x_2^v = r_2^T x = \begin{bmatrix} \dfrac{-1}{3} & \dfrac{-1}{3} & \dfrac{2}{3} \end{bmatrix} \begin{bmatrix} 6 \\ 9 \\ 9 \end{bmatrix} = 1$$

$$x_3^v = r_3^T x = \begin{bmatrix} \dfrac{-1}{3} & \dfrac{2}{3} & \dfrac{-1}{3} \end{bmatrix} \begin{bmatrix} 6 \\ 9 \\ 9 \end{bmatrix} = 1,$$

and the expansion is written

$$\mathbf{x} = x_1^v \mathbf{v}_1 + x_2^v \mathbf{v}_2 + x_3^v \mathbf{v}_3 = 4 \begin{bmatrix} 1 \\ 1 \\ 1 \end{bmatrix} + 1 \begin{bmatrix} 1 \\ 2 \\ 3 \end{bmatrix} + 1 \begin{bmatrix} 1 \\ 3 \\ 2 \end{bmatrix}.$$

We can represent the process in matrix form:

$$\mathbf{x}^v = \mathbf{B}^{-1} \mathbf{x} = \begin{bmatrix} \dfrac{5}{3} & -\dfrac{1}{3} & -\dfrac{1}{3} \\[2mm] -\dfrac{1}{3} & -\dfrac{1}{3} & \dfrac{2}{3} \\[2mm] -\dfrac{1}{3} & \dfrac{2}{3} & -\dfrac{1}{3} \end{bmatrix} \begin{bmatrix} 6 \\ 9 \\ 9 \end{bmatrix} = \begin{bmatrix} 4 \\ 1 \\ 1 \end{bmatrix}.$$

Recall that both $\mathbf{x}^v$ and $\mathbf{x}$ are representations of the same vector, but are expanded in terms of different basis sets. (It is assumed that $\mathbf{x}$ uses the standard basis set, unless otherwise indicated.)

5

Epilogue

This chapter has presented a few of the basic concepts of vector spaces, material that is critical to the understanding of how neural networks work. This subject of vector spaces is very large, and we have made no attempt to cover all its aspects. Instead, we have presented those concepts that we feel are most relevant to neural networks. The topics covered here will be revisited in almost every chapter that follows.

The next chapter will continue our investigation of the topics of linear algebra most relevant to neural networks. There we will concentrate on linear transformations and matrices.

Further Reading

[Brog91]   W. L. Brogan, *Modern Control Theory*, 3rd Ed., Englewood Cliffs, NJ: Prentice-Hall, 1991.

This is a well-written book on the subject of linear systems. The first half of the book is devoted to linear algebra. It also has good sections on the solution of linear differential equations and the stability of linear and nonlinear systems. It has many worked problems.

[Stra76]   G. Strang, *Linear Algebra and Its Applications*, New York: Academic Press, 1980.

Strang has written a good basic text on linear algebra. Many applications of linear algebra are integrated into the text.

5

Exercises

E5.1 Consider again the perceptron described in Problem P5.1. If $b \neq 0$, show that the decision boundary is not a vector space.

E5.2 What is the dimension of the vector space described in Problem P5.1?

E5.3 Consider the set of all continuous functions that satisfy the condition $f(0) = 0$. Show that this is a vector space.

E5.4 Show that the set of 2×2 matrices is a vector space.

E5.5 Which of the following sets of vectors are independent? Find the dimension of the vector space spanned by each set. (Verify your answers to parts (i) and (iv) using the MATLAB function **rank**.)

```
» 2 + 2
ans =
    4
```

i. $\begin{bmatrix} 1 \\ 2 \\ 3 \end{bmatrix} \quad \begin{bmatrix} 1 \\ 0 \\ 1 \end{bmatrix} \quad \begin{bmatrix} 1 \\ 2 \\ 1 \end{bmatrix}$

ii. $\sin t \qquad \cos t \qquad \cos(2t)$

iii. $1 + t \qquad 1 - t$

iv. $\begin{bmatrix} 1 \\ 2 \\ 2 \\ 1 \end{bmatrix} \quad \begin{bmatrix} 1 \\ 0 \\ 0 \\ 1 \end{bmatrix} \quad \begin{bmatrix} 3 \\ 4 \\ 4 \\ 3 \end{bmatrix}$

E5.6 Recall the apple and orange pattern recognition problem of Chapter 3. Find the angles between each of the prototype patterns (*orange* and *apple*) and the test input pattern (*oblong orange*). Verify that the angles make intuitive sense.

$$\mathbf{p}_1 = \begin{bmatrix} 1 \\ -1 \\ -1 \end{bmatrix} (orange) \qquad \mathbf{p}_2 = \begin{bmatrix} 1 \\ 1 \\ -1 \end{bmatrix} (apple) \qquad \mathbf{p} = \begin{bmatrix} -1 \\ -1 \\ -1 \end{bmatrix}$$

E5.7 Using the following basis vectors, find an orthogonal set using Gram-Schmidt orthogonalization. (Check your answer using MATLAB.)

$$\mathbf{y}_1 = \begin{bmatrix} 1 \\ 0 \\ 0 \end{bmatrix} \qquad \mathbf{y}_2 = \begin{bmatrix} 1 \\ 1 \\ 0 \end{bmatrix} \qquad \mathbf{y}_3 = \begin{bmatrix} 1 \\ 1 \\ 1 \end{bmatrix}$$

E5.8 Consider the vector space of all piecewise continuous functions on the interval [0, 1]. The set $\{f_1, f_2, f_3\}$, which is defined in Figure E15.1, contains three vectors from this vector space.

    i. Show that this set is linearly independent.

    ii. Generate an orthogonal set using the Gram-Schmidt procedure. The inner product is defined to be

$$(f, g) = \int_0^1 f(t) g(t)\, dt.$$

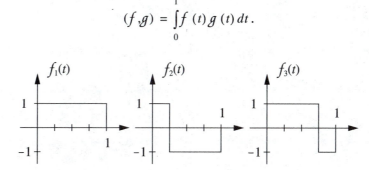

Figure E15.1 Basis Set for Problem E5.8

E5.9 Expand $\mathbf{x} = \begin{bmatrix} 1 & 2 & 2 \end{bmatrix}^T$ in terms of the following basis set. (Verify your answer using MATLAB.)

$$\mathbf{v}_1 = \begin{bmatrix} -1 \\ 1 \\ 0 \end{bmatrix} \qquad \mathbf{v}_2 = \begin{bmatrix} 1 \\ 1 \\ -2 \end{bmatrix} \qquad \mathbf{v}_3 = \begin{bmatrix} 1 \\ 1 \\ 0 \end{bmatrix}$$

E5.10 Find the value of a that makes $\|x - ay\|$ a minimum. (Use $\|x\| = (x, x)^{1/2}$.) Show that for this value of a the vector $z = x - ay$ is orthogonal to y and that

$$\|x - ay\|^2 + \|ay\|^2 = \|x\|^2 .$$

(The vector ay is the projection of x on y.) Draw a diagram for the case where x and y are two-dimensional. Explain how this concept is related to Gram-Schmidt orthogonalization.

6 Linear Transformations for Neural Networks

6

Objectives

This chapter will continue the work of Chapter 5 in laying out the mathematical foundations for our analysis of neural networks. In Chapter 5 we reviewed vector spaces; in this chapter we investigate linear transformations as they apply to neural networks.

As we have seen in previous chapters, the multiplication of an input vector by a weight matrix is one of the key operations that is performed by neural networks. This operation is an example of a linear transformation. We want to investigate general linear transformations and determine their fundamental characteristics. The concepts covered in this chapter, such as eigenvalues, eigenvectors and change of basis, will be critical to our understanding of such key neural network topics as performance learning (including the Widrow-Hoff rule and backpropagation) and Hopfield network convergence.

Theory and Examples

Recall the Hopfield network that was discussed in Chapter 3. (See Figure 6.1.) The output of the network is updated synchronously according to the equation

$$\mathbf{a}(t+1) = satlin(\mathbf{W}\mathbf{a}(t) + \mathbf{b}).\tag{6.1}$$

Notice that at each iteration the output of the network is again multiplied by the weight matrix **W**. What is the effect of this repeated operation? Can we determine whether or not the output of the network will converge to some steady state value, go to infinity, or oscillate? In this chapter we will lay the foundation for answering these questions, along with many other questions about neural networks discussed in this book.

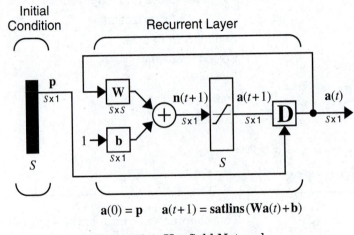

$$\mathbf{a}(0) = \mathbf{p} \qquad \mathbf{a}(t+1) = \mathbf{satlins}(\mathbf{W}\mathbf{a}(t)+\mathbf{b})$$

Figure 6.1 Hopfield Network

Linear Transformations

We begin with some general definitions.

Transformation   A *transformation* consists of three parts:

1.   a set of elements $X = \{x_i\}$, called the domain,

2.   a set of elements $Y = \{y_i\}$, called the range, and

3.   a rule relating each $x_i \in X$ to an element $y_i \in Y$.

Linear Transformation

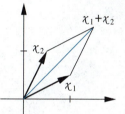

A transformation $\mathcal{A}$ is *linear* if:

1. for all $\chi_1, \chi_2 \in X$, $\mathcal{A}(\chi_1 + \chi_2) = \mathcal{A}(\chi_1) + \mathcal{A}(\chi_2)$,

2. for all $\chi \in X$, $a \in R$, $\mathcal{A}(a\chi) = a\mathcal{A}(\chi)$.

Consider, for example, the transformation obtained by rotating vectors in $\Re^2$ by an angle θ, as shown in the figure to the left. The next two figures illustrate that property 1 is satisfied for rotation. They show that if you want to rotate a sum of two vectors, you can rotate each vector first and then sum them. The fourth figure illustrates property 2. If you want to rotate a scaled vector, you can rotate it first and then scale it. Therefore rotation is a linear operation.

Matrix Representations

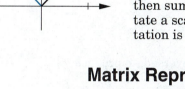

As we mentioned at the beginning of this chapter, matrix multiplication is an example of a linear transformation. We can also show that any linear transformation between two finite-dimensional vector spaces can be represented by a matrix (just as in the last chapter we showed that any general vector in a finite-dimensional vector space can be represented by a column of numbers). To show this we will use most of the concepts covered in the previous chapter.

Let $\{v_1, v_2, \ldots, v_n\}$ be a basis for vector space X, and let $\{u_1, u_2, \ldots, u_m\}$ be a basis for vector space Y. This means that for any two vectors $\chi \in X$ and $y \in Y$

$$\chi = \sum_{i=1}^{n} x_i v_i \text{ and } y = \sum_{i=1}^{m} y_i u_i. \tag{6.2}$$

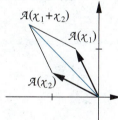

Let $\mathcal{A}$ be a linear transformation with domain X and range Y ($\mathcal{A}: X \to Y$). Then

$$\mathcal{A}(\chi) = y \tag{6.3}$$

can be written

$$\mathcal{A}\left(\sum_{j=1}^{n} x_j v_j\right) = \sum_{i=1}^{m} y_i u_i. \tag{6.4}$$

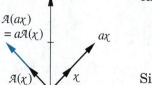

Since $\mathcal{A}$ is a linear operator, Eq. (6.4) can be written

$$\sum_{j=1}^{n} x_j \mathcal{A}(v_j) = \sum_{i=1}^{m} y_i u_i. \tag{6.5}$$

6

Since the vectors $\mathcal{A}\,(v_j)$ are elements of Y, they can be written as linear combinations of the basis vectors for Y:

$$\mathcal{A}\,(v_j) \;=\; \sum_{i=1}^{m} a_{ij} u_i .$$

(6.6)

(Note that the notation used for the coefficients of this expansion, a_{ij}, was not chosen by accident.) If we substitute Eq. (6.6) into Eq. (6.5) we obtain

$$\sum_{j=1}^{n} x_j \sum_{i=1}^{m} a_{ij} u_i \;=\; \sum_{i=1}^{m} y_i u_i .$$

(6.7)

The order of the summations can be reversed, to produce

$$\sum_{i=1}^{m} u_i \sum_{j=1}^{n} a_{ij} x_j \;=\; \sum_{i=1}^{m} y_i u_i .$$

(6.8)

This equation can be rearranged, to obtain

$$\sum_{i=1}^{m} u_i \left(\sum_{j=1}^{n} a_{ij} x_j - y_i \right) \;=\; 0 .$$

(6.9)

Recall that since the u_i form a basis set they must be independent. This means that each coefficient that multiplies u_i in Eq. (6.9) must be identically zero (see Eq. (5.4)), therefore

$$\sum_{j=1}^{n} a_{ij} x_j \;=\; y_i .$$

(6.10)

This is just matrix multiplication, as in

$$\begin{bmatrix} a_{11} & a_{12} & \cdots & a_{1n} \\ a_{21} & a_{22} & \cdots & a_{2n} \\ \vdots & \vdots & & \vdots \\ a_{m1} & a_{m2} & \cdots & a_{mn} \end{bmatrix} \begin{bmatrix} x_1 \\ x_2 \\ \vdots \\ x_n \end{bmatrix} = \begin{bmatrix} y_1 \\ y_2 \\ \vdots \\ y_m \end{bmatrix}$$

(6.11)

We can summarize these results: *For any linear transformation between two finite-dimensional vector spaces there is a matrix representation. When we multiply the matrix times the vector expansion for the domain vector x, we obtain the vector expansion for the transformed vector y.*

Keep in mind that the matrix representation is not unique (just as the representation of a general vector by a column of numbers is not unique — see

Chapter 5). If we change the basis set for the domain or for the range, the matrix representation will also change. We will use this fact to our advantage in later chapters.

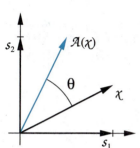

As an example of a matrix representation, consider the rotation transformation. Let's find a matrix representation for that transformation. The key step is given in Eq. (6.6). We must transform each basis vector for the domain and then expand it in terms of the basis vectors of the range. In this example the domain and the range are the same ($X = Y = \Re^2$), so to keep things simple we will use the standard basis for both ($u_i = v_i = s_i$), as shown in the adjacent figure.

The first step is to transform the first basis vector and expand the resulting transformed vector in terms of the basis vectors. If we rotate s_1 counterclockwise by the angle θ we obtain

$$\mathcal{A}(s_1) = \cos(\theta)s_1 + \sin(\theta)s_2 = \sum_{i=1}^{2} a_{i1}s_i = a_{11}s_1 + a_{21}s_2, \qquad (6.12)$$

as can be seen in the middle left figure. The two coefficients in this expansion make up the first column of the matrix representation.

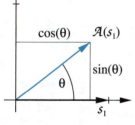

The next step is to transform the second basis vector. If we rotate s_2 counterclockwise by the angle θ we obtain

$$\mathcal{A}(s_2) = -\sin(\theta)s_1 + \cos(\theta)s_2 = \sum_{i=1}^{2} a_{i2}s_i = a_{12}s_1 + a_{22}s_2, \qquad (6.13)$$

as can be seen in the lower left figure. From this expansion we obtain the second column of the matrix representation. The complete matrix representation is thus given by

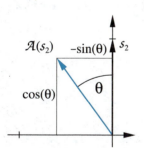

$$\mathbf{A} = \begin{bmatrix} \cos(\theta) & -\sin(\theta) \\ \sin(\theta) & \cos(\theta) \end{bmatrix}. \qquad (6.14)$$

Verify for yourself that when you multiply a vector by the matrix of Eq. (6.14), the vector is rotated by an angle θ.

In summary, to obtain the matrix representation of a transformation we use Eq. (6.6). We transform each basis vector for the domain and expand it in terms of the basis vectors of the range. The coefficients of each expansion produce one column of the matrix.

To graphically investigate the process of creating a matrix representation, use the Neural Network Design Demonstration Linear Transformations *(**nnd6lt**).*

6

Change of Basis

We notice from the previous section that the matrix representation of a linear transformation is not unique. The representation will depend on what basis sets are used for the domain and the range of the transformation. In this section we will illustrate exactly how a matrix representation changes as the basis sets are changed.

Consider a linear transformation $A : X \to Y$. Let $\{v_1, v_2, \ldots, v_n\}$ be a basis for vector space X, and let $\{u_1, u_2, \ldots, u_m\}$ be a basis for vector space Y. Therefore, any vector $\chi \in X$ can be written

$$\chi = \sum_{i=1}^{n} x_i v_i, \tag{6.15}$$

and any vector $y \in Y$ can be written

$$y = \sum_{i=1}^{m} y_i u_i. \tag{6.16}$$

So if

$$A(\chi) = y \tag{6.17}$$

the matrix representation will be

$$
\begin{bmatrix}
a_{11} & a_{12} & \cdots & a_{1n} \\
a_{21} & a_{22} & \cdots & a_{2n} \\
\vdots & \vdots & & \vdots \\
a_{m1} & a_{m2} & \cdots & a_{mn}
\end{bmatrix}
\begin{bmatrix}
x_1 \\
x_2 \\
\vdots \\
x_n
\end{bmatrix}
=
\begin{bmatrix}
y_1 \\
y_2 \\
\vdots \\
y_m
\end{bmatrix}, \tag{6.18}
$$

or

$$\mathbf{Ax} = \mathbf{y}. \tag{6.19}$$

Now suppose that we use different basis sets for X and Y. Let $\{t_1, t_2, \ldots, t_n\}$ be the new basis for X, and let $\{w_1, w_2, \ldots, w_m\}$ be the new basis for Y. With the new basis sets, the vector $\chi \in X$ is written

$$\chi = \sum_{i=1}^{n} x'_i t_i, \tag{6.20}$$

and the vector $y \in Y$ is written

$$y = \sum_{i=1}^{m} y'_i w_i. \tag{6.21}$$

This produces a new matrix representation:

$$\begin{bmatrix} a'_{11} & a'_{12} & \cdots & a'_{1n} \\ a'_{21} & a'_{22} & \cdots & a'_{2n} \\ \vdots & \vdots & & \vdots \\ a'_{m1} & a'_{m2} & \cdots & a'_{mn} \end{bmatrix} \begin{bmatrix} x'_1 \\ x'_2 \\ \vdots \\ x'_n \end{bmatrix} = \begin{bmatrix} y'_1 \\ y'_2 \\ \vdots \\ y'_m \end{bmatrix}, \tag{6.22}$$

or

$$\mathbf{A'x'} = \mathbf{y'}. \tag{6.23}$$

What is the relationship between $\mathbf{A}$ and $\mathbf{A'}$? To find out, we need to find the relationship between the two basis sets. First, since each t_i is an element of X, they can be expanded in terms of the original basis for X:

$$t_i = \sum_{j=1}^{n} t_{ji} v_j. \tag{6.24}$$

Next, since each w_i is an element of Y, they can be expanded in terms of the original basis for Y:

$$w_i = \sum_{j=1}^{m} w_{ji} u_j. \tag{6.25}$$

Therefore, the basis vectors can be written as columns of numbers:

$$\mathbf{t}_i = \begin{bmatrix} t_{1i} \\ t_{2i} \\ \vdots \\ t_{ni} \end{bmatrix} \qquad \mathbf{w}_i = \begin{bmatrix} w_{1i} \\ w_{2i} \\ \vdots \\ w_{mi} \end{bmatrix}. \tag{6.26}$$

Define a matrix whose columns are the $\mathbf{t}_i$:

$$\mathbf{B}_t = \begin{bmatrix} \mathbf{t}_1 & \mathbf{t}_2 & \cdots & \mathbf{t}_n \end{bmatrix}. \tag{6.27}$$

Then we can write Eq. (6.20) in matrix form:

$$\mathbf{x} = x'_1 \mathbf{t}_1 + x'_2 \mathbf{t}_2 + \cdots + x'_n \mathbf{t}_n = \mathbf{B}_t \mathbf{x'}. \tag{6.28}$$

6

This equation demonstrates the relationships between the two different representations for the vector χ. (Note that this is effectively the same as Eq. (5.43). You may want to revisit our discussion of reciprocal basis vectors in Chapter 5.)

Now define a matrix whose columns are the $\mathbf{w}_i$:

$$\mathbf{B}_w = \begin{bmatrix} \mathbf{w}_1 & \mathbf{w}_2 & \cdots & \mathbf{w}_m \end{bmatrix}. \tag{6.29}$$

This allows us to write Eq. (6.21) in matrix form,

$$\mathbf{y} = \mathbf{B}_w \mathbf{y}', \tag{6.30}$$

which then demonstrates the relationships between the two different representations for the vector y.

Now substitute Eq. (6.28) and Eq. (6.30) into Eq. (6.19):

$$\mathbf{A}\mathbf{B}_t \mathbf{x}' = \mathbf{B}_w \mathbf{y}'. \tag{6.31}$$

If we multiply both sides of this equation by $\mathbf{B}_w^{-1}$ we obtain

$$[\mathbf{B}_w^{-1} \mathbf{A}\mathbf{B}_t] \mathbf{x}' = \mathbf{y}'. \tag{6.32}$$

A comparison of Eq. (6.32) and Eq. (6.23) yields the following operation for a *change of basis*:

Change of Basis

$$\mathbf{A}' = [\mathbf{B}_w^{-1} \mathbf{A}\mathbf{B}_t]. \tag{6.33}$$

Similarity Transform

This key result, which describes the relationship between any two matrix representations of a given linear transformation, is called a *similarity transform* [Brog91]. It will be of great use to us in later chapters. It turns out that with the right choice of basis vectors we can obtain a matrix representation that reveals the key characteristics of the linear transformation it represents. This will be discussed in the next section.

As an example of changing basis sets, let's revisit the vector rotation example of the previous section. In that section a matrix representation was developed using the standard basis set $\{s_1, s_2\}$. Now let's find a new representation using the basis $\{t_1, t_2\}$, which is shown in the adjacent figure. (Note that in this example the same basis set is used for both the domain and the range.)

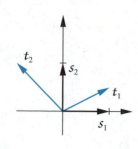

The first step is to expand t_1 and t_2 in terms of the standard basis set, as in Eq. (6.24) and Eq. (6.25). By inspection of the adjacent figure we find:

$$t_1 = s_1 + 0.5s_2, \tag{6.34}$$

$$t_2 = -s_1 + s_2. \tag{6.35}$$

Therefore we can write

$$\mathbf{t}_1 = \begin{bmatrix} 1 \\ 0.5 \end{bmatrix} \qquad \mathbf{t}_2 = \begin{bmatrix} -1 \\ 1 \end{bmatrix}. \tag{6.36}$$

Now we can form the matrix

$$\mathbf{B}_t = \begin{bmatrix} \mathbf{t}_1 & \mathbf{t}_2 \end{bmatrix} = \begin{bmatrix} 1 & -1 \\ 0.5 & 1 \end{bmatrix}, \tag{6.37}$$

and, because we are using the same basis set for both the domain and the range of the transformation,

$$\mathbf{B}_w = \mathbf{B}_t = \begin{bmatrix} 1 & -1 \\ 0.5 & 1 \end{bmatrix}. \tag{6.38}$$

We can now compute the new matrix representation from Eq. (6.33):

$$\mathbf{A}' = [\mathbf{B}_w^{-1} \mathbf{A} \mathbf{B}_t] = \begin{bmatrix} 2/3 & 2/3 \\ -1/3 & 2/3 \end{bmatrix} \begin{bmatrix} \cos\theta & -\sin\theta \\ \sin\theta & \cos\theta \end{bmatrix} \begin{bmatrix} 1 & -1 \\ 0.5 & 1 \end{bmatrix}$$

$$= \begin{bmatrix} 1/3\sin\theta + \cos\theta & -4/3\sin\theta \\ \frac{5}{6}\sin\theta & -1/3\sin\theta + \cos\theta \end{bmatrix}. \tag{6.39}$$

Take, for example, the case where $\theta = 30°$.

$$\mathbf{A}' = \begin{bmatrix} 1.033 & -0.667 \\ 0.417 & 0.699 \end{bmatrix}, \tag{6.40}$$

and

$$\mathbf{A} = \begin{bmatrix} 0.866 & -0.5 \\ 0.5 & 0.866 \end{bmatrix}. \tag{6.41}$$

To check that these matrices are correct, let's try a test vector

$$\mathbf{x} = \begin{bmatrix} 1 \\ 0.5 \end{bmatrix}, \text{ which corresponds to } \mathbf{x}' = \begin{bmatrix} 1 \\ 0 \end{bmatrix}. \tag{6.42}$$

(Note that the vector represented by $\mathbf{x}$ and $\mathbf{x}'$ is t_1, a member of the second basis set.) The transformed test vector would be

$$\mathbf{y} = \mathbf{Ax} = \begin{bmatrix} 0.866 & -0.5 \\ 0.5 & 0.866 \end{bmatrix} \begin{bmatrix} 1 \\ 0.5 \end{bmatrix} = \begin{bmatrix} 0.616 \\ 0.933 \end{bmatrix}, \tag{6.43}$$

which should correspond to

$$\mathbf{y}' = \mathbf{A}'\mathbf{x}' = \begin{bmatrix} 1.033 & -0.667 \\ 0.416 & 0.699 \end{bmatrix} \begin{bmatrix} 1 \\ 0 \end{bmatrix} = \begin{bmatrix} 1.033 \\ 0.416 \end{bmatrix}. \tag{6.44}$$

How can we test to see if $\mathbf{y}'$ does correspond to $\mathbf{y}$? Both should be representations of the same vector, y, in terms of two different basis sets; $\mathbf{y}$ uses the basis $\{s_1, s_2\}$ and $\mathbf{y}'$ uses the basis $\{t_1, t_2\}$. In Chapter 5 we used the reciprocal basis vectors to transform from one representation to another (see Eq. (5.43)). Using that concept we have

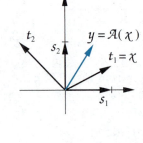

$$\mathbf{y}' = \mathbf{B}^{-1}\mathbf{y} = \begin{bmatrix} 1 & -1 \\ 0.5 & 1 \end{bmatrix}^{-1} \begin{bmatrix} 0.616 \\ 0.933 \end{bmatrix} = \begin{bmatrix} 2/3 & 2/3 \\ -1/3 & 2/3 \end{bmatrix} \begin{bmatrix} 0.616 \\ 0.933 \end{bmatrix} = \begin{bmatrix} 1.033 \\ 0.416 \end{bmatrix}, \tag{6.45}$$

which verifies our previous result. The vectors are displayed in the figure to the left. Verify graphically that the two representations, $\mathbf{y}$ and $\mathbf{y}'$, given by Eq. (6.43) and Eq. (6.44), are reasonable.

Eigenvalues and Eigenvectors

In this final section we want to discuss two key properties of linear transformations: eigenvalues and eigenvectors. Knowledge of these properties will allow us to answer some key questions about neural network performance, such as the question we posed at the beginning of this chapter, concerning the stability of Hopfield networks.

Eigenvalues
Eigenvectors
Let's first define what we mean by *eigenvalues* and *eigenvectors*. Consider a linear transformation $\mathcal{A}:X \to X$. (The domain is the same as the range.) Those vectors $z \in X$ that are not equal to zero and those scalars λ that satisfy

$$\mathcal{A}(z) = \lambda z \tag{6.46}$$

are called eigenvectors (z) and eigenvalues (λ), respectively. Notice that the term eigenvector is a little misleading, since it is not really a vector but a vector space, since if z satisfies Eq. (6.46), then az will also satisfy it.

Therefore an eigenvector of a given transformation represents a direction, such that any vector in that direction, when transformed, will continue to point in the same direction, but will be scaled by the eigenvalue. As an ex-

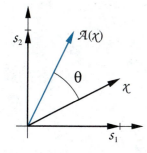

ample, consider again the rotation example used in the previous sections. Is there any vector that, when rotated by 30°, continues to point in the same direction? No; this is a case where there are no real eigenvalues. (If we allow complex scalars, then two eigenvalues exist, as we will see later.)

How can we compute the eigenvalues and eigenvectors? Suppose that a basis has been chosen for the n-dimensional vector space X. Then the matrix representation for Eq. (6.46) can be written

$$\mathbf{A}\mathbf{z} = \lambda\mathbf{z}, \tag{6.47}$$

or

$$[\mathbf{A} - \lambda\mathbf{I}]\,\mathbf{z} = \mathbf{0}. \tag{6.48}$$

This means that the columns of $[\mathbf{A} - \lambda\mathbf{I}]$ are dependent, and therefore the determinant of this matrix must be zero:

$$|[\mathbf{A} - \lambda\mathbf{I}]| = 0. \tag{6.49}$$

This determinant is an nth-order polynomial. Therefore Eq. (6.49) always has n roots, some of which may be complex and some of which may be repeated.

As an example, let's revisit the rotation example. If we use the standard basis set, the matrix of the transformation is

$$\mathbf{A} = \begin{bmatrix} \cos\theta & -\sin\theta \\ \sin\theta & \cos\theta \end{bmatrix}. \tag{6.50}$$

We can then write Eq. (6.49) as

$$\left\| \begin{bmatrix} \cos\theta - \lambda & -\sin\theta \\ \sin\theta & \cos\theta - \lambda \end{bmatrix} \right\| = 0 , \tag{6.51}$$

or

$$\lambda^2 - 2\lambda\cos\theta + ((\cos\theta)^2 + (\sin\theta)^2) = \lambda^2 - 2\lambda\cos\theta + 1 = 0. \tag{6.52}$$

The roots of this equation are

$$\lambda_1 = \cos\theta + j\sin\theta \qquad \lambda_2 = \cos\theta - j\sin\theta. \tag{6.53}$$

Therefore, as we predicted, this transformation has no real eigenvalues (if $\sin\theta \neq 0$). This means that when any real vector is transformed, it will point in a new direction.

Consider another matrix:

$$\mathbf{A} = \begin{bmatrix} -1 & 1 \\ 0 & -2 \end{bmatrix}. \qquad (6.54)$$

To find the eigenvalues we must solve

$$\left| \begin{bmatrix} -1-\lambda & 1 \\ 0 & -2-\lambda \end{bmatrix} \right| = 0, \qquad (6.55)$$

or

$$\lambda^2 + 3\lambda + 2 = (\lambda+1)(\lambda+2) = 0, \qquad (6.56)$$

and the eigenvalues are

$$\lambda_1 = -1 \qquad \lambda_2 = -2. \qquad (6.57)$$

To find the eigenvectors we must solve Eq. (6.48), which in this example becomes

$$\begin{bmatrix} -1-\lambda & 1 \\ 0 & -2-\lambda \end{bmatrix} \mathbf{z} = \begin{bmatrix} 0 \\ 0 \end{bmatrix}. \qquad (6.58)$$

We will solve this equation twice, once using λ_1 and once using λ_2. Beginning with λ_1 we have

$$\begin{bmatrix} 0 & 1 \\ 0 & -1 \end{bmatrix} \mathbf{z}_1 = \begin{bmatrix} 0 & 1 \\ 0 & -1 \end{bmatrix} \begin{bmatrix} z_{11} \\ z_{21} \end{bmatrix} = \begin{bmatrix} 0 \\ 0 \end{bmatrix} \qquad (6.59)$$

or

$$z_{21} = 0, \text{ no constraint on } z_{11}. \qquad (6.60)$$

Therefore the first eigenvector will be

$$\mathbf{z}_1 = \begin{bmatrix} 1 \\ 0 \end{bmatrix}, \qquad (6.61)$$

or any scalar multiple. For the second eigenvector we use λ_2:

$$\begin{bmatrix} 1 & 1 \\ 0 & 0 \end{bmatrix} \mathbf{z}_2 = \begin{bmatrix} 1 & 1 \\ 0 & 0 \end{bmatrix} \begin{bmatrix} z_{12} \\ z_{22} \end{bmatrix} = \begin{bmatrix} 0 \\ 0 \end{bmatrix}, \tag{6.62}$$

or

$$z_{22} = -z_{12}. \tag{6.63}$$

Therefore the second eigenvector will be

$$\mathbf{z}_2 = \begin{bmatrix} 1 \\ -1 \end{bmatrix}, \tag{6.64}$$

or any scalar multiple.

To verify our results we consider the following:

$$\mathbf{A}\mathbf{z}_1 = \begin{bmatrix} -1 & 1 \\ 0 & -2 \end{bmatrix} \begin{bmatrix} 1 \\ 0 \end{bmatrix} = \begin{bmatrix} -1 \\ 0 \end{bmatrix} = (-1) \begin{bmatrix} 1 \\ 0 \end{bmatrix} = \lambda_1 \mathbf{z}_1, \tag{6.65}$$

$$\mathbf{A}\mathbf{z}_2 = \begin{bmatrix} -1 & 1 \\ 0 & -2 \end{bmatrix} \begin{bmatrix} 1 \\ -1 \end{bmatrix} = \begin{bmatrix} -2 \\ 2 \end{bmatrix} = (-2) \begin{bmatrix} 1 \\ -1 \end{bmatrix} = \lambda_2 \mathbf{z}_2. \tag{6.66}$$

*To test your understanding of eigenvectors, use the Neural Network Design Demonstration Eigenvector Game (*nnd6eg*).*

Diagonalization

Whenever we have n distinct eigenvalues we are guaranteed that we can find n independent eigenvectors [Brog91]. Therefore the eigenvectors make up a basis set for the vector space of the transformation. Let's find the matrix of the previous transformation (Eq. (6.54)) using the eigenvectors as the basis vectors. From Eq. (6.33) we have

$$\mathbf{A}' = [\mathbf{B}^{-1}\mathbf{A}\mathbf{B}] = \begin{bmatrix} 1 & 1 \\ 0 & -1 \end{bmatrix} \begin{bmatrix} -1 & 1 \\ 0 & -2 \end{bmatrix} \begin{bmatrix} 1 & 1 \\ 0 & -1 \end{bmatrix} = \begin{bmatrix} -1 & 0 \\ 0 & -2 \end{bmatrix}. \tag{6.67}$$

Note that this is a diagonal matrix, with the eigenvalues on the diagonal. This is not a coincidence. Whenever we have distinct eigenvalues we can diagonalize the matrix representation by using the eigenvectors as the ba-

Diagonalization sis vectors. This *diagonalization* process is summarized in the following. Let

$$\mathbf{B} = \begin{bmatrix} \mathbf{z}_1 & \mathbf{z}_2 & \dots & \mathbf{z}_n \end{bmatrix}, \tag{6.68}$$

where $\{z_1, z_2, \ldots, z_n\}$ are the eigenvectors of a matrix $\mathbf{A}$. Then

$$[\mathbf{B}^{-1}\mathbf{A}\mathbf{B}] = \begin{bmatrix} \lambda_1 & 0 & \ldots & 0 \\ 0 & \lambda_2 & \ldots & 0 \\ \vdots & \vdots & & \vdots \\ 0 & 0 & \ldots & \lambda_n \end{bmatrix}, \tag{6.69}$$

where $\{\lambda_1, \lambda_2, \ldots, \lambda_n\}$ are the eigenvalues of the matrix $\mathbf{A}$.

This result will be very helpful as we analyze the performance of several neural networks in later chapters.

Summary of Results

Transformations

A *transformation* consists of three parts:

1. a set of elements $X = \{\chi_i\}$, called the domain,

2. a set of elements $Y = \{y_i\}$, called the range, and

3. a rule relating each $\chi_i \in X$ to an element $y_i \in Y$.

Linear Transformations

A transformation $\mathcal{A}$ is *linear* if:

1. for all $\chi_1, \chi_2 \in X$, $\mathcal{A}(\chi_1 + \chi_2) = \mathcal{A}(\chi_1) + \mathcal{A}(\chi_2)$,

2. for all $\chi \in X$, $a \in R$, $\mathcal{A}(a\chi) = a\mathcal{A}(\chi)$.

Matrix Representations

Let $\{v_1, v_2, \dots, v_n\}$ be a basis for vector space X, and let $\{u_1, u_2, \dots, u_m\}$ be a basis for vector space Y. Let $\mathcal{A}$ be a linear transformation with domain X and range Y:

$$\mathcal{A}(\chi) = y.$$

The coefficients of the matrix representation are obtained from

$$\mathcal{A}(v_j) = \sum_{i=1}^{m} a_{ij} u_i.$$

6

Change of Basis

$$\mathbf{B}_t = \left[\mathbf{t}_1\ \mathbf{t}_2\ \dots\ \mathbf{t}_n \right]$$

$$\mathbf{B}_w = \left[\mathbf{w}_1\ \mathbf{w}_2\ \dots\ \mathbf{w}_m \right]$$

$$\mathbf{A}' = [\mathbf{B}_w^{-1} \mathbf{A} \mathbf{B}_t]$$

Eigenvalues and Eigenvectors

$$\mathbf{A}\mathbf{z} = \lambda\mathbf{z}$$

$$|[\mathbf{A} - \lambda\mathbf{I}]| = 0$$

Diagonalization

$$\mathbf{B} = \begin{bmatrix} \mathbf{z}_1 & \mathbf{z}_2 & \dots & \mathbf{z}_n \end{bmatrix},$$

where $\{\mathbf{z}_1, \mathbf{z}_2, \dots, \mathbf{z}_n\}$ are the eigenvectors of a square matrix $\mathbf{A}$.

$$[\mathbf{B}^{-1}\mathbf{A}\mathbf{B}] = \begin{bmatrix} \lambda_1 & 0 & \dots & 0 \\ 0 & \lambda_2 & \dots & 0 \\ \vdots & \vdots & & \vdots \\ 0 & 0 & \dots & \lambda_n \end{bmatrix}$$

Solved Problems

P6.1 **Consider the single-layer network shown in Figure P6.1, which has a linear transfer function. Is the transformation from the input vector to the output vector a linear transformation?**

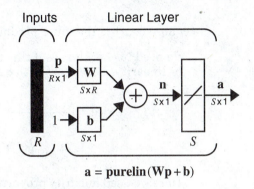

$$a = \text{purelin}(Wp + b)$$

Figure P6.1 Single-Neuron Perceptron

The network equation is

$$\mathbf{a} = \mathcal{A}(\mathbf{p}) = \mathbf{W}\mathbf{p} + \mathbf{b}.$$

In order for this transformation to be linear it must satisfy

1. $\mathcal{A}(\mathbf{p}_1 + \mathbf{p}_2) = \mathcal{A}(\mathbf{p}_1) + \mathcal{A}(\mathbf{p}_2)$,

2. $\mathcal{A}(a\mathbf{p}) = a\mathcal{A}(\mathbf{p})$.

Let's test condition 1 first.

$$\mathcal{A}(\mathbf{p}_1 + \mathbf{p}_2) = \mathbf{W}(\mathbf{p}_1 + \mathbf{p}_2) + \mathbf{b} = \mathbf{W}\mathbf{p}_1 + \mathbf{W}\mathbf{p}_2 + \mathbf{b}.$$

Compare this with

$$\mathcal{A}(\mathbf{p}_1) + \mathcal{A}(\mathbf{p}_2) = \mathbf{W}\mathbf{p}_1 + \mathbf{b} + \mathbf{W}\mathbf{p}_2 + \mathbf{b} = \mathbf{W}\mathbf{p}_1 + \mathbf{W}\mathbf{p}_2 + 2\mathbf{b}.$$

Clearly these two expressions will be equal only if $\mathbf{b} = \mathbf{0}$. Therefore this network performs a nonlinear transformation, even though it has a linear transfer function. This particular type of nonlinearity is called an affine transformation.

6

P6.2 We discussed projections in Chapter 5. Is a projection a linear transformation?

The projection of a vector χ onto a vector v is computed as

$$y = A(\chi) = \frac{(\chi, v)}{(v, v)} v ,$$

where (χ, v) is the inner product of χ with v.

We need to check to see if this transformation satisfies the two conditions for linearity. Let's start with condition 1:

$$A(\chi_1 + \chi_2) = \frac{(\chi_1 + \chi_2, v)}{(v, v)} v = \frac{(\chi_1, v) + (\chi_2, v)}{(v, v)} v = \frac{(\chi_1, v)}{(v, v)} v + \frac{(\chi_2, v)}{(v, v)} v$$

$$= A(\chi_1) + A(\chi_2) .$$

(Here we used linearity properties of inner products.) Checking condition 2:

$$A(a\chi) = \frac{(a\chi, v)}{(v, v)} v = \frac{a(\chi, v)}{(v, v)} v = a A(\chi) .$$

Therefore projection is a linear operation.

P6.3 Consider the transformation A created by reflecting a vector χ in $\mathfrak{R}^2$ about the line $x_1 + x_2 = 0$, as shown in Figure P6.2. Find the matrix of this transformation relative to the standard basis in $\mathfrak{R}^2$.

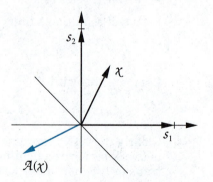

Figure P6.2 Reflection Transformation

The key to finding the matrix of a transformation is given in Eq. (6.6):

$$A(v_j) = \sum_{i=1}^{m} a_{ij}u_i.$$

We need to transform each basis vector of the domain and then expand the result in terms of the basis vectors for the range. Each time we do the expansion we get one column of the matrix representation. In this case the basis set for both the domain and the range is $\{s_1, s_2\}$. So let's transform s_1 first. If we reflect s_1 about the line $x_1 + x_2 = 0$, we find

$$A(s_1) = -s_2 = \sum_{i=1}^{2} a_{i1}s_i = a_{11}s_1 + a_{21}s_2 = 0s_1 + (-1)s_2$$

(as shown in the top left figure), which gives us the first column of the matrix. Next we transform s_2:

$$A(s_2) = -s_1 = \sum_{i=1}^{2} a_{i2}s_i = a_{12}s_1 + a_{22}s_2 = (-1)s_1 + 0s_2$$

(as shown in the second figure on the left), which gives us the second column of the matrix. The final result is

$$\begin{bmatrix} 0 & -1 \\ -1 & 0 \end{bmatrix}.$$

Let's test our result by transforming the vector $\mathbf{x} = \begin{bmatrix} 1 & 1 \end{bmatrix}^T$:

$$\mathbf{Ax} = \begin{bmatrix} 0 & -1 \\ -1 & 0 \end{bmatrix} \begin{bmatrix} 1 \\ 1 \end{bmatrix} = \begin{bmatrix} -1 \\ -1 \end{bmatrix}.$$

This is indeed the reflection of $\mathbf{x}$ about the line $x_1 + x_2 = 0$, as we can see in Figure P6.3.

$A(s_1) = -s_2$

$A(s_2) = -s_1$

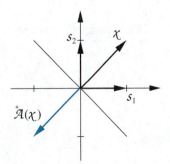

Figure P6.3 Test of Reflection Operation

6

(Can you guess the eigenvalues and eigenvectors of this transformation? Use the *Neural Network Design Demonstration Linear Transformations* (**nnd6lt**) to investigate this graphically. Compute the eigenvalues and eigenvectors, using the MATLAB function **eig**, and check your guess.)

P6.4 **Consider the space of complex numbers. Let this be the vector space** X**, and let the basis for** X **be** $\{1+j, 1-j\}$ **. Let** $\mathcal{A}: X \to X$ **be the conjugation operator (i.e.,** $\mathcal{A}(x) = x^*$**).**

    i. **Find the matrix of the transformation** $\mathcal{A}$ **relative to the basis set given above.**

    ii. **Find the eigenvalues and eigenvectors of the transformation.**

    iii. **Find the matrix representation for** $\mathcal{A}$ **relative to the eigenvectors as the basis vectors.**

i.   To find the matrix of the transformation, transform each of the basis vectors (by finding their conjugate):

$$\mathcal{A}(v_1) = \mathcal{A}(1+j) = 1-j = v_2 = a_{11}v_1 + a_{21}v_2 = 0v_1 + 1v_2,$$

$$\mathcal{A}(v_2) = \mathcal{A}(1-j) = 1+j = v_1 = a_{12}v_1 + a_{22}v_2 = 1v_1 + 0v_2.$$

This gives us the matrix representation

$$\mathbf{A} = \begin{bmatrix} 0 & 1 \\ 1 & 0 \end{bmatrix}.$$

ii.   To find the eigenvalues, we need to use Eq. (6.49):

$$|[\mathbf{A} - \lambda \mathbf{I}]| = \left\| \begin{bmatrix} -\lambda & 1 \\ 1 & -\lambda \end{bmatrix} \right\| = \lambda^2 - 1 = (\lambda - 1)(\lambda + 1) = 0.$$

So the eigenvalues are: $\lambda_1 = 1$, $\lambda_2 = -1$. To find the eigenvectors, use Eq. (6.48):

$$[\mathbf{A} - \lambda \mathbf{I}]\mathbf{z} = \begin{bmatrix} -\lambda & 1 \\ 1 & -\lambda \end{bmatrix} \mathbf{z} = \begin{bmatrix} 0 \\ 0 \end{bmatrix}.$$

For $\lambda = \lambda_1 = 1$ this gives us

$$\begin{bmatrix} -1 & 1 \\ 1 & -1 \end{bmatrix} \mathbf{z}_1 = \begin{bmatrix} -1 & 1 \\ 1 & -1 \end{bmatrix} \begin{bmatrix} z_{11} \\ z_{21} \end{bmatrix} = \begin{bmatrix} 0 \\ 0 \end{bmatrix},$$

or

$$z_{11} = z_{21}.$$

Therefore the first eigenvector will be

$$\mathbf{z}_1 = \begin{bmatrix} 1 \\ 1 \end{bmatrix},$$

or any scalar multiple. For the second eigenvector we use $\lambda = \lambda_2 = -1$:

$$\begin{bmatrix} 1 & 1 \\ 1 & 1 \end{bmatrix} \mathbf{z}_1 = \begin{bmatrix} 1 & 1 \\ 1 & 1 \end{bmatrix} \begin{bmatrix} z_{12} \\ z_{22} \end{bmatrix} = \begin{bmatrix} 0 \\ 0 \end{bmatrix},$$

or

$$z_{12} = -z_{22}.$$

Therefore the second eigenvector is

$$\mathbf{z}_2 = \begin{bmatrix} 1 \\ -1 \end{bmatrix},$$

or any scalar multiple.

Note that while these eigenvectors can be represented as columns of numbers, in reality they are complex numbers. For example:

$$z_1 = 1v_1 + 1v_2 = (1+j) + (1-j) = 2,$$

$$z_2 = 1v_1 + (-1)v_2 = (1+j) - (1-j) = 2j.$$

Checking that these are indeed eigenvectors:

$$A(z_1) = (2)^* = 2 = \lambda_1 z_1,$$

$$A(z_2) = (2j)^* = -2j = \lambda_2 z_2.$$

iii. To perform a change of basis we need to use Eq. (6.33):

$$\mathbf{A'} = [\mathbf{B}_w^{-1}\mathbf{A}\mathbf{B}_t] = [\mathbf{B}^{-1}\mathbf{A}\mathbf{B}],$$

where

$$B = \begin{bmatrix} \mathbf{z}_1 & \mathbf{z}_2 \end{bmatrix} = \begin{bmatrix} 1 & 1 \\ 1 & -1 \end{bmatrix}.$$

(We are using the same basis set for the range and the domain.) Therefore we have

$$A' = \begin{bmatrix} 0.5 & 0.5 \\ 0.5 & -0.5 \end{bmatrix} \begin{bmatrix} 0 & 1 \\ 1 & 0 \end{bmatrix} \begin{bmatrix} 1 & 1 \\ 1 & -1 \end{bmatrix} = \begin{bmatrix} 1 & 0 \\ 0 & -1 \end{bmatrix} = \begin{bmatrix} \lambda_1 & 0 \\ 0 & \lambda_2 \end{bmatrix}.$$

As expected from Eq. (6.69), we have diagonalized the matrix representation.

P6.5 **Diagonalize the following matrix:**

$$A = \begin{bmatrix} 2 & -2 \\ -1 & 3 \end{bmatrix}.$$

The first step is to find the eigenvalues:

$$|[A - \lambda I]| = \left| \begin{bmatrix} 2-\lambda & -2 \\ -1 & 3-\lambda \end{bmatrix} \right| = \lambda^2 - 5\lambda + 4 = (\lambda - 1)(\lambda - 4) = 0,$$

so the eigenvalues are $\lambda_1 = 1$, $\lambda_2 = 4$. To find the eigenvectors,

$$[A - \lambda I] \mathbf{z} = \begin{bmatrix} 2-\lambda & -2 \\ -1 & 3-\lambda \end{bmatrix} \mathbf{z} = \begin{bmatrix} 0 \\ 0 \end{bmatrix}.$$

For $\lambda = \lambda_1 = 1$

$$\begin{bmatrix} 1 & -2 \\ -1 & 2 \end{bmatrix} \mathbf{z}_1 = \begin{bmatrix} 1 & -2 \\ -1 & 2 \end{bmatrix} \begin{bmatrix} z_{11} \\ z_{21} \end{bmatrix} = \begin{bmatrix} 0 \\ 0 \end{bmatrix},$$

or

$$z_{11} = 2z_{21}.$$

Therefore the first eigenvector will be

$$\mathbf{z}_1 = \begin{bmatrix} 2 \\ 1 \end{bmatrix},$$

or any scalar multiple.

For $\lambda = \lambda_2 = 4$

$$\begin{bmatrix} -2 & -2 \\ -1 & -1 \end{bmatrix} \mathbf{z}_1 = \begin{bmatrix} -2 & -2 \\ -1 & -1 \end{bmatrix} \begin{bmatrix} z_{12} \\ z_{22} \end{bmatrix} = \begin{bmatrix} 0 \\ 0 \end{bmatrix} ,$$

or

$$z_{12} = -z_{22} .$$

Therefore the second eigenvector will be

$$\mathbf{z}_2 = \begin{bmatrix} 1 \\ -1 \end{bmatrix} ,$$

or any scalar multiple.

To diagonalize the matrix we use Eq. (6.69):

$$\mathbf{A}' = [\mathbf{B}^{-1}\mathbf{A}\mathbf{B}] ,$$

where

$$\mathbf{B} = \begin{bmatrix} \mathbf{z}_1 & \mathbf{z}_2 \end{bmatrix} = \begin{bmatrix} 2 & 1 \\ 1 & -1 \end{bmatrix} .$$

Therefore we have

$$\mathbf{A}' = \begin{bmatrix} \dfrac{1}{3} & \dfrac{1}{3} \\ \dfrac{1}{3} & -\dfrac{2}{3} \end{bmatrix} \begin{bmatrix} 2 & -2 \\ -1 & 3 \end{bmatrix} \begin{bmatrix} 2 & 1 \\ 1 & -1 \end{bmatrix} = \begin{bmatrix} 1 & 0 \\ 0 & 4 \end{bmatrix} = \begin{bmatrix} \lambda_1 & 0 \\ 0 & \lambda_2 \end{bmatrix} .$$

P6.6 **Consider a transformation $\mathcal{A} : R^3 \rightarrow R^2$ whose matrix representation relative to the standard basis sets is**

$$\mathbf{A} = \begin{bmatrix} 3 & -1 & 0 \\ 0 & 0 & 1 \end{bmatrix} .$$

Find the matrix for this transformation relative to the basis sets:

$$T = \left\{ \begin{bmatrix} 2 \\ 0 \\ 1 \end{bmatrix}, \begin{bmatrix} 0 \\ -1 \\ 0 \end{bmatrix}, \begin{bmatrix} 0 \\ -2 \\ 3 \end{bmatrix} \right\} \qquad W = \left\{ \begin{bmatrix} 1 \\ 0 \end{bmatrix}, \begin{bmatrix} 0 \\ -2 \end{bmatrix} \right\}.$$

The first step is to form the matrices

$$\mathbf{B}_t = \begin{bmatrix} 2 & 0 & 0 \\ 0 & -1 & -2 \\ 1 & 0 & 3 \end{bmatrix} \qquad \mathbf{B}_w = \begin{bmatrix} 1 & 0 \\ 0 & -2 \end{bmatrix}.$$

Now we use Eq. (6.33) to form the new matrix representation:

$$\mathbf{A}' = [\mathbf{B}_w^{-1} \mathbf{A} \mathbf{B}_t],$$

$$\mathbf{A}' = \begin{bmatrix} 1 & 0 \\ 0 & -\frac{1}{2} \end{bmatrix} \begin{bmatrix} 3 & -1 & 0 \\ 0 & 0 & 1 \end{bmatrix} \begin{bmatrix} 2 & 0 & 0 \\ 0 & -1 & -2 \\ 1 & 0 & 3 \end{bmatrix} = \begin{bmatrix} 6 & 1 & 2 \\ -\frac{1}{2} & 0 & -\frac{3}{2} \end{bmatrix}.$$

Therefore this is the matrix of the transformation with respect to the basis sets T and W.

P6.7 **Consider a transformation $\mathcal{A} : \mathfrak{R}^2 \to \mathfrak{R}^2$. One basis set for $\mathfrak{R}^2$ is given as $V = \{v_1, v_2\}$.**

i. Find the matrix of the transformation $\mathcal{A}$ relative to the basis set V if it is given that

$$\mathcal{A}(v_1) = v_1 + 2v_2,$$

$$\mathcal{A}(v_2) = v_1 + v_2.$$

ii. Consider a new basis set $W = \{w_1, w_2\}$. Find the matrix of the transformation $\mathcal{A}$ relative to the basis set W if it is given that

$$w_1 = v_1 + v_2,$$

$$w_2 = v_1 - v_2.$$

i. Each of the two equations gives us one column of the matrix, as defined in Eq. (6.6). Therefore the matrix is

$$A = \begin{bmatrix} 1 & 1 \\ 2 & 1 \end{bmatrix}.$$

ii. We can represent the W basis vectors as columns of numbers in terms of the V basis vectors:

$$\mathbf{w}_1 = \begin{bmatrix} 1 \\ 1 \end{bmatrix} \qquad \mathbf{w}_2 = \begin{bmatrix} 1 \\ -1 \end{bmatrix}.$$

We can now form the basis matrix that we need to perform the similarity transform:

$$\mathbf{B}_w = \begin{bmatrix} 1 & 1 \\ 1 & -1 \end{bmatrix}.$$

The new matrix representation can then be obtained from Eq. (6.33):

$$\mathbf{A'} = [\mathbf{B}_w^{-1} \mathbf{A} \mathbf{B}_w],$$

$$\mathbf{A'} = \begin{bmatrix} \frac{1}{2} & \frac{1}{2} \\ \frac{1}{2} & -\frac{1}{2} \end{bmatrix} \begin{bmatrix} 1 & 1 \\ 2 & 1 \end{bmatrix} \begin{bmatrix} 1 & 1 \\ 1 & -1 \end{bmatrix} = \begin{bmatrix} \frac{5}{2} & \frac{1}{2} \\ -\frac{1}{2} & -\frac{1}{2} \end{bmatrix}.$$

6

P6.8 **Consider the vector space P^2 of all polynomials of degree less than or equal to 2. One basis for this vector space is $V = \{1, t, t^2\}$. Consider the differentiation transformation $\mathcal{D}$.**

    i. Find the matrix of this transformation relative to the basis set V.

    ii. Find the eigenvalues and eigenvectors of the transformation.

i. The first step is to transform each of the basis vectors:

$$\mathcal{D}(1) = 0 = (0) 1 + (0) t + (0) t^2,$$

$$\mathcal{D}(t) = 1 = (1) 1 + (0) t + (0) t^2,$$

$$\mathcal{D}(t^2) = 2t = (0) 1 + (2) t + (0) t^2.$$

The matrix of the transformation is then given by

$$\mathbf{D} = \begin{bmatrix} 0 & 1 & 0 \\ 0 & 0 & 2 \\ 0 & 0 & 0 \end{bmatrix}.$$

ii. To find the eigenvalues we must solve

$$|[\mathbf{D} - \lambda\mathbf{I}]| = \begin{vmatrix} -\lambda & 1 & 0 \\ 0 & -\lambda & 2 \\ 0 & 0 & -\lambda \end{vmatrix} = -\lambda^3 = 0.$$

Therefore all three eigenvalues are zero. To find the eigenvectors we need to solve

$$[\mathbf{D} - \lambda\mathbf{I}]\,\mathbf{z} = \begin{bmatrix} -\lambda & 1 & 0 \\ 0 & -\lambda & 2 \\ 0 & 0 & -\lambda \end{bmatrix}\mathbf{z} = \begin{bmatrix} 0 \\ 0 \\ 0 \end{bmatrix}.$$

For $\lambda = 0$ we have

$$\begin{bmatrix} 0 & 1 & 0 \\ 0 & 0 & 2 \\ 0 & 0 & 0 \end{bmatrix}\begin{bmatrix} z_1 \\ z_2 \\ z_3 \end{bmatrix} = \begin{bmatrix} 0 \\ 0 \\ 0 \end{bmatrix}.$$

This means that

$$z_2 = z_3 = 0.$$

Therefore we have a single eigenvector:

$$\mathbf{z} = \begin{bmatrix} 1 \\ 0 \\ 0 \end{bmatrix}.$$

Therefore the only polynomial whose derivative is a scaled version of itself is a constant (a zeroth-order polynomial).

P6.9 **Consider a transformation** $\mathcal{A}:R^2 \to R^2$. **Two examples of transformed vectors are given in Figure P6.4. Find the matrix representation of this transformation relative to the standard basis set.**

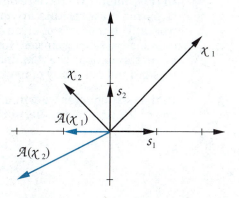

Figure P6.4 Transformation for Problem P6.9

For this problem we do not know how the basis vectors are transformed, so we cannot use Eq. (6.6) to find the matrix representation. However, we do know how two vectors are transformed, and we do know how those vectors can be represented in terms of the standard basis set. From Figure P6.4 we can write the following equations:

$$\mathbf{A}\begin{bmatrix} 2 \\ 2 \end{bmatrix} = \begin{bmatrix} -1 \\ 0 \end{bmatrix}, \ \mathbf{A}\begin{bmatrix} -1 \\ 1 \end{bmatrix} = \begin{bmatrix} -2 \\ -1 \end{bmatrix}.$$

We then put these two equations together to form

$$\mathbf{A}\begin{bmatrix} 2 & -1 \\ 2 & 1 \end{bmatrix} = \begin{bmatrix} -1 & -2 \\ 0 & -1 \end{bmatrix}.$$

So that

$$\mathbf{A} = \begin{bmatrix} -1 & -2 \\ 0 & -1 \end{bmatrix} \begin{bmatrix} 2 & -1 \\ 2 & 1 \end{bmatrix}^{-1} = \begin{bmatrix} -1 & -2 \\ 0 & -1 \end{bmatrix} \begin{bmatrix} \dfrac{1}{4} & \dfrac{1}{4} \\ -\dfrac{1}{2} & \dfrac{1}{2} \end{bmatrix} = \begin{bmatrix} \dfrac{3}{4} & -\dfrac{5}{4} \\ \dfrac{1}{2} & -\dfrac{1}{2} \end{bmatrix}.$$

This is the matrix representation of the transformation with respect to the standard basis set.

This procedure is used in the *Neural Network Design Demonstration Linear Transformations* (**nnd6lt**).

Epilogue

In this chapter we have reviewed those properties of linear transformations and matrices that are most important to our study of neural networks. The concepts of eigenvalues, eigenvectors, change of basis (similarity transformation) and diagonalization will be used again and again throughout the remainder of this text. Without this linear algebra background our study of neural networks could only be superficial.

In the next chapter we will use linear algebra to analyze the operation of one of the first neural network training algorithms — the Hebb rule.

Further Reading

[Brog91] W. L. Brogan, *Modern Control Theory*, 3rd Ed., Englewood Cliffs, NJ: Prentice-Hall, 1991.

This is a well-written book on the subject of linear systems. The first half of the book is devoted to linear algebra. It also has good sections on the solution of linear differential equations and the stability of linear and nonlinear systems. It has many worked problems.

[Stra76] G. Strang, *Linear Algebra and Its Applications*, New York: Academic Press, 1980.

Strang has written a good basic text on linear algebra. Many applications of linear algebra are integrated into the text.

6

Exercises

E6.1 Is the operation of transposing a matrix a linear transformation?

E6.2 Consider again the neural network shown in Figure P6.1. Show that if the bias vector **b** is equal to zero then the network performs a linear operation.

E6.3 Consider the linear transformation illustrated in Figure E6.1.

    i. Find the matrix representation of this transformation relative to the standard basis set.

    ii. Find the matrix of this transformation relative to the basis set $\{v_1, v_2\}$.

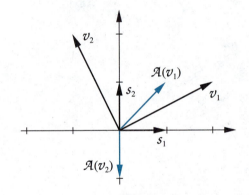

Figure E6.1 Example Transformation for Exercise E6.3

E6.4 Consider the space of complex numbers. Let this be the vector space X, and let the basis for X be $\{1 + j, 1 - j\}$. Let $\mathcal{A} : X \to X$ be the operation of multiplication by $(1 + j)$ (i.e., $\mathcal{A}(\chi) = (1 + j)\chi$).

    i. Find the matrix of the transformation $\mathcal{A}$ relative to the basis set given above.

    ii. Find the eigenvalues and eigenvectors of the transformation.

    iii. Find the matrix representation for $\mathcal{A}$ relative to the eigenvectors as the basis vectors.

    iv. Check your answers to parts (ii) and (iii) using MATLAB.

E6.5 Consider a transformation $A : P^2 \to P^3$, from the space of second-order polynomials to the space of third-order polynomials, which is defined by the following:

$$x = a_0 + a_1 t + a_2 t^2,$$

$$A(x) = a_0 (t+1) + a_1 (t+1)^2 + a_2 (t+1)^3.$$

Find the matrix representation of this transformation relative to the basis sets $V^2 = \{1, t, t^2\}$, $V^3 = \{1, t, t^2, t^3\}$.

E6.6 Consider the space of functions of the form $\alpha \sin(t + \phi)$. One basis set for this space is $V = \{\sin t, \cos t\}$. Consider the differentiation transformation $\mathcal{D}$.

  i. Find the matrix of the transformation $\mathcal{D}$ relative to the basis set V.

  ii. Find the eigenvalues and eigenvectors of the transformation. Show the eigenvectors as columns of numbers and as functions of t.

  iii. Find the matrix of the transformation relative to the eigenvectors as basis vectors.

E6.7 Consider the vector spaces P^2 and P^3 of second-order and third-order polynomials. Find the matrix representation of the integration transformation $I : P^2 \to P^3$, relative to the basis sets $V^2 = \{1, t, t^2\}$, $V^3 = \{1, t, t^2, t^3\}$.

E6.8 A certain linear transformation $A : \Re^2 \to \Re^2$ has a matrix representation relative to the standard basis set of

$$\mathbf{A} = \begin{bmatrix} 1 & 2 \\ 3 & 4 \end{bmatrix}.$$

Find the matrix representation of this transformation relative to the new basis set:

$$V = \left\{ \begin{bmatrix} 1 \\ 3 \end{bmatrix}, \begin{bmatrix} 2 \\ 5 \end{bmatrix} \right\}.$$

E6.9 We know that a certain linear transformation $A : R^2 \to R^2$ has eigenvalues and eigenvectors given by

6

$$\lambda_1 = 1 \qquad \mathbf{z}_1 = \begin{bmatrix} 1 \\ 1 \end{bmatrix} \qquad \lambda_2 = 2 \qquad \mathbf{z}_2 = \begin{bmatrix} 1 \\ 2 \end{bmatrix}.$$

(The eigenvectors are represented relative to the standard basis set.)

i. Find the matrix representation of the transformation $\mathcal{A}$ relative to the standard basis set.

ii. Find the matrix representation relative to the new basis

$$V = \left\{ \begin{bmatrix} 1 \\ 1 \end{bmatrix}, \begin{bmatrix} -1 \\ 1 \end{bmatrix} \right\}.$$

E6.10 Consider the following basis set for $\mathfrak{R}^2$:

$$V = \{\mathbf{v}_1, \mathbf{v}_2\} = \left\{ \begin{bmatrix} 1 \\ -1 \end{bmatrix}, \begin{bmatrix} 1 \\ -2 \end{bmatrix} \right\}.$$

(The basis vectors are represented relative to the standard basis set.)

i. Find the reciprocal basis vectors for this basis set.

ii. Consider a transformation $\mathcal{A}:\mathfrak{R}^2 \to \mathfrak{R}^2$. The matrix representation for $\mathcal{A}$ relative to the standard basis in $\mathfrak{R}^2$ is

$$\mathbf{A} = \begin{bmatrix} 0 & 1 \\ -2 & -3 \end{bmatrix}.$$

Find the expansion of $\mathbf{Av}_1$ in terms of the basis set V. (Use the reciprocal basis vectors.)

iii. Find the expansion of $\mathbf{Av}_2$ in terms of the basis set V.

iv. Find the matrix representation for $\mathcal{A}$ relative to the basis V. (This step should require no further computation.)

7 Supervised Hebbian Learning

Objectives

The Hebb rule was one of the first neural network learning laws. It was proposed by Donald Hebb in 1949 as a possible mechanism for synaptic modification in the brain and since then has been used to train artificial neural networks.

In this chapter we will use the linear algebra concepts of the previous two chapters to explain why Hebbian learning works. We will also show how the Hebb rule can be used to train neural networks for pattern recognition.

Theory and Examples

Donald O. Hebb was born in Chester, Nova Scotia, just after the turn of the century. He originally planned to become a novelist, and obtained a degree in English from Dalhousie University in Halifax in 1925. Since every first-rate novelist needs to have a good understanding of human nature, he began to study Freud after graduation and became interested in psychology. He then pursued a master's degree in psychology at McGill University, where he wrote a thesis on Pavlovian conditioning. He received his Ph.D. from Harvard in 1936, where his dissertation investigated the effects of early experience on the vision of rats. Later he joined the Montreal Neurological Institute, where he studied the extent of intellectual changes in brain surgery patients. In 1942 he moved to the Yerkes Laboratories of Primate Biology in Florida, where he studied chimpanzee behavior.

In 1949 Hebb summarized his two decades of research in *The Organization of Behavior* [Hebb49]. The main premise of this book was that behavior could be explained by the action of neurons. This was in marked contrast to the behaviorist school of psychology (with proponents such as B. F. Skinner), which emphasized the correlation between stimulus and response and discouraged the use of any physiological hypotheses. It was a confrontation between a top-down philosophy and a bottom-up philosophy. Hebb stated his approach: "The method then calls for learning as much as one can about what the parts of the brain do (primarily the physiologist's field), and relating the behavior as far as possible to this knowledge (primarily for the psychologist); then seeing what further information is to be had about how the total brain works, from the discrepancy between (1) actual behavior and (2) the behavior that would be predicted from adding up what is known about the action of the various parts."

The most famous idea contained in *The Organization of Behavior* was the postulate that came to be known as Hebbian learning:

Hebb's Postulate *"When an axon of cell A is near enough to excite a cell B and repeatedly or persistently takes part in firing it, some growth process or metabolic change takes place in one or both cells such that A's efficiency, as one of the cells firing B, is increased."*

This postulate suggested a physical mechanism for learning at the cellular level. Although Hebb never claimed to have firm physiological evidence for his theory, subsequent research has shown that some cells do exhibit Hebbian learning. Hebb's theories continue to influence current research in neuroscience.

As with most historic ideas, Hebb's postulate was not completely new, as he himself emphasized. It had been foreshadowed by several others, including Freud. Consider, for example, the following principle of association stated by psychologist and philosopher William James in 1890: "When two brain processes are active together or in immediate succession, one of them, on reoccurring tends to propagate its excitement into the other."

Linear Associator

Hebb's learning law can be used in combination with a variety of neural network architectures. We will use a very simple architecture for our initial presentation of Hebbian learning. In this way we can concentrate on the learning law rather than the architecture. The network we will use is the *linear associator*, which is shown in Figure 7.1. (This network was introduced independently by James Anderson [Ande72] and Teuvo Kohonen [Koho72].)

Linear Associator

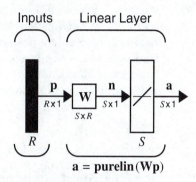

$$\mathbf{a} = \mathbf{purelin}(\mathbf{Wp})$$

Figure 7.1 Linear Associator

The output vector **a** is determined from the input vector **p** according to:

$$\mathbf{a} = \mathbf{Wp},\tag{7.1}$$

or

$$a_i = \sum_{j=1}^{Q} w_{ij} p_j.\tag{7.2}$$

Associative Memory

The linear associator is an example of a type of neural network called an *associative memory*. The task of an associative memory is to learn Q pairs of prototype input/output vectors:

$$\{\mathbf{p}_1, \mathbf{t}_1\}, \{\mathbf{p}_2, \mathbf{t}_2\}, \dots, \{\mathbf{p}_Q, \mathbf{t}_Q\}.\tag{7.3}$$

In other words, if the network receives an input $\mathbf{p} = \mathbf{p}_q$ then it should produce an output $\mathbf{a} = \mathbf{t}_q$, for $q = 1, 2, \dots, Q$. In addition, if the input is changed slightly (i.e., $\mathbf{p} = \mathbf{p}_q + \delta$) then the output should only be changed slightly (i.e., $\mathbf{a} = \mathbf{t}_q + \varepsilon$).

7

The Hebb Rule

How can we interpret Hebb's postulate mathematically, so that we can use it to train the weight matrix of the linear associator? First, let's rephrase the postulate: If two neurons on either side of a synapse are activated simultaneously, the strength of the synapse will increase. Notice from Eq. (7.2) that the connection (synapse) between input p_j and output a_i is the weight w_{ij}. Therefore Hebb's postulate would imply that if a positive p_j produces a positive a_i then w_{ij} should increase. This suggests that one mathematical interpretation of the postulate could be

The Hebb Rule

$$w_{ij}^{new} = w_{ij}^{old} + \alpha\, f_i(a_{iq})\, g_j(p_{jq}),\tag{7.4}$$

where p_{jq} is the jth element of the qth input vector $\mathbf{p}_q$; a_{iq} is the ith element of the network output when the qth input vector is presented to the network; and α is a positive constant, called the learning rate. This equation says that the change in the weight w_{ij} is proportional to a product of functions of the activities on either side of the synapse. For this chapter we will simplify Eq. (7.4) to the following form

$$w_{ij}^{new} = w_{ij}^{old} + \alpha a_{iq} p_{jq}.\tag{7.5}$$

Note that this expression actually extends Hebb's postulate beyond its strict interpretation. The change in the weight is proportional to a product of the activity on either side of the synapse. Therefore, not only do we increase the weight when both p_j and a_i are positive, but we also increase the weight when they are both negative. In addition, this implementation of the Hebb rule will decrease the weight whenever p_j and a_i have opposite sign.

The Hebb rule defined in Eq. (7.5) is an *unsupervised* learning rule. It does not require any information concerning the target output. In this chapter we are interested in using the Hebb rule for supervised learning, in which the target output is known for each input vector. (We will revisit the unsupervised Hebb rule in Chapter 13.) For the *supervised* Hebb rule we substitute the target output for the actual output. In this way, we are telling the algorithm what the network *should* do, rather than what it is currently doing. The resulting equation is

$$w_{ij}^{new} = w_{ij}^{old} + t_{iq} p_{jq},\tag{7.6}$$

where t_{iq} is the ith element of the qth target vector $\mathbf{t}_q$. (We have set the learning rate α to one, for simplicity.)

Notice that Eq. (7.6) can be written in vector notation:

$$\mathbf{W}^{new} = \mathbf{W}^{old} + \mathbf{t}_q \mathbf{p}_q^T.\tag{7.7}$$

If we assume that the weight matrix is initialized to zero and then each of the Q input/output pairs are applied once to Eq. (7.7), we can write

$$\mathbf{W} = \mathbf{t}_1 \mathbf{p}_1^T + \mathbf{t}_2 \mathbf{p}_2^T + \cdots + \mathbf{t}_Q \mathbf{p}_Q^T = \sum_{q=1}^{Q} \mathbf{t}_q \mathbf{p}_q^T. \tag{7.8}$$

This can be represented in matrix form:

$$\mathbf{W} = \begin{bmatrix} \mathbf{t}_1 & \mathbf{t}_2 & \cdots & \mathbf{t}_Q \end{bmatrix} \begin{bmatrix} \mathbf{p}_1^T \\ \mathbf{p}_2^T \\ \vdots \\ \mathbf{p}_Q^T \end{bmatrix} = \mathbf{T}\mathbf{P}^T, \tag{7.9}$$

where

$$\mathbf{T} = \begin{bmatrix} \mathbf{t}_1 & \mathbf{t}_2 & \cdots & \mathbf{t}_Q \end{bmatrix}, \quad \mathbf{P} = \begin{bmatrix} \mathbf{p}_1 & \mathbf{p}_2 & \cdots & \mathbf{p}_Q \end{bmatrix}. \tag{7.10}$$

Performance Analysis

Let's analyze the performance of Hebbian learning for the linear associator. First consider the case where the $\mathbf{p}_q$ vectors are orthonormal (orthogonal and unit length). If $\mathbf{p}_k$ is input to the network, then the network output can be computed

$$\mathbf{a} = \mathbf{W}\mathbf{p}_k = \left(\sum_{q=1}^{Q} \mathbf{t}_q \mathbf{p}_q^T \right) \mathbf{p}_k = \sum_{q=1}^{Q} \mathbf{t}_q (\mathbf{p}_q^T \mathbf{p}_k). \tag{7.11}$$

Since the $\mathbf{p}_q$ are orthonormal,

$$(\mathbf{p}_q^T \mathbf{p}_k) = 1 \qquad q = k$$
$$= 0 \qquad q \neq k. \tag{7.12}$$

Therefore Eq. (7.11) can be rewritten

$$\mathbf{a} = \mathbf{W}\mathbf{p}_k = \mathbf{t}_k. \tag{7.13}$$

The output of the network is equal to the target output. This shows that, if the input prototype vectors are orthonormal, the Hebb rule will produce the correct output for each input.

7

But what about non-orthogonal prototype vectors? Let's assume that each $\mathbf{p}_q$ vector is unit length, but that they are not orthogonal. Then Eq. (7.11) becomes

$$
\mathbf{a} = \mathbf{W}\mathbf{p}_k = \mathbf{t}_k + \underbrace{\left(\sum_{q \neq k} \mathbf{t}_q \, (\mathbf{p}_q^T \mathbf{p}_k) \right)}_{\text{\textit{Error}}}.
\tag{7.14}
$$

Because the vectors are not orthogonal, the network will not produce the correct output. The magnitude of the error will depend on the amount of correlation between the prototype input patterns.

As an example, suppose that the prototype input/output vectors are

$$
\left\{ \mathbf{p}_1 = \begin{bmatrix} 0.5 \\ -0.5 \\ 0.5 \\ -0.5 \end{bmatrix}, \mathbf{t}_1 = \begin{bmatrix} 1 \\ -1 \end{bmatrix} \right\}
\qquad
\left\{ \mathbf{p}_2 = \begin{bmatrix} 0.5 \\ 0.5 \\ -0.5 \\ -0.5 \end{bmatrix}, \mathbf{t}_2 = \begin{bmatrix} 1 \\ 1 \end{bmatrix} \right\}.
\tag{7.15}
$$

(Check that the two input vectors are orthonormal.)

The weight matrix would be

$$
\mathbf{W} = \mathbf{T}\mathbf{P}^T = \begin{bmatrix} 1 & 1 \\ -1 & 1 \end{bmatrix} \begin{bmatrix} 0.5 & -0.5 & 0.5 & -0.5 \\ 0.5 & 0.5 & -0.5 & -0.5 \end{bmatrix} = \begin{bmatrix} 1 & 0 & 0 & -1 \\ 0 & 1 & -1 & 0 \end{bmatrix}.
\tag{7.16}
$$

If we test this weight matrix on the two prototype inputs we find

$$
\mathbf{W}\mathbf{p}_1 = \begin{bmatrix} 1 & 0 & 0 & -1 \\ 0 & 1 & -1 & 0 \end{bmatrix} \begin{bmatrix} 0.5 \\ -0.5 \\ 0.5 \\ -0.5 \end{bmatrix} = \begin{bmatrix} 1 \\ -1 \end{bmatrix},
\tag{7.17}
$$

and

$$
\mathbf{W}\mathbf{p}_2 = \begin{bmatrix} 1 & 0 & 0 & -1 \\ 0 & 1 & -1 & 0 \end{bmatrix} \begin{bmatrix} 0.5 \\ 0.5 \\ -0.5 \\ -0.5 \end{bmatrix} = \begin{bmatrix} 1 \\ 1 \end{bmatrix}.
\tag{7.18}
$$

Success!! The outputs of the network are equal to the targets.

Now let's revisit the *apple* and *orange* recognition problem described in Chapter 3. Recall that the prototype inputs were

$$\mathbf{p}_1 = \begin{bmatrix} 1 \\ -1 \\ -1 \end{bmatrix} (orange) \qquad \mathbf{p}_2 = \begin{bmatrix} 1 \\ 1 \\ -1 \end{bmatrix} (apple) . \qquad (7.19)$$

(Note that they are not orthogonal.) If we normalize these inputs and choose as desired outputs –1 and 1, we obtain

$$\left\{ \mathbf{p}_1 = \begin{bmatrix} 0.5774 \\ -0.5774 \\ -0.5774 \end{bmatrix}, \mathbf{t}_1 = \begin{bmatrix} -1 \end{bmatrix} \right\} \qquad \left\{ \mathbf{p}_2 = \begin{bmatrix} 0.5774 \\ 0.5774 \\ -0.5774 \end{bmatrix}, \mathbf{t}_2 = \begin{bmatrix} 1 \end{bmatrix} \right\} . \qquad (7.20)$$

Our weight matrix becomes

$$\mathbf{W} = \mathbf{TP}^T = \begin{bmatrix} -1 & 1 \end{bmatrix} \begin{bmatrix} 0.5774 & -0.5774 & -0.5774 \\ 0.5774 & 0.5774 & -0.5774 \end{bmatrix} = \begin{bmatrix} 0 & 1.547 & 0 \end{bmatrix} . \qquad (7.21)$$

So, if we use our two prototype patterns,

$$\mathbf{Wp}_1 = \begin{bmatrix} 0 & 1.547 & 0 \end{bmatrix} \begin{bmatrix} 0.5774 \\ -0.5774 \\ -0.5774 \end{bmatrix} = \begin{bmatrix} -0.8932 \end{bmatrix} , \qquad (7.22)$$

$$\mathbf{Wp}_2 = \begin{bmatrix} 0 & 1.547 & 0 \end{bmatrix} \begin{bmatrix} 0.5774 \\ 0.5774 \\ -0.5774 \end{bmatrix} = \begin{bmatrix} 0.8932 \end{bmatrix} . \qquad (7.23)$$

The outputs are close, but do not quite match the target outputs.

Pseudoinverse Rule

When the prototype input patterns are not orthogonal, the Hebb rule produces some errors. There are several procedures that can be used to reduce these errors. In this section we will discuss one of those procedures, the pseudoinverse rule.

Recall that the task of the linear associator was to produce an output of $\mathbf{t}_q$ for an input of $\mathbf{p}_q$. In other words,

$$\mathbf{Wp}_q = \mathbf{t}_q \qquad q = 1, 2, \dots, Q . \qquad (7.24)$$

If it is not possible to choose a weight matrix so that these equations are exactly satisfied, then we want them to be approximately satisfied. One approach would be to choose the weight matrix to minimize the following performance index:

$$F(\mathbf{W}) = \sum_{q=1}^{Q} \| \mathbf{t}_q - \mathbf{W}\mathbf{p}_q \|^2 . \tag{7.25}$$

If the prototype input vectors $\mathbf{p}_q$ are orthonormal and we use the Hebb rule to find $\mathbf{W}$, then $F(\mathbf{W})$ will be zero. When the input vectors are not orthogonal and we use the Hebb rule, then $F(\mathbf{W})$ will be not be zero, and it is not clear that $F(\mathbf{W})$ will be minimized. It turns out that the weight matrix that will minimize $F(\mathbf{W})$ is obtained by using the pseudoinverse matrix, which we will define next.

First, let's rewrite Eq. (7.24) in matrix form:

$$\mathbf{W}\mathbf{P} = \mathbf{T}, \tag{7.26}$$

where

$$\mathbf{T} = \begin{bmatrix} \mathbf{t}_1 \ \mathbf{t}_2 \ \cdots \ \mathbf{t}_Q \end{bmatrix}, \mathbf{P} = \begin{bmatrix} \mathbf{p}_1 \ \mathbf{p}_2 \ \cdots \ \mathbf{p}_Q \end{bmatrix}. \tag{7.27}$$

Then Eq. (7.25) can be written

$$F(\mathbf{W}) = \| \mathbf{T} - \mathbf{W}\mathbf{P} \|^2 = \| \mathbf{E} \|^2 , \tag{7.28}$$

where

$$\mathbf{E} = \mathbf{T} - \mathbf{W}\mathbf{P}, \tag{7.29}$$

and

$$\| \mathbf{E} \|^2 = \sum_i \sum_j e_{ij}^2 . \tag{7.30}$$

Note that $F(\mathbf{W})$ can be made zero if we can solve Eq. (7.26). If the $\mathbf{P}$ matrix has an inverse, the solution is

$$\mathbf{W} = \mathbf{T}\mathbf{P}^{-1} . \tag{7.31}$$

However, this is rarely possible. Normally the $\mathbf{p}_q$ vectors (the columns of $\mathbf{P}$) will be independent, but R (the dimension of $\mathbf{p}_q$) will be larger than Q (the number of $\mathbf{p}_q$ vectors). Therefore, $\mathbf{P}$ will not be a square matrix, and no exact inverse will exist.

It has been shown [Albe72] that the weight matrix that minimizes Eq. (7.25) is given by the *pseudoinverse rule*:

$$\mathbf{W} = \mathbf{TP}^+, \qquad (7.32)$$

where $\mathbf{P}^+$ is the Moore-Penrose pseudoinverse. The pseudoinverse of a real matrix $\mathbf{P}$ is the unique matrix that satisfies

$$\mathbf{PP}^+\mathbf{P} = \mathbf{P},$$

$$\mathbf{P}^+\mathbf{PP}^+ = \mathbf{P}^+, \qquad (7.33)$$

$$\mathbf{P}^+\mathbf{P} = \left(\mathbf{P}^+\mathbf{P}\right)^T,$$

$$\mathbf{PP}^+ = \left(\mathbf{PP}^+\right)^T.$$

When the number, R, of rows of $\mathbf{P}$ is greater than the number of columns, Q, of $\mathbf{P}$, and the columns of $\mathbf{P}$ are independent, then the pseudoinverse can be computed by

$$\mathbf{P}^+ = \left(\mathbf{P}^T\mathbf{P}\right)^{-1}\mathbf{P}^T. \qquad (7.34)$$

To test the pseudoinverse rule (Eq. (7.32)), consider again the apple and orange recognition problem. Recall that the input/output prototype vectors are

$$\left\{ \mathbf{p}_1 = \begin{bmatrix} 1 \\ -1 \\ -1 \end{bmatrix}, \mathbf{t}_1 = \begin{bmatrix} -1 \end{bmatrix} \right\} \qquad \left\{ \mathbf{p}_2 = \begin{bmatrix} 1 \\ 1 \\ -1 \end{bmatrix}, \mathbf{t}_2 = \begin{bmatrix} 1 \end{bmatrix} \right\}. \qquad (7.35)$$

(Note that we do not need to normalize the input vectors when using the pseudoinverse rule.)

The weight matrix is calculated from Eq. (7.32):

$$\mathbf{W} = \mathbf{TP}^+ = \begin{bmatrix} -1 & 1 \end{bmatrix} \left(\begin{bmatrix} 1 & 1 \\ -1 & 1 \\ -1 & -1 \end{bmatrix} \right)^+, \qquad (7.36)$$

where the pseudoinverse is computed from Eq. (7.34):

$$\mathbf{P}^+ = \left(\mathbf{P}^T\mathbf{P}\right)^{-1}\mathbf{P}^T = \begin{bmatrix} 3 & 1 \\ 1 & 3 \end{bmatrix}^{-1} \begin{bmatrix} 1 & -1 & -1 \\ 1 & 1 & -1 \end{bmatrix} = \begin{bmatrix} 0.25 & -0.5 & -0.25 \\ 0.25 & 0.5 & -0.25 \end{bmatrix}. \qquad (7.37)$$

This produces the following weight matrix:

$$\mathbf{W} = \mathbf{TP}^+ = \begin{bmatrix} -1 & 1 \end{bmatrix} \begin{bmatrix} 0.25 & -0.5 & -0.25 \\ 0.25 & 0.5 & -0.25 \end{bmatrix} = \begin{bmatrix} 0 & 1 & 0 \end{bmatrix}. \tag{7.38}$$

Let's try this matrix on our two prototype patterns.

$$\mathbf{Wp}_1 = \begin{bmatrix} 0 & 1 & 0 \end{bmatrix} \begin{bmatrix} 1 \\ -1 \\ -1 \end{bmatrix} = \begin{bmatrix} -1 \end{bmatrix} \tag{7.39}$$

$$\mathbf{Wp}_2 = \begin{bmatrix} 0 & 1 & 0 \end{bmatrix} \begin{bmatrix} 1 \\ 1 \\ -1 \end{bmatrix} = \begin{bmatrix} 1 \end{bmatrix} \tag{7.40}$$

The network outputs exactly match the desired outputs. Compare this result with the performance of the Hebb rule. As you can see from Eq. (7.22) and Eq. (7.23), the Hebbian outputs are only close, while the pseudoinverse rule produces exact results.

Application

Now let's see how we might use the Hebb rule on a practical, although greatly oversimplified, pattern recognition problem. For this problem we will use a special type of associative memory — the autoassociative memory. In an *autoassociative memory* the desired output vector is equal to the input vector (i.e., $\mathbf{t}_q = \mathbf{p}_q$). We will use an autoassociative memory to store a set of patterns and then to recall these patterns, even when corrupted patterns are provided as input.

Autoassociative Memory

The patterns we want to store are shown to the left. (Since we are designing an autoassociative memory, these patterns represent the input vectors and the targets.) They represent the digits {0, 1, 2} displayed in a 6X5 grid. We need to convert these digits to vectors, which will become the prototype patterns for our network. Each white square will be represented by a "-1", and each dark square will be represented by a "1". Then, to create the input vectors, we will scan each 6X5 grid one column at a time. For example, the first prototype pattern will be

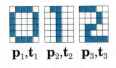

$\mathbf{p}_1,\mathbf{t}_1 \quad \mathbf{p}_2,\mathbf{t}_2 \quad \mathbf{p}_3,\mathbf{t}_3$

$$\mathbf{p}_1 = \begin{bmatrix} -1 & 1 & 1 & 1 & 1 & -1 & 1 & -1 & -1 & -1 & -1 & 1 & 1 & -1 & \dots & 1 & -1 \end{bmatrix}^T. \tag{7.41}$$

The vector $\mathbf{p}_1$ corresponds to the digit "0", $\mathbf{p}_2$ to the digit "1", and $\mathbf{p}_3$ to the digit "2". Using the Hebb rule, the weight matrix is computed

$$\mathbf{W} = \mathbf{p}_1 \mathbf{p}_1^T + \mathbf{p}_2 \mathbf{p}_2^T + \mathbf{p}_3 \mathbf{p}_3^T. \tag{7.42}$$

(Note that $\mathbf{p}_q$ replaces $\mathbf{t}_q$ in Eq. (7.8), since this is autoassociative memory.)

Because there are only two allowable values for the elements of the prototype vectors, we will modify the linear associator so that its output elements can only take on values of "–1" or "1". We can do this by replacing the linear transfer function with a symmetrical hard limit transfer function. The resulting network is displayed in Figure 7.2.

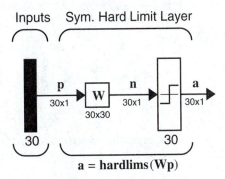

Figure 7.2 Autoassociative Network for Digit Recognition

Now let's investigate the operation of this network. We will provide the network with corrupted versions of the prototype patterns and then check the network output. In the first test, which is shown in Figure 7.3, the network is presented with a prototype pattern in which the lower half of the pattern is occluded. In each case the correct pattern is produced by the network.

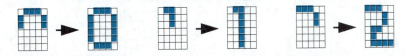

Figure 7.3 Recovery of 50% Occluded Patterns

In the next test we remove even more of the prototype patterns. Figure 7.4 illustrates the result of removing the lower two-thirds of each pattern. In this case only the digit "1" is recovered correctly. The other two patterns produce results that do not correspond to any of the prototype patterns. This is a common problem in associative memories. We would like to design networks so that the number of such spurious patterns would be minimized. We will come back to this topic again in Chapter 18, when we discuss recurrent associative memories.

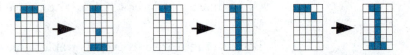

Figure 7.4 Recovery of 67% Occluded Patterns

In our final test we will present the autoassociative network with noisy versions of the prototype pattern. To create the noisy patterns we will randomly change seven elements of each pattern. The results are shown in Figure 7.5. For these examples all of the patterns were correctly recovered.

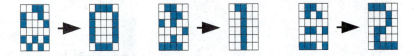

Figure 7.5 Recovery of Noisy Patterns

 To experiment with this type of pattern recognition problem, use the Neural Network Design Demonstration Hebb Rule (nnd7hr).

Variations of Hebbian Learning

There have been a number of variations on the basic Hebb rule. In fact, many of the learning laws that will be discussed in the remainder of this text have some relationship to the Hebb rule.

One of the problems of the Hebb rule is that it can lead to weight matrices having very large elements if there are many prototype patterns in the training set. Consider again the basic rule:

$$\mathbf{W}^{new} = \mathbf{W}^{old} + \mathbf{t}_q \mathbf{p}_q^T. \tag{7.43}$$

A positive parameter α, called the learning rate, can be used to limit the amount of increase in the weight matrix elements, if the learning rate is less than one, as in:

$$\mathbf{W}^{new} = \mathbf{W}^{old} + \alpha \mathbf{t}_q \mathbf{p}_q^T. \tag{7.44}$$

We can also add a decay term, so that the learning rule behaves like a smoothing filter, remembering the most recent inputs more clearly:

$$\mathbf{W}^{new} = \mathbf{W}^{old} + \alpha \mathbf{t}_q \mathbf{p}_q^T - \gamma \mathbf{W}^{old} = (1 - \gamma) \mathbf{W}^{old} + \alpha \mathbf{t}_q \mathbf{p}_q^T, \tag{7.45}$$

where γ is a positive constant less than one. As γ approaches zero, the learning law becomes the standard rule. As γ approaches one, the learning law quickly forgets old inputs and remembers only the most recent patterns. This keeps the weight matrix from growing without bound.

The idea of filtering the weight changes and of having an adjustable learning rate are important ones, and we will discuss them again in Chapter 10 and Chapters 12 – 16.

If we modify Eq. (7.44) by replacing the desired output with the difference between the desired output and the actual output, we get another important learning rule:

$$\mathbf{W}^{new} = \mathbf{W}^{old} + \alpha \, (\mathbf{t}_q - \mathbf{a}_q) \, \mathbf{p}_q^T. \tag{7.46}$$

This is sometimes known as the delta rule, since it uses the difference between desired and actual output. It is also known as the Widrow-Hoff algorithm, after the researchers who introduced it. The delta rule adjusts the weights so as to minimize the mean square error (see Chapter 10). For this reason it will produce the same results as the pseudoinverse rule, which minimizes the sum of squares of errors (see Eq. (7.25)). The advantage of the delta rule is that it can update the weights after each new input pattern is presented, whereas the pseudoinverse rule computes the weights in one step, after all of the input/target pairs are known. This sequential updating allows the delta rule to adapt to a changing environment. The delta rule will be discussed in detail in Chapter 10.

The basic Hebb rule will be discussed again, in a different context, in Chapter 13. In the present chapter we have used a supervised form of the Hebb rule. We have assumed that the desired outputs of the network, $\mathbf{t}_q$, are known, and can be used in the learning rule. In the unsupervised Hebb rule, which is discussed in Chapter 13, the *actual* network output is used instead of the *desired* network output, as in:

$$\mathbf{W}^{new} = \mathbf{W}^{old} + \alpha \mathbf{a}_q \mathbf{p}_q^T, \tag{7.47}$$

where $\mathbf{a}_q$ is the output of the network when $\mathbf{p}_q$ is given as the input (see also Eq. (7.5)). This unsupervised form of the Hebb rule, which does not require knowledge of the desired output, is actually a more direct interpretation of Hebb's postulate than is the supervised form discussed in this chapter.

Summary of Results

Hebb's Postulate

"When an axon of cell A is near enough to excite a cell B and repeatedly or persistently takes part in firing it, some growth process or metabolic change takes place in one or both cells such that A's efficiency, as one of the cells firing B, is increased."

Linear Associator

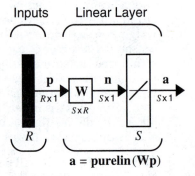

$$\mathbf{a} = \mathbf{purelin}(\mathbf{Wp})$$

The Hebb Rule

$$w_{ij}^{new} = w_{ij}^{old} + t_{qi}p_{qj}$$

$$\mathbf{W} = \mathbf{t}_1\mathbf{p}_1^T + \mathbf{t}_2\mathbf{p}_2^T + \cdots + \mathbf{t}_Q\mathbf{p}_Q^T$$

$$\mathbf{W} = \begin{bmatrix} \mathbf{t}_1 \ \mathbf{t}_2 \ \cdots \ \mathbf{t}_Q \end{bmatrix} \begin{bmatrix} \mathbf{p}_1^T \\ \mathbf{p}_2^T \\ \vdots \\ \mathbf{p}_Q^T \end{bmatrix} = \mathbf{T}\mathbf{P}^T$$

Pseudoinverse Rule

$$\mathbf{W} = \mathbf{T}\mathbf{P}^+$$

When the number, R, of rows of $\mathbf{P}$ is greater than the number of columns, Q, of $\mathbf{P}$ and the columns of $\mathbf{P}$ are independent, then the pseudoinverse can be computed by

$$\mathbf{P}^{+} = (\mathbf{P}^{T}\mathbf{P})^{-1}\mathbf{P}^{T}.$$

Variations of Hebbian Learning

Filtered Learning

(See Chapter 14)

$$\mathbf{W}^{new} = (1 - \gamma)\,\mathbf{W}^{old} + \alpha \mathbf{t}_{q}\mathbf{p}_{q}^{T}$$

Delta Rule

(See Chapter 10)

$$\mathbf{W}^{new} = \mathbf{W}^{old} + \alpha\,(\mathbf{t}_{q} - \mathbf{a}_{q})\,\mathbf{p}_{q}^{T}$$

Unsupervised Hebb

(See Chapter 13)

$$\mathbf{W}^{new} = \mathbf{W}^{old} + \alpha \mathbf{a}_{q}\mathbf{p}_{q}^{T}$$

7

Solved Problems

P7.1 **Consider the linear associator shown in Figure P7.1.**

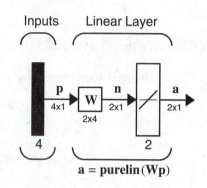

$$a = \text{purelin}(Wp)$$

Figure P7.1   Single-Neuron Perceptron

Let the input/output prototype vectors be

$$\left\{ p_1 = \begin{bmatrix} 1 \\ -1 \\ 1 \\ -1 \end{bmatrix}, t_1 = \begin{bmatrix} 1 \\ -1 \end{bmatrix} \right\} \qquad \left\{ p_2 = \begin{bmatrix} 1 \\ 1 \\ -1 \\ -1 \end{bmatrix}, t_2 = \begin{bmatrix} 1 \\ 1 \end{bmatrix} \right\}.$$

   i. **Use the Hebb rule to find the appropriate weight matrix for this linear associator.**

  ii. **Repeat part (i) using the pseudoinverse rule.**

 iii. **Apply the input p_1 to the linear associator using the weight matrix of part (i), then using the weight matrix of part (ii).**

i.   The first step is to create the **P** and **T** matrices of Eq. (7.10):

$$P = \begin{bmatrix} 1 & 1 \\ -1 & 1 \\ 1 & -1 \\ -1 & -1 \end{bmatrix}, \qquad T = \begin{bmatrix} 1 & 1 \\ -1 & 1 \end{bmatrix}.$$

Then the weight matrix can be computed using Eq. (7.9):

$$\mathbf{W}^h = \mathbf{TP}^T = \begin{bmatrix} 1 & 1 \\ -1 & 1 \end{bmatrix} \begin{bmatrix} 1 & -1 & 1 & -1 \\ 1 & 1 & -1 & -1 \end{bmatrix} = \begin{bmatrix} 2 & 0 & 0 & -2 \\ 0 & 2 & -2 & 0 \end{bmatrix}.$$

ii. For the pseudoinverse rule we use Eq. (7.32):

$$\mathbf{W} = \mathbf{TP}^+.$$

Since the number of rows of $\mathbf{P}$, four, is greater than the number of columns of $\mathbf{P}$, two, and the columns of $\mathbf{P}$ are independent, then the pseudoinverse can be computed by Eq. (7.34):

$$\mathbf{P}^+ = (\mathbf{P}^T\mathbf{P})^{-1}\mathbf{P}^T.$$

$$\mathbf{P}^+ = \left(\begin{bmatrix} 1 & -1 & 1 & -1 \\ 1 & 1 & -1 & -1 \end{bmatrix} \begin{bmatrix} 1 & 1 \\ -1 & 1 \\ 1 & -1 \\ -1 & -1 \end{bmatrix} \right)^{-1} \begin{bmatrix} 1 & -1 & 1 & -1 \\ 1 & 1 & -1 & -1 \end{bmatrix} = \left(\begin{bmatrix} 4 & 0 \\ 0 & 4 \end{bmatrix} \right)^{-1} \begin{bmatrix} 1 & -1 & 1 & -1 \\ 1 & 1 & -1 & -1 \end{bmatrix}$$

$$= \begin{bmatrix} \frac{1}{4} & 0 \\ 0 & \frac{1}{4} \end{bmatrix} \begin{bmatrix} 1 & -1 & 1 & -1 \\ 1 & 1 & -1 & -1 \end{bmatrix} = \begin{bmatrix} \frac{1}{4} & -\frac{1}{4} & \frac{1}{4} & -\frac{1}{4} \\ \frac{1}{4} & \frac{1}{4} & -\frac{1}{4} & -\frac{1}{4} \end{bmatrix}$$

The weight matrix can now be computed:

$$\mathbf{W}^p = \mathbf{TP}^+ = \begin{bmatrix} 1 & 1 \\ -1 & 1 \end{bmatrix} \begin{bmatrix} \frac{1}{4} & -\frac{1}{4} & \frac{1}{4} & -\frac{1}{4} \\ \frac{1}{4} & \frac{1}{4} & -\frac{1}{4} & -\frac{1}{4} \end{bmatrix} = \begin{bmatrix} \frac{1}{2} & 0 & 0 & -\frac{1}{2} \\ 0 & \frac{1}{2} & -\frac{1}{2} & 0 \end{bmatrix}.$$

iii. We now test the two weight matrices.

$$\mathbf{W}^h\mathbf{p}_1 = \begin{bmatrix} 2 & 0 & 0 & -2 \\ 0 & 2 & -2 & 0 \end{bmatrix} \begin{bmatrix} 1 \\ -1 \\ 1 \\ -1 \end{bmatrix} = \begin{bmatrix} 4 \\ -4 \end{bmatrix} \neq \mathbf{t}_1$$

7

$$\mathbf{W}^{p}\mathbf{p}_1 = \begin{bmatrix} \frac{1}{2} & 0 & 0 & -\frac{1}{2} \\ 0 & \frac{1}{2} & -\frac{1}{2} & 0 \end{bmatrix} \begin{bmatrix} 1 \\ -1 \\ 1 \\ -1 \end{bmatrix} = \begin{bmatrix} 1 \\ -1 \end{bmatrix} = \mathbf{t}_1$$

Why didn't the Hebb rule produce the correct results? Well, consider again Eq. (7.11). Since $\mathbf{p}_1$ and $\mathbf{p}_2$ are orthogonal (check that they are) this equation can be written

$$\mathbf{W}^{h}\mathbf{p}_1 = \mathbf{t}_1 (\mathbf{p}_1^{T}\mathbf{p}_1),$$

but the $\mathbf{p}_1$ vector is not normalized, so $(\mathbf{p}_1^{T}\mathbf{p}_1) \neq 1$. Therefore the output of the network will not be $\mathbf{t}_1$.

The pseudoinverse rule, on the other hand, is guaranteed to minimize

$$\sum_{q=1}^{2} \|\mathbf{t}_q - \mathbf{W}\mathbf{p}_q\|^2,$$

which in this case can be made equal to zero.

P7.2 **Consider the prototype patterns shown to the left.**

  i. Are these patterns orthogonal?

  ii. Design an autoassociator for these patterns. Use the Hebb rule.

  iii. What response does the network give to the test input pattern, $\mathbf{p}_t$, shown to the left?

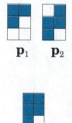

$\mathbf{p}_1$ $\quad$ $\mathbf{p}_2$

$\mathbf{p}_t$

i. The first thing we need to do is to convert the patterns into vectors. Let's assign any solid square the value 1 and any open square the value –1. Then to convert from the two-dimensional pattern to a vector we will scan the pattern column by column. (We could use rows if we wished.) The two prototype vectors then become:

$$\mathbf{p}_1 = \begin{bmatrix} 1 & 1 & -1 & 1 & -1 & -1 \end{bmatrix}^{T} \qquad \mathbf{p}_2 = \begin{bmatrix} -1 & 1 & 1 & 1 & 1 & -1 \end{bmatrix}^{T}.$$

To test orthogonality we take the inner product of $\mathbf{p}_1$ and $\mathbf{p}_2$:

$$\mathbf{p}_1^T \mathbf{p}_2 = \begin{bmatrix} 1 & 1 & -1 & 1 & -1 & -1 \end{bmatrix} \begin{bmatrix} -1 \\ 1 \\ 1 \\ 1 \\ 1 \\ -1 \end{bmatrix} = 0 \; .$$

Therefore they are orthogonal. (Although they are not normalized since

$$\mathbf{p}_1^T \mathbf{p}_1 = \mathbf{p}_2^T \mathbf{p}_2 = 6 \, .)$$

ii. We will use an autoassociator like the one in Figure 7.2, except that the number of inputs and outputs to the network will be six. To find the weight matrix we use the Hebb rule:

$$\mathbf{W} = \mathbf{T}\mathbf{P}^T ,$$

where

$$\mathbf{P} = \mathbf{T} = \begin{bmatrix} 1 & -1 \\ 1 & 1 \\ -1 & 1 \\ 1 & 1 \\ -1 & 1 \\ -1 & -1 \end{bmatrix} .$$

Therefore the weight matrix is

$$\mathbf{W} = \mathbf{T}\mathbf{P}^T = \begin{bmatrix} 1 & -1 \\ 1 & 1 \\ -1 & 1 \\ 1 & 1 \\ -1 & 1 \\ -1 & -1 \end{bmatrix} \begin{bmatrix} 1 & 1 & -1 & 1 & -1 & -1 \\ -1 & 1 & 1 & 1 & 1 & -1 \end{bmatrix} = \begin{bmatrix} 2 & 0 & -2 & 0 & -2 & 0 \\ 0 & 2 & 0 & 2 & 0 & -2 \\ -2 & 0 & 2 & 0 & 2 & 0 \\ 0 & 2 & 0 & 2 & 0 & -2 \\ -2 & 0 & 2 & 0 & 2 & 0 \\ 0 & -2 & 0 & -2 & 0 & 2 \end{bmatrix} .$$

iii. To apply the test pattern to the network we convert it to a vector:

$$\mathbf{p}_t = \begin{bmatrix} 1 & 1 & 1 & 1 & 1 & -1 \end{bmatrix}^T .$$

The network response is then

$$\mathbf{a} = \mathbf{hardlims}\,(\mathbf{Wp}_t) = \mathbf{hardlims}\left(\begin{bmatrix} 2 & 0 & -2 & 0 & -2 & 0 \\ 0 & 2 & 0 & 2 & 0 & -2 \\ -2 & 0 & 2 & 0 & 2 & 0 \\ 0 & 2 & 0 & 2 & 0 & -2 \\ -2 & 0 & 2 & 0 & 2 & 0 \\ 0 & -2 & 0 & -2 & 0 & 2 \end{bmatrix}\begin{bmatrix} 1 \\ 1 \\ 1 \\ 1 \\ 1 \\ -1 \end{bmatrix}\right)$$

$$\mathbf{a} = \mathbf{hardlims}\left(\begin{bmatrix} -2 \\ 6 \\ 2 \\ 6 \\ 2 \\ -6 \end{bmatrix}\right) = \begin{bmatrix} -1 \\ 1 \\ 1 \\ 1 \\ 1 \\ -1 \end{bmatrix} = \mathbf{p}_2\,.$$

Is this a satisfactory response? How would we want the network to respond to this input pattern? The network should produce the prototype pattern that is closest to the input pattern. In this case the test input pattern, $\mathbf{p}_t$, has a Hamming distance of 1 from $\mathbf{p}_2$, and a distance of 2 from $\mathbf{p}_1$. Therefore the network did produce the correct response. (See Chapter 3 for a discussion of Hamming distance.)

Note that in this example the prototype vectors were not normalized. This did not cause the same problem with network performance that we saw in Problem P7.1, because of the *hardlims* nonlinearity. It forces the network output to be either 1 or -1. In fact, most of the interesting and useful properties of neural networks are due to the effects of nonlinearities.

P7.3 **Consider an autoassociation problem in which there are three prototype patterns (shown below as $\mathbf{p}_1$, $\mathbf{p}_2$, $\mathbf{p}_3$). Design autoassociative networks to recognize these patterns, using both the Hebb rule and the pseudoinverse rule. Check their performance on the test pattern $\mathbf{p}_t$ shown below.**

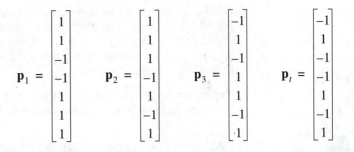

$$\mathbf{p}_1 = \begin{bmatrix} 1 \\ 1 \\ -1 \\ -1 \\ 1 \\ 1 \\ 1 \end{bmatrix} \qquad \mathbf{p}_2 = \begin{bmatrix} 1 \\ 1 \\ 1 \\ -1 \\ 1 \\ -1 \\ 1 \end{bmatrix} \qquad \mathbf{p}_3 = \begin{bmatrix} -1 \\ 1 \\ -1 \\ 1 \\ 1 \\ -1 \\ 1 \end{bmatrix} \qquad \mathbf{p}_t = \begin{bmatrix} -1 \\ 1 \\ -1 \\ -1 \\ 1 \\ -1 \\ 1 \end{bmatrix}$$

This problem is a little tedious to work out by hand, so let's use MATLAB. First we create the prototype vectors.

```
p1=[ 1  1 -1 -1  1  1  1]';
p2=[ 1  1  1 -1  1  1  1]';
p3=[-1  1 -1  1  1 -1  1]';
P=[p1 p2 p3];
```

Now we can compute the weight matrix using the Hebb rule.

```
wh=P*P';
```

To check the network we create the test vector.

```
pt=[-1  1 -1 -1  1 -1  1]';
```

The network response is then calculated.

```
ah=hardlims(wh*pt);
ah'
ans =
      1      1     -1     -1      1     -1      1
```

Notice that this response does not match any of the prototype vectors. This is not surprising since the prototype patterns are not orthogonal. Let's try the pseudoinverse rule.

```
pseu=inv(P'*P)*P';
wp=P*pseu;
ap=hardlims(wp*pt);
ap'
ans =
     -1      1     -1      1      1     -1      1
```

7

Note that the network response is equal to $\mathbf{p}_3$. Is this the correct response? As usual, we want the response to be the prototype pattern closest to the input pattern. In this case $\mathbf{p}_t$ is a Hamming distance of 2 from both $\mathbf{p}_1$ and $\mathbf{p}_2$, but only a distance of 1 from $\mathbf{p}_3$. Therefore the pseudoinverse rule produces the correct response.

Try other test inputs to see if there are additional cases where the pseudo-inverse rule produces better results than the Hebb rule.

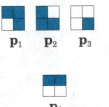

$\mathbf{p}_1 \quad \mathbf{p}_2 \quad \mathbf{p}_3$

$\mathbf{p}_t$

P7.4 **Consider the three prototype patterns shown to the left.**

    i. **Use the Hebb rule to design a perceptron network that will recognize these three patterns.**

    ii. **Find the response of the network to the pattern $\mathbf{p}_t$ shown to the left. Is the response correct?**

i. We can convert the patterns to vectors, as we did in previous problems, to obtain:

$$\mathbf{p}_1 = \begin{bmatrix} 1 \\ -1 \\ 1 \\ 1 \end{bmatrix} \qquad \mathbf{p}_2 = \begin{bmatrix} 1 \\ 1 \\ -1 \\ 1 \end{bmatrix} \qquad \mathbf{p}_3 = \begin{bmatrix} -1 \\ -1 \\ -1 \\ 1 \end{bmatrix} \qquad \mathbf{p}_t = \begin{bmatrix} 1 \\ -1 \\ 1 \\ -1 \end{bmatrix}.$$

We now need to choose the desired output vectors for each prototype input vector. Since there are three prototype vectors that we need to distinguish, we will need two elements in the output vector. We can choose the three desired outputs to be:

$$\mathbf{t}_1 = \begin{bmatrix} -1 \\ -1 \end{bmatrix} \qquad \mathbf{t}_2 = \begin{bmatrix} -1 \\ 1 \end{bmatrix} \qquad \mathbf{t}_3 = \begin{bmatrix} 1 \\ -1 \end{bmatrix}.$$

(Note that this choice was arbitrary. Any distinct combination of 1 and –1 could have been chosen for each vector.)

The resulting network is shown in Figure P7.2.

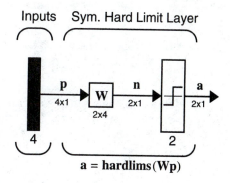

Figure P7.2 Perceptron Network for Problem P7.4

The next step is to determine the weight matrix using the Hebb rule.

$$
\mathbf{W} = \mathbf{TP}^T = \begin{bmatrix} -1 & -1 & 1 \\ -1 & 1 & -1 \end{bmatrix} \begin{bmatrix} 1 & -1 & 1 & 1 \\ 1 & 1 & -1 & 1 \\ -1 & -1 & -1 & 1 \end{bmatrix} = \begin{bmatrix} -3 & -1 & -1 & -1 \\ 1 & 3 & -1 & -1 \end{bmatrix}
$$

ii. The response of the network to the test input pattern is calculated as follows.

$$
\mathbf{a} = \mathbf{hardlims}\,(\mathbf{Wp}_t) = \mathbf{hardlims}\left(\begin{bmatrix} -3 & -1 & -1 & -1 \\ 1 & 3 & -1 & -1 \end{bmatrix} \begin{bmatrix} 1 \\ -1 \\ 1 \\ -1 \end{bmatrix} \right)
$$

$$
= \mathbf{hardlims}\left(\begin{bmatrix} -2 \\ -2 \end{bmatrix} \right) = \begin{bmatrix} -1 \\ -1 \end{bmatrix} \rightarrow \mathbf{p}_1 \,.
$$

So the response of the network indicates that the test input pattern is closest to $\mathbf{p}_1$. Is this correct? Yes, the Hamming distance to $\mathbf{p}_1$ is 1, while the distance to $\mathbf{p}_2$ and $\mathbf{p}_3$ is 3.

P7.5 **Suppose that we have a linear autoassociator that has been designed for Q orthogonal prototype vectors of length R using the Hebb rule. The vector elements are either 1 or –1.**

    i. Show that the Q prototype patterns are eigenvectors of the weight matrix.

ii. What are the other $(R - Q)$ **eigenvectors of the weight matrix?**

i. Suppose the prototype vectors are:

$$\mathbf{p}_1, \mathbf{p}_2, \cdots, \mathbf{p}_Q.$$

Since this is an autoassociator, these are both the input vectors and the desired output vectors. Therefore

$$\mathbf{T} = \begin{bmatrix} \mathbf{p}_1 & \mathbf{p}_2 & \cdots & \mathbf{p}_Q \end{bmatrix} \qquad \mathbf{P} = \begin{bmatrix} \mathbf{p}_1 & \mathbf{p}_2 & \cdots & \mathbf{p}_Q \end{bmatrix}.$$

If we then use the Hebb rule to calculate the weight matrix we find

$$\mathbf{W} = \mathbf{T}\mathbf{P}^T = \sum_{q=1}^{Q} \mathbf{p}_q \mathbf{p}_q^T,$$

from Eq. (7.8). Now, if we apply one of the prototype vectors as input to the network we obtain

$$\mathbf{a} = \mathbf{W}\mathbf{p}_k = \left(\sum_{q=1}^{Q} \mathbf{p}_q \mathbf{p}_q^T \right) \mathbf{p}_k = \sum_{q=1}^{Q} \mathbf{p}_q (\mathbf{p}_q^T \mathbf{p}_k).$$

Because the patterns are orthogonal, this reduces to

$$\mathbf{a} = \mathbf{p}_k (\mathbf{p}_k^T \mathbf{p}_k).$$

And since every element of $\mathbf{p}_k$ must be either -1 or 1, we find that

$$\mathbf{a} = \mathbf{p}_k Q.$$

To summarize the results:

$$\mathbf{W}\mathbf{p}_k = Q\mathbf{p}_k,$$

which implies that $\mathbf{p}_k$ is an eigenvector of $\mathbf{W}$ and Q is the corresponding eigenvalue. Each prototype vector is an eigenvector with the same eigenvalue.

ii. Note that the repeated eigenvalue Q has a Q-dimensional eigenspace associated with it: the subspace spanned by the Q prototype vectors. Now consider the subspace that is orthogonal to this eigenspace. Every vector in this subspace should be orthogonal to each prototype vector. The dimension of the orthogonal subspace will be $R - Q$. Consider the following arbitrary basis set for this orthogonal space:

$$\mathbf{z}_1, \mathbf{z}_2, \ldots, \mathbf{z}_{R-Q}.$$

If we apply any one of these basis vectors to the network we obtain:

$$\mathbf{a} = \mathbf{W}\mathbf{z}_k = \left(\sum_{q=1}^{Q} \mathbf{p}_q \mathbf{p}_q^T \right) \mathbf{z}_k = \sum_{q=1}^{Q} \mathbf{p}_q (\mathbf{p}_q^T \mathbf{z}_k) = 0,$$

since each $\mathbf{z}_k$ is orthogonal to every $\mathbf{p}_q$. This implies that each $\mathbf{z}_k$ is an eigenvector of $\mathbf{W}$ with eigenvalue 0.

To summarize, the weight matrix $\mathbf{W}$ has two eigenvalues, Q and 0. This means that any vector in the space spanned by the prototype vectors will be amplified by Q, whereas any vector that is orthogonal to the prototype vectors will be set to 0. We will revisit this concept when we discuss the performance of the Hopfield network in Chapter 18.

P7.6 **The networks we have used so far in this chapter have not included a bias vector. Consider the problem of designing a perceptron network (Figure P7.3) to recognize the following patterns:**

$$\mathbf{p}_1 = \begin{bmatrix} 1 \\ 1 \end{bmatrix} \qquad \mathbf{p}_2 = \begin{bmatrix} 2 \\ 2 \end{bmatrix}.$$

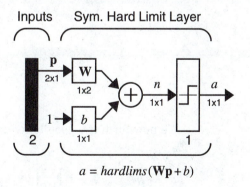

$$a = hardlims(\mathbf{W}\mathbf{p}+b)$$

Figure P7.3 Single-Neuron Perceptron

    i. Why is a bias required to solve this problem?

    ii. Use the pseudoinverse rule to design a network with bias to solve this problem.

i.   Recall from Chapters 3 and 4 that the decision boundary for the perceptron network is the line defined by:

$$\mathbf{W}\mathbf{p} + b = 0 .$$

If there is no bias, then $b = 0$ and the boundary is defined by:

$$\mathbf{W}\mathbf{p} = 0 ,$$

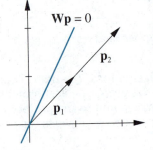

which is a line that must pass through the origin. Now consider the two vectors, $\mathbf{p}_1$ and $\mathbf{p}_2$, which are given in this problem. They are shown graphically in the figure to the left, along with an arbitrary decision boundary that passes through the origin. It is clear that no decision boundary that passes through the origin could separate these two vectors. Therefore a bias is required to solve this problem.

ii. To use the pseudoinverse rule (or the Hebb rule) when there is a bias term, we should treat the bias as another weight, with an input of 1 (as is shown in all of the network figures). We then augment the input vectors with a 1 as the last element:

$$\mathbf{p}'_1 = \begin{bmatrix} 1 \\ 1 \\ 1 \end{bmatrix} \qquad \mathbf{p}'_2 = \begin{bmatrix} 2 \\ 2 \\ 1 \end{bmatrix} .$$

Let's choose the desired outputs to be

$$t_1 = 1 \qquad t_2 = -1 ,$$

so that

$$\mathbf{P} = \begin{bmatrix} 1 & 2 \\ 1 & 2 \\ 1 & 1 \end{bmatrix}, \ \mathbf{T} = \begin{bmatrix} 1 & -1 \end{bmatrix} .$$

We now form the pseudoinverse matrix:

$$\mathbf{P}^+ = \left(\begin{bmatrix} 1 & 1 & 1 \\ 2 & 2 & 1 \end{bmatrix} \begin{bmatrix} 1 & 2 \\ 1 & 2 \\ 1 & 1 \end{bmatrix} \right)^{-1} \begin{bmatrix} 1 & 1 & 1 \\ 2 & 2 & 1 \end{bmatrix} = \begin{bmatrix} 3 & 5 \\ 5 & 9 \end{bmatrix}^{-1} \begin{bmatrix} 1 & 1 & 1 \\ 2 & 2 & 1 \end{bmatrix} = \begin{bmatrix} -0.5 & -0.5 & 2 \\ 0.5 & 0.5 & -1 \end{bmatrix} .$$

The augmented weight matrix is then computed:

$$\mathbf{W}' = \mathbf{T}\mathbf{P}^+ = \begin{bmatrix} 1 & -1 \end{bmatrix} \begin{bmatrix} -0.5 & -0.5 & 2 \\ 0.5 & 0.5 & -1 \end{bmatrix} = \begin{bmatrix} -1 & -1 & 3 \end{bmatrix} .$$

We can then pull out the standard weight matrix and bias:

$$\mathbf{W} = \begin{bmatrix} -1 & -1 \end{bmatrix} \qquad b = 3 .$$

The decision boundary for this weight and bias is shown in the Figure P7.4. This boundary does separate the two prototype vectors.

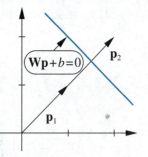

Figure P7.4 Decision Boundary for Solved Problem P7.6

P7.7 **In all of our pattern recognition examples thus far, we have represented patterns as vectors by using "1" and "–1" to represent dark and light pixels (picture elements), respectively. What if we were to use "1" and "0" instead? How should the Hebb rule be changed?**

First, let's introduce some notation to distinguish the two different representations (usually referred to as the bipolar {–1, 1} representation and the binary {0, 1} representation). The bipolar representation of the prototype input/output vectors will be denoted

$$\{\mathbf{p}_1, \mathbf{t}_1\}, \{\mathbf{p}_2, \mathbf{t}_2\}, \ldots, \{\mathbf{p}_Q, \mathbf{t}_Q\} ,$$

and the binary representation will be denoted

$$\{\mathbf{p'}_1, \mathbf{t'}_1\}, \{\mathbf{p'}_2, \mathbf{t'}_2\}, \ldots, \{\mathbf{p'}_Q, \mathbf{t'}_Q\} .$$

The relationship between the two representations is given by:

$$\mathbf{p'}_q = \frac{1}{2}\mathbf{p}_q + \frac{1}{2}\mathbf{1} \qquad \mathbf{p}_q = 2\mathbf{p'}_q - \mathbf{1} ,$$

where **1** is a vector of ones.

Next, we determine the form of the binary associative network. We will use the network shown in Figure P7.5. It is different than the bipolar associative network, as shown in Figure 7.2, in two ways. First, it uses the *hardlim* nonlinearity rather than *hardlims*, since the output should be either 0 or 1. Secondly, it uses a bias vector. It requires a bias vector because all binary vectors will fall into one quadrant of the vector space, so a boundary that passes through the origin will not always be able to divide the patterns. (See Problem P7.6.)

The next step is to determine the weight matrix and the bias vector for this network. If we want the binary network of Figure P7.5 to have the same effective response as a bipolar network (as in Figure 7.2), then the net input, **n**, should be the same for both networks:

$$\mathbf{W'p'} + \mathbf{b} = \mathbf{Wp}.$$

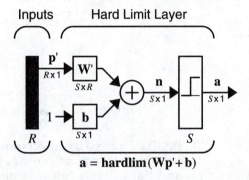

$$\mathbf{a} = \mathbf{hardlim}(\mathbf{Wp'} + \mathbf{b})$$

Figure P7.5 Binary Associative Network

This will guarantee that whenever the bipolar network produces a "1" the binary network will produce a "1", and whenever the bipolar network produces a "–1" the binary network will produce a "0".

If we then substitute for **p'** as a function of **p** we find:

$$\mathbf{W'}\left(\frac{1}{2}\mathbf{p} + \frac{1}{2}\mathbf{1}\right) + \mathbf{b} = \frac{1}{2}\mathbf{W'p} + \frac{1}{2}\mathbf{W'1} + \mathbf{b} = \mathbf{Wp}.$$

Therefore, to produce the same results as the bipolar network, we should choose

$$\mathbf{W'} = 2\mathbf{W} \qquad \mathbf{b} = -\mathbf{W1},$$

where **W** is the bipolar weight matrix.

Epilogue

We had two main objectives for this chapter. First, we wanted to introduce one of the most influential neural network learning rules: the Hebb rule. This was one of the first neural learning rules ever proposed, and yet it continues to influence even the most recent developments in network learning theory. Second, we wanted to show how the performance of this learning rule could be explained using the linear algebra concepts discussed in the two preceding chapters. This is one of the key objectives of this text. We want to show how certain important mathematical concepts underlie the operation of all artificial neural networks. We plan to continue to weave together the mathematical ideas with the neural network applications, and hope in the process to increase our understanding of both.

We will again revisit the Hebb rule in Chapters 13 and 18. In Chapter 18 we will use the Hebb rule in the design of a *recurrent* associative memory network — the Hopfield network.

The next two chapters introduce some mathematics that are critical to our understanding of the two learning laws covered in Chapters 10 and 11. Those learning laws fall under a subheading called *performance* learning, because they attempt to optimize the performance of the network. In order to understand these performance learning laws, we need to introduce some basic concepts in optimization. As with the material on the Hebb rule, our understanding of these topics in optimization will be greatly aided by our previous work in linear algebra.

7

Further Reading

[Albe72]   A. Albert, *Regression and the Moore-Penrose Pseudoinverse*, New York: Academic Press, 1972.

Albert's text is the major reference for the theory and basic properties of the pseudoinverse. Proofs are included for all major pseudoinverse theorems.

[Ande72]   J. Anderson, "A simple neural network generating an interactive memory," *Mathematical Biosciences*, vol. 14, pp. 197–220, 1972.

Anderson proposed a "linear associator" model for associative memory. The model was trained, using a generalization of the Hebb postulate, to learn an association between input and output vectors. The physiological plausibility of the network was emphasized. Kohonen published a closely related paper at the same time [Koho72], although the two researchers were working independently.

[Hebb49]   D. O. Hebb, *The Organization of Behavior*, New York: Wiley, 1949.

The main premise of this seminal book is that behavior can be explained by the action of neurons. In it, Hebb proposes one of the first learning laws, which postulated a mechanism for learning at the cellular level.

[Koho72]   T. Kohonen, "Correlation matrix memories," *IEEE Transactions on Computers*, vol. 21, pp. 353–359, 1972.

Kohonen proposed a correlation matrix model for associative memory. The model was trained, using the outer product rule (also known as the Hebb rule), to learn an association between input and output vectors. The mathematical structure of the network was emphasized. Anderson published a closely related paper at the same time [Ande72], although the two researchers were working independently.

Exercises

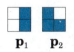

p₁ **p₂**

E7.1 Consider the prototype patterns given to the left.

    i. Are $\mathbf{p}_1$ and $\mathbf{p}_2$ orthogonal?

    ii. Use the Hebb rule to design an autoassociator network for these patterns.

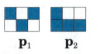

$\mathbf{p}_t$

    iii. Test the operation of the network using the test input pattern $\mathbf{p}_t$ shown to the left. Does the network perform as you expected? Explain.

E7.2 Repeat Exercise E7.1 using the pseudoinverse rule.

E7.3 Use the Hebb rule to determine the weight matrix for a perceptron network (shown in Figure E7.1) to recognize the patterns shown to the left.

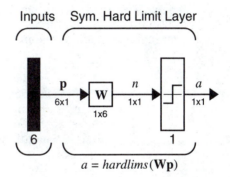

Figure E7.1 Perceptron Network for Exercise E7.3

E7.4 In Problem P7.7 we demonstrated how networks can be trained using the Hebb rule when the prototype vectors are given in binary (as opposed to bipolar) form. Repeat Exercise E7.1 using the binary representation for the prototype vectors. Show that the response of this binary network is equivalent to the response of the original bipolar network.

E7.5 Show that an autoassociator network will continue to perform if we zero the diagonal elements of a weight matrix that has been determined by the Hebb rule. In other words, suppose that the weight matrix is determined from:

$$\mathbf{W} = \mathbf{PP}^T - Q\mathbf{I},$$

where Q is the number of prototype vectors. (Hint: show that the prototype vectors continue to be eigenvectors of the new weight matrix.)

E7.6 We have three input/output prototype vector pairs:

$$\left\{ \mathbf{p}_1 = \begin{bmatrix} 1 \\ 0 \end{bmatrix}, t_1 = 1 \right\}, \left\{ \mathbf{p}_2 = \begin{bmatrix} 1 \\ 1 \end{bmatrix}, t_2 = -1 \right\}, \left\{ \mathbf{p}_3 = \begin{bmatrix} 0 \\ 1 \end{bmatrix}, t_3 = 1 \right\}.$$

    i. Show that this problem cannot be solved unless the network uses a bias.

    ii. Use the pseudoinverse rule to design a network for these prototype vectors. Verify that the network correctly transforms the prototype vectors.

E7.7 One question we might ask about the Hebb and pseudoinverse rules is: How many prototype patterns can be stored in one weight matrix? Test this experimentally using the digit recognition problem that was discussed on page 7-10. Begin with the digits "0" and "1". Add one digit at a time up to "6", and test how often the correct digit is reconstructed after randomly changing 2, 4 and 6 pixels.

    i. First use the Hebb rule to create the weight matrix for the digits "0" and "1". Then randomly change 2 pixels of each digit and apply the noisy digits to the network. Repeat this process 10 times, and record the percentage of times in which the correct pattern (without noise) is produced at the output of the network. Repeat as 4 and 6 pixels of each digit are modified. The entire process is then repeated when the digits "0", "1" and "2" are used. This continues, one digit at a time, until you test the network when all of the digits "0" through "6" are used. When you have completed all of the tests, you will be able to plot three curves showing percentage error versus number of digits stored, one curve each for 2, 4 and 6 pixel errors.

    ii. Repeat part (i) using the pseudoinverse rule, and compare the results of the two rules.

8 Performance Surfaces and Optimum Points

Objectives

This chapter lays the foundation for a type of neural network training technique called performance learning. There are several different classes of network learning laws, including associative learning (as in the Hebbian learning of Chapter 7) and competitive learning (which we will discuss in Chapter 14). Performance learning is another important class of learning law, in which the network parameters are adjusted to optimize the performance of the network. In the next two chapters we will lay the groundwork for the development of performance learning, which will then be presented in detail in Chapters 10–12. The main objective of the present chapter is to investigate performance surfaces and to determine conditions for the existence of minima and maxima of the performance surface. Chapter 9 will follow this up with a discussion of procedures to locate the minima or maxima.

8

Theory and Examples

Performance Learning There are several different learning laws that fall under the category of *performance learning*. Two of these will be presented in this text. These learning laws are distinguished by the fact that during training the network parameters (weights and biases) are adjusted in an effort to optimize the "performance" of the network.

There are two steps involved in this optimization process. The first step is to define what we mean by "performance." In other words, we must find a quantitative measure of network performance, called the *performance index*, which is small when the network performs well and large when the network performs poorly. In this chapter, and in Chapter 9, we will assume that the performance index is given. In Chapters 10 and 11 we will discuss the choice of performance index.

Performance Index

The second step of the optimization process is to search the parameter space (adjust the network weights and biases) in order to reduce the performance index. In this chapter we will investigate the characteristics of performance surfaces and set some conditions that will guarantee that a surface does have a minimum point (the optimum we are searching for). Thus, in this chapter we will obtain some understanding of what performance surfaces look like. Then, in Chapter 9 we will develop procedures for locating the optimum points.

Taylor Series

Taylor Series Expansion Let us say that the performance index that we want to minimize is represented by $F(x)$, where x is the scalar parameter we are adjusting. We will assume that the performance index is an analytic function, so that all of its derivatives exist. Then it can be represented by its *Taylor series expansion* about some nominal point x^*:

$$F(x) = F(x^*) + \frac{d}{dx}F(x)\Big|_{x = x^*}(x - x^*)$$

$$+ \frac{1}{2}\frac{d^2}{dx^2}F(x)\Big|_{x = x^*}(x - x^*)^2 + \cdots \tag{8.1}$$

$$+ \frac{1}{n!}\frac{d^n}{dx^n}F(x)\Big|_{x = x^*}(x - x^*)^n + \cdots$$

We will use the Taylor series expansion to approximate the performance index, by limiting the expansion to a finite number of terms. For example, let

$$F(x) = \cos(x) . \tag{8.2}$$

The Taylor series expansion for $F(x)$ about the point $x^* = 0$ is

$$F(x) = \cos(x) = \cos(0) - \sin(0)(x-0) - \frac{1}{2}\cos(0)(x-0)^2$$
$$+ \frac{1}{6}\sin(0)(x-0)^3 + \cdots \tag{8.3}$$

$$= 1 - \frac{1}{2}x^2 + \frac{1}{24}x^4 + \cdots$$

The zeroth-order approximation of $F(x)$ (using only the zeroth power of x) is

$$F(x) \approx F_0(x) = 1 . \tag{8.4}$$

The second-order approximation is

$$F(x) \approx F_2(x) = 1 - \frac{1}{2}x^2 . \tag{8.5}$$

(Note that in this case the first-order approximation is the same as the zeroth-order approximation, since the first derivative is zero.)

The fourth-order approximation is

$$F(x) \approx F_4(x) = 1 - \frac{1}{2}x^2 + \frac{1}{24}x^4 . \tag{8.6}$$

A graph showing $F(x)$ and these three approximations is shown in Figure 8.1.

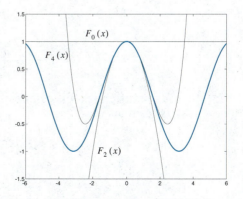

Figure 8.1 Cosine Function and Taylor Series Approximations

From the figure we can see that all three approximations are accurate if x is very close to $x^* = 0$. However, as x moves farther away from x^* only the higher-order approximations are accurate. The second-order approximation is accurate over a wider range than the zeroth-order approximation, and the fourth-order approximation is accurate over a wider range than the second-order approximation. An investigation of Eq. (8.1) explains this behavior. Each succeeding term in the series involves a higher power of $(x - x^*)$. As x gets closer to x^*, these terms will become geometrically smaller.

We will use the Taylor series approximations of the performance index to investigate the shape of the performance index in the neighborhood of possible optimum points.

To experiment with Taylor series expansions of the cosine function, use the Neural Network Design Demonstration Taylor Series (**nnd8ts**).

Vector Case

Of course the neural network performance index will not be a function of a scalar x. It will be a function of all of the network parameters (weights and biases), of which there may be a very large number. Therefore, we need to extend the Taylor series expansion to functions of many variables. Consider the following function of n variables:

$$F(\mathbf{x}) = F(x_1, x_2, \ldots, x_n).$$ (8.7)

The Taylor series expansion for this function, about the point x^*, will be

$$F(\mathbf{x}) = F(\mathbf{x}^*) + \frac{\partial}{\partial x_1} F(\mathbf{x}) \Big|_{\mathbf{x} = \mathbf{x}^*} (x_1 - x_1^*) + \frac{\partial}{\partial x_2} F(\mathbf{x}) \Big|_{\mathbf{x} = \mathbf{x}^*} (x_2 - x_2^*)$$

$$+ \cdots + \frac{\partial}{\partial x_n} F(\mathbf{x}) \Big|_{\mathbf{x} = \mathbf{x}^*} (x_n - x_n^*) + \frac{1}{2} \frac{\partial^2}{\partial x_1^2} F(\mathbf{x}) \Big|_{\mathbf{x} = \mathbf{x}^*} (x_1 - x_1^*)^2$$ (8.8)

$$+ \frac{1}{2} \frac{\partial^2}{\partial x_1 \partial x_2} F(\mathbf{x}) \Big|_{\mathbf{x} = \mathbf{x}^*} (x_1 - x_1^*)(x_2 - x_2^*) + \cdots$$

This notation is a bit cumbersome. It is more convenient to write it in matrix form, as in:

$$F(\mathbf{x}) = F(\mathbf{x}^*) + \nabla F(\mathbf{x})^T \Big|_{\mathbf{x} = \mathbf{x}^*} (\mathbf{x} - \mathbf{x}^*)$$

$$+ \frac{1}{2} (\mathbf{x} - \mathbf{x}^*)^T \nabla^2 F(\mathbf{x}) \Big|_{\mathbf{x} = \mathbf{x}^*} (\mathbf{x} - \mathbf{x}^*) + \cdots$$ (8.9)

Gradient   where $\nabla F(\mathbf{x})$ is the *gradient*, and is defined as

$$\nabla F(\mathbf{x}) = \left[\frac{\partial}{\partial x_1} F(\mathbf{x}) \quad \frac{\partial}{\partial x_2} F(\mathbf{x}) \quad \cdots \quad \frac{\partial}{\partial x_n} F(\mathbf{x}) \right]^T, \tag{8.10}$$

Hessian and $\nabla^2 F(\mathbf{x})$ is the *Hessian*, and is defined as:

$$\nabla^2 F(\mathbf{x}) = \begin{bmatrix} \frac{\partial^2}{\partial x_1^2} F(\mathbf{x}) & \frac{\partial^2}{\partial x_1 \partial x_2} F(\mathbf{x}) & \cdots & \frac{\partial^2}{\partial x_1 \partial x_n} F(\mathbf{x}) \\ \frac{\partial^2}{\partial x_2 \partial x_1} F(\mathbf{x}) & \frac{\partial^2}{\partial x_2^2} F(\mathbf{x}) & \cdots & \frac{\partial^2}{\partial x_2 \partial x_n} F(\mathbf{x}) \\ \vdots & \vdots & & \vdots \\ \frac{\partial^2}{\partial x_n \partial x_1} F(\mathbf{x}) & \frac{\partial^2}{\partial x_n \partial x_2} F(\mathbf{x}) & \cdots & \frac{\partial^2}{\partial x_n^2} F(\mathbf{x}) \end{bmatrix}. \tag{8.11}$$

The gradient and the Hessian are very important to our understanding of performance surfaces. In the next section we discuss the practical meaning of these two concepts.

To experiment with Taylor series expansions of a function of two variables, use the Neural Network Design Demonstration Vector Taylor Series (**nnd8ts2**).

Directional Derivatives

The ith element of the gradient, $\partial F(\mathbf{x}) / \partial x_i$, is the first derivative of the performance index F along the x_i axis. The ith element of the diagonal of the Hessian matrix, $\partial^2 F(\mathbf{x}) / (\partial x_i^2)$, is the second derivative of the performance index F along the x_i axis. What if we want to know the derivative of the function in an arbitrary direction? We let $\mathbf{p}$ be a vector in the direction along which we wish to know the derivative. This *directional deriva-tive* can be computed from

Directional Derivative

$$\frac{\mathbf{p}^T \nabla F(\mathbf{x})}{\|\mathbf{p}\|}. \tag{8.12}$$

The second derivative along $\mathbf{p}$ can also be computed:

$$\frac{\mathbf{p}^T \nabla^2 F(\mathbf{x}) \mathbf{p}}{\|\mathbf{p}\|^2}. \tag{8.13}$$

8

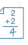

To illustrate these concepts, consider the function

$$F(\mathbf{x}) = x_1^2 + 2x_2^2. \tag{8.14}$$

Suppose that we want to know the derivative of the function at the point $\mathbf{x}^* = \begin{bmatrix} 0.5 & 0.5 \end{bmatrix}^T$ in the direction $\mathbf{p} = \begin{bmatrix} 2 & -1 \end{bmatrix}^T$. First we evaluate the gradient at $\mathbf{x}^*$:

$$\nabla F(\mathbf{x})\Big|_{\mathbf{x} = \mathbf{x}^*} = \begin{bmatrix} \dfrac{\partial}{\partial x_1} F(\mathbf{x}) \\ \dfrac{\partial}{\partial x_2} F(\mathbf{x}) \end{bmatrix}_{\mathbf{x} = \mathbf{x}^*} = \begin{bmatrix} 2x_1 \\ 4x_2 \end{bmatrix}_{\mathbf{x} = \mathbf{x}^*} = \begin{bmatrix} 1 \\ 2 \end{bmatrix}. \tag{8.15}$$

The derivative in the direction $\mathbf{p}$ can then be computed:

$$\frac{\mathbf{p}^T \nabla F(\mathbf{x})}{\|\mathbf{p}\|} = \frac{\begin{bmatrix} 2 & -1 \end{bmatrix} \begin{bmatrix} 1 \\ 2 \end{bmatrix}}{\left\| \begin{bmatrix} 2 \\ -1 \end{bmatrix} \right\|} = \frac{\begin{bmatrix} 0 \end{bmatrix}}{\sqrt{5}} = 0. \tag{8.16}$$

Therefore the function has zero slope in the direction $\mathbf{p}$ from the point $\mathbf{x}^*$. Why did this happen? What can we say about those directions that have zero slope? If we consider the definition of directional derivative in Eq. (8.12), we can see that the numerator is an inner product between the direction vector and the gradient. Therefore any direction that is orthogonal to the gradient will have zero slope.

Which direction has the greatest slope? The maximum slope will occur when the inner product of the direction vector and the gradient is a maximum. This happens when the direction vector is the same as the gradient. (Notice that the magnitude of the direction vector has no effect, since we normalize by its magnitude.) This effect is illustrated in Figure 8.2, which shows a contour plot and a 3-D plot of $F(\mathbf{x})$. On the contour plot we see five vectors starting from our nominal point $\mathbf{x}^*$ and pointing in different directions. At the end of each vector the first directional derivative is displayed. The maximum derivative occurs in the direction of the gradient. The zero derivative is in the direction orthogonal to the gradient (tangent to the contour line).

To experiment with directional derivatives, use the Neural Network Design Demonstration Directional Derivatives *(**nnd8dd**).*

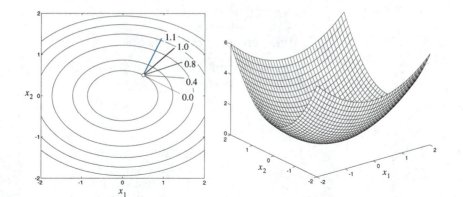

Figure 8.2 Quadratic Function and Directional Derivatives

Minima

Recall that the objective of performance learning will be to optimize the network performance index. In this section we want to define what we mean by an optimum point. We will assume that the optimum point is a minimum of the performance index. The definitions can be easily modified for maximization problems.

Strong Minimum

Strong Minimum

The point x* is a strong minimum of $F(\mathbf{x})$ **if a scalar** $\delta > 0$ **exists, such that** $F(\mathbf{x}) < F(\mathbf{x} + \Delta\mathbf{x})$ **for all** $\Delta\mathbf{x}$ **such that** $\delta > \|\Delta\mathbf{x}\| > 0$.

In other words, if we move away from a strong minimum a small distance in *any* direction the function will increase.

Global Minimum

Global Minimum

The point x* is a unique global minimum of $F(\mathbf{x})$ **if** $F(\mathbf{x}) < F(\mathbf{x} + \Delta\mathbf{x})$ **for all** $\Delta\mathbf{x} \neq \mathbf{0}$.

For a simple strong minimum, $\mathbf{x}^*$, the function may be smaller than $F(\mathbf{x}^*)$ at some points outside a small neighborhood of $\mathbf{x}^*$. Therefore this is sometimes called a local minimum. For a global minimum the function will be larger than the minimum point at every other point in the parameter space.

Weak Minimum

Weak Minimum

The point x* is a weak minimum of $F(\mathbf{x})$ **if it is not a strong minimum, and a scalar** $\delta > 0$ **exists, such that** $F(\mathbf{x}) \leq F(\mathbf{x} + \Delta\mathbf{x})$ **for all** $\Delta\mathbf{x}$ **such that** $\delta > \|\Delta\mathbf{x}\| > 0$.

8

No matter which direction we move away from a weak minimum, the function cannot decrease, although there may be some directions in which the function does not change.

As an example of local and global minimum points, consider the following scalar function:

$$F(x) = 3x^4 - 7x^2 - \frac{1}{2}x + 6. \tag{8.17}$$

This function is displayed in Figure 8.3. Notice that it has two strong minimum points: at approximately –1.1 and 1.1. For both of these points the function increases in a local neighborhood. The minimum at 1.1 is a global minimum, since there is no other point for which the function is as small.

There is no weak minimum for this function. We will show a two-dimensional example of a weak minimum later.

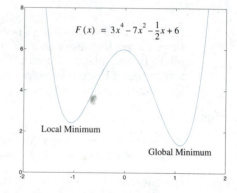

Figure 8.3 Scalar Example of Local and Global Minima

Now let's consider some vector cases. First, consider the following function:

$$F(\mathbf{x}) = (x_2 - x_1)^4 + 8x_1 x_2 - x_1 + x_2 + 3. \tag{8.18}$$

Contour Plot In Figure 8.4 we have a *contour plot* (a series of curves along which the function value remains constant) and a 3-D surface plot for this function (for function values less than 12). We can see that the function has two strong local minimum points: one at (–0.42, 0.42), and the other at (0.55, –0.55). The global minimum point is at (0.55, –0.55).

Saddle Point There is also another interesting feature of this function at (–0.13, 0.13). It is called a *saddle point* because of the shape of the surface in the neighborhood of the point. It is characterized by the fact that along the line $x_1 = -x_2$ the saddle point is a local maximum, but along a line orthogonal to that line it is a local minimum. We will investigate this example in more detail in Problems P8.2 and P8.5.

This function is used in the Neural Network Design Demonstration Vector Taylor Series (`nnd8ts2`*).*

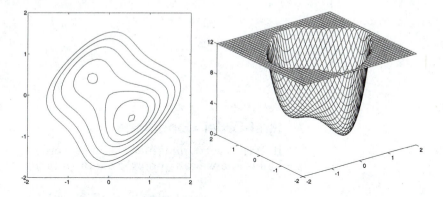

Figure 8.4 Vector Example of Minima and Saddle Point

As a final example, consider the function defined in Eq. (8.19):

$$F(\mathbf{x}) = (x_1^2 - 1.5 x_1 x_2 + 2 x_2^2) x_1^2 \qquad (8.19)$$

The contour and 3-D plots of this function are given in Figure 8.5. Here we can see that any point along the line $x_1 = 0$ is a weak minimum.

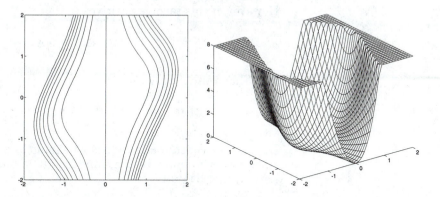

Figure 8.5 Weak Minimum Example

Necessary Conditions for Optimality

Now that we have defined what we mean by an optimum (minimum) point, let's identify some conditions that would have to be satisfied by such a point. We will again use the Taylor series expansion to derive these conditions:

$$F(\mathbf{x}) = F(\mathbf{x}^* + \Delta\mathbf{x}) = F(\mathbf{x}^*) + \nabla F(\mathbf{x})^T \Big|_{\mathbf{x} = \mathbf{x}^*} \Delta\mathbf{x}$$

$$(8.20)$$

$$+ \frac{1}{2}\Delta\mathbf{x}^T \nabla^2 F(\mathbf{x}) \Big|_{\mathbf{x} = \mathbf{x}^*} \Delta\mathbf{x} + \cdots,$$

where

$$\Delta\mathbf{x} = \mathbf{x} - \mathbf{x}^*. \qquad (8.21)$$

First-Order Conditions

If $\|\Delta\mathbf{x}\|$ is very small then the higher order terms in Eq. (8.20) will be negligible and we can approximate the function as

$$F(\mathbf{x}^* + \Delta\mathbf{x}) \cong F(\mathbf{x}^*) + \nabla F(\mathbf{x})^T \Big|_{\mathbf{x} = \mathbf{x}^*} \Delta\mathbf{x}. \qquad (8.22)$$

The point $\mathbf{x}^*$ is a candidate minimum point, which means that the function should go up (or at least not go down) if $\Delta\mathbf{x}$ is not zero. For this to happen the second term in Eq. (8.22) should not be negative. In other words

$$\nabla F(\mathbf{x})^T \Big|_{\mathbf{x} = \mathbf{x}^*} \Delta\mathbf{x} \geq 0. \qquad (8.23)$$

However, if this term is positive,

$$\nabla F(\mathbf{x})^T \Big|_{\mathbf{x} = \mathbf{x}^*} \Delta\mathbf{x} > 0, \qquad (8.24)$$

then this would imply that

$$F(\mathbf{x}^* + \Delta\mathbf{x}) \cong F(\mathbf{x}^*) - \nabla F(\mathbf{x})^T \Big|_{\mathbf{x} = \mathbf{x}^*} \Delta\mathbf{x} < F(\mathbf{x}^*). \qquad (8.25)$$

But this is a contradiction, since $\mathbf{x}^*$ should be a minimum point. Therefore, since Eq. (8.23) must be true, and Eq. (8.24) must be false, the only alternative must be that

$$\nabla F(\mathbf{x})^T \Big|_{\mathbf{x} = \mathbf{x}^*} \Delta\mathbf{x} = 0. \qquad (8.26)$$

Since this must be true for any $\Delta\mathbf{x}$, we have

$$\nabla F(\mathbf{x}) \Big|_{\mathbf{x} = \mathbf{x}^*} = \mathbf{0}. \qquad (8.27)$$

Stationary Points Therefore the gradient must be zero at a minimum point. This is a first-order, necessary (but not sufficient) condition for $\mathbf{x}^*$ to be a local minimum point. Any points that satisfy Eq. (8.27) are called *stationary points*.

Second-Order Conditions

Assume that we have a stationary point $\mathbf{x}^*$. Since the gradient of $F(\mathbf{x})$ is zero at all stationary points, the Taylor series expansion will be

$$F(\mathbf{x}^* + \Delta\mathbf{x}) = F(\mathbf{x}^*) + \frac{1}{2}\Delta\mathbf{x}^T\nabla^2 F(\mathbf{x})\Big|_{\mathbf{X} = \mathbf{x}^*}\Delta\mathbf{x} + \cdots. \tag{8.28}$$

As before, we will consider only those points in a small neighborhood of $\mathbf{x}^*$, so that $\|\Delta\mathbf{x}\|$ is small and $F(\mathbf{x})$ can be approximated by the first two terms in Eq. (8.28). Therefore a strong minimum will exist at $\mathbf{x}^*$ if

$$\Delta\mathbf{x}^T\nabla^2 F(\mathbf{x})\Big|_{\mathbf{X} = \mathbf{x}^*}\Delta\mathbf{x} > 0. \tag{8.29}$$

Positive Definite Matrix

For this to be true for arbitrary $\Delta\mathbf{x} \neq \mathbf{0}$ requires that the Hessian matrix be positive definite. (By definition, a matrix $\mathbf{A}$ is *positive definite* if

$$\mathbf{z}^T\mathbf{A}\mathbf{z} > 0 \tag{8.30}$$

Positive Semidefinite

for any vector $\mathbf{z} \neq \mathbf{0}$. It is *positive semidefinite* if

$$\mathbf{z}^T\mathbf{A}\mathbf{z} \geq 0 \tag{8.31}$$

for any vector $\mathbf{z}$. We can check these conditions by testing the eigenvalues of the matrix. If all eigenvalues are positive, then the matrix is positive definite. If all eigenvalues are nonnegative, then the matrix is positive semidefinite.)

Sufficient Condition

A positive definite Hessian matrix is a second-order, *sufficient* condition for a strong minimum to exist. It is not a necessary condition. A minimum can still be strong if the second-order term of the Taylor series is zero, but the third-order term is positive. Therefore the second-order, *necessary* condition for a strong minimum is that the Hessian matrix be positive semidefinite.

To illustrate these conditions, consider the following function of two variables:

$$F(\mathbf{x}) = x_1^4 + x_2^2. \tag{8.32}$$

First, we want to locate any stationary points, so we need to evaluate the gradient:

$$\nabla F(\mathbf{x}) = \begin{bmatrix} 4x_1^3 \\ 2x_2 \end{bmatrix} = \mathbf{0}. \tag{8.33}$$

Therefore the only stationary point is the point $\mathbf{x}^* = \mathbf{0}$. We now need to test the second-order condition, which requires the Hessian matrix:

$$\nabla^2 F(\mathbf{x})\Big|_{\mathbf{x}=\mathbf{0}} = \begin{bmatrix} 12x_1^2 & 0 \\ 0 & 2 \end{bmatrix}\Bigg|_{\mathbf{x}=\mathbf{0}} = \begin{bmatrix} 0 & 0 \\ 0 & 2 \end{bmatrix}. \tag{8.34}$$

This matrix is positive semidefinite, which is a necessary condition for $\mathbf{x}^* = \mathbf{0}$ to be a strong minimum point. We cannot guarantee from first-order and second-order conditions that it is a minimum point, but we have not eliminated it as a possibility. Actually, even though the Hessian matrix is only positive semidefinite, $\mathbf{x}^* = \mathbf{0}$ is a strong minimum point, but we cannot prove it from the conditions we have discussed.

Just to summarize, the necessary conditions for $\mathbf{x}^*$ to be a minimum, strong or weak, of $F(\mathbf{x})$ are:

$$\nabla F(\mathbf{x})\Big|_{\mathbf{x}=\mathbf{x}^*} = \mathbf{0} \text{ and } \nabla^2 F(\mathbf{x})\Big|_{\mathbf{x}=\mathbf{x}^*} \text{ positive semidefinite.}$$

The sufficient conditions for $\mathbf{x}^*$ to be a strong minimum point of $F(\mathbf{x})$ are:

$$\nabla F(\mathbf{x})\Big|_{\mathbf{x}=\mathbf{x}^*} = \mathbf{0} \text{ and } \nabla^2 F(\mathbf{x})\Big|_{\mathbf{x}=\mathbf{x}^*} \text{ positive definite.}$$

Quadratic Functions

We will find throughout this text that one type of performance index is universal — the quadratic function. This is true because there are many applications in which the quadratic function appears, but also because many functions can be approximated by quadratic functions in small neighborhoods, especially near local minimum points. For this reason we want to spend a little time investigating the characteristics of the quadratic function.

Quadratic Function The general form of a *quadratic function* is

$$F(\mathbf{x}) = \frac{1}{2}\mathbf{x}^T\mathbf{A}\mathbf{x} + \mathbf{d}^T\mathbf{x} + c, \tag{8.35}$$

where the matrix $\mathbf{A}$ is symmetric. (If the matrix is not symmetric it can be replaced by a symmetric matrix that produces the same $F(\mathbf{x})$. Try it!)

To find the gradient for this function, we will use the following useful properties of the gradient:

$$\nabla(\mathbf{h}^T\mathbf{x}) = \nabla(\mathbf{x}^T\mathbf{h}) = \mathbf{h}, \tag{8.36}$$

where $\mathbf{h}$ is a constant vector, and

$$\nabla \mathbf{x}^T \mathbf{Q} \mathbf{x} \ = \ \mathbf{Q} \mathbf{x} + \mathbf{Q}^T \mathbf{x} \ = \ 2\mathbf{Q} \mathbf{x} \ \text{(for symmetric } \mathbf{Q}). \tag{8.37}$$

We can now compute the gradient of $F(\mathbf{x})$:

$$\nabla F(\mathbf{x}) \ = \ \mathbf{A} \mathbf{x} + \mathbf{d}, \tag{8.38}$$

and in a similar way we can find the Hessian:

$$\nabla^2 F(\mathbf{x}) \ = \ \mathbf{A}. \tag{8.39}$$

All higher derivatives of the quadratic function are zero. Therefore the first three terms of the Taylor series expansion (as in Eq. (8.20)) give an exact representation of the function. We can also say that all analytic functions behave like quadratics over a small neighborhood (i.e., when $\|\Delta \mathbf{x}\|$ is small).

Eigensystem of the Hessian

We now want to investigate the general shape of the quadratic function. It turns out that we can tell a lot about the shape by looking at the eigenvalues and eigenvectors of the Hessian matrix. Consider a quadratic function that has a stationary point at the origin, and whose value there is zero:

$$F(\mathbf{x}) \ = \ \frac{1}{2}\mathbf{x}^T \mathbf{A} \mathbf{x}. \tag{8.40}$$

The shape of this function can be seen more clearly if we perform a change of basis (see Chapter 6). We want to use the eigenvectors of the Hessian matrix, $\mathbf{A}$, as the new basis vectors. Since $\mathbf{A}$ is symmetric, its eigenvectors will be mutually orthogonal. (See [Brog91].) This means that if we make up a matrix with the eigenvectors as the columns, as in Eq. (6.68):

$$\mathbf{B} \ = \ \left[\mathbf{z}_1 \ \mathbf{z}_2 \ ... \ \mathbf{z}_n \right], \tag{8.41}$$

the inverse of the matrix will be the same as the transpose:

$$\mathbf{B}^{-1} \ = \ \mathbf{B}^T. \tag{8.42}$$

(This assumes that we have normalized the eigenvectors.)

If we now perform a change of basis, so that the eigenvectors are the basis vectors (as in Eq. (6.69)), the new $\mathbf{A}$ matrix will be

$$\mathbf{A}' \ = \ [\mathbf{B}^T \mathbf{A} \mathbf{B}] \ = \ \begin{bmatrix} \lambda_1 & 0 & ... & 0 \\ 0 & \lambda_2 & ... & 0 \\ \vdots & \vdots & & \vdots \\ 0 & 0 & ... & \lambda_n \end{bmatrix} = \Lambda, \tag{8.43}$$

where the λ_i are the eigenvalues of $\mathbf{A}$. We can also write this equation as

$$\mathbf{A} = \mathbf{B\Lambda B}^T. \tag{8.44}$$

We will now use the concept of the directional derivative to explain the physical meaning of the eigenvalues and eigenvectors of $\mathbf{A}$, and to explain how they determine the shape of the surface of the quadratic function.

Recall from Eq. (8.13) that the second derivative of a function $F(\mathbf{x})$ in the direction of a vector $\mathbf{p}$ is given by

$$\frac{\mathbf{p}^T \nabla^2 F(\mathbf{x}) \mathbf{p}}{\|\mathbf{p}\|^2} = \frac{\mathbf{p}^T \mathbf{A} \mathbf{p}}{\|\mathbf{p}\|^2}. \tag{8.45}$$

Now define

$$\mathbf{p} = \mathbf{Bc}, \tag{8.46}$$

where $\mathbf{c}$ is the representation of the vector $\mathbf{p}$ with respect to the eigenvectors of $\mathbf{A}$. (See Eq. (6.28) and the discussion that follows.) With this definition, and Eq. (8.44), we can rewrite Eq. (8.45):

$$\frac{\mathbf{p}^T \mathbf{A} \mathbf{p}}{\|\mathbf{p}\|^2} = \frac{\mathbf{c}^T \mathbf{B}^T (\mathbf{B\Lambda B}^T) \mathbf{Bc}}{\mathbf{c}^T \mathbf{B}^T \mathbf{Bc}} = \frac{\mathbf{c}^T \mathbf{\Lambda c}}{\mathbf{c}^T \mathbf{c}} = \frac{\sum_{i=1}^{n} \lambda_i c_i^2}{\sum_{i=1}^{n} c_i^2}. \tag{8.47}$$

This result tells us several useful things. First, note that this second derivative is just a weighted average of the eigenvalues. Therefore it can never be larger that the largest eigenvalue, or smaller than the smallest eigenvalue. In other words,

$$\lambda_{min} \le \frac{\mathbf{p}^T \mathbf{A} \mathbf{p}}{\|\mathbf{p}\|^2} \le \lambda_{max}. \tag{8.48}$$

Under what condition, if any, will this second derivative be equal to the largest eigenvalue? What if we choose

$$\mathbf{p} = \mathbf{z}_{max}, \tag{8.49}$$

where $\mathbf{z}_{max}$ is the eigenvector associated with the largest eigenvalue, λ_{max}? For this case the $\mathbf{c}$ vector will be

$$\mathbf{c} = \mathbf{B}^T \mathbf{p} = \mathbf{B}^T \mathbf{z}_{max} = \begin{bmatrix} 0 & 0 & \dots & 0 & 1 & 0 & \dots & 0 \end{bmatrix}^T, \tag{8.50}$$

where the one occurs only in the position that corresponds to the largest eigenvalue (i.e., $c_{max} = 1$). This is because the eigenvectors are orthonormal.

If we now substitute $\mathbf{z}_{max}$ for $\mathbf{p}$ in Eq. (8.47) we obtain

$$\frac{\mathbf{z}_{max}^{T}\mathbf{A}\mathbf{z}_{max}}{\|\mathbf{z}_{max}\|^2} = \frac{\sum\limits_{i=1}^{n}\lambda_i c_i^2}{\sum\limits_{i=1}^{n}c_i^2} = \lambda_{max}. \tag{8.51}$$

So the maximum second derivative occurs in the direction of the eigenvector that corresponds to the largest eigenvalue. In fact, in each of the eigenvector directions the second derivatives will be equal to the corresponding eigenvalue. In other directions the second derivative will be a weighted average of the eigenvalues. The eigenvalues are the second derivatives in the directions of the eigenvectors.

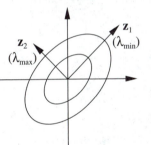

The eigenvectors define a new coordinate system in which the quadratic cross terms vanish. The eigenvectors are known as the principal axes of the function contours. The figure to the left illustrates these concepts in two dimensions. This figure illustrates the case where the first eigenvalue is smaller than the second eigenvalue. Therefore the minimum curvature (second derivative) will occur in the direction of the first eigenvector. This means that we will cross contour lines more slowly in this direction. The maximum curvature will occur in the direction of the second eigenvector, therefore we will cross contour lines more quickly in that direction.

One caveat about this figure: it is only valid when both eigenvalues have the same sign, so that we have either a strong minimum or a strong maximum. For these cases the contour lines are always elliptical. We will provide examples later where the eigenvalues have opposite signs and where one of the eigenvalues is zero.

For our first example, consider the following function:

$$F(\mathbf{x}) = x_1^2 + x_2^2 = \frac{1}{2}\mathbf{x}^T\begin{bmatrix} 2 & 0 \\ 0 & 2 \end{bmatrix}\mathbf{x}. \tag{8.52}$$

The Hessian matrix and its eigenvalues and eigenvectors are

$$\nabla^2 F(\mathbf{x}) = \begin{bmatrix} 2 & 0 \\ 0 & 2 \end{bmatrix}, \lambda_1 = 2, \mathbf{z}_1 = \begin{bmatrix} 1 \\ 0 \end{bmatrix}, \lambda_2 = 2, \mathbf{z}_2 = \begin{bmatrix} 0 \\ 1 \end{bmatrix}. \tag{8.53}$$

(Actually, any two independent vectors could be the eigenvectors in this case. There is a repeated eigenvalue, and its eigenvector is the plane.)

8

Since all the eigenvalues are equal, the curvature should be the same in all directions, and therefore the function should have circular contours. Figure 8.6 shows the contour and 3-D plots for this function, a circular hollow.

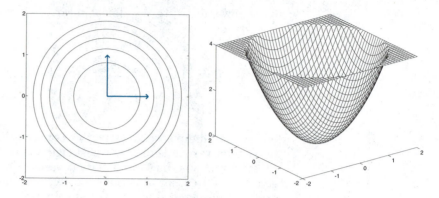

Figure 8.6 Circular Hollow

Let's try an example with distinct eigenvalues. Consider the following quadratic function:

$$F(\mathbf{x}) = x_1^2 + x_1 x_2 + x_2^2 = \frac{1}{2}\mathbf{x}^T \begin{bmatrix} 2 & 1 \\ 1 & 2 \end{bmatrix} \mathbf{x} \tag{8.54}$$

The Hessian matrix and its eigenvalues and eigenvectors are

$$\nabla^2 F(\mathbf{x}) = \begin{bmatrix} 2 & 1 \\ 1 & 2 \end{bmatrix}, \; \lambda_1 = 1, \; \mathbf{z}_1 = \begin{bmatrix} 1 \\ -1 \end{bmatrix}, \; \lambda_2 = 3, \; \mathbf{z}_2 = \begin{bmatrix} 1 \\ 1 \end{bmatrix}. \tag{8.55}$$

(As we discussed in Chapter 6, the eigenvectors are not unique, they can be multiplied by any scalar.) In this case the maximum curvature is in the direction of $\mathbf{z}_2$ so we should cross contour lines more quickly in that direction. Figure 8.7 shows the contour and 3-D plots for this function, an elliptical hollow.

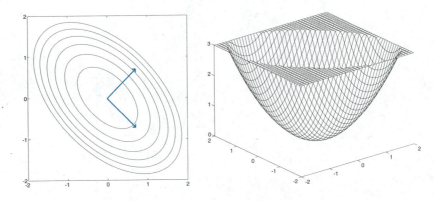

Figure 8.7 Elliptical Hollow

What happens when the eigenvalues have opposite signs? Consider the following function:

$$F(\mathbf{x}) = -\frac{1}{4}x_1^2 - \frac{3}{2}x_1 x_2 - \frac{1}{4}x_2^2 = \frac{1}{2}\mathbf{x}^T \begin{bmatrix} -0.5 & -1.5 \\ -1.5 & -0.5 \end{bmatrix} \mathbf{x}. \tag{8.56}$$

The Hessian matrix and its eigenvalues and eigenvectors are

$$\nabla^2 F(\mathbf{x}) = \begin{bmatrix} -0.5 & -1.5 \\ -1.5 & -0.5 \end{bmatrix}, \; \lambda_1 = 1, \; \mathbf{z}_1 = \begin{bmatrix} -1 \\ 1 \end{bmatrix}, \; \lambda_2 = -2, \; \mathbf{z}_2 = \begin{bmatrix} -1 \\ -1 \end{bmatrix}. \tag{8.57}$$

The first eigenvalue is positive, so there is positive curvature in the direction of $\mathbf{z}_1$. The second eigenvalue is negative, so there is negative curvature in the direction of $\mathbf{z}_2$. Also, since the magnitude of the second eigenvalue is greater than the magnitude of the first eigenvalue, we will cross contour lines faster in the direction of $\mathbf{z}_2$.

Figure 8.8 shows the contour and 3-D plots for this function, an elongated saddle. Note that the stationary point,

$$\mathbf{x}^* = \begin{bmatrix} 0 \\ 0 \end{bmatrix}, \tag{8.58}$$

is no longer a strong minimum point, since the Hessian matrix is not positive definite. Since the eigenvalues are of opposite sign, we know that the Hessian is indefinite (see [Brog91]). The stationary point is therefore a saddle point. It is a minimum of the function along the first eigenvector (positive eigenvalue), but it is a maximum of the function along the second eigenvector (negative eigenvalue).

8

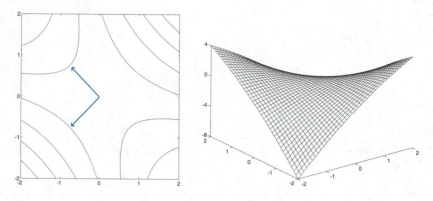

Figure 8.8 Elongated Saddle

As a final example, let's try a case where one of the eigenvalues is zero. An example of this is given by the following function:

$$F(\mathbf{x}) = \frac{1}{2}x_1^2 - x_1 x_2 + \frac{1}{2}x_2^2 = \frac{1}{2}\mathbf{x}^T \begin{bmatrix} 1 & -1 \\ -1 & 1 \end{bmatrix} \mathbf{x}. \tag{8.59}$$

The Hessian matrix and its eigenvalues and eigenvectors are

$$\nabla^2 F(\mathbf{x}) = \begin{bmatrix} 1 & -1 \\ -1 & 1 \end{bmatrix}, \lambda_1 = 1, \mathbf{z}_1 = \begin{bmatrix} -1 \\ 1 \end{bmatrix}, \lambda_2 = 0, \mathbf{z}_2 = \begin{bmatrix} -1 \\ -1 \end{bmatrix}. \tag{8.60}$$

The second eigenvalue is zero, so we would expect to have zero curvature along $\mathbf{z}_2$. Figure 8.9 shows the contour and 3-D plots for this function, a stationary valley. In this case the Hessian matrix is positive semidefinite, and we have a weak minimum along the line

$$x_1 = x_2, \tag{8.61}$$

corresponding to the second eigenvector.

For quadratic functions the Hessian matrix must be positive definite in order for a strong minimum to exist. For higher-order functions it is possible to have a strong minimum with a positive semidefinite Hessian matrix, as we discussed previously in the section on minima.

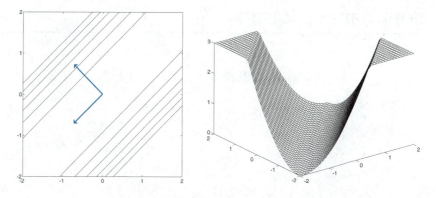

Figure 8.9 Stationary Valley

 To experiment with other quadratic functions, use the Neural Network Design Demonstration Quadratic Function (**nnd8qf**).

At this point we can summarize some characteristics of the quadratic function.

1. If the eigenvalues of the Hessian matrix are all positive, the function will have a single strong minimum.

2. If the eigenvalues are all negative, the function will have a single strong maximum.

3. If some eigenvalues are positive and other eigenvalues are negative, the function will have a single saddle point.

4. If the eigenvalues are all nonnegative, but some eigenvalues are zero, then the function will either have a weak minimum (as in Figure 8.9) or will have no stationary point (see Solved Problem P8.7).

5. If the eigenvalues are all nonpositive, but some eigenvalues are zero, then the function will either have a weak maximum or will have no stationary point.

We should note that in this discussion we have assumed, for simplicity, that the stationary point of the quadratic function was at the origin, and that it had a zero value there. This requires that the terms $\mathbf{d}$ and c in Eq. (8.35) both be zero. If c is nonzero then the function is simply increased in magnitude by c at every point. The shape of the contours do not change. When $\mathbf{d}$ is nonzero, and $\mathbf{A}$ is invertible, the shape of the contours are not changed, but the stationary point of the function moves to

$$\mathbf{x}^* = -\mathbf{A}^{-1}\mathbf{d}. \tag{8.62}$$

If $\mathbf{A}$ is not invertible (has some zero eigenvalues) and $\mathbf{d}$ is nonzero then no stationary points will exist (see Solved Problem P8.7).

Summary of Results

Taylor Series

$$F(\mathbf{x}) = F(\mathbf{x}^*) + \nabla F(\mathbf{x})^T \Big|_{\mathbf{x} = \mathbf{x}^*} (\mathbf{x} - \mathbf{x}^*)$$

$$+ \frac{1}{2}(\mathbf{x} - \mathbf{x}^*)^T \nabla^2 F(\mathbf{x}) \Big|_{\mathbf{x} = \mathbf{x}^*} (\mathbf{x} - \mathbf{x}^*) + \cdots$$

Gradient

$$\nabla F(\mathbf{x}) = \left[\frac{\partial}{\partial x_1} F(\mathbf{x}) \quad \frac{\partial}{\partial x_2} F(\mathbf{x}) \quad \cdots \quad \frac{\partial}{\partial x_n} F(\mathbf{x}) \right]^T$$

Hessian Matrix

$$\nabla^2 F(\mathbf{x}) = \begin{bmatrix} \dfrac{\partial^2}{\partial x_1^2} F(\mathbf{x}) & \dfrac{\partial^2}{\partial x_1 \partial x_2} F(\mathbf{x}) & \cdots & \dfrac{\partial^2}{\partial x_1 \partial x_n} F(\mathbf{x}) \\[2ex] \dfrac{\partial^2}{\partial x_2 \partial x_1} F(\mathbf{x}) & \dfrac{\partial^2}{\partial x_2^2} F(\mathbf{x}) & \cdots & \dfrac{\partial^2}{\partial x_2 \partial x_n} F(\mathbf{x}) \\[2ex] \vdots & \vdots & & \vdots \\[2ex] \dfrac{\partial^2}{\partial x_n \partial x_1} F(\mathbf{x}) & \dfrac{\partial^2}{\partial x_n \partial x_2} F(\mathbf{x}) & \cdots & \dfrac{\partial^2}{\partial x_n^2} F(\mathbf{x}) \end{bmatrix}$$

Directional Derivatives

First Directional Derivative

$$\frac{\mathbf{p}^T \nabla F(\mathbf{x})}{\|\mathbf{p}\|}$$

Second Directional Derivative

$$\frac{\mathbf{p}^T \nabla^2 F(\mathbf{x}) \mathbf{p}}{\|\mathbf{p}\|^2}$$

Minima

Strong Minimum

The point $\mathbf{x}^*$ is a strong minimum of $F(\mathbf{x})$ if a scalar $\delta > 0$ exists, such that $F(\mathbf{x}) < F(\mathbf{x} + \Delta\mathbf{x})$ for all $\Delta\mathbf{x}$ such that $\delta > \|\Delta\mathbf{x}\| > 0$.

Global Minimum

The point $\mathbf{x}^*$ is a unique global minimum of $F(\mathbf{x})$ if $F(\mathbf{x}) < F(\mathbf{x} + \Delta\mathbf{x})$ for all $\Delta\mathbf{x} \neq \mathbf{0}$.

Weak Minimum

The point $\mathbf{x}^*$ is a weak minimum of $F(\mathbf{x})$ if it is not a strong minimum, and a scalar $\delta > 0$ exists, such that $F(\mathbf{x}) \leq F(\mathbf{x} + \Delta\mathbf{x})$ for all $\Delta\mathbf{x}$ such that $\delta > \|\Delta\mathbf{x}\| > 0$.

Necessary Conditions for Optimality

First-Order Condition

$$\nabla F(\mathbf{x}) \Big|_{\mathbf{x} = \mathbf{x}^*} = \mathbf{0} \text{ (Stationary Points)}$$

Second-Order Condition

$$\nabla^2 F(\mathbf{x}) \Big|_{\mathbf{x} = \mathbf{x}^*} \geq 0 \text{ (Positive Semidefinite Hessian Matrix)}$$

Quadratic Functions

$$F(\mathbf{x}) = \frac{1}{2}\mathbf{x}^T \mathbf{A}\mathbf{x} + \mathbf{d}^T \mathbf{x} + c$$

Gradient

$$\nabla F(\mathbf{x}) = \mathbf{A}\mathbf{x} + \mathbf{d}$$

Hessian

$$\nabla^2 F(\mathbf{x}) = \mathbf{A}$$

Directional Derivatives

$$\lambda_{min} \leq \frac{\mathbf{p}^T \mathbf{A}\mathbf{p}}{\|\mathbf{p}\|^2} \leq \lambda_{max}$$

8

Solved Problems

P8.1 **In Figure 8.1 we illustrated 3 approximations to the cosine function about the point $x^* = 0$. Repeat that procedure about the point $x^* = \pi/2$.**

The function we want to approximate is

$$F(x) = \cos(x).$$

The Taylor series expansion for $F(x)$ about the point $x^* = \pi/2$ is

$$F(x) = \cos(x) = \cos\left(\frac{\pi}{2}\right) - \sin\left(\frac{\pi}{2}\right)\left(x - \frac{\pi}{2}\right) - \frac{1}{2}\cos\left(\frac{\pi}{2}\right)\left(x - \frac{\pi}{2}\right)^2$$

$$+ \frac{1}{6}\sin\left(\frac{\pi}{2}\right)\left(x - \frac{\pi}{2}\right)^3 + \cdots$$

$$= -\left(x - \frac{\pi}{2}\right) + \frac{1}{6}\left(x - \frac{\pi}{2}\right)^3 - \frac{1}{120}\left(x - \frac{\pi}{2}\right)^5 + \cdots$$

The zeroth-order approximation of $F(x)$ is

$$F(x) \approx F_0(x) = 0.$$

The first-order approximation is

$$F(\mathbf{x}) \approx F_1(x) = -\left(x - \frac{\pi}{2}\right) = \frac{\pi}{2} - x.$$

(Note that in this case the second-order approximation is the same as the first-order approximation, since the second derivative is zero.)

The third-order approximation is

$$F(\mathbf{x}) \approx F_3(x) = -\left(x - \frac{\pi}{2}\right) + \frac{1}{6}\left(x - \frac{\pi}{2}\right)^3.$$

A graph showing $F(x)$ and these three approximations is shown in Figure P8.1. Note that in this case the zeroth-order approximation is very poor, while the first-order approximation is accurate over a reasonably wide range. Compare this result with Figure 8.1. In that case we were expanding about a local maximum point, $x^* = 0$, so the first derivative was zero.

Check the Taylor series expansions at other points using the Neural Network Design Demonstration Taylor Series (**nnd8ts**).

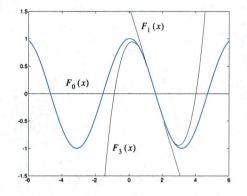

Figure P8.1 Cosine Approximation About $x = \pi/2$

P8.2 **Recall the function that is displayed in Figure 8.4, on page 8-9. We know that this function has two strong minima. Find the second-order Taylor series expansions for this function about the two minima.**

The equation for this function is

$$F(\mathbf{x}) = (x_2 - x_1)^4 + 8x_1 x_2 - x_1 + x_2 + 3.$$

To find the second-order Taylor series expansion, we need to find the gradient and the Hessian for $F(\mathbf{x})$. For the gradient we have

$$\nabla F(\mathbf{x}) = \begin{bmatrix} \dfrac{\partial}{\partial x_1} F(\mathbf{x}) \\[2mm] \dfrac{\partial}{\partial x_2} F(\mathbf{x}) \end{bmatrix} = \begin{bmatrix} -4(x_2 - x_1)^3 + 8x_2 - 1 \\[2mm] 4(x_2 - x_1)^3 + 8x_1 + 1 \end{bmatrix},$$

and the Hessian matrix is

$$\nabla^2 F(\mathbf{x}) = \begin{bmatrix} \dfrac{\partial^2}{\partial x_1^2} F(\mathbf{x}) & \dfrac{\partial^2}{\partial x_1 \partial x_2} F(\mathbf{x}) \\[3mm] \dfrac{\partial^2}{\partial x_2 \partial x_1} F(\mathbf{x}) & \dfrac{\partial^2}{\partial x_2^2} F(\mathbf{x}) \end{bmatrix}$$

$$= \begin{bmatrix} 12(x_2 - x_1)^2 & -12(x_2 - x_1)^2 + 8 \\[2mm] -12(x_2 - x_1)^2 + 8 & 12(x_2 - x_1)^2 \end{bmatrix}$$

8

One strong minimum occurs at $\mathbf{x}^1 = \begin{bmatrix} -0.42 & 0.42 \end{bmatrix}^T$, and the other at $\mathbf{x}^2 = \begin{bmatrix} 0.55 & -0.55 \end{bmatrix}^T$. If we perform the second-order Taylor series expansion of $F(\mathbf{x})$ about these two points we obtain:

$$F^1(\mathbf{x}) = F(\mathbf{x}^1) + \nabla F(\mathbf{x})^T \Big|_{\mathbf{x}=\mathbf{x}^1} (\mathbf{x}-\mathbf{x}^1) + \frac{1}{2}(\mathbf{x}-\mathbf{x}^1)^T \nabla^2 F(\mathbf{x}) \Big|_{\mathbf{x}=\mathbf{x}^1} (\mathbf{x}-\mathbf{x}^1)$$

$$= 2.93 + \frac{1}{2}\left(\mathbf{x} - \begin{bmatrix} -0.42 \\ 0.42 \end{bmatrix}\right)^T \begin{bmatrix} 8.42 & -0.42 \\ -0.42 & 8.42 \end{bmatrix} \left(\mathbf{x} - \begin{bmatrix} -0.42 \\ 0.42 \end{bmatrix}\right).$$

If we simplify this expression we find

$$F^1(\mathbf{x}) = 4.49 - \begin{bmatrix} -3.7128 & 3.7128 \end{bmatrix}\mathbf{x} + \frac{1}{2}\mathbf{x}^T \begin{bmatrix} 8.42 & -0.42 \\ -0.42 & 8.42 \end{bmatrix}\mathbf{x}.$$

Repeating this process for $\mathbf{x}^2$ results in

$$F^2(\mathbf{x}) = 7.41 - \begin{bmatrix} 11.781 & -11.781 \end{bmatrix}\mathbf{x} + \frac{1}{2}\mathbf{x}^T \begin{bmatrix} 14.71 & -6.71 \\ -6.71 & 14.71 \end{bmatrix}\mathbf{x}.$$

The original function and the two approximations are plotted in the following figures.

 *Check the Taylor series expansions at other points using the Neural Network Design Demonstration Vector Taylor Series (**nnd8ts2**).*

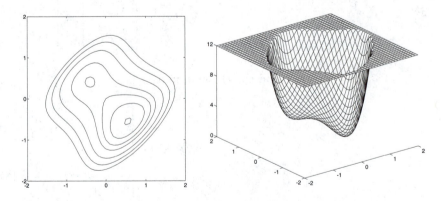

Figure P8.2 Function $F(\mathbf{x})$ for Problem P8.2

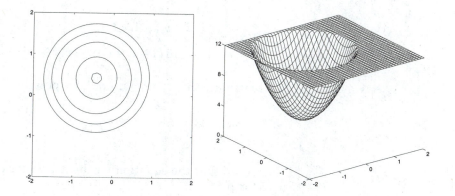

Figure P8.3 Function $F^1(\mathbf{x})$ for Problem P8.2

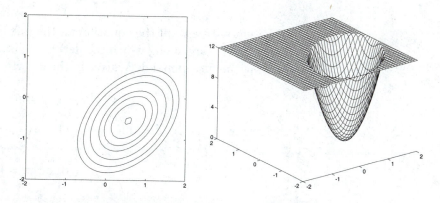

Figure P8.4 Function $F^2(\mathbf{x})$ for Problem P8.2

P8.3 **For the function** $F(\mathbf{x})$ **given below, find the equation for the line that is tangent to the contour line at** $\mathbf{x} = \begin{bmatrix} 0 & 0 \end{bmatrix}^T$.

$$F(\mathbf{x}) = (2 + x_1)^2 + 5(1 - x_1 - x_2^2)^2$$

To solve this problem we can use the directional derivative. What is the derivative of $F(\mathbf{x})$ along a line that is tangent to a contour line? Since the contour is a line along which the function does not change, the derivative of $F(\mathbf{x})$ should be zero in the direction of the contour. So we can get the equation for the tangent to the contour line by setting the directional derivative equal to zero.

First we need to find the gradient:

$$\nabla F(\mathbf{x}) = \begin{bmatrix} 2(2+x_1) + 10(1-x_1-x_2^2)(-1) \\ 10(1-x_1-x_2^2)(-2x_2) \end{bmatrix} = \begin{bmatrix} -6 + 12x_1 + 10x_2^2 \\ -20x_2 + 20x_1x_2 + 20x_2^3 \end{bmatrix}.$$

If we evaluate this at $\mathbf{x}^* = \begin{bmatrix} 0 & 0 \end{bmatrix}^T$, we obtain

$$\nabla F(\mathbf{x}^*) = \begin{bmatrix} -6 \\ 0 \end{bmatrix}.$$

Now recall that the equation for the derivative of $F(\mathbf{x})$ in the direction of a vector $\mathbf{p}$ is

$$\frac{\mathbf{p}^T \nabla F(\mathbf{x})}{\|\mathbf{p}\|}.$$

Therefore if we want the equation for the line that passes through $\mathbf{x}^* = \begin{bmatrix} 0 & 0 \end{bmatrix}^T$ and along which the derivative is zero, we can set the numerator of the directional derivative in the direction of $\Delta\mathbf{x}$ to zero:

$$\Delta\mathbf{x}^T \nabla F(\mathbf{x}^*) = 0,$$

where $\Delta\mathbf{x} = \mathbf{x} - \mathbf{x}^*$. For this case we have

$$\mathbf{x}^T \begin{bmatrix} -6 \\ 0 \end{bmatrix} = 0, \text{ or } x_1 = 0.$$

This result is illustrated in Figure P8.5.

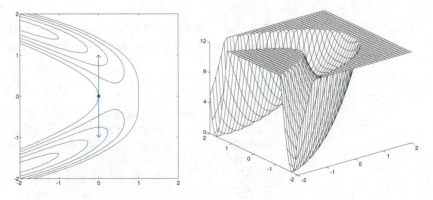

Figure P8.5 Plot of $F(\mathbf{x})$ for Problem P8.3

P8.4 **Consider the following fourth-order polynomial:**

$$F(x) = x^4 - \frac{2}{3}x^3 - 2x^2 + 2x + 4.$$

Find any stationary points and test them to see if they are minima.

To find the stationary points we set the derivative of $F(x)$ to zero:

$$\frac{d}{dx}F(x) = 4x^3 - 2x^2 - 4x + 2 = 0.$$

We can use MATLAB to find the roots of this polynomial:

```
coef=[4 -2 -4 2];
stapoints=roots(coef);
stapoints'
ans =
   1.0000   -1.0000   0.5000
```

Now we need to check the second derivative at each of these points. The second derivative of $F(x)$ is

$$\frac{d^2}{dx^2}F(x) = 12x^2 - 4x - 4.$$

If we evaluate this at each of the stationary points we find

$$\left(\frac{d^2}{dx^2}F(1) = 4\right), \left(\frac{d^2}{dx^2}F(-1) = 12\right), \left(\frac{d^2}{dx^2}F(0.5) = -3\right).$$

Therefore we should have strong local minima at 1 and –1 (since the second derivatives were positive), and a strong local maximum at 0.5 (since the second derivative was negative). To find the global minimum we would have to evaluate the function at the two local minima:

$$(F(1) = 4.333), (F(-1) = 1.667).$$

Therefore the global minimum occurs at –1. But are we sure that this is a global minimum? What happens to the function as $x \to \infty$ or $x \to -\infty$? In this case, because the highest power of x has a positive coefficient and is an even power (x^4), the function goes to ∞ at both limits. So we can safely say that the global minimum occurs at –1. The function is plotted in Figure P8.6.

8

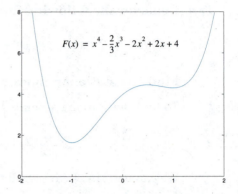

Figure P8.6 Graph of $F(x)$ for Problem P8.4

P8.5 Look back to the function of Problem P8.2. This function has three stationary points:

$$\mathbf{x}^1 = \begin{bmatrix} -0.42 \\ 0.42 \end{bmatrix}, \mathbf{x}^2 = \begin{bmatrix} -0.13 \\ 0.13 \end{bmatrix}, \mathbf{x}^3 = \begin{bmatrix} 0.55 \\ -0.55 \end{bmatrix}.$$

Test whether or not any of these points could be local minima.

From Problem P8.2 we know that the Hessian matrix for the function is

$$\nabla^2 F(\mathbf{x}) = \begin{bmatrix} 12(x_2 - x_1)^2 & -12(x_2 - x_1)^2 + 8 \\ -12(x_2 - x_1)^2 + 8 & 12(x_2 - x_1)^2 \end{bmatrix}.$$

To test the definiteness of this matrix we can check the eigenvalues. If the eigenvalues are all positive, the Hessian is positive definite, which guarantees a strong minimum. If the eigenvalues are nonnegative, the Hessian is positive semidefinite, which is consistent with either a strong or a weak minimum. If one eigenvalue is positive and the other eigenvalue is negative, the Hessian is indefinite, which would signal a saddle point.

If we evaluate the Hessian at $\mathbf{x}^1$, we find

$$\nabla^2 F(\mathbf{x}^1) = \begin{bmatrix} 8.42 & -0.42 \\ -0.42 & 8.42 \end{bmatrix}.$$

The eigenvalues of this matrix are

$$\lambda_1 = 8.84, \lambda_2 = 8.0,$$

therefore $\mathbf{x}^1$ must be a strong minimum point.

If we evaluate the Hessian at $\mathbf{x}^2$, we find

$$\nabla^2 F(\mathbf{x}^2) = \begin{bmatrix} 0.87 & 7.13 \\ 7.13 & 0.87 \end{bmatrix}.$$

The eigenvalues of this matrix are

$$\lambda_1 = -6.26, \ \lambda_2 = 8.0,$$

therefore $\mathbf{x}^2$ must be a saddle point. In one direction the curvature is negative, and in another direction the curvature is positive. The negative curvature is in the direction of the first eigenvector, and the positive curvature is in the direction of the second eigenvector. The eigenvectors are

$$\mathbf{z}_1 = \begin{bmatrix} 1 \\ -1 \end{bmatrix} \text{ and } \mathbf{z}_2 = \begin{bmatrix} 1 \\ 1 \end{bmatrix}.$$

(Note that this is consistent with our previous discussion of this function on page 8-8.)

If we evaluate the Hessian at $\mathbf{x}^3$, we find

$$\nabla^2 F(\mathbf{x}^3) = \begin{bmatrix} 14.7 & -6.71 \\ -6.71 & 14.7 \end{bmatrix}.$$

The eigenvalues of this matrix are

$$\lambda_1 = 21.42, \ \lambda_2 = 8.0,$$

therefore $\mathbf{x}^3$ must be a strong minimum point.

Check these results using the Neural Network Design Demonstration Vector Taylor Series (`nnd8ts2`).

P8.6 **Let's apply the concepts in this chapter to a neural network problem. Consider the linear network shown in Figure P8.7. Suppose that the desired inputs/outputs for the network are**

$$\{ (p_1 = 2), (t_1 = 0.5) \}, \{ (p_2 = -1), (t_2 = 0) \}.$$

Sketch the following performance index for this network:

$$F(\mathbf{x}) = (t_1 - a_1(\mathbf{x}))^2 + (t_2 - a_2(\mathbf{x}))^2.$$

8

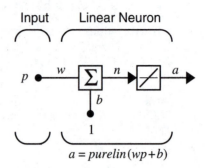

$$a = purelin(wp+b)$$

Figure P8.7 Linear Network for Problem P8.6

The parameters of this network are w and b, which make up the parameter vector

$$\mathbf{x} = \begin{bmatrix} w \\ b \end{bmatrix}.$$

We want to sketch the performance index $F(\mathbf{x})$. First we will show that the performance index is a quadratic function. Then we will find the eigenvectors and eigenvalues of the Hessian matrix and use them to sketch the contour plot of the function.

Begin by writing $F(\mathbf{x})$ as an explicit function of the parameter vector $\mathbf{x}$:

$$F(\mathbf{x}) = e_1^2 + e_2^2,$$

where

$$(e_1 = t_1 - (wp_1 + b)), \ (e_2 = t_2 - (wp_2 + b)).$$

This can be written in matrix form:

$$F(\mathbf{x}) = \mathbf{e}^T\mathbf{e},$$

where

$$\mathbf{e} = \mathbf{t} - \begin{bmatrix} p_1 & 1 \\ p_2 & 1 \end{bmatrix}\mathbf{x} = \mathbf{t} - \mathbf{G}\mathbf{x}.$$

The performance index can now be rewritten:

$$F(\mathbf{x}) = [\mathbf{t} - \mathbf{G}\mathbf{x}]^T[\mathbf{t} - \mathbf{G}\mathbf{x}] = \mathbf{t}^T\mathbf{t} - 2\mathbf{t}^T\mathbf{G}\mathbf{x} + \mathbf{x}^T\mathbf{G}^T\mathbf{G}\mathbf{x}.$$

If we compare this with Eq. (8.35):

$$F(\mathbf{x}) = \frac{1}{2}\mathbf{x}^T\mathbf{A}\mathbf{x} + \mathbf{d}^T\mathbf{x} + c,$$

we can see that the performance index for this linear network is a quadratic function, with

$$c = \mathbf{t}^T\mathbf{t}, \mathbf{d} = -2\mathbf{G}^T\mathbf{t}, \text{ and } \mathbf{A} = 2\mathbf{G}^T\mathbf{G}.$$

The gradient of the quadratic function is given in Eq. (8.38):

$$\nabla F(\mathbf{x}) = \mathbf{A}\mathbf{x} + \mathbf{d} = 2\mathbf{G}^T\mathbf{G}\mathbf{x} - 2\mathbf{G}^T\mathbf{t}.$$

The stationary point (also the center of the function contours) will occur where the gradient is equal to zero:

$$\mathbf{x}^* = -\mathbf{A}^{-1}\mathbf{d} = [\mathbf{G}^T\mathbf{G}]^{-1}\mathbf{G}^T\mathbf{t}.$$

For

$$\mathbf{G} = \begin{bmatrix} p_1 & 1 \\ p_2 & 1 \end{bmatrix} = \begin{bmatrix} 2 & 1 \\ -1 & 1 \end{bmatrix} \text{ and } \mathbf{t} = \begin{bmatrix} 0.5 \\ 0 \end{bmatrix}$$

we have

$$\mathbf{x}^* = [\mathbf{G}^T\mathbf{G}]^{-1}\mathbf{G}^T\mathbf{t} = \begin{bmatrix} 5 & 1 \\ 1 & 2 \end{bmatrix}^{-1} \begin{bmatrix} 1 \\ 0.5 \end{bmatrix} = \begin{bmatrix} 0.167 \\ 0.167 \end{bmatrix}.$$

(Therefore the optimal network parameters are $w = 0.167$ and $b = 0.167$.)

The Hessian matrix of the quadratic function is given by Eq. (8.39):

$$\nabla^2 F(\mathbf{x}) = \mathbf{A} = 2\mathbf{G}^T\mathbf{G} = \begin{bmatrix} 10 & 2 \\ 2 & 4 \end{bmatrix}.$$

To sketch the contour plot we need the eigenvectors and eigenvalues of the Hessian. For this case we find

$$\left\{ (\lambda_1 = 10.6), \left(\mathbf{z}_1 = \begin{bmatrix} 1 \\ 0.3 \end{bmatrix} \right) \right\}, \left\{ (\lambda_2 = 3.4), \left(\mathbf{z}_2 = \begin{bmatrix} 0.3 \\ -1 \end{bmatrix} \right) \right\}.$$

Therefore we know that $\mathbf{x}^*$ is a strong minimum. Also, since the first eigenvalue is larger than the second, we know that the contours will be elliptical and that the long axis of the ellipses will be in the direction of the second eigenvector. The contours will be centered at **x*** . This is demonstrated in Figure P8.8.

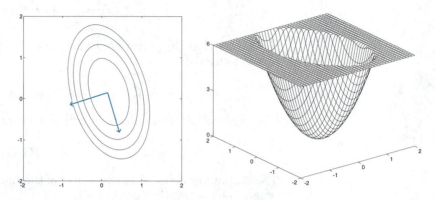

Figure P8.8 Graph of Function for Problem P8.6

P8.7 **There are quadratic functions that do not have stationary points. This problem illustrates one such case. Consider the following function:**

$$F(\mathbf{x}) = \begin{bmatrix} 1 & -1 \end{bmatrix} \mathbf{x} + \frac{1}{2}\mathbf{x}^T \begin{bmatrix} 1 & 1 \\ 1 & 1 \end{bmatrix} \mathbf{x}.$$

Sketch the contour plot of this function.

As with Problem P8.6, we need to find the eigenvalues and eigenvectors of the Hessian matrix. By inspection of the quadratic function we see that the Hessian matrix is

$$\nabla^2 F(\mathbf{x}) = \mathbf{A} = \begin{bmatrix} 1 & 1 \\ 1 & 1 \end{bmatrix}. \tag{8.63}$$

The eigenvalues and eigenvectors are

$$\left\{ (\lambda_1 = 0), \left(\mathbf{z}_1 = \begin{bmatrix} 1 \\ -1 \end{bmatrix} \right) \right\}, \left\{ (\lambda_2 = 2), \left(\mathbf{z}_2 = \begin{bmatrix} 1 \\ 1 \end{bmatrix} \right) \right\}.$$

Notice that the first eigenvalue is zero, so there is no curvature along the first eigenvector. The second eigenvalue is positive, so there is positive curvature along the second eigenvector. If we had no linear term in $F(\mathbf{x})$, the plot of the function would show a stationary valley, as in Figure 8.9. In this case we must find out if the linear term creates a slope in the direction of the valley (the direction of the first eigenvector).

The linear term is

$$F_{lin}(\mathbf{x}) = \begin{bmatrix} 1 & -1 \end{bmatrix} \mathbf{x}.$$

From Eq. (8.36) we know that the gradient of this term is

$$\nabla F_{lin}(\mathbf{x}) = \begin{bmatrix} 1 \\ -1 \end{bmatrix},$$

which means that the linear term is increasing most rapidly in the direction of this gradient. Since the quadratic term has no curvature in this direction, the overall function will have a linear slope in this direction. Therefore $F(\mathbf{x})$ will have positive curvature in the direction of the second eigenvector and a linear slope in the direction of the first eigenvector. The contour plot and the 3-D plot for this function are given in Figure P8.9.

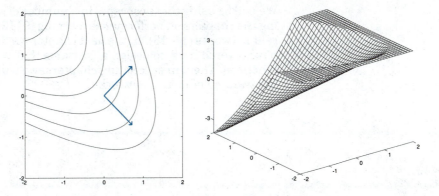

Figure P8.9 Falling Valley Function for Problem P8.7

Whenever any of the eigenvalues of the Hessian matrix are zero it is impossible to solve for the stationary point of the quadratic function using

$$\mathbf{x}^* = -\mathbf{A}^{-1}\mathbf{d},$$

since the Hessian matrix does not have an inverse. This lack of an inverse could mean that we have a weak minimum point, as illustrated in Figure 8.9, or that there is no stationary point, as this example shows.

8

Epilogue

Performance learning is one of the most important classes of neural network learning rules. With performance learning, network parameters are adjusted to optimize network performance. In this chapter we have introduced tools that we will need to understand performance learning rules. After reading this chapter and solving the exercises, you should be able to:

   i. Perform a Taylor series expansion and use it to approximate a function.

  ii. Calculate a directional derivative.

 iii. Find stationary points and test whether they could be minima.

  iv. Sketch contour plots of quadratic functions.

We will be using these concepts in a number of succeeding chapters, including the chapters on performance learning (9–12) and the chapters on recurrent networks (17–18). In the next chapter we will build on the concepts we have covered here, to design algorithms that will optimize performance functions. Then, in succeeding chapters, we will apply these algorithms to the training of neural networks.

Further Reading

[Brog91]   W. L. Brogan, *Modern Control Theory,* 3rd Ed., Englewood Cliffs, NJ: Prentice-Hall, 1991.

This is a well-written book on the subject of linear systems. The first half of the book is devoted to linear algebra. It also has good sections on the solution of linear differential equations and the stability of linear and nonlinear systems. It has many worked problems.

[Gill81]   P. E. Gill, W. Murray, and M. H. Wright, *Practical Optimization*, New York: Academic Press, 1981.

As the title implies, this text emphasizes the practical implementation of optimization algorithms. It provides motivation for the optimization methods, as well as details of implementation that affect algorithm performance.

[Himm72]   D. M. Himmelblau, *Applied Nonlinear Programming*, New York: McGraw-Hill, 1972.

This is a comprehensive text on nonlinear optimization. It covers both constrained and unconstrained optimization problems. The text is very complete, with many examples worked out in detail.

[Scal85]   L. E. Scales, *Introduction to Non-Linear Optimization*, New York: Springer-Verlag, 1985.

A very readable text describing the major optimization algorithms, this text emphasizes methods of optimization rather than existence theorems and proofs of convergence. Algorithms are presented with intuitive explanations, along with illustrative figures and examples. Pseudo-code is presented for most algorithms.

8

Exercises

E8.1 Consider the following scalar function:

$$F(x) = \frac{1}{x^3 - \frac{3}{4}x - \frac{1}{2}}.$$

    i. Find the second-order Taylor series approximation for $F(x)$ about the point $x = -0.5$.

    ii. Find the second-order Taylor series approximation for $F(x)$ about the point $x = 1.1$.

    iii. Plot $F(x)$ and the two approximations and discuss their accuracy.

E8.2 Consider the following function of two variables:

$$F(\mathbf{x}) = e^{(2x_1^2 + 2x_2^2 + x_1 - 5x_2 + 10)}.$$

    i. Find the second-order Taylor series approximation for $F(\mathbf{x})$ about the point $\mathbf{x} = \begin{bmatrix} 0 & 0 \end{bmatrix}^T$.

    ii. Find the stationary point for this approximation.

    iii. Find the stationary point for $F(\mathbf{x})$. (Note that the exponent of $F(\mathbf{x})$ is simply a quadratic function.)

    iv. Explain the difference between the two stationary points. (Use MATLAB to plot the two functions.)

E8.3 For the following functions find the first and second directional derivatives from the point $\mathbf{x} = \begin{bmatrix} 1 & 1 \end{bmatrix}^T$ in the direction $\mathbf{p} = \begin{bmatrix} -1 & 1 \end{bmatrix}^T$.

    i. $F(\mathbf{x}) = \frac{7}{2}x_1^2 - 6x_1 x_2 - x_2^2$

    ii. $F(\mathbf{x}) = 5x_1^2 - 6x_1 x_2 + 5x_2^2 + 4x_1 + 4x_2$

    iii. $F(\mathbf{x}) = \frac{9}{2}x_1^2 - 2x_1 x_2 + 3x_2^2 + 2x_1 - x_2$

    iv. $F(\mathbf{x}) = -\frac{1}{2}(7x_1^2 + 12x_1 x_2 - 2x_2^2)$

E8.4 For the following function,

$$F(x) = x^4 - \frac{1}{2}x^2 + 1,$$

    i. find the stationary points,

    ii. test the stationary points to find minimum and maximum points, and

    iii. plot the function using MATLAB to verify your answers.

E8.5 Consider the following function of two variables:

$$F(\mathbf{x}) = (x_1 + x_2)^4 - 12x_1x_2 + x_1 + x_2 + 1.$$

    i. Verify that the function has three stationary points at

$$\mathbf{x}^1 = \begin{bmatrix} -0.6504 \\ -0.6504 \end{bmatrix}, \mathbf{x}^2 = \begin{bmatrix} 0.085 \\ 0.085 \end{bmatrix}, \mathbf{x}^3 = \begin{bmatrix} 0.5655 \\ 0.5655 \end{bmatrix}.$$

    ii. Test the stationary points to find any minima, maxima or saddle points.

    iii. Find the second-order Taylor series approximations for the function at each of the stationary points.

    iv. Plot the function and the approximations using MATLAB.

E8.6 For the functions of Exercise E8.3:

    i. find the stationary points,

    ii. test the stationary points to find minima, maxima or saddle points,

    iii. provide rough sketches of the contour plots, using the eigenvalues and eigenvectors of the Hessian matrices, and

    iv. plot the functions using MATLAB to verify your answers.

E8.7 Recall the function in Problem P8.7. For that function there was no stationary point. It is possible to modify the function, by changing only the **d** vector, so that a stationary point will exist. Find a new nonzero **d** vector that will create a weak minimum.

9 Performance Optimization

Objectives

We initiated our discussion of performance optimization in Chapter 8. There we introduced the Taylor series expansion as a tool for analyzing the performance surface, and then used it to determine conditions that must be satisfied by optimum points. In this chapter we will again use the Taylor series expansion, in this case to develop algorithms to locate the optimum points. We will discuss three different categories of optimization algorithm: steepest descent, Newton's method and conjugate gradient. In Chapters 10–12 we will apply all of these algorithms to the training of neural networks.

9

Theory and Examples

In the previous chapter we began our investigation of performance surfaces. Now we are in a position to develop algorithms to search the parameter space and locate minimum points of the surface (find the optimum weights and biases for a given neural network).

It is interesting to note that most of the algorithms presented in this chapter were developed hundreds of years ago. The basic principles of optimization were discovered during the 17th century, by such scientists and mathematicians as Kepler, Fermat, Newton and Leibniz. From 1950 on, these principles were rediscovered to be implemented on "high speed" (in comparison to the pen and paper available to Newton) digital computers. The success of these efforts stimulated significant research on new algorithms, and the field of optimization theory became recognized as a major branch of mathematics. Now neural network researchers have access to a vast storehouse of optimization theory and practice that can be applied to the training of neural networks. We have only begun to tap this rich resource.

The objective of this chapter, then, is to develop algorithms to optimize a performance index $F(\mathbf{x})$. For our purposes the word "optimize" will mean to find the value of $\mathbf{x}$ that minimizes $F(\mathbf{x})$. All of the optimization algorithms we will discuss are iterative. We begin from some initial guess, $\mathbf{x}_0$, and then update our guess in stages according to an equation of the form

$$\mathbf{x}_{k+1} = \mathbf{x}_k + \alpha_k \mathbf{p}_k, \tag{9.1}$$

or

$$\Delta \mathbf{x}_k = (\mathbf{x}_{k+1} - \mathbf{x}_k) = \alpha_k \mathbf{p}_k, \tag{9.2}$$

where the vector $\mathbf{p}_k$ represents a search direction, and the positive scalar α_k is the learning rate, which determines the length of the step.

The algorithms we will discuss in this chapter are distinguished by the choice of the search direction, $\mathbf{p}_k$. We will discuss three different possibilities. There are also a variety of ways to select the learning rate, α_k, and we will discuss several of these.

Steepest Descent

When we update our guess of the optimum (minimum) point using Eq. (9.1), we would like to have the function decrease at each iteration. In other words,

$$F(\mathbf{x}_{k+1}) < F(\mathbf{x}_k). \tag{9.3}$$

How can we choose a direction, $\mathbf{p}_k$, so that for sufficiently small learning rate, α_k, we will move "downhill" in this way? Consider the first-order Taylor series expansion (see Eq. (8.9)) of $F(\mathbf{x})$ about the old guess $\mathbf{x}_k$:

$$F(\mathbf{x}_{k+1}) = F(\mathbf{x}_k + \Delta\mathbf{x}_k) \approx F(\mathbf{x}_k) + \mathbf{g}_k^T \Delta\mathbf{x}_k, \tag{9.4}$$

where $\mathbf{g}_k$ is the gradient evaluated at the old guess $\mathbf{x}_k$:

$$\mathbf{g}_k \equiv \nabla F(\mathbf{x})\big|_{\mathbf{x} = \mathbf{x}_k}. \tag{9.5}$$

For $F(\mathbf{x}_{k+1})$ to be less than $F(\mathbf{x}_k)$, the second term on the right-hand side of Eq. (9.4) must be negative:

$$\mathbf{g}_k^T \Delta\mathbf{x}_k = \alpha_k \mathbf{g}_k^T \mathbf{p}_k < 0. \tag{9.6}$$

We will select an α_k that is small, but greater than zero. This implies:

$$\mathbf{g}_k^T \mathbf{p}_k < 0. \tag{9.7}$$

Descent Direction   Any vector $\mathbf{p}_k$ that satisfies this equation is called a *descent direction*. The function must go down if we take a small enough step in this direction. This brings up another question. What is the direction of steepest descent? (In what direction will the function decrease most rapidly?) This will occur when

$$\mathbf{g}_k^T \mathbf{p}_k \tag{9.8}$$

is most negative. (We assume that the length of $\mathbf{p}_k$ does not change, only the direction.) This is an inner product between the gradient and the direction vector. It will be most negative when the direction vector is the negative of the gradient. (Review our discussion of directional derivatives on page 8-6.) Therefore a vector that points in the steepest descent direction is

$$\mathbf{p}_k = -\mathbf{g}_k. \tag{9.9}$$

Steepest Descent   Using this in the iteration of Eq. (9.1) produces the method of *steepest descent*:

$$\mathbf{x}_{k+1} = \mathbf{x}_k - \alpha_k \mathbf{g}_k. \tag{9.10}$$

For steepest descent there are two general methods for determining the learning rate, α_k. One approach is to minimize the performance index **Learning Rate** $F(\mathbf{x})$ with respect to α_k at each iteration. In this case we are minimizing along the line

$$\mathbf{x}_k - \alpha_k \mathbf{g}_k. \tag{9.11}$$

9

The other method for selecting α_k is to use a fixed value (e.g., $\alpha_k = 0.02$), or to use variable, but predetermined, values (e.g., $\alpha_k = 1/k$). We will discuss the choice of α_k in more detail in the following examples.

Let's apply the steepest descent algorithm to the following function,

$$F(\mathbf{x}) = x_1^2 + 25x_2^2, \tag{9.12}$$

starting from the initial guess

$$\mathbf{x}_0 = \begin{bmatrix} 0.5 \\ 0.5 \end{bmatrix}. \tag{9.13}$$

The first step is to find the gradient:

$$\nabla F(\mathbf{x}) = \begin{bmatrix} \dfrac{\partial}{\partial x_1} F(\mathbf{x}) \\ \dfrac{\partial}{\partial x_2} F(\mathbf{x}) \end{bmatrix} = \begin{bmatrix} 2x_1 \\ 50x_2 \end{bmatrix}. \tag{9.14}$$

If we evaluate the gradient at the initial guess we find

$$\mathbf{g}_0 = \nabla F(\mathbf{x}) \big|_{\mathbf{x} = \mathbf{x}_0} = \begin{bmatrix} 1 \\ 25 \end{bmatrix}. \tag{9.15}$$

Assume that we use a fixed learning rate of $\alpha = 0.01$. The first iteration of the steepest descent algorithm would be

$$\mathbf{x}_1 = \mathbf{x}_0 - \alpha \mathbf{g}_0 = \begin{bmatrix} 0.5 \\ 0.5 \end{bmatrix} - 0.01 \begin{bmatrix} 1 \\ 25 \end{bmatrix} = \begin{bmatrix} 0.49 \\ 0.25 \end{bmatrix}. \tag{9.16}$$

The second iteration of steepest descent produces

$$\mathbf{x}_2 = \mathbf{x}_1 - \alpha \mathbf{g}_1 = \begin{bmatrix} 0.49 \\ 0.25 \end{bmatrix} - 0.01 \begin{bmatrix} 0.98 \\ 12.5 \end{bmatrix} = \begin{bmatrix} 0.4802 \\ 0.125 \end{bmatrix}. \tag{9.17}$$

If we continue the iterations we obtain the trajectory illustrated in Figure 9.1.

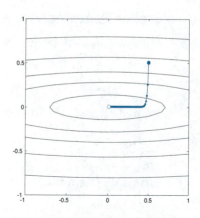

Figure 9.1 Trajectory for Steepest Descent with $\alpha = 0.01$

Note that the steepest descent trajectory, for small learning rate, follows a path that is always orthogonal to the contour lines. This is because the gradient is orthogonal to the contour lines. (See the discussion on page 8-6.)

How would a change in the learning rate change the performance of the algorithm? If we increase the learning rate to $\alpha = 0.035$, we obtain the trajectory illustrated in Figure 9.2. Note that the trajectory now oscillates. If we make the learning rate too large the algorithm will become unstable; the oscillations will increase instead of decaying.

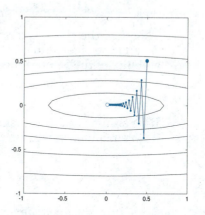

Figure 9.2 Trajectory for Steepest Descent with $\alpha = 0.035$

We would like to make the learning rate large, since then we will be taking large steps and would expect to converge faster. However, as we can see from this example, if we make the learning rate too large the algorithm will become unstable. Is there some way to predict the maximum allowable learning rate? This is not possible for arbitrary functions, but for quadratic functions we can set an upper limit.

9

Stable Learning Rates

Suppose that the performance index is a quadratic function:

$$F(\mathbf{x}) = \frac{1}{2}\mathbf{x}^T\mathbf{A}\mathbf{x} + \mathbf{d}^T\mathbf{x} + c. \tag{9.18}$$

From Eq. (8.38) the gradient of the quadratic function is

$$\nabla F(\mathbf{x}) = \mathbf{A}\mathbf{x} + \mathbf{d}. \tag{9.19}$$

If we now insert this expression into our expression for the steepest descent algorithm (assuming a constant learning rate), we obtain

$$\mathbf{x}_{k+1} = \mathbf{x}_k - \alpha\mathbf{g}_k = \mathbf{x}_k - \alpha(\mathbf{A}\mathbf{x}_k + \mathbf{d}) \tag{9.20}$$

or

$$\mathbf{x}_{k+1} = [\mathbf{I} - \alpha\mathbf{A}]\mathbf{x}_k - \alpha\mathbf{d}. \tag{9.21}$$

This is a linear dynamic system, which will be stable if the eigenvalues of the matrix $[\mathbf{I} - \alpha\mathbf{A}]$ are less than one in magnitude (see [Brog91]). We can express the eigenvalues of this matrix in terms of the eigenvalues of the Hessian matrix $\mathbf{A}$. Let $\{\lambda_1, \lambda_2, \ldots, \lambda_n\}$ and $\{\mathbf{z}_1, \mathbf{z}_2, \ldots, \mathbf{z}_n\}$ be the eigenvalues and eigenvectors of the Hessian matrix. Then

$$[\mathbf{I} - \alpha\mathbf{A}]\mathbf{z}_i = \mathbf{z}_i - \alpha\mathbf{A}\mathbf{z}_i = \mathbf{z}_i - \alpha\lambda_i\mathbf{z}_i = (1 - \alpha\lambda_i)\mathbf{z}_i. \tag{9.22}$$

Therefore the eigenvectors of $[\mathbf{I} - \alpha\mathbf{A}]$ are the same as the eigenvectors of $\mathbf{A}$, and the eigenvalues of $[\mathbf{I} - \alpha\mathbf{A}]$ are $(1 - \alpha\lambda_i)$. Our condition for the stability of the steepest descent algorithm is then

$$|(1 - \alpha\lambda_i)| < 1. \tag{9.23}$$

If we assume that the quadratic function has a strong minimum point, then its eigenvalues must be positive numbers. Eq. (9.23) then reduces to

$$\alpha < \frac{2}{\lambda_i}. \tag{9.24}$$

Since this must be true for all the eigenvalues of the Hessian matrix we have

$$\alpha < \frac{2}{\lambda_{max}}. \tag{9.25}$$

The maximum stable learning rate is inversely proportional to the maximum curvature of the quadratic function. The curvature tells us how fast the gradient is changing. If the gradient is changing too fast we may jump past the minimum point so far that the gradient at the new location will be larger in magnitude (but opposite direction) than the gradient at the old location. This will cause the steps to increase in size at each iteration.

Let's apply this result to our previous example. The Hessian matrix for that quadratic function is

$$\mathbf{A} = \begin{bmatrix} 2 & 0 \\ 0 & 50 \end{bmatrix}. \tag{9.26}$$

The eigenvalues and eigenvectors of $\mathbf{A}$ are

$$\left\{ (\lambda_1 = 2), \left(\mathbf{z}_1 = \begin{bmatrix} 1 \\ 0 \end{bmatrix} \right) \right\}, \left\{ \lambda_2 = 50, \left(\mathbf{z}_2 = \begin{bmatrix} 0 \\ 1 \end{bmatrix} \right) \right\}. \tag{9.27}$$

Therefore the maximum allowable learning rate is

$$\alpha < \frac{2}{\lambda_{max}} = \frac{2}{50} = 0.04. \tag{9.28}$$

This result is illustrated experimentally in Figure 9.3, which shows the steepest descent trajectories when the learning rate is just below ($\alpha = 0.039$) and just above ($\alpha = 0.041$), the maximum stable value.

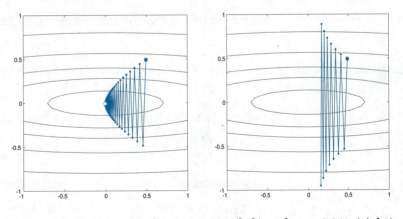

Figure 9.3 Trajectories for $\alpha = 0.039$ (left) and $\alpha = 0.041$ (right).

This example has illustrated several points. The learning rate is limited by the largest eigenvalue (second derivative) of the Hessian matrix. The algorithm tends to converge most quickly in the direction of the eigenvector corresponding to this largest eigenvalue, and we don't want to overshoot the minimum point by too far in that direction. (Note that in our examples the initial step is almost parallel to the x_2 axis, which is $\mathbf{z}_2$.) However, the algorithm will tend to converge most slowly in the direction of the eigenvector that corresponds to the smallest eigenvalue ($\mathbf{z}_1$ for our example). In the end it is the smallest eigenvalue, in combination with the learning rate, that determines how quickly the algorithm will converge. When there is a great difference in magnitude between the largest and smallest eigenvalues, the steepest descent algorithm will converge slowly.

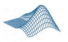

To experiment with steepest descent on this quadratic function, use the Neural Network Design Demonstration Steepest Descent for a Quadratic (`nnd9sdq`).

Minimizing Along a Line

Another approach for selecting the learning rate is to minimize the performance index with respect to α_k at each iteration. In other words, choose α_k to minimize

$$F(\mathbf{x}_k + \alpha_k\mathbf{p}_k) .\tag{9.29}$$

To do this for arbitrary functions requires a line search, which we will discuss in Chapter 12. For quadratic functions it is possible to perform the linear minimization analytically. The derivative of Eq. (9.29) with respect to α_k, for quadratic $F(\mathbf{x})$, can be shown to be

$$\frac{d}{d\alpha_k}F(\mathbf{x}_k + \alpha_k\mathbf{p}_k) = \nabla F(\mathbf{x})^T\Big|_{\mathbf{x}=\mathbf{x}_k}\mathbf{p}_k + \alpha_k\mathbf{p}_k^T\nabla^2 F(\mathbf{x})\Big|_{\mathbf{x}=\mathbf{x}_k}\mathbf{p}_k.\tag{9.30}$$

If we set this derivative equal to zero and solve for α_k, we obtain

$$\alpha_k = -\frac{\nabla F(\mathbf{x})^T\Big|_{\mathbf{x}=\mathbf{x}_k}\mathbf{p}_k}{\mathbf{p}_k^T\nabla^2 F(\mathbf{x})\Big|_{\mathbf{x}=\mathbf{x}_k}\mathbf{p}_k} = -\frac{\mathbf{g}_k^T\mathbf{p}_k}{\mathbf{p}_k^T\mathbf{A}_k\mathbf{p}_k},\tag{9.31}$$

where $\mathbf{A}_k$ is the Hessian matrix evaluated at the old guess $\mathbf{x}_k$:

$$\mathbf{A}_k \equiv \nabla^2 F(\mathbf{x})\Big|_{\mathbf{x}=\mathbf{x}_k}.\tag{9.32}$$

(For quadratic functions the Hessian matrix is not a function of k.)

Let's apply steepest descent with line minimization to the following quadratic function:

$$F(\mathbf{x}) = \frac{1}{2}\mathbf{x}^T\begin{bmatrix} 2 & 1 \\ 1 & 2 \end{bmatrix}\mathbf{x},\tag{9.33}$$

starting from the initial guess

$$\mathbf{x}_0 = \begin{bmatrix} 0.8 \\ -0.25 \end{bmatrix}. \tag{9.34}$$

The gradient of this function is

$$\nabla F(\mathbf{x}) = \begin{bmatrix} 2x_1 + x_2 \\ x_1 + 2x_2 \end{bmatrix}. \tag{9.35}$$

The search direction for steepest descent is the negative of the gradient. For the first iteration this will be

$$\mathbf{p}_0 = -\mathbf{g}_0 = -\nabla F(\mathbf{x}) \big|_{\mathbf{x} = \mathbf{x}_0} = \begin{bmatrix} -1.35 \\ -0.3 \end{bmatrix}. \tag{9.36}$$

From Eq. (9.31), the learning rate for the first iteration will be

$$\alpha_0 = -\frac{\begin{bmatrix} 1.35 & 0.3 \end{bmatrix} \begin{bmatrix} -1.35 \\ -0.3 \end{bmatrix}}{\begin{bmatrix} -1.35 & -0.3 \end{bmatrix} \begin{bmatrix} 2 & 1 \\ 1 & 2 \end{bmatrix} \begin{bmatrix} -1.35 \\ -0.3 \end{bmatrix}} = 0.413. \tag{9.37}$$

The first step of steepest descent will then produce

$$\mathbf{x}_1 = \mathbf{x}_0 - \alpha_0 \mathbf{g}_0 = \begin{bmatrix} 0.8 \\ -0.25 \end{bmatrix} - 0.413 \begin{bmatrix} 1.35 \\ 0.3 \end{bmatrix} = \begin{bmatrix} 0.24 \\ -0.37 \end{bmatrix}. \tag{9.38}$$

The first five iterations of the algorithm are illustrated in Figure 9.4.

Note that the successive steps of the algorithm are orthogonal. Why does this happen? First, when we minimize along a line we will always stop at a point that is tangent to a contour line. Then, since the gradient is orthogonal to the contour line, the next step, which is along the negative of the gradient, will be orthogonal to the previous step.

We can show this analytically by using the chain rule on Eq. (9.30):

$$\frac{d}{d\alpha_k} F(\mathbf{x}_k + \alpha_k \mathbf{p}_k) = \frac{d}{d\alpha_k} F(\mathbf{x}_{k+1}) = \nabla F(\mathbf{x})^T \big|_{\mathbf{x} = \mathbf{x}_{k+1}} \frac{d}{d\alpha_k} [\mathbf{x}_k + \alpha_k \mathbf{p}_k] \tag{9.39}$$

$$= \nabla F(\mathbf{x})^T \big|_{\mathbf{x} = \mathbf{x}_{k+1}} \mathbf{p}_k = \mathbf{g}_{k+1}^T \mathbf{p}_k.$$

9

Therefore at the minimum point, where this derivative is zero, the gradient is orthogonal to the previous search direction. Since the next search direction is the negative of this gradient, the consecutive search directions must be orthogonal. (Note that this result implies that when minimizing in any direction, the gradient at the minimum point will be orthogonal to the search direction, even if we are not using steepest descent. We will use this result in our discussion of conjugate directions.)

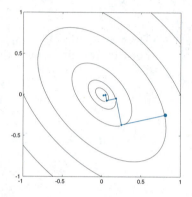

Figure 9.4 Steepest Descent with Minimization Along a Line

To experiment with steepest descent with minimization along a line, use the Neural Network Design Demonstration Method Comparison (nnd9mc).

Later in this chapter we will find that we can improve performance if we adjust the search directions, so that instead of being orthogonal they are *conjugate*. (We will define this term later.) If conjugate directions are used the function can be exactly minimized in at most n steps, where n is the dimension of $\mathbf{x}$. (There are certain types of quadratic functions that are minimized in one step by the steepest descent algorithm. Can you think of such a function? How is its Hessian matrix characterized?)

Newton's Method

The derivation of the steepest descent algorithm was based on the first-order Taylor series expansion (Eq. (9.4)). Newton's method is based on the second-order Taylor series:

$$F(\mathbf{x}_{k+1}) = F(\mathbf{x}_k + \Delta\mathbf{x}_k) \approx F(\mathbf{x}_k) + \mathbf{g}_k^T\Delta\mathbf{x}_k + \frac{1}{2}\Delta\mathbf{x}_k^T\mathbf{A}_k\Delta\mathbf{x}_k. \qquad (9.40)$$

The principle behind Newton's method is to locate the stationary point of this quadratic approximation to $F(\mathbf{x})$. If we use Eq. (8.38) to take the gradient of this quadratic function with respect to $\Delta\mathbf{x}_k$ and set it equal to zero, we find

$$\mathbf{g}_k + \mathbf{A}_k \Delta \mathbf{x}_k = 0. \tag{9.41}$$

Solving for $\Delta \mathbf{x}_k$ produces

$$\Delta \mathbf{x}_k = -\mathbf{A}_k^{-1} \mathbf{g}_k. \tag{9.42}$$

Newton's Method *Newton's method* is then defined:

$$\mathbf{x}_{k+1} = \mathbf{x}_k - \mathbf{A}_k^{-1} \mathbf{g}_k. \tag{9.43}$$

To illustrate the operation of Newton's method, let's apply it to our previous example function of Eq. (9.12):

$$F(\mathbf{x}) = x_1^2 + 25 x_2^2. \tag{9.44}$$

The gradient and Hessian matrices are

$$\nabla F(\mathbf{x}) = \begin{bmatrix} \dfrac{\partial}{\partial x_1} F(\mathbf{x}) \\ \dfrac{\partial}{\partial x_2} F(\mathbf{x}) \end{bmatrix} = \begin{bmatrix} 2x_1 \\ 50x_2 \end{bmatrix}, \ \nabla^2 F(\mathbf{x}) = \begin{bmatrix} 2 & 0 \\ 0 & 50 \end{bmatrix}. \tag{9.45}$$

If we start from the same initial guess

$$\mathbf{x}_0 = \begin{bmatrix} 0.5 \\ 0.5 \end{bmatrix}, \tag{9.46}$$

the first step of Newton's method would be

$$\mathbf{x}_1 = \begin{bmatrix} 0.5 \\ 0.5 \end{bmatrix} - \begin{bmatrix} 2 & 0 \\ 0 & 50 \end{bmatrix}^{-1} \begin{bmatrix} 1 \\ 25 \end{bmatrix} = \begin{bmatrix} 0.5 \\ 0.5 \end{bmatrix} - \begin{bmatrix} 0.5 \\ 0.5 \end{bmatrix} = \begin{bmatrix} 0 \\ 0 \end{bmatrix}. \tag{9.47}$$

This method will always find the minimum of a quadratic function in one step. This is because Newton's method is designed to approximate a function as quadratic and then locate the stationary point of the quadratic approximation. If the original function is quadratic (with a strong minimum) it will be minimized in one step. The trajectory of Newton's method for this problem is given in Figure 9.5.

If the function $F(\mathbf{x})$ is not quadratic, then Newton's method will not generally converge in one step. In fact, we cannot be sure that it will converge at all, since this will depend on the function and the initial guess.

9

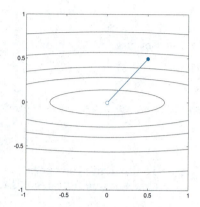

Figure 9.5 Trajectory for Newton's Method

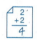

Recall the function given by Eq. (8.18):

$$F(\mathbf{x}) = (x_2 - x_1)^4 + 8x_1x_2 - x_1 + x_2 + 3. \tag{9.48}$$

We know from Chapter 8 (see Problem P8.5) that this function has three stationary points:

$$\mathbf{x}^1 = \begin{bmatrix} -0.42 \\ 0.42 \end{bmatrix}, \mathbf{x}^2 = \begin{bmatrix} -0.13 \\ 0.13 \end{bmatrix}, \mathbf{x}^3 = \begin{bmatrix} 0.55 \\ -0.55 \end{bmatrix}. \tag{9.49}$$

The first point is a strong local minimum, the second point is a saddle point, and the third point is a strong global minimum.

If we apply Newton's method to this problem, starting from the initial guess $\mathbf{x}_0 = \begin{bmatrix} 1.5 & 0 \end{bmatrix}^T$, our first iteration will be as shown in Figure 9.6. The graph on the left-hand side of the figure is a contour plot of the original function. On the right we see the quadratic approximation to the function at the initial guess.

The function is not minimized in one step, which is not surprising since the function is not quadratic. However, we do take a step toward the global minimum, and if we continue for two more iterations the algorithm will converge to within 0.01 of the global minimum. Newton's method converges quickly in many applications because analytic functions can be accurately approximated by quadratic functions in a small neighborhood of a strong minimum. So as we move closer to the minimum point, Newton's method will more accurately predict its location. In this case we can see that the contour plot of the quadratic approximation is similar to the contour plot of the original function near the initial guess.

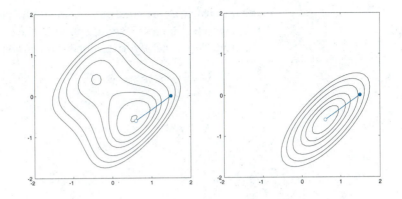

Figure 9.6 One Iteration of Newton's Method from $\mathbf{x}_0 = \begin{bmatrix} 1.5 & 0 \end{bmatrix}^T$

In Figure 9.7 we see one iteration of Newton's method from the initial guess $\mathbf{x}_0 = \begin{bmatrix} -1.5 & 0 \end{bmatrix}^T$. In this case we are converging to the local minimum. Clearly Newton's method cannot distinguish between a local minimum and a global minimum, since it approximates the function as a quadratic, and the quadratic function can have only one minimum. Newton's method, like steepest descent, relies on the local features of the surface (the first and second derivatives). It cannot know the global character of the function.

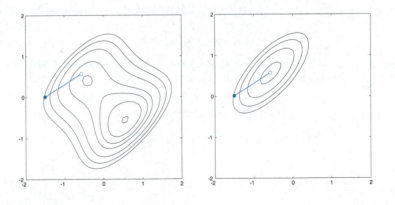

Figure 9.7 One Iteration of Newton's Method from $\mathbf{x}_0 = \begin{bmatrix} -1.5 & 0 \end{bmatrix}^T$

In Figure 9.8 we see one iteration of Newton's method from the initial guess $\mathbf{x}_0 = \begin{bmatrix} 0.75 & 0.75 \end{bmatrix}^T$. Now we are converging toward the saddle point of the function. Note that Newton's method locates the stationary point of the quadratic approximation to the function at the current guess. It does not distinguish between minima, maxima and saddle points. For this problem

9

the quadratic approximation has a saddle point (indefinite Hessian matrix), which is near the saddle point of the original function. If we continue the iterations, the algorithm does converge to the saddle point of $F(\mathbf{x})$.

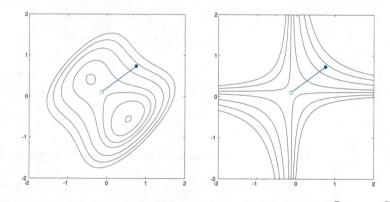

Figure 9.8 One Iteration of Newton's Method from $\mathbf{x}_0 = \begin{bmatrix} 0.75 & 0.75 \end{bmatrix}^T$

In each of the cases we have looked at so far the stationary point of the quadratic approximation has been close to a corresponding stationary point of $F(\mathbf{x})$. This is not always the case. In fact, Newton's method can produce very unpredictable results.

In Figure 9.9 we see one iteration of Newton's method from the initial guess $\mathbf{x}_0 = \begin{bmatrix} 1.15 & 0.75 \end{bmatrix}^T$. In this case the quadratic approximation predicts a saddle point, however, the saddle point is located very close to the local minimum of $F(\mathbf{x})$. If we continue the iterations, the algorithm will converge to the local minimum. Notice that the initial guess was actually farther away from the local minimum than it was for the previous case, in which the algorithm converged to the saddle point.

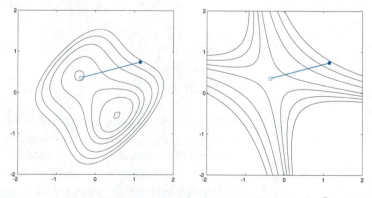

Figure 9.9 One Iteration of Newton's Method from $\mathbf{x}_0 = \begin{bmatrix} 1.15 & 0.75 \end{bmatrix}^T$

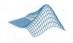 *To experiment with Newton's method and steepest descent on this function, use the Neural Network Design Demonstrations Newton's Method* (**nnd9nm**) *and Steepest Descent* (**nnd9sd**).

This is a good place to summarize some of the properties of Newton's method that we have observed.

While Newton's method usually produces faster convergence than steepest descent, the behavior of Newton's method can be quite complex. In addition to the problem of convergence to saddle points (which is very unlikely with steepest descent), it is possible for the algorithm to oscillate or diverge. Steepest descent is guaranteed to converge, if the learning rate is not too large or if we perform a linear minimization at each stage.

In Chapter 12 we will discuss a variation of Newton's method that is well suited to neural network training. It eliminates the divergence problem by using steepest descent steps whenever divergence begins to occur.

Another problem with Newton's method is that it requires the computation and storage of the Hessian matrix, as well as its inverse. If we compare steepest descent, Eq. (9.10), with Newton's method, Eq. (9.43), we see that their search directions will be identical when

$$\mathbf{A}_k = \mathbf{A}_k^{-1} = \mathbf{I}. \tag{9.50}$$

This observation has lead to a class of optimization algorithms know as quasi-Newton or one-step-secant methods. These methods replace $\mathbf{A}_k^{-1}$ with a positive definite matrix, $\mathbf{H}_k$, which is updated at each iteration without matrix inversion. The algorithms are typically designed so that for quadratic functions $\mathbf{H}_k$ will converge to $\mathbf{A}^{-1}$. (The Hessian is constant for quadratic functions.) See [Gill81], [Scal85] or [Batt92] for a discussion of these methods.

Conjugate Gradient

Quadratic Termination

Newton's method has a property called *quadratic termination*, which means that it minimizes a quadratic function exactly in a finite number of iterations. Unfortunately, it requires calculation and storage of the second derivatives. When the number of parameters, n, is large, it may be impractical to compute all of the second derivatives. (Note that the gradient has n elements, while the Hessian has n^2 elements.) This is especially true with neural networks, where practical applications can require several hundred to many thousand weights. For these cases we would like to have methods that require only first derivatives but still have quadratic termination.

Recall the performance of the steepest descent algorithm, with linear searches at each iteration. The search directions at consecutive iterations were orthogonal (see Figure 9.4). For quadratic functions with elliptical

9

contours this produces a zig-zag trajectory of short steps. Perhaps quadratic search directions are not the best choice. Is there a set of search directions that will guarantee quadratic termination? One possibility is conjugate directions.

Suppose that we wish to locate the minimum of the following quadratic function:

$$F(\mathbf{x}) = \frac{1}{2}\mathbf{x}^T\mathbf{A}\mathbf{x} + \mathbf{d}^T\mathbf{x} + c. \tag{9.51}$$

Conjugate   A set of vectors $\{\mathbf{p}_k\}$ is mutually *conjugate* with respect to a positive definite Hessian matrix $\mathbf{A}$ if and only if

$$\mathbf{p}_k^T\mathbf{A}\mathbf{p}_j = 0 \qquad k \neq j. \tag{9.52}$$

As with orthogonal vectors, there are an infinite number of mutually conjugate sets of vectors that span a given n-dimensional space. One set of conjugate vectors consists of the eigenvectors of $\mathbf{A}$. Let $\{\lambda_1, \lambda_2, \ldots, \lambda_n\}$ and $\{\mathbf{z}_1, \mathbf{z}_2, \ldots, \mathbf{z}_n\}$ be the eigenvalues and eigenvectors of the Hessian matrix. To see that the eigenvectors are conjugate, replace $\mathbf{p}_k$ with $\mathbf{z}_k$ in Eq. (9.52):

$$\mathbf{z}_k^T\mathbf{A}\mathbf{z}_j = \lambda_j\mathbf{z}_k^T\mathbf{z}_j = 0 \qquad k \neq j, \tag{9.53}$$

where the last equality holds because the eigenvectors of a symmetric matrix are mutually orthogonal. Therefore the eigenvectors are both conjugate and orthogonal. (Can you find a quadratic function where all orthogonal vectors are also conjugate?)

It is not surprising that we can minimize a quadratic function exactly by searching along the eigenvectors of the Hessian matrix, since they form the principal axes of the function contours. (See the discussion on pages 8-13 through 8-19.) Unfortunately this is not of much practical help, since to find the eigenvectors we must first find the Hessian matrix. We want to find an algorithm that does not require the computation of second derivatives.

It can be shown (see [Scal85] or [Gill81]) that if we make a sequence of exact linear searches along any set of conjugate directions $\{\mathbf{p}_1, \mathbf{p}_2, \ldots, \mathbf{p}_n\}$, then the exact minimum of any quadratic function, with n parameters, will be reached in at most n searches. The question is "How can we construct these conjugate search directions?" First, we want to restate the conjugacy condition, which is given in Eq. (9.52), without use of the Hessian matrix. Recall that for quadratic functions

$$\nabla F(\mathbf{x}) = \mathbf{A}\mathbf{x} + \mathbf{d}, \tag{9.54}$$

$$\nabla^2 F(\mathbf{x}) = \mathbf{A}. \tag{9.55}$$

By combining these equations we find that the change in the gradient at iteration $k+1$ is

$$\Delta \mathbf{g}_k = \mathbf{g}_{k+1} - \mathbf{g}_k = (\mathbf{A}\mathbf{x}_{k+1} + \mathbf{d}) - (\mathbf{A}\mathbf{x}_k + \mathbf{d}) = \mathbf{A}\Delta\mathbf{x}_k, \tag{9.56}$$

where, from Eq. (9.2), we have

$$\Delta \mathbf{x}_k = (\mathbf{x}_{k+1} - \mathbf{x}_k) = \alpha_k \mathbf{p}_k, \tag{9.57}$$

and α_k is chosen to minimize $F(\mathbf{x})$ in the direction $\mathbf{p}_k$.

We can now restate the conjugacy conditions (Eq. (9.52)):

$$\alpha_k \mathbf{p}_k^T \mathbf{A} \mathbf{p}_j = \Delta \mathbf{x}_k^T \mathbf{A} \mathbf{p}_j = \Delta \mathbf{g}_k^T \mathbf{p}_j = 0 \qquad k \neq j. \tag{9.58}$$

Note that we no longer need to know the Hessian matrix. We have restated the conjugacy conditions in terms of the changes in the gradient at successive iterations of the algorithm. The search directions will be conjugate if they are orthogonal to the changes in the gradient.

Note that the first search direction, $\mathbf{p}_0$, is arbitrary, and $\mathbf{p}_1$ can be any vector that is orthogonal to $\Delta \mathbf{g}_0$. Therefore there are an infinite number of sets of conjugate vectors. It is common to begin the search in the steepest descent direction:

$$\mathbf{p}_0 = -\mathbf{g}_0. \tag{9.59}$$

Then, at each iteration we need to construct a vector $\mathbf{p}_k$ that is orthogonal to $\{\Delta \mathbf{g}_0, \Delta \mathbf{g}_1, \ldots, \Delta \mathbf{g}_{k-1}\}$. It is a procedure similar to Gram-Schmidt orthogonalization, which we discussed in Chapter 5. It can be simplified (see [Scal85]) to iterations of the form

$$\mathbf{p}_k = -\mathbf{g}_k + \beta_k \mathbf{p}_{k-1}. \tag{9.60}$$

The scalars β_k can be chosen by several different methods, which produce equivalent results for quadratic functions. The most common choices (see [Scal85]) are

$$\beta_k = \frac{\Delta \mathbf{g}_{k-1}^T \mathbf{g}_k}{\Delta \mathbf{g}_{k-1}^T \mathbf{p}_{k-1}}, \tag{9.61}$$

due to Hestenes and Steifel,

9

$$\beta_k = \frac{\mathbf{g}_k^T \mathbf{g}_k}{\mathbf{g}_{k-1}^T \mathbf{g}_{k-1}} \qquad (9.62)$$

due to Fletcher and Reeves, and

$$\beta_k = \frac{\Delta \mathbf{g}_{k-1}^T \mathbf{g}_k}{\mathbf{g}_{k-1}^T \mathbf{g}_{k-1}} \qquad (9.63)$$

due to Polak and Ribiére.

Conjugate Gradient   To summarize our discussion, the *conjugate gradient* method consists of the following steps:

1. Select the first search direction to be the negative of the gradient, as in Eq. (9.59).

2. Take a step according to Eq. (9.57), selecting the learning rate α_k to minimize the function along the search direction. We will discuss general linear minimization techniques in Chapter 12. For quadratic functions we can use Eq. (9.31).

3. Select the next search direction according to Eq. (9.60), using Eq. (9.61), Eq. (9.62), or Eq. (9.63) to calculate β_k.

4. If the algorithm has not converged, return to step 2.

To illustrate the performance of the algorithm, recall the example we used to demonstrate steepest descent with linear minimization:

$$F(\mathbf{x}) = \frac{1}{2}\mathbf{x}^T \begin{bmatrix} 2 & 1 \\ 1 & 2 \end{bmatrix} \mathbf{x}, \qquad (9.64)$$

with initial guess

$$\mathbf{x}_0 = \begin{bmatrix} 0.8 \\ -0.25 \end{bmatrix}. \qquad (9.65)$$

The gradient of this function is

$$\nabla F(\mathbf{x}) = \begin{bmatrix} 2x_1 + x_2 \\ x_1 + 2x_2 \end{bmatrix}. \qquad (9.66)$$

As with steepest descent, the first search direction is the negative of the gradient:

$$\mathbf{p}_0 = -\mathbf{g}_0 = -\nabla F(\mathbf{x})^T\big|_{\mathbf{x} = \mathbf{x}_0} = \begin{bmatrix} -1.35 \\ -0.3 \end{bmatrix}. \tag{9.67}$$

From Eq. (9.31), the learning rate for the first iteration will be

$$\alpha_0 = -\frac{\begin{bmatrix} 1.35 & 0.3 \end{bmatrix} \begin{bmatrix} -1.35 \\ -0.3 \end{bmatrix}}{\begin{bmatrix} -1.35 & -0.3 \end{bmatrix} \begin{bmatrix} 2 & 1 \\ 1 & 2 \end{bmatrix} \begin{bmatrix} -1.35 \\ -0.3 \end{bmatrix}} = 0.413. \tag{9.68}$$

The first step of conjugate gradient is therefore:

$$\mathbf{x}_1 = \mathbf{x}_0 + \alpha_0 \mathbf{p}_0 = \begin{bmatrix} 0.8 \\ -0.25 \end{bmatrix} + 0.413 \begin{bmatrix} -1.35 \\ -0.3 \end{bmatrix} = \begin{bmatrix} 0.24 \\ -0.37 \end{bmatrix}, \tag{9.69}$$

which is equivalent to the first step of steepest descent with minimization along a line.

Now we need to find the second search direction from Eq. (9.60). This requires the gradient at $\mathbf{x}_1$:

$$\mathbf{g}_1 = \nabla F(\mathbf{x})\big|_{\mathbf{x} = \mathbf{x}_1} = \begin{bmatrix} 2 & 1 \\ 1 & 2 \end{bmatrix} \begin{bmatrix} 0.24 \\ -0.37 \end{bmatrix} = \begin{bmatrix} 0.11 \\ -0.5 \end{bmatrix}. \tag{9.70}$$

We can now find β_1:

$$\beta_1 = \frac{\mathbf{g}_1^T \mathbf{g}_1}{\mathbf{g}_0^T \mathbf{g}_0} = \frac{\begin{bmatrix} 0.11 & -0.5 \end{bmatrix} \begin{bmatrix} 0.11 \\ -0.5 \end{bmatrix}}{\begin{bmatrix} 1.35 & 0.3 \end{bmatrix} \begin{bmatrix} 1.35 \\ 0.3 \end{bmatrix}} = \frac{0.2621}{1.9125} = 0.137, \tag{9.71}$$

using the method of Fletcher and Reeves (Eq. (9.62)). The second search direction is then computed from Eq. (9.60):

$$\mathbf{p}_1 = -\mathbf{g}_1 + \beta_1 \mathbf{p}_0 = \begin{bmatrix} -0.11 \\ 0.5 \end{bmatrix} + 0.137 \begin{bmatrix} -1.35 \\ -0.3 \end{bmatrix} = \begin{bmatrix} -0.295 \\ 0.459 \end{bmatrix}. \tag{9.72}$$

From Eq. (9.31), the learning rate for the second iteration will be

9

$$\alpha_1 = -\frac{\begin{bmatrix} 0.11 & -0.5 \end{bmatrix} \begin{bmatrix} -0.295 \\ 0.459 \end{bmatrix}}{\begin{bmatrix} -0.295 & 0.459 \end{bmatrix} \begin{bmatrix} 2 & 1 \\ 1 & 2 \end{bmatrix} \begin{bmatrix} -0.295 \\ 0.459 \end{bmatrix}} = \frac{0.262}{0.325} = 0.807 . \tag{9.73}$$

The second step of conjugate gradient is therefore

$$\mathbf{x}_2 = \mathbf{x}_1 + \alpha_1 \mathbf{p}_1 = \begin{bmatrix} 0.24 \\ -0.37 \end{bmatrix} + 0.807 \begin{bmatrix} -0.295 \\ 0.459 \end{bmatrix} = \begin{bmatrix} 0 \\ 0 \end{bmatrix} . \tag{9.74}$$

As predicted, the algorithm converges exactly to the minimum in two iterations (since this is a two-dimensional quadratic function), as illustrated in Figure 9.10. Compare this result with the steepest descent algorithm, as shown in Figure 9.4. The conjugate gradient algorithm adjusts the second search direction so that it will pass through the minimum of the function (center of the function contours), instead of using an orthogonal search direction, as in steepest descent.

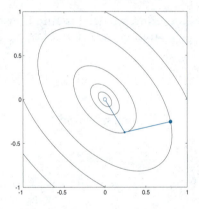

Figure 9.10 Conjugate Gradient Algorithm

We will return to the conjugate gradient algorithm in Chapter 12. In that chapter we will discuss how the algorithm should be adjusted for non-quadratic functions.

To experiment with the conjugate gradient algorithm and compare it with steepest descent, use the Neural Network Design Demonstration Method Comparison (**nnd9mc**).

Summary of Results

General Minimization Algorithm

$$\mathbf{x}_{k+1} = \mathbf{x}_k + \alpha_k \mathbf{p}_k$$

or

$$\Delta \mathbf{x}_k = (\mathbf{x}_{k+1} - \mathbf{x}_k) = \alpha_k \mathbf{p}_k$$

Steepest Descent Algorithm

$$\mathbf{x}_{k+1} = \mathbf{x}_k - \alpha_k \mathbf{g}_k$$

Where $\mathbf{g}_k \equiv \nabla F(\mathbf{x})\big|_{\mathbf{x} = \mathbf{x}_k}$

Stable Learning Rate ($\alpha_k = \alpha$, constant)

$$\alpha < \frac{2}{\lambda_{max}}$$

$\{\lambda_1, \lambda_2, \dots, \lambda_n\}$ Eigenvalues of Hessian matrix $\mathbf{A}$

Learning Rate to Minimize Along the Line $\mathbf{x}_{k+1} = \mathbf{x}_k + \alpha_k \mathbf{p}_k$

$$\alpha_k = -\frac{\mathbf{g}_k^T \mathbf{p}_k}{\mathbf{p}_k^T \mathbf{A} \mathbf{p}_k} \quad \text{(For quadratic functions)}$$

After Minimizing Along the Line $\mathbf{x}_{k+1} = \mathbf{x}_k + \alpha_k \mathbf{p}_k$

$$\mathbf{g}_{k+1}^T \mathbf{p}_k = 0$$

Newton's Method

$$\mathbf{x}_{k+1} = \mathbf{x}_k - \mathbf{A}_k^{-1} \mathbf{g}_k$$

Where $\mathbf{A}_k \equiv \nabla^2 F(\mathbf{x})\big|_{\mathbf{x} = \mathbf{x}_k}$

9

Conjugate Gradient Algorithm

$$\Delta \mathbf{x}_k = \alpha_k \mathbf{p}_k$$

Learning rate α_k is chosen to minimize along the line $\mathbf{x}_{k+1} = \mathbf{x}_k + \alpha_k \mathbf{p}_k$.

$$\mathbf{p}_0 = -\mathbf{g}_0$$

$$\mathbf{p}_k = -\mathbf{g}_k + \beta_k \mathbf{p}_{k-1}$$

$$\beta_k = \frac{\Delta \mathbf{g}_{k-1}^T \mathbf{g}_k}{\Delta \mathbf{g}_{k-1}^T \mathbf{p}_{k-1}} \quad \text{or} \quad \beta_k = \frac{\mathbf{g}_k^T \mathbf{g}_k}{\mathbf{g}_{k-1}^T \mathbf{g}_{k-1}} \quad \text{or} \quad \beta_k = \frac{\Delta \mathbf{g}_{k-1}^T \mathbf{g}_k}{\mathbf{g}_{k-1}^T \mathbf{g}_{k-1}}$$

Where $\mathbf{g}_k \equiv \nabla F(\mathbf{x})\big|_{\mathbf{x} = \mathbf{x}_k}$ and $\Delta \mathbf{g}_k = \mathbf{g}_{k+1} - \mathbf{g}_k$.

Solved Problems

P9.1 We want to find the minimum of the following function:

$$F(\mathbf{x}) = 5x_1^2 - 6x_1x_2 + 5x_2^2 + 4x_1 + 4x_2.$$

i. Sketch a contour plot of this function.

ii. Sketch the trajectory of the steepest descent algorithm on the contour plot of part (i) if the initial guess is $\mathbf{x}_0 = \begin{bmatrix} -1 & -2.5 \end{bmatrix}^T$. Assume a very small learning rate is used.

iii. What is the maximum stable learning rate?

i. To sketch the contour plot we first need to find the Hessian matrix. For quadratic functions we can do this by putting the function into the standard form (see Eq. (8.35)):

$$F(\mathbf{x}) = \frac{1}{2}\mathbf{x}^T\mathbf{A}\mathbf{x} + \mathbf{d}^T\mathbf{x} + c = \frac{1}{2}\mathbf{x}^T\begin{bmatrix} 10 & -6 \\ -6 & 10 \end{bmatrix}\mathbf{x} + \begin{bmatrix} 4 & 4 \end{bmatrix}\mathbf{x}.$$

From Eq. (8.39) the Hessian matrix is

$$\nabla^2 F(\mathbf{x}) = \mathbf{A} = \begin{bmatrix} 10 & -6 \\ -6 & 10 \end{bmatrix}.$$

The eigenvalues and eigenvectors of this matrix are

$$\lambda_1 = 4, \mathbf{z}_1 = \begin{bmatrix} 1 \\ 1 \end{bmatrix}, \lambda_2 = 16, \mathbf{z}_2 = \begin{bmatrix} 1 \\ -1 \end{bmatrix}.$$

From the discussion on quadratic functions in Chapter 8 (see page 8-15) we know that the function contours are elliptical. The maximum curvature of $F(\mathbf{x})$ is in the direction of $\mathbf{z}_2$, since λ_2 is larger than λ_1, and the minimum curvature is in the direction of $\mathbf{z}_1$ (the long axis of the ellipses).

Next we need to find the center of the contours (the stationary point). This occurs when the gradient is equal to zero. From Eq. (8.38) we find

$$\nabla F(\mathbf{x}) = \mathbf{A}\mathbf{x} + \mathbf{d} = \begin{bmatrix} 10 & -6 \\ -6 & 10 \end{bmatrix}\mathbf{x} + \begin{bmatrix} 4 \\ 4 \end{bmatrix} = \begin{bmatrix} 0 \\ 0 \end{bmatrix}.$$

Therefore

$$\mathbf{x}^* = -\begin{bmatrix} 10 & -6 \\ -6 & 10 \end{bmatrix}^{-1} \begin{bmatrix} 4 \\ 4 \end{bmatrix} = \begin{bmatrix} -1 \\ -1 \end{bmatrix}.$$

The contours will be elliptical, centered at $\mathbf{x}^*$, with long axis in the direction of $\mathbf{z}_1$. The contour plot is shown in Figure P9.1.

ii. We know that the gradient is always orthogonal to the contour line, therefore the steepest descent trajectory, if we take small enough steps, will follow a path that is orthogonal to each contour line it intersects. We can therefore trace the trajectory without performing any computations. The result is shown in Figure P9.1.

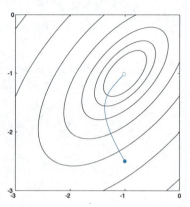

Figure P9.1 Contour Plot and Steep. Desc. Trajectory for Problem P9.1

iii. From Eq. (9.25) we know that the maximum stable learning rate for a quadratic function is determined by the maximum eigenvalue of the Hessian matrix:

$$\alpha < \frac{2}{\lambda_{max}}.$$

The maximum eigenvalue for this problem is $\lambda_2 = 16$, therefore for stability

$$\alpha < \frac{2}{16} = 0.125.$$

This result is verified experimentally in Figure P9.2, which shows the steepest descent trajectories when the learning rate is just below ($\alpha = 0.12$) and just above ($\alpha = 0.13$) the maximum stable value.

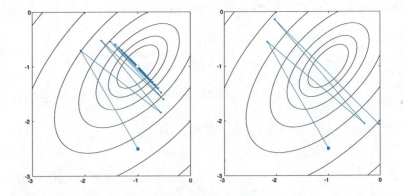

Figure P9.2 Trajectories for $\alpha = 0.12$ (left) and $\alpha = 0.13$ (right)

P9.2 **Consider again the quadratic function of Problem P9.1. Take two steps of the steepest descent algorithm, minimizing along a line at each step. Use the following initial condition:**

$$\mathbf{x}_0 = \begin{bmatrix} 0 & -2 \end{bmatrix}^T.$$

In Problem P9.1 we found the gradient of the function to be

$$\nabla F(\mathbf{x}) = \mathbf{A}\mathbf{x} + \mathbf{d} = \begin{bmatrix} 10 & -6 \\ -6 & 10 \end{bmatrix}\mathbf{x} + \begin{bmatrix} 4 \\ 4 \end{bmatrix}.$$

If we evaluate this at $\mathbf{x}_0$, we find

$$\mathbf{g}_0 = \nabla F(\mathbf{x}_0) = \mathbf{A}\mathbf{x}_0 + \mathbf{d} = \begin{bmatrix} 10 & -6 \\ -6 & 10 \end{bmatrix}\begin{bmatrix} 0 \\ -2 \end{bmatrix} + \begin{bmatrix} 4 \\ 4 \end{bmatrix} = \begin{bmatrix} 16 \\ -16 \end{bmatrix}.$$

Therefore the first search direction is

$$\mathbf{p}_0 = -\mathbf{g}_0 = \begin{bmatrix} -16 \\ 16 \end{bmatrix}.$$

To minimize along a line, for a quadratic function, we can use Eq. (9.31):

$$\alpha_0 = -\frac{\mathbf{g}_0^T\mathbf{p}_0}{\mathbf{p}_0^T\mathbf{A}\mathbf{p}_0} = -\frac{\begin{bmatrix} 16 & -16 \end{bmatrix}\begin{bmatrix} -16 \\ 16 \end{bmatrix}}{\begin{bmatrix} -16 & 16 \end{bmatrix}\begin{bmatrix} 10 & -6 \\ -6 & 10 \end{bmatrix}\begin{bmatrix} -16 \\ 16 \end{bmatrix}} = -\frac{-512}{8192} = 0.0625.$$

9

Therefore the first iteration of steepest descent will be

$$\mathbf{x}_1 = \mathbf{x}_0 - \alpha_0 \mathbf{g}_0 = \begin{bmatrix} 0 \\ -2 \end{bmatrix} - 0.0625 \begin{bmatrix} 16 \\ -16 \end{bmatrix} = \begin{bmatrix} -1 \\ -1 \end{bmatrix}.$$

To begin the second iteration we need to find the gradient at $\mathbf{x}_1$:

$$\mathbf{g}_1 = \nabla F(\mathbf{x}_1) = \mathbf{A}\mathbf{x}_1 + \mathbf{d} = \begin{bmatrix} 10 & -6 \\ -6 & 10 \end{bmatrix} \begin{bmatrix} -1 \\ -1 \end{bmatrix} + \begin{bmatrix} 4 \\ 4 \end{bmatrix} = \begin{bmatrix} 0 \\ 0 \end{bmatrix}.$$

Therefore we have reached a stationary point; the algorithm has converged. From Problem P9.1 we know that $\mathbf{x}_1$ is indeed the minimum point of this quadratic function. The trajectory is shown in Figure P9.3.

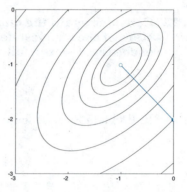

Figure P9.3 Steepest Descent with Linear Minimization for Problem P9.2

This is an unusual case, where the steepest descent algorithm located the minimum in one iteration. Notice that this occurred because the initial guess was located in the direction of one of the eigenvectors of the Hessian matrix, with respect to the minimum point. For those cases where every direction is an eigenvector, the steepest descent algorithm will always locate the minimum in one iteration. What would this imply about the eigenvalues of the Hessian matrix?

P9.3 **Recall Problem P8.6, in which we derived a performance index for a linear neural network. The network, which is displayed again in Figure P9.4, was to be trained for the following input/output pairs:**

$$\{ (p_1 = 2), (t_1 = 0.5) \}, \{ (p_2 = -1), (t_2 = 0) \}$$

The performance index for the network was defined to be

$$F(\mathbf{x}) = (t_1 - a_1(\mathbf{x}))^2 + (t_2 - a_2(\mathbf{x}))^2,$$

which was displayed in Figure P8.8.

i. **Use the steepest descent algorithm to locate the optimal parameters for this network (recall that** $\mathbf{x} = \begin{bmatrix} w & b \end{bmatrix}^T$ **), starting from the initial guess** $\mathbf{x}_0 = \begin{bmatrix} 1 & 1 \end{bmatrix}^T$. **Use a learning rate of** $\alpha = 0.05$.

ii. **What is the maximum stable learning rate?**

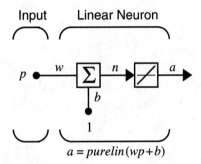

$$a = purelin(wp+b)$$

Figure P9.4 Linear Network for Problems P9.3 and P8.6

i. In Problem P8.6 we found that the performance index could be written in quadratic form:

$$F(\mathbf{x}) = \frac{1}{2}\mathbf{x}^T \mathbf{A}\mathbf{x} + \mathbf{d}^T \mathbf{x} + c,$$

where

$$c = \mathbf{t}^T \mathbf{t} = \begin{bmatrix} 0.5 & 0 \end{bmatrix} \begin{bmatrix} 0.5 \\ 0 \end{bmatrix} = 0.25,$$

$$\mathbf{d} = -2\mathbf{G}^T \mathbf{t} = -2 \begin{bmatrix} 2 & -1 \\ 1 & 1 \end{bmatrix} \begin{bmatrix} 0.5 \\ 0 \end{bmatrix} = \begin{bmatrix} -2 \\ -1 \end{bmatrix},$$

$$\mathbf{A} = 2\mathbf{G}^T \mathbf{G} = \begin{bmatrix} 10 & 2 \\ 2 & 4 \end{bmatrix}.$$

The gradient at $\mathbf{x}_0$ is

$$\mathbf{g}_0 = \nabla F(\mathbf{x}_0) = \mathbf{A}\mathbf{x}_0 + \mathbf{d} = \begin{bmatrix} 10 & 2 \\ 2 & 4 \end{bmatrix} \begin{bmatrix} 1 \\ 1 \end{bmatrix} + \begin{bmatrix} -2 \\ -1 \end{bmatrix} = \begin{bmatrix} 10 \\ 5 \end{bmatrix}.$$

The first iteration of steepest descent will be

$$\mathbf{x}_1 = \mathbf{x}_0 - \alpha\mathbf{g}_0 = \begin{bmatrix} 1 \\ 1 \end{bmatrix} - 0.05 \begin{bmatrix} 10 \\ 5 \end{bmatrix} = \begin{bmatrix} 0.5 \\ 0.75 \end{bmatrix}.$$

The second iteration will be

$$\mathbf{x}_2 = \mathbf{x}_1 - \alpha\mathbf{g}_1 = \begin{bmatrix} 0.5 \\ 0.75 \end{bmatrix} - 0.05 \begin{bmatrix} 4.5 \\ 3 \end{bmatrix} = \begin{bmatrix} 0.275 \\ 0.6 \end{bmatrix}.$$

The remaining iterations are displayed in Figure P9.5. The algorithm converges to the minimum point $\mathbf{x}^* = \begin{bmatrix} 0.167 & 0.167 \end{bmatrix}^T$. Therefore the optimal value for both the weight and the bias of this network is 0.167.

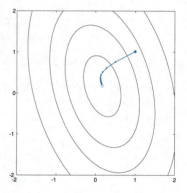

Figure P9.5 Steepest Descent Trajectory for Problem P9.3 with $\alpha = 0.05$

Note that in order to train this network we needed to know all of the input/output pairs. We then performed iterations of the steepest descent algorithm until convergence was achieved. In Chapter 10 we will introduce an adaptive algorithm, based on steepest descent, for training linear networks. With this adaptive algorithm the network parameters are updated after each input/output pair is presented. We will show how this allows the network to adapt to a changing environment.

ii. The maximum eigenvalue of the Hessian matrix for this problem is $\lambda_1 = 10.6$ (see Problem P8.6), therefore for stability

$$\alpha < \frac{2}{10.6} = 0.1887.$$

P9.4 **Consider the function**

$$F(\mathbf{x}) = e^{(x_1^2 - x_1 + 2x_2^2 + 4)} .$$

Take one iteration of Newton's method from the initial guess $\mathbf{x}_0 = \begin{bmatrix} 1 & -2 \end{bmatrix}^T$. How close is this result to the minimum point of $F(\mathbf{x})$? Explain.

The first step is to find the gradient and the Hessian matrix. The gradient is given by

$$\nabla F(\mathbf{x}) = \begin{bmatrix} \dfrac{\partial}{\partial x_1} F(\mathbf{x}) \\ \dfrac{\partial}{\partial x_2} F(\mathbf{x}) \end{bmatrix} = e^{(x_1^2 - x_1 + 2x_2^2 + 4)} \begin{bmatrix} (2x_1 - 1) \\ (4x_2) \end{bmatrix},$$

and the Hessian matrix is given by

$$\nabla^2 F(\mathbf{x}) = \begin{bmatrix} \dfrac{\partial^2}{\partial x_1^2} F(\mathbf{x}) & \dfrac{\partial^2}{\partial x_1 \partial x_2} F(\mathbf{x}) \\ \dfrac{\partial^2}{\partial x_2 \partial x_1} F(\mathbf{x}) & \dfrac{\partial^2}{\partial x_2^2} F(\mathbf{x}) \end{bmatrix}$$

$$= e^{(x_1^2 - x_1 + 2x_2^2 + 4)} \begin{bmatrix} 4x_1^2 - 4x_1 + 3 & (2x_1 - 1)(4x_2) \\ (2x_1 - 1)(4x_2) & 16x_2^2 + 4 \end{bmatrix}.$$

If we evaluate these at the initial guess we find

$$\mathbf{g}_0 = \nabla F(\mathbf{x}) \big|_{\mathbf{x} = \mathbf{x}_0} = \begin{bmatrix} 0.163 \times 10^6 \\ -1.302 \times 10^6 \end{bmatrix},$$

and

$$\mathbf{A}_0 = \nabla^2 F(\mathbf{x}) \big|_{\mathbf{x} = \mathbf{x}_0} = \begin{bmatrix} 0.049 \times 10^7 & -0.130 \times 10^7 \\ -0.130 \times 10^7 & 1.107 \times 10^7 \end{bmatrix}.$$

Therefore the first iteration of Newton's method, from Eq. (9.43), will be

9

$$\mathbf{x}_1 = \mathbf{x}_0 - \mathbf{A}_0^{-1}\mathbf{g}_0 = \begin{bmatrix} 1 \\ -2 \end{bmatrix} - \begin{bmatrix} 0.049\times10^7 & -0.130\times10^7 \\ -0.130\times10^7 & 1.107\times10^7 \end{bmatrix}^{-1} \begin{bmatrix} 0.163\times10^6 \\ -1.302\times10^6 \end{bmatrix} = \begin{bmatrix} 0.971 \\ -1.886 \end{bmatrix}$$

How close is this to the true minimum point of $F(\mathbf{x})$? First, note that the exponent of $F(\mathbf{x})$ is a quadratic function:

$$x_1^2 - x_1 + 2x_2^2 + 4 = \frac{1}{2}\mathbf{x}^T\mathbf{A}\mathbf{x} + \mathbf{d}^T\mathbf{x} + c = \frac{1}{2}\mathbf{x}^T\begin{bmatrix} 2 & 0 \\ 0 & 4 \end{bmatrix}\mathbf{x} + \begin{bmatrix} -1 & 0 \end{bmatrix}\mathbf{x} + 4.$$

The minimum point of $F(\mathbf{x})$ will be the same as the minimum point of the exponent, which is

$$\mathbf{x}^* = -\mathbf{A}^{-1}\mathbf{d} = -\begin{bmatrix} 2 & 0 \\ 0 & 4 \end{bmatrix}^{-1}\begin{bmatrix} -1 \\ 0 \end{bmatrix} = \begin{bmatrix} 0.5 \\ 0 \end{bmatrix}.$$

Therefore Newton's method has taken only a very small step toward the true minimum point. This is because $F(\mathbf{x})$ cannot be accurately approximated by a quadratic function in the neighborhood of $\mathbf{x}_0 = \begin{bmatrix} 1 & -2 \end{bmatrix}^T$.

For this problem Newton's method will converge to the true minimum point, but it will take many iterations. The trajectory for Newton's method is illustrated in Figure P9.6.

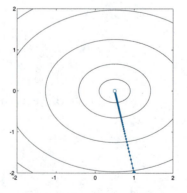

Figure P9.6 Newton's Method Trajectory for Problem P9.4

P9.5 **Compare the performance of Newton's method and steepest descent on the following function:**

$$F(\mathbf{x}) = \frac{1}{2}\mathbf{x}^T \begin{bmatrix} 1 & -1 \\ -1 & 1 \end{bmatrix} \mathbf{x}.$$

Start from the initial guess

$$\mathbf{x}_0 = \begin{bmatrix} 1 \\ 0 \end{bmatrix}.$$

Recall that this function is an example of a stationary valley (see Eq. (8.59) and Figure 8.9). The gradient is

$$\nabla F(\mathbf{x}) = \mathbf{A}\mathbf{x} + \mathbf{d} = \begin{bmatrix} 1 & -1 \\ -1 & 1 \end{bmatrix} \mathbf{x}$$

and the Hessian matrix is

$$\nabla^2 F(\mathbf{x}) = \mathbf{A} = \begin{bmatrix} 1 & -1 \\ -1 & 1 \end{bmatrix}.$$

Newton's method is given by

$$\mathbf{x}_{k+1} = \mathbf{x}_k - \mathbf{A}_k^{-1} \mathbf{g}_k.$$

Note, however, that we cannot actually perform this algorithm, because the Hessian matrix is singular. We know from our discussion of this function in Chapter 8 that this function does not have a strong minimum, but it does have a weak minimum along the line $x_1 = x_2$.

What about steepest descent? If we start from the initial guess, with learning rate $\alpha = 0.1$, the first two iterations will be

$$\mathbf{x}_1 = \mathbf{x}_0 - \alpha \mathbf{g}_0 = \begin{bmatrix} 1 \\ 0 \end{bmatrix} - 0.1 \begin{bmatrix} 1 \\ -1 \end{bmatrix} = \begin{bmatrix} 0.9 \\ -0.1 \end{bmatrix},$$

$$\mathbf{x}_2 = \mathbf{x}_1 - \alpha \mathbf{g}_1 = \begin{bmatrix} 0.9 \\ -0.1 \end{bmatrix} - 0.1 \begin{bmatrix} 2 \\ -2 \end{bmatrix} = \begin{bmatrix} 0.8 \\ -0.2 \end{bmatrix}.$$

9

The complete trajectory is shown in Figure P9.7. This is a case where the steepest descent algorithm performs better than Newton's method. Steepest descent converges to a minimum point (weak minimum), while Newton's method fails to converge. In Chapter 12 we will discuss a technique that combines steepest descent with Newton's method, to overcome the problem of singular (or almost singular) Hessian matrices.

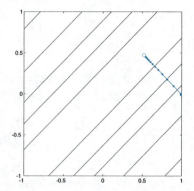

Figure P9.7 Steepest Descent Trajectory for Problem P9.5 with $\alpha = 0.1$

P9.6 Consider the following function:

$$F(\mathbf{x}) = x_1^3 + x_1 x_2 - x_1^2 x_2^2$$

    i. Perform one iteration of Newton's method from the initial guess $\mathbf{x}_0 = \begin{bmatrix} 1 & 1 \end{bmatrix}^T$.

    ii. Find the second-order Taylor series expansion of $F(\mathbf{x})$ about $\mathbf{x}_0$. Is this quadratic function minimized at the point $\mathbf{x}_1$ found in part (i)? Explain.

i.   The gradient of $F(\mathbf{x})$ is

$$\nabla F(\mathbf{x}) = \begin{bmatrix} \dfrac{\partial}{\partial x_1} F(\mathbf{x}) \\[2mm] \dfrac{\partial}{\partial x_2} F(\mathbf{x}) \end{bmatrix} = \begin{bmatrix} 3x_1^2 + x_2 - 2x_1 x_2^2 \\[2mm] x_1 - 2x_1^2 x_2 \end{bmatrix},$$

and the Hessian matrix is

$$\nabla^2 F(\mathbf{x}) = \begin{bmatrix} 6x_1 - 2x_2^2 & 1 - 4x_1 x_2 \\ 1 - 4x_1 x_2 & -2x_1^2 \end{bmatrix}.$$

If we evaluate these at the initial guess we find

$$\mathbf{g}_0 = \nabla F(\mathbf{x})\big|_{\mathbf{x} = \mathbf{x}_0} = \begin{bmatrix} 2 \\ -1 \end{bmatrix},$$

$$\mathbf{A}_0 = \nabla^2 F(\mathbf{x})\big|_{\mathbf{x} = \mathbf{x}_0} = \begin{bmatrix} 4 & -3 \\ -3 & -2 \end{bmatrix}.$$

The first iteration of Newton's method is then

$$\mathbf{x}_1 = \mathbf{x}_0 - \mathbf{A}_0^{-1} \mathbf{g}_0 = \begin{bmatrix} 1 \\ 1 \end{bmatrix} - \begin{bmatrix} 4 & -3 \\ -3 & -2 \end{bmatrix}^{-1} \begin{bmatrix} 2 \\ -1 \end{bmatrix} = \begin{bmatrix} 0.5882 \\ 1.1176 \end{bmatrix}.$$

ii. From Eq. (9.40), the second-order Taylor series expansion of $F(\mathbf{x})$ about $\mathbf{x}_0$ is

$$F(\mathbf{x}) = F(\mathbf{x}_0 + \Delta \mathbf{x}_0) \approx F(\mathbf{x}_0) + \mathbf{g}_0^T \Delta \mathbf{x}_0 + \frac{1}{2} \Delta \mathbf{x}_0^T \mathbf{A}_0 \Delta \mathbf{x}_0.$$

If we substitute the values for $\mathbf{x}_0$, $\mathbf{g}_0$ and $\mathbf{A}_0$, we find

$$F(\mathbf{x}) \approx 1 + \begin{bmatrix} 2 & -1 \end{bmatrix} \left\{ \mathbf{x} - \begin{bmatrix} 1 \\ 1 \end{bmatrix} \right\} + \frac{1}{2} \left\{ \mathbf{x} - \begin{bmatrix} 1 \\ 1 \end{bmatrix} \right\}^T \begin{bmatrix} 4 & -3 \\ -3 & -2 \end{bmatrix} \left\{ \mathbf{x} - \begin{bmatrix} 1 \\ 1 \end{bmatrix} \right\}.$$

This can be reduced to

$$F(\mathbf{x}) \approx -2 + \begin{bmatrix} 1 & 4 \end{bmatrix} \mathbf{x} + \frac{1}{2} \mathbf{x}^T \begin{bmatrix} 4 & -3 \\ -3 & -2 \end{bmatrix} \mathbf{x}.$$

This function has a stationary point at $\mathbf{x}_1$. The question is whether or not the stationary point is a strong minimum. This can be determined from the eigenvalues of the Hessian matrix. If both eigenvalues are positive, it is a strong minimum. If both eigenvalues are negative, it is a strong maximum. If the two eigenvalues have opposite signs, it is a saddle point. In this case the eigenvalues of $\mathbf{A}_0$ are

$$\lambda_1 = 5.24 \text{ and } \lambda_2 = -3.24.$$

9

Therefore the quadratic approximation to $F(\mathbf{x})$ at $\mathbf{x}_0$ is not minimized at $\mathbf{x}_1$, since it is a saddle point. Figure P9.8 displays the contour plots of $F(\mathbf{x})$ and its quadratic approximation.

This sort of problem was also illustrated in Figure 9.8 and Figure 9.9. Newton's method does locate the stationary point of the quadratic approximation of the function at the current guess. It does not distinguish between minima, maxima and saddle points.

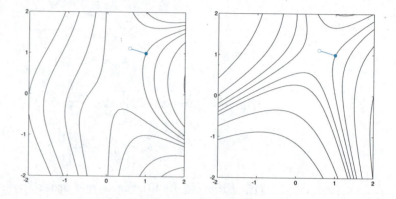

Figure P9.8 One Iteration of Newton's Method from $\mathbf{x}_0 = \begin{bmatrix} 1 & 1 \end{bmatrix}^T$

P9.7 Repeat Problem P9.3 (i) using the conjugate gradient algorithm.

Recall that the function to be minimized was

$$F(\mathbf{x}) = 0.25 + \begin{bmatrix} -2 & -1 \end{bmatrix}\mathbf{x} + \frac{1}{2}\mathbf{x}^T\begin{bmatrix} 10 & 2 \\ 2 & 4 \end{bmatrix}\mathbf{x}.$$

The gradient at $\mathbf{x}_0$ is

$$\mathbf{g}_0 = \nabla F(\mathbf{x}_0) = \mathbf{A}\mathbf{x}_0 + \mathbf{d} = \begin{bmatrix} 10 & 2 \\ 2 & 4 \end{bmatrix}\begin{bmatrix} 1 \\ 1 \end{bmatrix} + \begin{bmatrix} -2 \\ -1 \end{bmatrix} = \begin{bmatrix} 10 \\ 5 \end{bmatrix}.$$

The first search direction is then

$$\mathbf{p}_0 = -\mathbf{g}_0 = \begin{bmatrix} -10 \\ -5 \end{bmatrix}.$$

To minimize along a line, for a quadratic function, we can use Eq. (9.31):

$$\alpha_0 = -\frac{\mathbf{g}_0^T \mathbf{p}_0}{\mathbf{p}_0^T \mathbf{A} \mathbf{p}_0} = -\frac{\begin{bmatrix} 10 & 5 \end{bmatrix} \begin{bmatrix} -10 \\ -5 \end{bmatrix}}{\begin{bmatrix} -10 & -5 \end{bmatrix} \begin{bmatrix} 10 & 2 \\ 2 & 4 \end{bmatrix} \begin{bmatrix} -10 \\ -5 \end{bmatrix}} = \frac{-125}{1300} = 0.0962 .$$

Therefore the first iteration of conjugate gradient will be

$$\mathbf{x}_1 = \mathbf{x}_0 + \alpha_0 \mathbf{p}_0 = \begin{bmatrix} 1 \\ 1 \end{bmatrix} + 0.0962 \begin{bmatrix} -10 \\ -5 \end{bmatrix} = \begin{bmatrix} 0.038 \\ 0.519 \end{bmatrix} .$$

Now we need to find the second search direction from Eq. (9.60). This requires the gradient at $\mathbf{x}_1$:

$$\mathbf{g}_1 = \nabla F(\mathbf{x}) \big|_{\mathbf{x} = \mathbf{x}_1} = \begin{bmatrix} 10 & 2 \\ 2 & 4 \end{bmatrix} \begin{bmatrix} 0.038 \\ 0.519 \end{bmatrix} + \begin{bmatrix} -2 \\ -1 \end{bmatrix} = \begin{bmatrix} -0.577 \\ 1.154 \end{bmatrix} .$$

We can now find β_1:

$$\beta_1 = \frac{\Delta \mathbf{g}_0^T \mathbf{g}_1}{\mathbf{g}_0^T \mathbf{g}_0} = \frac{\begin{bmatrix} -10.577 & -3.846 \end{bmatrix} \begin{bmatrix} -0.577 \\ 1.154 \end{bmatrix}}{\begin{bmatrix} 10 & 5 \end{bmatrix} \begin{bmatrix} 10 \\ 5 \end{bmatrix}} = \frac{1.665}{125} = 0.0133 ,$$

using the method of Polak and Ribiére (Eq. (9.63)). (The other two methods for computing β_1 will produce the same results for a quadratic function. You may want to try them.) The second search direction is then computed from Eq. (9.60):

$$\mathbf{p}_1 = -\mathbf{g}_1 + \beta_1 \mathbf{p}_0 = \begin{bmatrix} 0.577 \\ -1.154 \end{bmatrix} + 0.0133 \begin{bmatrix} -10 \\ -5 \end{bmatrix} = \begin{bmatrix} 0.444 \\ -1.220 \end{bmatrix} .$$

From Eq. (9.31), the learning rate for the second iteration will be

$$\alpha_1 = -\frac{\begin{bmatrix} -0.577 & 1.154 \end{bmatrix} \begin{bmatrix} 0.444 \\ -1.220 \end{bmatrix}}{\begin{bmatrix} 0.444 & -1.220 \end{bmatrix} \begin{bmatrix} 10 & 2 \\ 2 & 4 \end{bmatrix} \begin{bmatrix} 0.444 \\ -1.220 \end{bmatrix}} = -\frac{-1.664}{5.758} = 0.2889 .$$

The second step of conjugate gradient is therefore

9

$$\mathbf{x}_2 = \mathbf{x}_1 + \alpha_1 \mathbf{p}_1 = \begin{bmatrix} 0.038 \\ 0.519 \end{bmatrix} + 0.2889 \begin{bmatrix} 0.444 \\ -1.220 \end{bmatrix} = \begin{bmatrix} 0.1667 \\ 0.1667 \end{bmatrix}.$$

As expected, the minimum is reached in two iterations. The trajectory is illustrated in Figure P9.9.

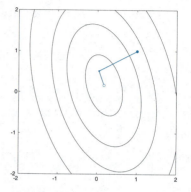

Figure P9.9 Conjugate Gradient Trajectory for Problem P9.7

P9.8 Show that conjugate vectors are independent.

Suppose that we have a set of vectors, $\{\mathbf{p}_0, \mathbf{p}_1, \dots, \mathbf{p}_{n-1}\}$, which are conjugate with respect to the Hessian matrix $\mathbf{A}$. If these vectors are dependent, then, from Eq. (5.4), it must be true that

$$\sum_{j=0}^{n-1} a_j \mathbf{p}_j = \mathbf{0},$$

for some set of constants $a_0, a_1, \dots, a_{n-1}$, at least one of which is nonzero. If we multiply both sides of this equation by $\mathbf{p}_k^T \mathbf{A}$, we obtain

$$\mathbf{p}_k^T \mathbf{A} \sum_{j=0}^{n-1} a_j \mathbf{p}_j = \sum_{j=0}^{n-1} a_j \mathbf{p}_k^T \mathbf{A} \mathbf{p}_j = a_k \mathbf{p}_k^T \mathbf{A} \mathbf{p}_k = 0,$$

where the second equality comes from the definition of conjugate vectors in Eq. (9.52). If $\mathbf{A}$ is positive definite (a unique strong minimum exists), then $\mathbf{p}_k^T \mathbf{A} \mathbf{p}_k$ must be strictly positive. This implies that a_k must be zero for all k. Therefore conjugate directions must be independent.

Epilogue

In this chapter we have introduced three different optimization algorithms: steepest descent, Newton's method and conjugate gradient. The basis for these algorithms is the Taylor series expansion. Steepest descent is derived by using a first-order expansion, whereas Newton's method and conjugate gradient are designed for second-order (quadratic) functions.

Steepest descent has the advantage that it is very simple, requiring calculation only of the gradient. It is also guaranteed to converge to a stationary point if the learning rate is small enough. The disadvantage of steepest descent is that training times are generally longer than for other algorithms. This is especially true when the eigenvalues of the Hessian matrix, for quadratic functions, have a wide range of magnitudes.

Newton's method is generally much faster than steepest descent. For quadratic functions it will locate a stationary point in one iteration. One disadvantage is that it requires calculation and storage of the Hessian matrix, as well as its inverse. In addition, the convergence properties of Newton's method are quite complex. In Chapter 12 we will introduce a modification of Newton's method that overcomes some of the disadvantages of the standard algorithm.

The conjugate gradient algorithm is something of a compromise between steepest descent and Newton's method. It will locate the minimum of a quadratic function in a finite number of iterations, but it does not require calculation and storage of the Hessian matrix. It is well suited to problems with large numbers of parameters, where it is impractical to compute and store the Hessian.

In later chapters we will apply each of these optimization algorithms to the training of neural networks. In Chapter 10 we will demonstrate how an approximate steepest descent algorithm, Widrow-Hoff learning, can be used to train linear networks. In Chapter 11 we generalize Widrow-Hoff learning to train multilayer networks. In Chapter 12 the conjugate gradient algorithm, and a variation of Newton's method, are used to speed up the training of multilayer networks.

9

Further Reading

[Batt92]   R. Battiti, "First and Second Order Methods for Learning: Between Steepest Descent and Newton's Method," *Neural Computation*, Vol. 4, No. 2, pp. 141-166, 1992.

This article reviews the latest developments in unconstrained optimization using first and second derivatives. The techniques discussed are those that are most suitable for neural network applications.

[Brog91]   W. L. Brogan, *Modern Control Theory,* 3rd Ed., Englewood Cliffs, NJ: Prentice-Hall, 1991.

This is a well-written book on the subject of linear systems. The first half of the book is devoted to linear algebra. It also has good sections on the solution of linear differential equations and the stability of linear and nonlinear systems. It has many worked problems.

[Gill81]   P. E. Gill, W. Murray and M. H. Wright, *Practical Optimization*, New York: Academic Press, 1981.

As the title implies, this text emphasizes the practical implementation of optimization algorithms. It provides motivation for the optimization methods, as well as details of implementation that affect algorithm performance.

[Himm72]   D. M. Himmelblau, *Applied Nonlinear Programming*, New York: McGraw-Hill, 1972.

This is a comprehensive text on nonlinear optimization. It covers both constrained and unconstrained optimization problems. The text is very complete, with many examples worked out in detail.

[Scal85]   L. E. Scales, *Introduction to Non-Linear Optimization*, New York: Springer-Verlag, 1985.

A very readable text describing the major optimization algorithms, this text emphasizes methods of optimization rather than existence theorems and proofs of convergence. Algorithms are presented with intuitive explanations, along with illustrative figures and examples. Pseudo-code is presented for most algorithms.

Exercises

E9.1 In Problem P9.1 we found the maximum stable learning rate for the steepest descent algorithm when applied to a particular quadratic function. Will the algorithm always diverge when a larger learning rate is used, or are there any conditions for which the algorithm will still converge?

E9.2 We want to find the minimum of the following function:

$$F(\mathbf{x}) = \frac{1}{2}\mathbf{x}^T \begin{bmatrix} 6 & -2 \\ -2 & 6 \end{bmatrix} \mathbf{x} + \begin{bmatrix} -1 & -1 \end{bmatrix} \mathbf{x}.$$

    i. Sketch a contour plot of this function.

    ii. Sketch the trajectory of the steepest descent algorithm on the contour plot of part (i), if the initial guess is $\mathbf{x}_0 = \begin{bmatrix} 0 & 0 \end{bmatrix}^T$. Assume a very small learning rate is used.

    iii. Perform two iterations of steepest descent with learning rate $\alpha = 0.1$.

    iv. What is the maximum stable learning rate?

    v. What is the maximum stable learning rate for the initial guess given in part (ii)? (See Exercise E9.1.)

    vi. Write a MATLAB M-file to implement the steepest descent algorithm for this problem, and use it to check your answers to parts (i). through (v).

```
» 2 + 2
ans =
    4
```

E9.3 For the quadratic function

$$F(\mathbf{x}) = x_1^2 + 2x_2^2,$$

    i. Find the minimum of the function along the line

$$\mathbf{x} = \begin{bmatrix} 1 \\ 1 \end{bmatrix} + \alpha \begin{bmatrix} -1 \\ -2 \end{bmatrix}.$$

    ii. Verify that the gradient of $F(\mathbf{x})$ at the minimum point from part (i) is orthogonal to the line along which the minimization occurred.

9

E9.4 For the functions given in Exercise E8.3 perform two iterations of the steepest descent algorithm with linear minimization, starting from the initial guess $\mathbf{x}_0 = \begin{bmatrix} 1 & 1 \end{bmatrix}^T$. Write MATLAB M-files to check your answer.

E9.5 Consider the following function

$$F(\mathbf{x}) = [1 + (x_1 + x_2 - 5)^2][1 + (3x_1 - 2x_2)^2]$$

    i. Perform one iteration of Newton's method, starting from the initial guess $\mathbf{x}_0 = \begin{bmatrix} 10 & 10 \end{bmatrix}^T$.

    ii. Repeat part (i), starting from the initial guess $\mathbf{x}_0 = \begin{bmatrix} 2 & 2 \end{bmatrix}^T$.

    iii. Find the minimum of the function, and compare with your results from the previous two parts.

E9.6 Recall the function presented in Exercise E8.5. Write MATLAB M-files to implement the steepest descent algorithm and Newton's method for that function. Test the performance of the algorithms for various initial guesses.

E9.7 Repeat Exercise E9.4 using the conjugate gradient algorithm. Use each of the three methods (Eq. (9.61)–Eq. (9.63)) at least once.

E9.8 Prove or disprove the following statement:

If $\mathbf{p}_1$ is conjugate to $\mathbf{p}_2$ and $\mathbf{p}_2$ is conjugate to $\mathbf{p}_3$,
then $\mathbf{p}_1$ is conjugate to $\mathbf{p}_3$.

10 Widrow-Hoff Learning

Objectives

In the previous two chapters we laid the foundation for *performance learning*, in which a network is trained to optimize its performance. In this chapter we apply the principles of performance learning to a single-layer linear neural network.

Widrow-Hoff learning is an approximate steepest descent algorithm, in which the performance index is mean square error. This algorithm is important to our discussion for two reasons. First, it is widely used today in many signal processing applications, several of which we will discuss in this chapter. In addition, it is the precursor to the backpropagation algorithm for multilayer networks, which is presented in Chapter 11

10

Theory and Examples

Bernard Widrow began working in neural networks in the late 1950s, at about the same time that Frank Rosenblatt developed the perceptron learning rule. In 1960 Widrow, and his graduate student Marcian Hoff, introduced the ADALINE (ADAptive LInear NEuron) network, and a learning rule which they called the LMS (Least Mean Square) algorithm [WiHo60].

Their ADALINE network is very similar to the perceptron, except that its transfer function is linear, instead of hard-limiting. Both the ADALINE and the perceptron suffer from the same inherent limitation: they can only solve linearly separable problems (recall our discussion in Chapters 3 and 4). The LMS algorithm, however, is more powerful than the perceptron learning rule. While the perceptron rule is guaranteed to converge to a solution that correctly categorizes the training patterns, the resulting network can be sensitive to noise, since patterns often lie close to the decision boundaries. The LMS algorithm minimizes mean square error, and therefore tries to move the decision boundaries as far from the training patterns as possible.

The LMS algorithm has found many more practical uses than the perceptron learning rule. This is especially true in the area of digital signal processing. For example, most long distance phone lines use ADALINE networks for echo cancellation. We will discuss these applications in detail later in the chapter.

Because of the great success of the LMS algorithm in signal processing applications, and because of the lack of success in adapting the algorithm to multilayer networks, Widrow stopped work on neural networks in the early 1960s and began to work full time on adaptive signal processing. He returned to the neural network field in the 1980s and began research on the use of neural networks in adaptive control, using temporal backpropagation, a descendant of his original LMS algorithm.

ADALINE Network

The ADALINE network is shown in Figure 10.1. Notice that it has the same basic structure as the perceptron network we discussed in Chapter 4. The only difference is that it has a linear transfer function.

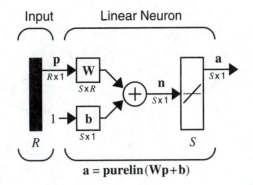

$$a = \mathbf{purelin}(\mathbf{Wp}+\mathbf{b})$$

Figure 10.1 ADALINE Network

The output of the network is given by

$$a = \mathbf{purelin}(\mathbf{Wp} + \mathbf{b}) = \mathbf{Wp} + \mathbf{b}. \tag{10.1}$$

Recall from our discussion of the perceptron network that the ith element of the network output vector can be written

$$a_i = purelin(n_i) = purelin({_i}\mathbf{w}^T\mathbf{p} + b_i) = {_i}\mathbf{w}^T\mathbf{p} + b_i, \tag{10.2}$$

where ${_i}\mathbf{w}$ is made up of the elements of the ith row of $\mathbf{W}$:

$$ {_i}\mathbf{w} = \begin{bmatrix} w_{i,1} \\ w_{i,2} \\ \vdots \\ w_{i,R} \end{bmatrix}. \tag{10.3}$$

Single ADALINE

To simplify our discussion, let's consider a single ADALINE with two inputs. The diagram for this network is shown in Figure 10.2.

The output of the network is given by

$$a = purelin(n) = purelin({_1}\mathbf{w}^T\mathbf{p} + b) = {_1}\mathbf{w}^T\mathbf{p} + b$$

$$= {_1}\mathbf{w}^T\mathbf{p} + b = w_{1,1}p_1 + w_{1,2}p_2 + b. \tag{10.4}$$

10

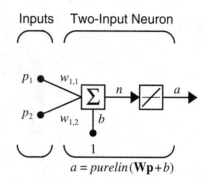

Figure 10.2 Two-Input Linear Neuron

You may recall from Chapter 4 that the perceptron has a *decision boundary*, which is determined by the input vectors for which the net input n is zero. Now, does the ADALINE also have such a boundary? Clearly it does. If we set $n = 0$ then ${}_1\mathbf{w}^T\mathbf{p} + b = 0$ specifies such a line, as shown in Figure 10.3.

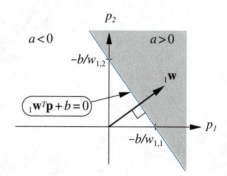

Figure 10.3 Decision Boundary for Two-Input ADALINE

The neuron output is greater than 0 in the gray area. In the white area the output is less than zero. Now, what does this imply about the ADALINE? It says that the ADALINE can be used to classify objects into two categories. However, it can do so only if the objects are linearly separable. Thus, in this respect, the ADALINE has the same limitation as the perceptron.

Mean Square Error

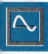

Now that we have examined the characteristics of the ADALINE network, we are ready to begin our development of the LMS algorithm. As with the perceptron rule, the LMS algorithm is an example of supervised training, in which the learning rule is provided with a set of examples of proper network behavior:

$$\{\mathbf{p}_1, \mathbf{t}_1\}, \{\mathbf{p}_2, \mathbf{t}_2\}, \dots, \{\mathbf{p}_Q, \mathbf{t}_Q\}, \tag{10.5}$$

where $\mathbf{p}_q$ is an input to the network, and $\mathbf{t}_q$ is the corresponding target output. As each input is applied to the network, the network output is compared to the target.

The LMS algorithm will adjust the weights and biases of the ADALINE in order to minimize the mean square error, where the error is the difference between the target output and the network output. In this section we want to discuss this performance index. We will consider first the single-neuron case.

To simply our development, we will lump all of the parameters we are adjusting, including the bias, into one vector:

$$\mathbf{x} = \begin{bmatrix} {}_1\mathbf{w} \\ b \end{bmatrix}. \tag{10.6}$$

Similarly, we include the bias input "1" as a component of the input vector

$$\mathbf{z} = \begin{bmatrix} \mathbf{p} \\ 1 \end{bmatrix}. \tag{10.7}$$

Now the network output, which we usually write in the form

$$a = {}_1\mathbf{w}^T \mathbf{p} + b, \tag{10.8}$$

can be written as

$$a = \mathbf{x}^T \mathbf{z}. \tag{10.9}$$

This allows us to conveniently write out an expression for the ADALINE network *mean square error*:

$$F(\mathbf{x}) = E[e^2] = E[(t-a)^2] = E[(t-\mathbf{x}^T\mathbf{z})^2], \tag{10.10}$$

where the expectation is taken over all sets of input/target pairs. (Here we use $E[\ ]$ to denote expected value. We use a generalized definition of expectation, which becomes a time-average for deterministic signals. See [WiSt85].) We can expand this expression as follows:

$$
\begin{aligned}
F(\mathbf{x}) &= E[t^2 - 2t\mathbf{x}^T\mathbf{z} + \mathbf{x}^T\mathbf{z}\mathbf{z}^T\mathbf{x}] \\
&= E[t^2] - 2\mathbf{x}^T E[t\mathbf{z}] + \mathbf{x}^T E[\mathbf{z}\mathbf{z}^T]\mathbf{x}.
\end{aligned}
\tag{10.11}
$$

10

This can be written in the following convenient form:

$$F(\mathbf{x}) = c - 2\mathbf{x}^T\mathbf{h} + \mathbf{x}^T\mathbf{R}\mathbf{x}, \tag{10.12}$$

where

$$c = E[t^2], \ \mathbf{h} = E[t\mathbf{z}] \ \text{and} \ \mathbf{R} = E[\mathbf{z}\mathbf{z}^T]. \tag{10.13}$$

Correlation Matrix

Here the vector $\mathbf{h}$ gives the cross-correlation between the input vector and its associated target, while $\mathbf{R}$ is the input *correlation matrix*. The diagonal elements of this matrix are equal to the mean square values of the elements of the input vectors.

Take a close look at Eq. (10.12), and compare it with the general form of the quadratic function given in Eq. (8.35) and repeated here:

$$F(\mathbf{x}) = c + \mathbf{d}^T\mathbf{x} + \frac{1}{2}\mathbf{x}^T\mathbf{A}\mathbf{x}. \tag{10.14}$$

We can see that the mean square error performance index for the ADALINE network is a quadratic function, where

$$\mathbf{d} = -2\mathbf{h} \ \text{and} \ \mathbf{A} = 2\mathbf{R}. \tag{10.15}$$

This is a very important result, because we know from Chapter 8 that the characteristics of the quadratic function depend primarily on the Hessian matrix $\mathbf{A}$. For example, if the eigenvalues of the Hessian are all positive, then the function will have one unique global minimum.

In this case the Hessian matrix is twice the correlation matrix $\mathbf{R}$, and it can be shown that all correlation matrices are either positive definite or positive semidefinite, which means that they can never have negative eigenvalues. We are left with two possibilities. If the correlation matrix has only positive eigenvalues, the performance index will have one unique global minimum (see Figure 8.7). If the correlation matrix has some zero eigenvalues, the performance index will either have a weak minimum (see Figure 8.9) or no minimum (see Problem P8.7), depending on the vector $\mathbf{d} = -2\mathbf{h}$.

Now let's locate the stationary point of the performance index. From our previous discussion of quadratic functions we know that the gradient is

$$\nabla F(\mathbf{x}) = \nabla\left(c + \mathbf{d}^T\mathbf{x} + \frac{1}{2}\mathbf{x}^T\mathbf{A}\mathbf{x}\right) = \mathbf{d} + \mathbf{A}\mathbf{x} = -2\mathbf{h} + 2\mathbf{R}\mathbf{x}. \tag{10.16}$$

The stationary point of $F(\mathbf{x})$ can be found by setting the gradient equal to zero:

$$-2\mathbf{h} + 2\mathbf{R}\mathbf{x} = 0. \tag{10.17}$$

Therefore, if the correlation matrix is positive definite there will be a unique stationary point, which will be a strong minimum:

$$\mathbf{x}^* = \mathbf{R}^{-1}\mathbf{h}.\qquad(10.18)$$

It is worth noting here that the existence of a unique solution depends only on the correlation matrix $\mathbf{R}$. Therefore the characteristics of the input vectors determine whether or not a unique solution exists.

LMS Algorithm

Now that we have analyzed our performance index, the next step is to design an algorithm to locate the minimum point. If we could calculate the statistical quantities $\mathbf{h}$ and $\mathbf{R}$, we could find the minimum point directly from Eq. (10.18). If we did not want to calculate the inverse of $\mathbf{R}$, we could use the steepest descent algorithm, with the gradient calculated from Eq. (10.16). In general, however, it is not desirable or convenient to calculate $\mathbf{h}$ and $\mathbf{R}$. For this reason we will use an approximate steepest descent algorithm, in which we use an estimated gradient.

The key insight of Widrow and Hoff was that they could estimate the mean square error $F(\mathbf{x})$ by

$$\hat{F}(\mathbf{x}) = (t(k) - a(k))^2 = e^2(k),\qquad(10.19)$$

where the expectation of the squared error has been replaced by the squared error at iteration k. Then, at each iteration we have a gradient estimate of the form:

$$\hat{\nabla}F(\mathbf{x}) = \nabla e^2(k).\qquad(10.20)$$

The first R elements of $\nabla e^2(k)$ are derivatives with respect to the network weights, while the $(R+1)$st element is the derivative with respect to the bias. Thus we have

$$[\nabla e^2(k)]_j = \frac{\partial e^2(k)}{\partial w_{1,j}} = 2e(k)\frac{\partial e(k)}{\partial w_{1,j}} \text{ for } j = 1, 2, \dots, R,\qquad(10.21)$$

and

$$[\nabla e^2(k)]_{R+1} = \frac{\partial e^2(k)}{\partial b} = 2e(k)\frac{\partial e(k)}{\partial b}.\qquad(10.22)$$

Now consider the partial derivative terms at the ends of these equations. First evaluate the partial derivative of $e(k)$ with respect to the weight $w_{1,j}$:

10

$$\frac{\partial e(k)}{\partial w_{1,j}} = \frac{\partial [t(k) - a(k)]}{\partial w_{1,j}} = \frac{\partial}{\partial w_{1,j}} [t(k) - ({}_{1}\mathbf{w}^{T}\mathbf{p}(k) + b)]$$

$$= \frac{\partial}{\partial w_{1,j}} \left[t(k) - \left(\sum_{i=1}^{R} w_{1,i}p_{i}(k) + b \right) \right]$$

(10.23)

where $p_i(k)$ is the ith element of the input vector at the kth iteration. This simplifies to

$$\frac{\partial e(k)}{\partial w_{1,j}} = -p_j(k) .$$

(10.24)

In a similar way we can obtain the final element of the gradient:

$$\frac{\partial e(k)}{\partial b} = -1 .$$

(10.25)

Note that $p_j(k)$ and 1 are the elements of the input vector $\mathbf{z}$, so the gradient of the squared error at iteration k can be written

$$\hat{\nabla} F(\mathbf{x}) = \nabla e^2(k) = -2e(k)\mathbf{z}(k) .$$

(10.26)

Now we can see the beauty of approximating the mean square error by the single error at iteration k, as in Eq. (10.19). To calculate this approximate gradient we need only multiply the error times the input.

This approximation to $\nabla F(\mathbf{x})$ can now be used in the steepest descent algorithm. From Eq. (9.10) the steepest descent algorithm, with constant learning rate, is

$$\mathbf{x}_{k+1} = \mathbf{x}_k - \alpha \nabla F(\mathbf{x}) \big|_{\mathbf{x} = \mathbf{x}_k} .$$

(10.27)

If we substitute $\hat{\nabla} F(\mathbf{x})$, from Eq. (10.26), for $\nabla F(\mathbf{x})$ we find

$$\mathbf{x}_{k+1} = \mathbf{x}_k + 2\alpha e(k)\mathbf{z}(k) ,$$

(10.28)

or

$${}_{1}\mathbf{w}(k+1) = {}_{1}\mathbf{w}(k) + 2\alpha e(k)\mathbf{p}(k) ,$$

(10.29)

and

$$b(k+1) = b(k) + 2\alpha e(k) .$$

(10.30)

These last two equations make up the least mean square (LMS) algorithm. This is also referred to as the delta rule or the Widrow-Hoff learning algorithm.

The preceding results can be modified to handle the case where we have multiple outputs, and therefore multiple neurons, as in Figure 10.1. To update the ith row of the weight matrix use

$$_i\mathbf{w}(k+1) = {}_i\mathbf{w}(k) + 2\alpha e_i(k)\mathbf{p}(k),\tag{10.31}$$

where $e_i(k)$ is the ith element of the error at iteration k. To update the ith element of the bias we use

$$b_i(k+1) = b_i(k) + 2\alpha e_i(k).\tag{10.32}$$

LMS Algorithm   The *LMS algorithm* can be written conveniently in matrix notation:

$$\mathbf{W}(k+1) = \mathbf{W}(k) + 2\alpha\mathbf{e}(k)\mathbf{p}^T(k),\tag{10.33}$$

and

$$\mathbf{b}(k+1) = \mathbf{b}(k) + 2\alpha\mathbf{e}(k).\tag{10.34}$$

Note that the error $\mathbf{e}$ and the bias $\mathbf{b}$ are now vectors.

Analysis of Convergence

The stability of the steepest descent algorithm was investigated in Chapter 9. There we found that the maximum stable learning rate for quadratic functions is $\alpha < 2/\lambda_{max}$, where λ_{max} is the largest eigenvalue of the Hessian matrix. Now we want to investigate the convergence of the LMS algorithm, which is approximate steepest descent. We will find that the result is the same.

To begin, note that in the LMS algorithm, Eq. (10.28), $\mathbf{x}_k$ is a function only of $\mathbf{z}(k-1), \mathbf{z}(k-2), \dots, \mathbf{z}(0)$. If we assume that successive input vectors are statistically independent, then $\mathbf{x}_k$ is independent of $\mathbf{z}(k)$. We will show in the following development that for stationary input processes meeting this condition, the expected value of the weight vector will converge to

$$\mathbf{x}^* = \mathbf{R}^{-1}\mathbf{h}.\tag{10.35}$$

This is the minimum mean square error $\{E[e_k^2]\}$ solution, as we saw in Eq. (10.18).

Recall the LMS algorithm (Eq. (10.28)):

$$\mathbf{x}_{k+1} = \mathbf{x}_k + 2\alpha e(k)\mathbf{z}(k).\tag{10.36}$$

Now take the expectation of both sides:

$$E[\mathbf{x}_{k+1}] = E[\mathbf{x}_k] + 2\alpha E[e(k)\mathbf{z}(k)].\tag{10.37}$$

10

Substitute $t(k) - \mathbf{x}_k^T \mathbf{z}(k)$ for the error to give

$$E[\mathbf{x}_{k+1}] = E[\mathbf{x}_k] + 2\alpha \{ E[t(k)\mathbf{z}(k)] - E[(\mathbf{x}_k^T \mathbf{z}(k))\mathbf{z}(k)] \} . \quad (10.38)$$

Finally, substitute $\mathbf{z}^T(k)\mathbf{x}_k$ for $\mathbf{x}_k^T \mathbf{z}(k)$ and rearrange terms to give

$$E[\mathbf{x}_{k+1}] = E[\mathbf{x}_k] + 2\alpha \{ E[t_k \mathbf{z}(k)] - E[(\mathbf{z}(k)\mathbf{z}^T(k))\mathbf{x}_k] \} . \quad (10.39)$$

Since $\mathbf{x}_k$ is independent of $\mathbf{z}(k)$:

$$E[\mathbf{x}_{k+1}] = E[\mathbf{x}_k] + 2\alpha \{ \mathbf{h} - \mathbf{R}E[\mathbf{x}_k] \} . \quad (10.40)$$

This can be written as

$$E[\mathbf{x}_{k+1}] = [\mathbf{I} - 2\alpha\mathbf{R}]E[\mathbf{x}_k] + 2\alpha\mathbf{h} . \quad (10.41)$$

This dynamic system will be stable if all of the eigenvalues of $[\mathbf{I} - 2\alpha\mathbf{R}]$ fall inside the unit circle (see [Brog91]). Recall from Chapter 9 that the eigenvalues of $[\mathbf{I} - 2\alpha\mathbf{R}]$ will be $1 - 2\alpha\lambda_i$, where the λ_i are the eigenvalues of $\mathbf{R}$. Therefore, the system will be stable if

$$1 - 2\alpha\lambda_i > -1 . \quad (10.42)$$

Since $\lambda_i > 0$, $1 - 2\alpha\lambda_i$ is always less than 1. The condition on stability is therefore

$$\alpha < 1/\lambda_i \quad \text{for all } i, \quad (10.43)$$

or

$$0 < \alpha < 1/\lambda_{max} . \quad (10.44)$$

Note that this condition is equivalent to the condition we derived in Chapter 9 for the steepest descent algorithm, although in that case we were using the eigenvalues of the Hessian matrix $\mathbf{A}$. Now we are using the eigenvalues of the input correlation matrix $\mathbf{R}$. (Recall that $\mathbf{A} = 2\mathbf{R}$.)

If this condition on stability is satisfied, the steady state solution is

$$E[\mathbf{x}_{ss}] = [\mathbf{I} - 2\alpha\mathbf{R}]E[\mathbf{x}_{ss}] + 2\alpha\mathbf{h} , \quad (10.45)$$

or

$$E[\mathbf{x}_{ss}] = \mathbf{R}^{-1}\mathbf{h} = \mathbf{x}^* . \quad (10.46)$$

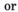

Thus the LMS solution, obtained by applying one input vector at a time, is the same as the minimum mean square error solution of Eq. (10.18).

To test the ADALINE network and the LMS algorithm consider again the apple/orange recognition problem originally discussed in Chapter 3. For simplicity we will assume that the ADALINE network has a zero bias.

The LMS weight update algorithm of Eq. (10.29) will be used to calculate the new weights at each step in the network training:

$$\mathbf{W}(k+1) = \mathbf{W}(k) + 2\alpha e(k)\mathbf{p}^T(k) . \tag{10.47}$$

First let's compute the maximum stable learning rate α. We can get such a value by finding the eigenvalues of the input correlation matrix. Recall that the orange and apple vectors and their associated targets are

$$\left\{ \mathbf{p}_1 = \begin{bmatrix} 1 \\ -1 \\ -1 \end{bmatrix}, t_1 = \begin{bmatrix} -1 \end{bmatrix} \right\} \qquad \left\{ \mathbf{p}_2 = \begin{bmatrix} 1 \\ 1 \\ -1 \end{bmatrix}, t_2 = \begin{bmatrix} 1 \end{bmatrix} \right\} . \tag{10.48}$$

If we assume that the input vectors are generated randomly with equal probability, we can compute the input correlation matrix:

$$\mathbf{R} = E[\mathbf{p}\mathbf{p}^T] = \frac{1}{2}\mathbf{p}_1\mathbf{p}_1^T + \frac{1}{2}\mathbf{p}_2\mathbf{p}_2^T$$

$$= \frac{1}{2}\begin{bmatrix} 1 \\ -1 \\ -1 \end{bmatrix}\begin{bmatrix} 1 & -1 & -1 \end{bmatrix} + \frac{1}{2}\begin{bmatrix} 1 \\ 1 \\ -1 \end{bmatrix}\begin{bmatrix} 1 & 1 & -1 \end{bmatrix} = \begin{bmatrix} 1 & 0 & -1 \\ 0 & 1 & 0 \\ -1 & 0 & 1 \end{bmatrix} . \tag{10.49}$$

The eigenvalues of $\mathbf{R}$ are

$$\lambda_1 = 1.0, \qquad \lambda_2 = 0.0, \qquad \lambda_3 = 2.0 . \tag{10.50}$$

Thus, the maximum stable learning rate is

$$\alpha < \frac{1}{\lambda_{max}} = \frac{1}{2.0} = 0.5 . \tag{10.51}$$

To be conservative we will pick $\alpha = 0.2$. (Note that in practical applications it might not be practical to calculate $\mathbf{R}$, and α could be selected by trial and error. Other techniques for choosing α are given in [WiSt85].)

We will start, arbitrarily, with all the weights set to zero, and then will apply inputs $\mathbf{p}_1$, $\mathbf{p}_2$, $\mathbf{p}_1$, $\mathbf{p}_2$, etc., in that order, calculating the new weights after each input is presented. (The presentation of the weights in alternat-

10

ing order is not necessary. A random sequence would be fine.) Presenting $\mathbf{p}_1$, the orange, and using its target of –1 we get

$$a(0) = \mathbf{W}(0)\,\mathbf{p}(0) = \mathbf{W}(0)\,\mathbf{p}_1 = \begin{bmatrix} 0 & 0 & 0 \end{bmatrix} \begin{bmatrix} 1 \\ -1 \\ -1 \end{bmatrix} = 0 \,, \qquad (10.52)$$

and

$$e(0) = t(0) - a(0) = t_1 - a(0) = -1 - 0 = -1 \,. \qquad (10.53)$$

Now we can calculate the new weight matrix:

$$\mathbf{W}(1) = \mathbf{W}(0) + 2\alpha e(0)\,\mathbf{p}^T(0)$$

$$= \begin{bmatrix} 0 & 0 & 0 \end{bmatrix} + 2(0.2)(-1) \begin{bmatrix} 1 \\ -1 \\ -1 \end{bmatrix}^T = \begin{bmatrix} -0.4 & 0.4 & 0.4 \end{bmatrix} \,. \qquad (10.54)$$

According to plan, we will next present the apple, $\mathbf{p}_2$, and its target of 1:

$$a(1) = \mathbf{W}(1)\,\mathbf{p}(1) = \mathbf{W}(1)\,\mathbf{p}_2 = \begin{bmatrix} -0.4 & 0.4 & 0.4 \end{bmatrix} \begin{bmatrix} 1 \\ 1 \\ -1 \end{bmatrix} = -0.4 \,, \qquad (10.55)$$

and so the error is

$$e(1) = t(1) - a(1) = t_2 - a(1) = 1 - (-0.4) = 1.4 \,. \qquad (10.56)$$

Now we calculate the new weights:

$$\mathbf{W}(2) = \mathbf{W}(1) + 2\alpha e(1)\,\mathbf{p}^T(1)$$

$$= \begin{bmatrix} -0.4 & 0.4 & 0.4 \end{bmatrix} + 2(0.2)(1.4) \begin{bmatrix} 1 \\ 1 \\ -1 \end{bmatrix}^T = \begin{bmatrix} 0.16 & 0.96 & -0.16 \end{bmatrix} \,. \qquad (10.57)$$

Next we present the orange again:

$$a(2) = \mathbf{W}(2)\,\mathbf{p}(2) = \mathbf{W}(2)\,\mathbf{p}_1 = \begin{bmatrix} 0.16 & 0.96 & -0.16 \end{bmatrix} \begin{bmatrix} 1 \\ -1 \\ -1 \end{bmatrix} = -0.64 \,. \qquad (10.58)$$

The error is

$$e(2) = t(2) - a(2) = t_1 - a(2) = -1 - (-0.64) = -0.36 . \qquad (10.59)$$

The new weights are

$$\mathbf{W}(3) = \mathbf{W}(2) + 2\alpha e(2)\mathbf{p}^T(2) = \begin{bmatrix} 0.016 & 1.1040 & -0.0160 \end{bmatrix} . \qquad (10.60)$$

If we continue this procedure, the algorithm converges to

$$\mathbf{W}(\infty) = \begin{bmatrix} 0 & 1 & 0 \end{bmatrix} . \qquad (10.61)$$

Compare this result with the result of the perceptron learning rule in Chapter 4. You will notice that the ADALINE has produced the same decision boundary that we designed in Chapter 3 for the apple/orange problem. This boundary falls halfway between the two reference patterns. The perceptron rule did not produce such a boundary. This is because the perceptron rule stops as soon as the patterns are correctly classified, even though some patterns may be close to the boundaries. The LMS algorithm minimizes the mean square error. Therefore it tries to move the decision boundaries as far from the reference patterns as possible.

Adaptive Filtering

As we mentioned at the beginning of this chapter, the ADALINE network has the same major limitation as the perceptron network; it can only solve linearly separable problems. In spite of this, the ADALINE has been much more widely used than the perceptron network. In fact, it is safe to say that it is one of the most widely used neural networks in practical applications. One of the major application areas of the ADALINE has been adaptive filtering, where it is still used extensively. In this section we will demonstrate an adaptive filtering example.

Tapped Delay Line   In order to use the ADALINE network as an adaptive filter, we need to introduce a new building block, the tapped delay line. A *tapped delay line* with R outputs is shown in Figure 10.4.

The input signal enters from the left. At the output of the tapped delay line we have an R-dimensional vector, consisting of the input signal at the current time and at delays of from 1 to $R-1$ time steps.

10

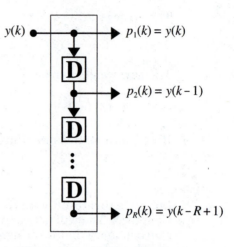

Figure 10.4 Tapped Delay Line

Adaptive Filter   If we combine a tapped delay line with an ADALINE network, we can create an *adaptive filter*, as is shown in Figure 10.5. The output of the filter is given by

$$a(k) = purelin(\mathbf{W}\mathbf{p} + b) = \sum_{i=1}^{R} w_{1,i} y(k - i + 1) + b. \qquad (10.62)$$

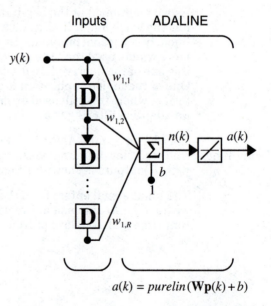

$$a(k) = purelin(\mathbf{W}\mathbf{p}(k) + b)$$

Figure 10.5 Adaptive Filter ADALINE

If you are familiar with digital signal processing, you will recognize the network of Figure 10.5 as a finite impulse response (FIR) filter [WiSt85]. It is beyond the scope of this text to review the field of digital signal processing, but we can demonstrate the usefulness of this adaptive filter through a simple, but practical, example.

Adaptive Noise Cancellation

An adaptive filter can be used in a variety of novel ways. In the following example we will use it for noise cancellation. Take some time to look at this example, for it is a little different from what you might expect. For instance, the output "error" that the network tries to minimize is actually an approximation to the signal we are trying to recover!

Let's suppose that a doctor, in trying to review the electroencephalogram (EEG) of a distracted graduate student, finds that the signal he would like to see has been contaminated by a 60-Hz noise source. He is examining the patient on-line and wants to view the best signal that can be obtained. Figure 10.6 shows how an adaptive filter can be used to remove the contaminating signal.

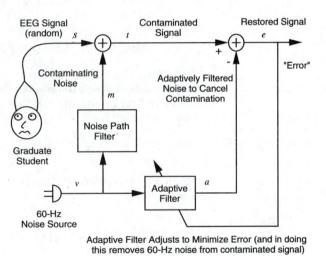

Figure 10.6 Noise Cancellation System

As shown, a sample of the original 60-Hz signal is fed to an adaptive filter, whose elements are adjusted so as to minimize the "error" e. The desired output of the filter is the contaminated EEG signal t. The adaptive filter will do its best to reproduce this contaminated signal, but it only knows about the original noise source, v. Thus, it can only reproduce the part of t that is linearly correlated with v, which is m. In effect, the adaptive filter will attempt to mimic the noise path filter, so that the output of the filter

a will be close to the contaminating noise m. In this way the error e will be close to the original uncontaminated EEG signal s.

In this simple case of a single sine wave noise source, a neuron with two weights and no bias is sufficient to implement the filter. The inputs to the filter are the current and previous values of the noise source. Such a two-input filter can attenuate and phase-shift the noise v in the desired way. The filter is shown in Figure 10.7.

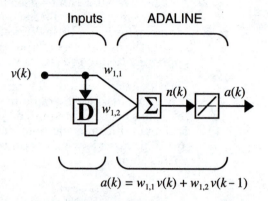

$$a(k) = w_{1,1} v(k) + w_{1,2} v(k-1)$$

Figure 10.7 Adaptive Filter for Noise Cancellation

We can apply the mathematical relationships developed in the previous sections of this chapter to analyze this system. In order to do so, we will first need to find the input correlation matrix $\mathbf{R}$ and the input/target cross-correlation vector $\mathbf{h}$:

$$\mathbf{R} = [\mathbf{zz}^T] \quad \text{and} \quad \mathbf{h} = E[t\mathbf{z}] \ . \tag{10.63}$$

In our case the input vector is given by the current and previous values of the noise source:

$$\mathbf{z}(k) = \begin{bmatrix} v(k) \\ v(k-1) \end{bmatrix}, \tag{10.64}$$

while the target is the sum of the current signal and filtered noise:

$$t(k) = s(k) + m(k) \ . \tag{10.65}$$

Now expand the expressions for $\mathbf{R}$ and $\mathbf{h}$ to give

$$\mathbf{R} = \begin{bmatrix} E[v^2(k)] & E[v(k)v(k-1)] \\ E[v(k-1)v(k)] & E[v^2(k-1)] \end{bmatrix}, \tag{10.66}$$

and

$$\mathbf{h} = \begin{bmatrix} E[(s(k) + m(k))v(k)] \\ E[(s(k) + m(k))v(k-1)] \end{bmatrix}. \tag{10.67}$$

To obtain specific values for these two quantities we must define the noise signal v, the EEG signal s and the filtered noise m. For this exercise we will assume: the EEG signal is a white (uncorrelated from one time step to the next) random signal uniformly distributed between the values -0.2 and $+0.2$, the noise source (60-Hz sine wave sampled at 180 Hz) is given by

$$v(k) = 1.2 \sin\left(\frac{2\pi k}{3}\right), \tag{10.68}$$

and the filtered noise that contaminates the EEG is the noise source attenuated by a factor of 10 and shifted in phase by $\pi/2$:

$$m(k) = 0.12 \sin\left(\frac{2\pi k}{3} + \frac{\pi}{2}\right). \tag{10.69}$$

Now calculate the elements of the input correlation matrix $\mathbf{R}$:

$$E[v^2(k)] = (1.2)^2 \frac{1}{3} \sum_{k=1}^{3} \left(\sin\left(\frac{2\pi k}{3}\right)\right)^2 = (1.2)^2 0.5 = 0.72, \tag{10.70}$$

$$E[v^2(k-1)] = E[v^2(k)] = 0.72, \tag{10.71}$$

$$E[v(k)v(k-1)] = \frac{1}{3} \sum_{k=1}^{3} \left(1.2 \sin\frac{2\pi k}{3}\right)\left(1.2 \sin\frac{2\pi(k-1)}{3}\right)$$

$$= (1.2)^2 0.5 \cos\left(\frac{2\pi}{3}\right) = -0.36 \tag{10.72}$$

(where we have used some trigonometric identities).

Thus $\mathbf{R}$ is

$$\mathbf{R} = \begin{bmatrix} 0.72 & -0.36 \\ -0.36 & 0.72 \end{bmatrix}. \tag{10.73}$$

The terms of $\mathbf{h}$ can be found in a similar manner. We will consider the top term in Eq. (10.67) first:

$$E[(s(k) + m(k))v(k)] = E[s(k)v(k)] + E[m(k)v(k)]. \tag{10.74}$$

10

Here the first term on the right is zero because $s(k)$ and $v(k)$ are independent and zero mean. The second term is also zero:

$$E[m(k)v(k)] = \frac{1}{3}\sum_{k=1}^{3}\left(0.12\,\sin\left(\frac{2\pi k}{3}+\frac{\pi}{2}\right)\right)\left(1.2\sin\frac{2\pi k}{3}\right) = 0 \quad (10.75)$$

Thus, the first element of **h** is zero.

Next consider the second element of **h**:

$$E[(s(k)+m(k))v(k-1)] = E[s(k)v(k-1)]$$
$$+ E[m(k)v(k-1)] . \quad (10.76)$$

As with the first element of **h**, the first term on the right is zero because $s(k)$ and $v(k-1)$ are independent and zero mean. The second term is evaluated as follows:

$$E[m(k)v(k-1)] = \frac{1}{3}\sum_{k=1}^{3}\left(0.12\,\sin\left(\frac{2\pi k}{3}+\frac{\pi}{2}\right)\right)\left(1.2\,\sin\frac{2\pi(k-1)}{3}\right) \quad (10.77)$$

$$= -0.0624 .$$

Thus, **h** is

$$\mathbf{h} = \begin{bmatrix} 0 \\ -0.0624 \end{bmatrix} . \quad (10.78)$$

The minimum mean square error solution for the weights is given by Eq. (10.18):

$$\mathbf{x}^* = \mathbf{R}^{-1}\mathbf{h} = \begin{bmatrix} 0.72 & -0.36 \\ -0.36 & 0.72 \end{bmatrix}^{-1}\begin{bmatrix} 0 \\ -0.0624 \end{bmatrix} = \begin{bmatrix} -0.0578 \\ -0.1156 \end{bmatrix} . \quad (10.79)$$

Now, what kind of error will we have at the minimum solution? To find this error recall Eq. (10.12):

$$F(\mathbf{x}) = c - 2\mathbf{x}^T\mathbf{h} + \mathbf{x}^T\mathbf{R}\mathbf{x} . \quad (10.80)$$

We have just found $\mathbf{x}^*$, **h** and **R**, so we only need to find c:

$$c = E[t^2(k)] = E[(s(k)+m(k))^2] \quad (10.81)$$

$$= E[s^2(k)] + 2E[s(k)m(k)] + E[m^2(k)] .$$

The middle term is zero because $s(k)$ and $m(k)$ are independent and zero mean. The first term, the expected value of the random signal, can be calculated as follows:

$$E[s^2(k)] = \frac{1}{0.4}\int_{-0.2}^{0.2} s^2 ds = \frac{1}{3(0.4)}s^3\Big|_{-0.2}^{0.2} = 0.0133 \,. \tag{10.82}$$

The mean square value of the filtered noise is

$$E[m^2(k)] = \frac{1}{3}\sum_{k=1}^{3}\left\{0.12 \sin\left(\frac{2\pi}{3}+\frac{\pi}{2}\right)\right\}^2 = 0.0072 \,, \tag{10.83}$$

so that

$$c = 0.0133 + 0.0072 = 0.0205 \,. \tag{10.84}$$

Substituting $\mathbf{x}^*$, $\mathbf{h}$ and $\mathbf{R}$ into Eq. (10.80), we find that the minimum mean square error is

$$F(\mathbf{x}^*) = 0.0205 - 2(0.0072) + 0.0072 = 0.0133 \,. \tag{10.85}$$

The minimum mean square error is the same as the mean square value of the EEG signal. This is what we expected, since the "error" of this adaptive noise canceller is in fact the reconstructed EEG signal.

Figure 10.8 illustrates the trajectory of the LMS algorithm in the weight space with learning rate $\alpha = 0.1$. The system weights $w_{1,1}$ and $w_{1,2}$ in this simulation were initialized arbitrarily to 0 and –2, respectively. You can see from this figure that the LMS trajectory looks like a noisy version of steepest descent.

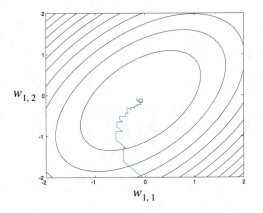

Figure 10.8 LMS Trajectory for $\alpha = 0.1$

10

Note that the contours in this figure reflect the fact that the eigenvalues and eigenvectors of the Hessian matrix ($\mathbf{A} = 2\mathbf{R}$) are

$$\lambda_1 = 2.16, \; \mathbf{z}_1 = \begin{bmatrix} -0.7071 \\ 0.7071 \end{bmatrix}, \; \lambda_2 = 0.72, \; \mathbf{z}_2 = \begin{bmatrix} -0.7071 \\ -0.7071 \end{bmatrix}. \tag{10.86}$$

(Refer back to our discussion in Chapter 8 on the eigensystem of the Hessian matrix.)

If the learning rate is decreased, the LMS trajectory is smoother than that shown in Figure 10.8, but the learning proceeds more slowly. If the learning rate is increased, the trajectory is more jagged and oscillatory. In fact, as noted earlier in this chapter, if the learning rate is increased too much the system does not converge at all. The maximum stable learning rate is $\alpha < 2/2.16 = 0.926$.

In order to judge the performance of our noise canceller, consider Figure 10.9. This figure illustrates how the filter adapts to cancel the noise. The top graph shows the restored and original EEG signals. At first the restored signal is a poor approximation of the original EEG signal. It takes about 0.2 second (with $\alpha = 0.1$) for the filter to adjust to give a reasonable restored signal. The mean square difference between the original and restored signal over the last half of the experiment was 0.002. This compares favorably with the signal mean square value of 0.0133. The difference between the original and restored signal is shown in the lower graph.

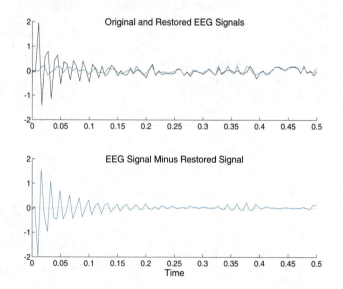

Figure 10.9 Adaptive Filter Cancellation of Contaminating Noise

You might wonder why the error does not go to zero. This is because the LMS algorithm is approximate steepest descent; it uses an estimate of the gradient, not the true gradient, to update the weights. The estimate of the gradient is a noisy version of the true gradient. This will cause the weights to continue to change slightly, even after the mean square error is at the minimum point. You can see this effect in Figure 10.8.

To experiment with the use of this adaptive noise cancellation filter, use the Neural Network Design Demonstration Adaptive Noise Cancellation (**nnd10nc**). *A more complex noise source and actual EEG data are used in the Demonstration* Electroencephalogram Noise Cancellation (**nnd10eeg**).

Echo Cancellation

Another very important practical application of adaptive noise cancellation is echo cancellation. Echoes are common in long distance telephone lines because of impedance mismatch at the "hybrid" device that forms the junction between the long distance line and the customer's local line. You may have experienced this effect on international telephone calls.

Figure 10.10 illustrates how an adaptive noise cancellation filter can be used to reduce these echoes [WiWi85]. At the end of the long distance line the incoming signal is sent to an adaptive filter, as well as to the hybrid device. The target output of the filter is the output of the hybrid. The filter thus tries to cancel the part of the hybrid output that is correlated with the input signal — the echo.

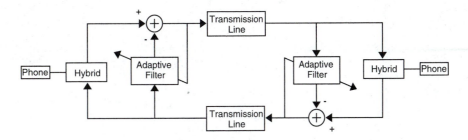

Figure 10.10 Echo Cancellation System

10

Summary of Results

ADALINE

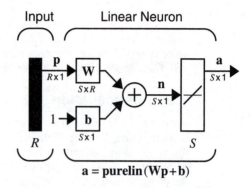

$$a = \mathbf{purelin}(\mathbf{Wp+b})$$

Mean Square Error

$$F(\mathbf{x}) = E[e^2] = E[(t-a)^2] = E[(t-\mathbf{x}^T\mathbf{z})^2]$$

$$F(\mathbf{x}) = c - 2\mathbf{x}^T\mathbf{h} + \mathbf{x}^T\mathbf{R}\mathbf{x},$$

$$c = E[t^2], \mathbf{h} = E[t\mathbf{z}] \text{ and } \mathbf{R} = E[\mathbf{z}\mathbf{z}^T]$$

Unique minimum, if it exists, is $\mathbf{x}^* = \mathbf{R}^{-1}\mathbf{h}$.

Where $\mathbf{x} = \begin{bmatrix} {}_1\mathbf{w} \\ b \end{bmatrix}$ and $\mathbf{z} = \begin{bmatrix} \mathbf{p} \\ 1 \end{bmatrix}$.

LMS Algorithm

$$\mathbf{W}(k+1) = \mathbf{W}(k) + 2\alpha\mathbf{e}(k)\mathbf{p}^T(k)$$

$$\mathbf{b}(k+1) = \mathbf{b}(k) + 2\alpha\mathbf{e}(k)$$

Convergence Point

$$\mathbf{x}^* = \mathbf{R}^{-1}\mathbf{h}$$

Stable Learning Rate

$$0 < \alpha < 1/\lambda_{max} \quad \text{where } \lambda_{max} \text{ is the maximum eigenvalue of } \mathbf{R}$$

Tapped Delay Line

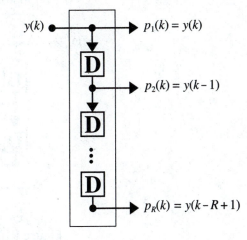

Adaptive Filter ADALINE

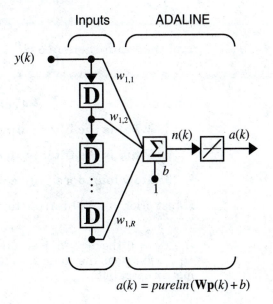

$$a(k) = purelin(\mathbf{W}\mathbf{p}(k) + b)$$

$$a(k) = purelin(\mathbf{W}\mathbf{p} + b) = \sum_{i=1}^{R} w_{1,i}\, y(k-i+1) + b$$

10

Solved Problems

P10.1 Consider the ADALINE filter in Figure P10.1.

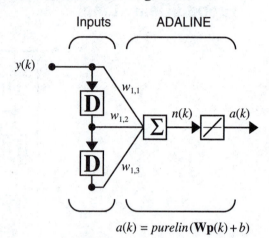

$$a(k) = purelin(\mathbf{W}p(k) + b)$$

Figure P10.1 ADALINE Filter

Suppose that

$$w_{1,1} = 2, \quad w_{1,2} = -1, \quad w_{1,3} = 3,$$

and the input sequence is

$$\{y(k)\} = \{\dots, 0, 0, 0, 5, -4, 0, 0, 0, \dots\}$$

where $y(0) = 5$, $y(1) = -4$, **etc.**

  i. What is the filter output just prior to $k = 0$?

  ii. What is the filter output from $k = 0$ **to** $k = 5$?

  iii. How long does $y(0)$ **contribute to the output?**

i. Just prior to $k = 0$ three zeros have entered the filter, and the output is zero.

ii. At $k = 0$ the digit "5" has entered the filter, and it will be multiplied by $w_{1,1}$, which has the value 2, so that $a(0) = 10$. This can be viewed as the matrix operation:

$$a(0) = \mathbf{W}\mathbf{p}(0) = \begin{bmatrix} w_{1,1} & w_{1,2} & w_{1,3} \end{bmatrix} \begin{bmatrix} y(0) \\ y(-1) \\ y(-2) \end{bmatrix} = \begin{bmatrix} 2 & -1 & 3 \end{bmatrix} \begin{bmatrix} 5 \\ 0 \\ 0 \end{bmatrix} = 10.$$

Similarly, one can calculate the next outputs as

$$a(1) = \mathbf{W}\mathbf{p}(1) = \begin{bmatrix} 2 & -1 & 3 \end{bmatrix} \begin{bmatrix} -4 \\ 5 \\ 0 \end{bmatrix} = -13$$

$$a(2) = \mathbf{W}\mathbf{p}(2) = \begin{bmatrix} 2 & -1 & 3 \end{bmatrix} \begin{bmatrix} 0 \\ -4 \\ 5 \end{bmatrix} = 19$$

$$a(3) = \mathbf{W}\mathbf{p}(3) = \begin{bmatrix} 2 & -1 & 3 \end{bmatrix} \begin{bmatrix} 0 \\ 0 \\ -4 \end{bmatrix} = -12, \ a(4) = \mathbf{W}\mathbf{p}(4) = \begin{bmatrix} 2 & -1 & 3 \end{bmatrix} \begin{bmatrix} 0 \\ 0 \\ 0 \end{bmatrix} = 0.$$

All remaining outputs will be zero.

iii. The effects of $y(0)$ last from $k = 0$ through $k = 2$, so it will have an influence for three time intervals. This corresponds to the length of the impulse response of this filter.

P10.2 **Suppose that we want to design an ADALINE network to distinguish between various categories of input vectors. Let us first try the categories listed below:**

$$\text{Category I:} \quad \mathbf{p}_1 = \begin{bmatrix} 1 & 1 \end{bmatrix}^T \text{ and } \mathbf{p}_2 = \begin{bmatrix} -1 & -1 \end{bmatrix}^T$$

$$\text{Category II:} \quad \mathbf{p}_3 = \begin{bmatrix} 2 & 2 \end{bmatrix}^T.$$

    i. Can an ADALINE network be designed to make such a distinction?

    ii. If the answer to part (i) is yes, what set of weights and bias might be used?

Next consider a different set of categories.

$$\text{Category III:} \quad \mathbf{p}_1 = \begin{bmatrix} 1 & 1 \end{bmatrix}^T \text{ and } \mathbf{p}_2 = \begin{bmatrix} 1 & -1 \end{bmatrix}^T$$

10

Category IV: $\mathbf{p}_3 = \begin{bmatrix} 1 & 0 \end{bmatrix}^T$.

   iii. **Can an ADALINE network be designed to make such a distinction?**

   iv. **If the answer to part (iii) is yes, what set of weights and bias might be used?**

i. The input vectors are plotted in Figure P10.2.

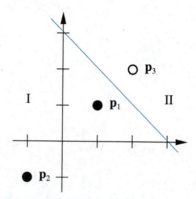

Figure P10.2 Input Vectors for Problem P10.1 (i)

The blue line in this figure is a decision boundary that separates the two categories successfully. Since they are linearly separable, an ADALINE network will do the job.

ii. The decision boundary passes through the points $(3, 0)$ and $(0, 3)$. We know these points to be the intercepts $-b/w_{1,1}$ and $-b/w_{1,2}$. Thus, a solution

$$ b = 3 , \; w_{1,1} = -1 , \; w_{1,2} = -1 , $$

is satisfactory. Note that if the output of the ADALINE is positive or zero the input vector is classified as Category I, and if the output is negative the input vector is classified as Category II. This solution also provides for error, since the decision boundary bisects the line between $\mathbf{p}_1$ and $\mathbf{p}_3$.

iii. The input vectors to be distinguished are shown in Figure P10.3. The vectors in the figure are not linearly separable, so an ADALINE network cannot distinguish between them.

iv. As noted in part (iii), an ADALINE cannot do the job, so there are no values for the weights and bias that are satisfactory.

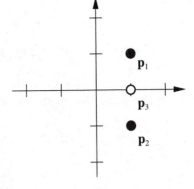

Figure P10.3 Input Vectors for Problem P10.1 (iii)

P10.3 Suppose that we have the following input/target pairs:

$$\left\{ \mathbf{p}_1 = \begin{bmatrix} 1 \\ 1 \end{bmatrix}, t_1 = 1 \right\} , \left\{ \mathbf{p}_2 = \begin{bmatrix} 1 \\ -1 \end{bmatrix}, t_2 = -1 \right\} .$$

These patterns occur with equal probability, and they are used to train an ADALINE network with no bias. What does the mean square error performance surface look like?

First we need to calculate the various terms of the quadratic function. Recall from Eq. (10.11) that the performance index can be written as

$$F(\mathbf{x}) = c - 2\mathbf{x}^T \mathbf{h} + \mathbf{x}^T \mathbf{R} \mathbf{x} .$$

Therefore we need to calculate c, $\mathbf{h}$ and $\mathbf{R}$.

The probability of each input occurring is 0.5, so the probability of each target is also 0.5. Thus, the expected value of the square of the targets is

$$c = E[t^2] = (1)^2 (0.5) + (-1)^2 (0.5) = 1 .$$

In a similar way, the cross-correlation between the input and the target can be calculated:

$$\mathbf{h} = E[t\mathbf{z}] = (0.5)(1) \begin{bmatrix} 1 \\ 1 \end{bmatrix} + (0.5)(-1) \begin{bmatrix} 1 \\ -1 \end{bmatrix} = \begin{bmatrix} 0 \\ 1 \end{bmatrix} .$$

Finally, the input correlation matrix $\mathbf{R}$ is

10

$$\mathbf{R} = E\,[\mathbf{z}\mathbf{z}^T] = \mathbf{p}_1\mathbf{p}_1^T(0.5) + \mathbf{p}_2\mathbf{p}_2^T(0.5)$$

$$= (0.5)\left[\begin{bmatrix}1\\1\end{bmatrix}\begin{bmatrix}1 & 1\end{bmatrix} + \begin{bmatrix}1\\-1\end{bmatrix}\begin{bmatrix}1 & -1\end{bmatrix}\right] = \begin{bmatrix}1 & 0\\0 & 1\end{bmatrix}$$

Therefore the mean square error performance index is

$$F(\mathbf{x}) = c - 2\mathbf{x}^T\mathbf{h} + \mathbf{x}^T\mathbf{R}\mathbf{x}$$

$$= 1 - 2\begin{bmatrix}w_{1,1} & w_{1,2}\end{bmatrix}\begin{bmatrix}0\\1\end{bmatrix} + \begin{bmatrix}w_{1,1} & w_{1,2}\end{bmatrix}\begin{bmatrix}1 & 0\\0 & 1\end{bmatrix}\begin{bmatrix}w_{1,1}\\w_{1,2}\end{bmatrix}$$

$$= 1 - 2w_{1,2} + w_{1,1}^2 + w_{1,2}^2$$

The Hessian matrix of $F(\mathbf{x})$, which is equal to $2\mathbf{R}$, has both eigenvalues at 2. Therefore the contours of the performance surface will be circular. To find the center of the contours (the minimum point), we need to solve Eq. (10.18):

$$\mathbf{x}^* = \mathbf{R}^{-1}\mathbf{h} = \begin{bmatrix}1 & 0\\0 & 1\end{bmatrix}^{-1}\begin{bmatrix}0\\1\end{bmatrix} = \begin{bmatrix}0\\1\end{bmatrix}.$$

Thus we have a minimum at $w_{1,1} = 0$, $w_{1,2} = 1$. The resulting mean square error performance surface is shown in Figure P10.4.

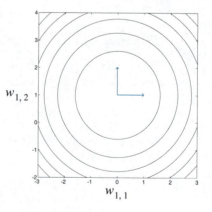

Figure P10.4 Contour Plot of $F(\mathbf{x})$ for Problem P10.3

P10.4 **Consider the system of Problem P10.3 again. Train the network using the LMS algorithm, with the initial guess set to zero and a learning rate $\alpha = 0.25$. Apply each reference pattern only once during training. Draw the decision boundary at each stage.**

Assume the input vector $\mathbf{p}_1$ is presented first. The output, error and new weights are calculated as follows:

$$a(0) = purelin\left[\begin{bmatrix} 0 & 0 \end{bmatrix}\begin{bmatrix} 1 \\ 1 \end{bmatrix}\right] = 0,$$

$$e(0) = t(0) - a(0) = 1 - 0 = 1,$$

$$\mathbf{W}(1) = \mathbf{W}(0) + 2\alpha e(0)\mathbf{p}(0)^T = \begin{bmatrix} 0 & 0 \end{bmatrix} + 2\left(\frac{1}{4}\right)(1)\begin{bmatrix} 1 & 1 \end{bmatrix} = \begin{bmatrix} \frac{1}{2} & \frac{1}{2} \end{bmatrix}.$$

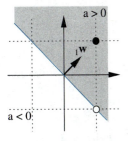

The decision boundary associated with these weights is shown to the left.

Now apply the second input vector:

$$a(1) = purelin\left\{\begin{bmatrix} \frac{1}{2} & \frac{1}{2} \end{bmatrix}\begin{bmatrix} 1 \\ -1 \end{bmatrix}\right\} = 0,$$

$$e(1) = t(1) - a(1) = -1 - 0 = -1,$$

$$\mathbf{W}(2) = \mathbf{W}(1) + 2\alpha e(1)\mathbf{p}(1)^T = \begin{bmatrix} \frac{1}{2} & \frac{1}{2} \end{bmatrix} + 2\left(\frac{1}{4}\right)(-1)\begin{bmatrix} 1 & -1 \end{bmatrix} = \begin{bmatrix} 0 & 1 \end{bmatrix}.$$

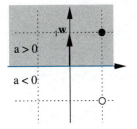

The decision boundary associated with these weights is shown to the left. This boundary shows real promise. It is exactly halfway between the input vectors. You might verify for yourself that each input vector, when applied, yields its correct associated target. (What set of weights would be optimal if the targets associated with the two input vectors were exchanged?)

P10.5 **Now consider the convergence of the system of Problems P10.3 and P10.4. What is the maximum stable learning rate for the LMS algorithm?**

The LMS convergence is determined by the learning rate α, which should not exceed the reciprocal of the largest eigenvalue of $\mathbf{R}$. We can determine this limit by finding these eigenvalues using MATLAB.

```
» 2 + 2
ans =
    4
```

10

```
[V,D] = eig (R)
V =
        1       0
        0       1

D=
        1       0
        0       1
```

The diagonal terms of matrix D give the eigenvalues, 1 and 1, while the columns of V show the eigenvectors. Note, incidentally, that the eigenvectors have the same direction as those shown in Figure P10.4.

The largest eigenvalue, $\lambda_{max} = 1$, sets the upper limit on the learning rate at

$$\alpha < 1/\lambda_{max} = 1/1 = 1.$$

The suggested learning rate in the previous problem was 0.25, and you found (perhaps) that the LMS algorithm converged quickly. What do you suppose happens when the learning rate is 1.0 or larger?

P10.6 **Consider the adaptive filter ADALINE shown in Figure P10.5. The purpose of this filter is to predict the next value of the input signal from the two previous values. Suppose that the input signal is a stationary random process, with autocorrelation function given by**

$$C_y(n) = E[y(k)y(k+n)]$$

$$C_y(0) = 3, C_y(1) = -1, C_y(2) = -1.$$

    i. Sketch the contour plot of the performance index (mean square error).

    ii. What is the maximum stable value of the learning rate (α) for the LMS algorithm?

    iii. Assume that a very small value is used for α. Sketch the path of the weights for the LMS algorithm, starting with initial guess $W(0) = \begin{bmatrix} 0.75 & 0 \end{bmatrix}^T$. Explain your procedure for sketching the path.

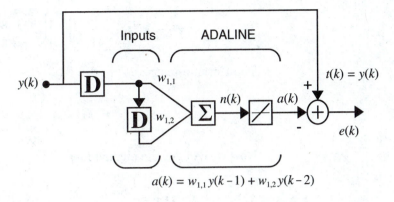

$$a(k) = w_{1,1} y(k-1) + w_{1,2} y(k-2)$$

Figure P10.5 Adaptive Predictor

i. To sketch the contour plot we first need to find the performance index and the eigenvalues and eigenvectors of the Hessian matrix. First note that the input vector is given by

$$\mathbf{z}(k) = \mathbf{p}(k) = \begin{bmatrix} y(k-1) \\ y(k-2) \end{bmatrix}.$$

Now consider the performance index. Recall from Eq. (10.12) that

$$F(\mathbf{x}) = c - 2\mathbf{x}^T \mathbf{h} + \mathbf{x}^T \mathbf{R} \mathbf{x}.$$

We can calculate the constants in the performance index as shown below:

$$c = E[t^2(k)] = E[y^2(k)] = C_y(0) = 3,$$

$$\mathbf{R} = E[\mathbf{z}\mathbf{z}^T] = E\begin{bmatrix} y^2(k-1) & y(k-1)y(k-2) \\ y(k-1)y(k-2) & y^2(k-2) \end{bmatrix}$$

$$= \begin{bmatrix} C_y(0) & C_y(1) \\ C_y(1) & C_y(0) \end{bmatrix} = \begin{bmatrix} 3 & -1 \\ -1 & 3 \end{bmatrix}$$

$$\mathbf{h} = E[t\,\mathbf{z}] = E\begin{bmatrix} y(k)y(k-1) \\ y(k)y(k-2) \end{bmatrix} = \begin{bmatrix} C_y(1) \\ C_y(2) \end{bmatrix} = \begin{bmatrix} -1 \\ -1 \end{bmatrix}.$$

The optimal weights are

10

$$\mathbf{x}^* = \mathbf{R}^{-1}\mathbf{h} = \begin{bmatrix} 3 & -1 \\ -1 & 3 \end{bmatrix}\begin{bmatrix} -1 \\ -1 \end{bmatrix} = \begin{bmatrix} 3/8 & 1/8 \\ 4/8 & 3/8 \end{bmatrix}\begin{bmatrix} -1 \\ -1 \end{bmatrix} = \begin{bmatrix} -1/2 \\ -1/2 \end{bmatrix}.$$

The Hessian matrix is

$$\nabla^2 F(\mathbf{x}) = \mathbf{A} = 2\mathbf{R} = \begin{bmatrix} 6 & -2 \\ -2 & 6 \end{bmatrix}.$$

Now we can get the eigenvalues:

$$\left| \mathbf{A} - \lambda\mathbf{I} \right| = \begin{vmatrix} 6-\lambda & -2 \\ -2 & 6-\lambda \end{vmatrix} = \lambda^2 - 12\lambda + 32 = (\lambda-8)(\lambda-4).$$

Thus,

$$\lambda_1 = 4, \qquad \lambda_2 = 8.$$

To find the eigenvectors we use

$$\left[\mathbf{A} - \lambda\mathbf{I}\right]\mathbf{v} = 0.$$

For $\lambda_1 = 4$,

$$\begin{bmatrix} 2 & -2 \\ -2 & 2 \end{bmatrix}\mathbf{v}_1 = 0 \qquad \mathbf{v}_1 = \begin{bmatrix} -1 \\ -1 \end{bmatrix},$$

and for $\lambda_2 = 8$,

$$\begin{bmatrix} -2 & -2 \\ -2 & 2 \end{bmatrix}\mathbf{v}_2 = 0 \qquad \mathbf{v}_2 = \begin{bmatrix} -1 \\ 1 \end{bmatrix}.$$

Therefore the contours of $F(\mathbf{x})$ will be elliptical, with the long axis of each ellipse along the first eigenvector, since the first eigenvalue has the smallest magnitude. The ellipses will be centered at $\mathbf{x}^*$. The contour plot is shown in Figure P10.6.

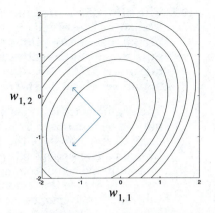

Figure P10.6 Error Contour for Problem P10.6

You might check your sketch by writing a MATLAB M-file to plot the contours.

ii. The maximum stable learning rate is the reciprocal of the maximum eigenvalue of $\mathbf{R}$, which is the same as twice the reciprocal of the largest eigenvalue of the Hessian matrix $\nabla^2 F(\mathbf{x}) = \mathbf{A}$:

$$\alpha < 2/\lambda_{max} = 2/8 = 0.25.$$

iii. The LMS algorithm is approximate steepest descent, so the trajectory for small learning rates will move perpendicular to the contour lines, as shown in Figure P10.7.

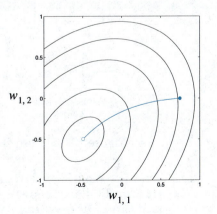

Figure P10.7 LMS Weight Trajectory

10

P10.7 **The pilot of an airplane is talking into a microphone in his cockpit. The sound received by the air traffic controller in the tower is garbled because the pilot's voice signal has been contaminated by engine noise that reaches his microphone. Can you suggest an adaptive ADALINE filter that might help reduce the noise in the signal received by the control tower? Explain your system.**

The engine noise that has been inadvertently added to the microphone input can be minimized by using the adaptive filtering system shown in Figure P10.8. A sample of the engine noise is supplied to an adaptive filter through a microphone in the cockpit. The desired output of the filter is the contaminated signal coming from the pilot's microphone. The filter attempts to reduce the "error" signal to a minimum. It can do this only by subtracting the component of the contaminated signal that is linearly correlated with the engine noise (and presumably uncorrelated with the pilot's voice). The result is that a clear voice signal is sent to the control tower, in spite of the fact that the engine noise got into the pilot's microphone along with his voice signal. (See [WiSt85] for discussion of similar noise cancellation systems.)

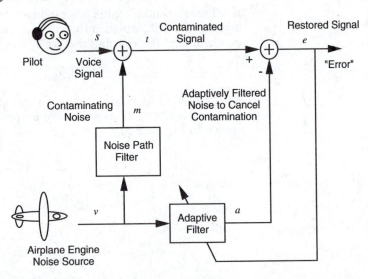

Figure P10.8 Filtering Engine Noise from Pilot's Voice Signal

P10.8 **This is a classification problem like that described in Problems P4.3 and P4.5, except that here we will use an ADALINE network and the LMS learning rule rather than the perceptron learning rule. First we will describe the problem.**

We have a classification problem with four classes of input vector. The four classes are

$$\text{class 1:} \left\{ \mathbf{p}_1 = \begin{bmatrix} 1 \\ 1 \end{bmatrix}, \mathbf{p}_2 = \begin{bmatrix} 1 \\ 2 \end{bmatrix} \right\}, \text{class 2:} \left\{ \mathbf{p}_3 = \begin{bmatrix} 2 \\ -1 \end{bmatrix}, \mathbf{p}_4 = \begin{bmatrix} 2 \\ 0 \end{bmatrix} \right\},$$

$$\text{class 3:} \left\{ \mathbf{p}_5 = \begin{bmatrix} -1 \\ 2 \end{bmatrix}, \mathbf{p}_6 = \begin{bmatrix} -2 \\ 1 \end{bmatrix} \right\}, \text{class 4:} \left\{ \mathbf{p}_7 = \begin{bmatrix} -1 \\ -1 \end{bmatrix}, \mathbf{p}_8 = \begin{bmatrix} -2 \\ -2 \end{bmatrix} \right\}.$$

Train an ADALINE network to solve this problem using the LMS learning rule. Assume that each pattern occurs with probability $1/8$.

Let's begin by displaying the input vectors, as in Figure P10.9. The light circles ○ indicate class 1 vectors, the light squares □ indicate class 2 vectors, the dark circles ● indicate class 3 vectors, and the dark squares ■ indicate class 4 vectors. These input vectors can be plotted as shown in Figure P10.9.

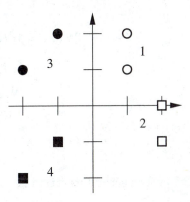

Figure P10.9 Input Vectors for Problem P10.8

We will use target vectors similar to the ones we introduced in Problem P4.3, except that we will replace any targets of 0 by targets of –1. (The perceptron could only output 0 or 1.) Thus, the training set will be:

$$\left\{ \mathbf{p}_1 = \begin{bmatrix} 1 \\ 1 \end{bmatrix}, \mathbf{t}_1 = \begin{bmatrix} -1 \\ -1 \end{bmatrix} \right\} \left\{ \mathbf{p}_2 = \begin{bmatrix} 1 \\ 2 \end{bmatrix}, \mathbf{t}_2 = \begin{bmatrix} -1 \\ -1 \end{bmatrix} \right\} \left\{ \mathbf{p}_3 = \begin{bmatrix} 2 \\ -1 \end{bmatrix}, \mathbf{t}_3 = \begin{bmatrix} -1 \\ 1 \end{bmatrix} \right\}$$

$$\left\{ \mathbf{p}_4 = \begin{bmatrix} 2 \\ 0 \end{bmatrix}, \mathbf{t}_4 = \begin{bmatrix} -1 \\ 1 \end{bmatrix} \right\} \left\{ \mathbf{p}_5 = \begin{bmatrix} -1 \\ 2 \end{bmatrix}, \mathbf{t}_5 = \begin{bmatrix} 1 \\ -1 \end{bmatrix} \right\} \left\{ \mathbf{p}_6 = \begin{bmatrix} -2 \\ 1 \end{bmatrix}, \mathbf{t}_6 = \begin{bmatrix} 1 \\ -1 \end{bmatrix} \right\}$$

$$\left\{ \mathbf{p}_7 = \begin{bmatrix} -1 \\ -1 \end{bmatrix}, \mathbf{t}_7 = \begin{bmatrix} 1 \\ 1 \end{bmatrix} \right\} \left\{ \mathbf{p}_8 = \begin{bmatrix} -2 \\ -2 \end{bmatrix}, \mathbf{t}_8 = \begin{bmatrix} 1 \\ 1 \end{bmatrix} \right\}$$

10

Also, we will begin as in Problem P4.5 with the following initial weights and biases:

$$\mathbf{W}(0) = \begin{bmatrix} 1 & 0 \\ 0 & 1 \end{bmatrix}, \mathbf{b}(0) = \begin{bmatrix} 1 \\ 1 \end{bmatrix}.$$

Now we are almost ready to train an ADALINE network using the LMS rule. We will use a learning rate of $\alpha = 0.04$, and we will present the input vectors in order according to their subscripts. The first iteration is

$$\mathbf{a}(0) = purelin\,(\mathbf{W}(0)\,\mathbf{p}(0) + \mathbf{b}(0)) = purelin\left(\begin{bmatrix} 1 & 0 \\ 0 & 1 \end{bmatrix}\begin{bmatrix} 1 \\ 1 \end{bmatrix} + \begin{bmatrix} 1 \\ 1 \end{bmatrix} \right) = \begin{bmatrix} 2 \\ 2 \end{bmatrix}$$

$$\mathbf{e}(0) = \mathbf{t}(0) - \mathbf{a}(0) = \begin{bmatrix} -1 \\ -1 \end{bmatrix} - \begin{bmatrix} 2 \\ 2 \end{bmatrix} = \begin{bmatrix} -3 \\ -3 \end{bmatrix}$$

$$\mathbf{W}(1) = \mathbf{W}(0) + 2\alpha\mathbf{e}(0)\,\mathbf{p}^T(0)$$

$$= \begin{bmatrix} 1 & 0 \\ 0 & 1 \end{bmatrix} + 2\,(0.04)\begin{bmatrix} -3 \\ -3 \end{bmatrix}\begin{bmatrix} 1 & 1 \end{bmatrix} = \begin{bmatrix} 0.76 & -0.24 \\ -0.24 & 0.76 \end{bmatrix}$$

$$\mathbf{b}(1) = \mathbf{b}(0) + 2\alpha\mathbf{e}(0) = \begin{bmatrix} 1 \\ 1 \end{bmatrix} + 2\,(0.04)\begin{bmatrix} -3 \\ -3 \end{bmatrix} = \begin{bmatrix} 0.76 \\ 0.76 \end{bmatrix}.$$

The second iteration is

$$\mathbf{a}(1) = purelin\,(\mathbf{W}(1)\,\mathbf{p}(1) + \mathbf{b}(1))$$

$$= purelin\left(\begin{bmatrix} 0.76 & -0.24 \\ -0.24 & 0.76 \end{bmatrix}\begin{bmatrix} 1 \\ 2 \end{bmatrix} + \begin{bmatrix} 0.76 \\ 0.76 \end{bmatrix} \right) = \begin{bmatrix} 1.04 \\ 2.04 \end{bmatrix}$$

$$\mathbf{e}(1) = \mathbf{t}(1) - \mathbf{a}(1) = \begin{bmatrix} -1 \\ -1 \end{bmatrix} - \begin{bmatrix} 1.04 \\ 2.04 \end{bmatrix} = \begin{bmatrix} -2.04 \\ -3.04 \end{bmatrix}$$

$$\mathbf{W}(2) = \mathbf{W}(1) + 2\alpha\mathbf{e}(1)\,\mathbf{p}^T(1)$$

$$= \begin{bmatrix} 0.76 & -0.24 \\ -0.24 & 0.76 \end{bmatrix} + 2\,(0.04)\begin{bmatrix} -2.04 \\ -3.04 \end{bmatrix}\begin{bmatrix} 1 & 2 \end{bmatrix} = \begin{bmatrix} 0.5968 & -0.5664 \\ -0.4832 & 0.2736 \end{bmatrix}$$

$$\mathbf{b}(2) = \mathbf{b}(1) + 2\alpha\mathbf{e}(1) = \begin{bmatrix} 0.76 \\ 0.76 \end{bmatrix} + 2\,(0.04)\begin{bmatrix} -2.04 \\ -3.04 \end{bmatrix} = \begin{bmatrix} 0.5968 \\ 0.5168 \end{bmatrix}.$$

If we continue until the weights converge we find

$$\mathbf{W}(\infty) = \begin{bmatrix} -0.5948 & -0.0523 \\ 0.1667 & -0.6667 \end{bmatrix}, \ \mathbf{b}(\infty) = \begin{bmatrix} 0.0131 \\ 0.1667 \end{bmatrix}.$$

The resulting decision boundaries are shown in Figure P10.10. Compare this result with the final decision boundaries created by the perceptron learning rule in Problem P4.5 (Figure P4.7). The perceptron rule stops training when all the patterns are classified correctly. The LMS algorithm moves the boundaries as far from the patterns as possible.

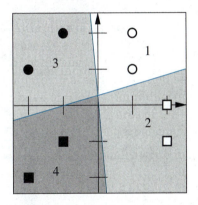

Figure P10.10 Final Decision Boundaries for Problem P10.8

P10.9 **Repeat the work of Widrow and Hoff on a pattern recognition problem from their classic 1960 paper [WiHo60]. They wanted to design a recognition system that would classify the six patterns shown in Figure P10.11.**

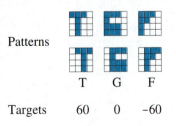

Patterns		
T	G	F

Targets	60	0	-60

Figure P10.11 Patterns and Their Classification Targets

10

These patterns represent the letters T, G and F, in an original form on the top and in a shifted form on the bottom. The targets for these letters (in their original and shifted forms) are +60, 0 and –60, respectively. (The values of 60, 0 and –60 were nice for use on the face of a meter that Widrow and Hoff used to display their network output.) The objective is to train a network so that it will classify the six patterns into the appropriate T, G or F groups.

The blue squares in the letters will be assigned the value +1, and the white squares will be assigned the value –1. First we convert each of the letters into a single 16-element vector. We choose to do this by starting at the upper left corner, going down the left column, then going down the second column, etc. For example, the vector corresponding to the unshifted letter T is

$$\mathbf{p}_1 = \begin{bmatrix} 1 & -1 & -1 & -1 & 1 & 1 & 1 & 1 & -1 & -1 & -1 & -1 & -1 & -1 & -1 \end{bmatrix}^T$$

We have such an input vector for each of the six letters.

The ADALINE network that we will use is shown in Figure P10.12.

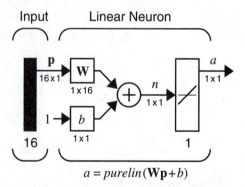

$$a = purelin(\mathbf{W}\mathbf{p} + b)$$

Figure P10.12 Adaptive Pattern Classifier

(Widrow and Hoff built their own machine to realize this ADALINE. According to them, it was "about the size of a lunch pail.")

Now we will present the six vectors to the network in a random sequence and adjust the weights of the network after each presentation using the LMS algorithm with a learning rate of $\alpha = 0.03$. After each adjustment of weights, all six vectors will be presented to the network to generate their outputs and corresponding errors. The sum of the squares of the errors will be examined as a measure of the quality of the network.

Figure P10.13 illustrates the convergence of the network. The network is trained to recognize these six characters in about 60 presentations, or roughly 10 for each of the possible input vectors.

The results shown in Figure P10.13 are quite like those obtained and published by Widrow and Hoff some 35 years ago. Widrow and Hoff did good science. One can indeed duplicate their work, even decades later (without a lunch pail).

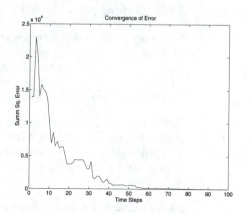

Figure P10.13 Error Convergence with Learning Rate of 0.03

 To experiment with this character recognition problem, use the Neural Network Design Demonstration Linear Pattern Classification (nnd10lc). *Notice the sensitivity of the network to noise in the input pattern.*

Epilogue

In this chapter we have presented the ADALINE neural network and the LMS learning rule. The ADALINE network is very similar to the perceptron network of Chapter 4, and it has the same fundamental limitation: it can only classify linearly separable patterns. In spite of this limitation on the network, the LMS algorithm is in fact more powerful than the perceptron learning rule. Because it minimizes mean square error, the algorithm is able to create decision boundaries that are more robust to noise than those of the perceptron learning rule.

The ADALINE network and the LMS algorithm have found many practical applications. Even though they were first presented in the late 1950s, they are still very much in use in adaptive filtering applications. Echo cancellers using the LMS algorithm are currently employed on many long distance telephone lines.

In addition to its importance as a practical solution to many adaptive filtering problems, the LMS algorithm is also important because it is the forerunner of the backpropagation algorithm, which we will discuss in Chapters 11 and 12. Like the LMS algorithm, backpropagation is an approximate steepest descent algorithm that minimizes mean square error. The only difference between the two algorithms is in the manner in which the derivatives are calculated. Backpropagation is a generalization of the LMS algorithm that can be used for multilayer networks. These more complex networks are not limited to linearly separable problems. They can solve arbitrary classification problems.

Further Reading

[AnRo89]   J. A. Anderson, E. Rosenfeld, *Neurocomputing: Foundations of Research*, Cambridge, MA: MIT Press, 1989.

Neurocomputing is a fundamental reference book. It contains over forty of the most important neurocomputing writings. Each paper is accompanied by an introduction that summarizes its results and gives a perspective on the position of the paper in the history of the field.

[StDo84]   W. D. Stanley, G. R. Dougherty, R. Dougherty, *Digital Signal Processing*, Reston VA: Reston, 1984

[WiHo60]   B. Widrow, M. E. Hoff, "Adaptive switching circuits," *1960 IRE WESCON Convention Record*, New York: IRE Part 4, pp. 96–104.

This seminal paper describes an adaptive perceptron-like network that can learn quickly and accurately. The authors assumed that the system had inputs, a desired output classification for each input, and that the system could calculate the error between the actual and desired output. The weights are adjusted, using a gradient descent method, so as to minimize the mean square error. (Least mean square error or LMS algorithm.)

This paper is reprinted in [AnRo88].

[WiSt 85]   B. Widrow and S. D. Stearns, *Adaptive Signal Processing*, Englewood Cliffs, NJ: Prentice-Hall, 1985.

This informative book describes the theory and application of adaptive signal processing. The authors include a review of the mathematical background that is needed, give details on their adaptive algorithms, and then discuss practical information about many applications.

[WiWi 88]   B. Widrow and R. Winter, "Neural nets for adaptive filtering and adaptive pattern recognition," *IEEE Computer Magazine*, March 1988, pp. 25–39.

This is a particularly readable paper that summarizes applications of adaptive multilayer neural networks. The networks are applied to system modeling, statistical prediction, echo cancellation, inverse modeling and pattern recognition.

10

Exercises

E10.1 An adaptive filter ADALINE is shown in Figure E10.1. Suppose that the weights of the network are given by

$$w_{1,1} = 1, \; w_{1,2} = -4, \; w_{1,3} = 2,$$

and the input to the filter is

$$\{y(k)\} = \{\dots, 0, 0, 0, 1, 1, 2, 0, 0, \dots\}.$$

Find the response $\{a(k)\}$ of the filter.

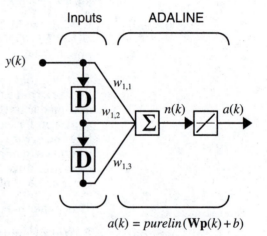

$$a(k) = purelin(\mathbf{W}\mathbf{p}(k) + b)$$

Figure E10.1 Adaptive Filter ADALINE for Exercise E10.1

E10.2 In Figure E10.2 two classes of patterns are given.

    i. Use the LMS algorithm to train an ADALINE network to distinguish between class I and class II patterns (we want the network to identify horizontal and vertical lines).

    ii. Can you explain why the ADALINE network might have difficulty with this problem?

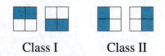

Figure E10.2 Pattern Classification Problem for Exercise E10.2

E10.3 Suppose that we have the following two reference patterns and their targets:

$$\left\{ \mathbf{p}_1 = \begin{bmatrix} 1 \\ 1 \end{bmatrix}, t_1 = 1 \right\}, \left\{ \mathbf{p}_2 = \begin{bmatrix} 1 \\ -1 \end{bmatrix}, t_1 = -1 \right\}.$$

In Problem P10.3 these input vectors to an ADALINE were assumed to occur with equal probability. Now suppose that the probability of vector $\mathbf{p}_1$ is 0.75 and that the probability of vector $\mathbf{p}_2$ is 0.25. Does this change of probabilities change the mean square error surface? If yes, what does the surface look like now? What is the maximum stable learning rate?

E10.4 In this exercise we will modify the reference pattern $\mathbf{p}_2$ from Problem P10.3:

$$\left\{ \mathbf{p}_1 = \begin{bmatrix} 1 \\ 1 \end{bmatrix}, t_1 = 1 \right\}, \left\{ \mathbf{p}_2 = \begin{bmatrix} -1 \\ -1 \end{bmatrix}, t_1 = -1 \right\}.$$

i. Assume that the patterns occur with equal probability. Find the mean square error and sketch the contour plot.

ii. Find the maximum stable learning rate.

iii. Write a MATLAB M-file to implement the LMS algorithm for this problem. Take 40 steps of the algorithm for a stable learning rate. Use the zero vector as the initial guess. Sketch the trajectory on the contour plot.

iv. Take 40 steps of the algorithm after setting the initial values of both parameters to 1. Sketch the final decision boundary.

v. Compare the final parameters from parts (iii) and (iv). Explain your results.

E10.5 We again use the reference patterns and targets from Problem P10.3, and assume that they occur with equal probability. This time we want to train an ADALINE network with a bias. We now have three parameters to find: $w_{1,1}$, $w_{1,2}$ and b.

i. Find the mean square error and the maximum stable learning rate.

ii. Write a MATLAB M-file to implement the LMS algorithm for this problem. Take 40 steps of the algorithm for a stable learning rate. Use the zero vector as the initial guess. Sketch the final decision boundary.

iii. Take 40 steps of the algorithm after setting the initial values of all parameters to 1. Sketch the final decision boundary.

iv. Compare the final parameters and the decision boundaries from parts (iii) and (iv). Explain your results.

10

E10.6 Consider the adaptive predictor in Figure E10.3.

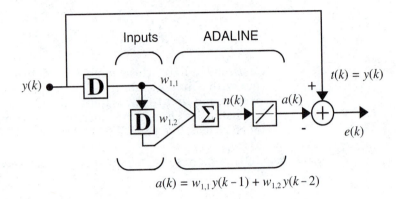

$$a(k) = w_{1,1} y(k-1) + w_{1,2} y(k-2)$$

Figure E10.3 Adaptive Predictor for Exercise E10.6

Assume that $y(k)$ is a stationary process with autocorrelation function

$$C_y(n) = E[y(k)(y(k+n))].$$

i. Write an expression for the mean square error in terms of $C_y(n)$.

ii. Give a specific expression for the mean square error when

$$y(k) = \sin\left(\frac{k\pi}{5}\right).$$

iii. Find the eigenvalues and eigenvectors of the Hessian matrix for the mean square error. Locate the minimum point and sketch a rough contour plot.

iv. Find the maximum stable learning rate for the LMS algorithm.

v. Take three steps of the LMS algorithm by hand, using a stable learning rate. Use the zero vector as the initial guess.

vi. Write a MATLAB M-file to implement the LMS algorithm for this problem. Take 40 steps of the algorithm for a stable learning rate and sketch the trajectory on the contour plot. Use the zero vector as the initial guess. Verify that the algorithm is converging to the optimal point.

vii. Verify experimentally that the algorithm is unstable for learning rates greater than that found in part (iv).

E10.7 Repeat Problem P10.9, but use the numerals "1", "2" and "4", instead of the letters "T", "G" and "F". Test the trained network on each reference pattern and on noisy patterns. Discuss the sensitivity of the network. (*Use the Neural Network Design Demonstration Linear Pattern Classification* (**nnd10lc**).)

11 Backpropagation

Objectives

In this chapter we continue our discussion of performance learning, which we began in Chapter 8, by presenting a generalization of the LMS algorithm of Chapter 10. This generalization, called backpropagation, can be used to train multilayer networks. As with the LMS learning law, backpropagation is an approximate steepest descent algorithm, in which the performance index is mean square error. The difference between the LMS algorithm and backpropagation is only in the way in which the derivatives are calculated. For a single-layer linear network the error is an explicit linear function of the network weights, and its derivatives with respect to the weights can be easily computed. In multilayer networks with nonlinear transfer functions, the relationship between the network weights and the error is more complex. In order to calculate the derivatives, we need to use the chain rule of calculus. In fact, this chapter is in large part a demonstration of how to use the chain rule.

11

Theory and Examples

The perceptron learning rule of Frank Rosenblatt and the LMS algorithm of Bernard Widrow and Marcian Hoff were designed to train single-layer perceptron-like networks. As we have discussed in previous chapters, these single-layer networks suffer from the disadvantage that they are only able to solve linearly separable classification problems. Both Rosenblatt and Widrow were aware of these limitations and proposed multilayer networks that could overcome them, but they were not able to generalize their algorithms to train these more powerful networks.

Apparently the first description of an algorithm to train multilayer networks was contained in the thesis of Paul Werbos in 1974 [Werbo74]. This thesis presented the algorithm in the context of general networks, with neural networks as a special case, and was not disseminated in the neural network community. It was not until the mid 1980s that the backpropagation algorithm was rediscovered and widely publicized. It was rediscovered independently by David Rumelhart, Geoffrey Hinton and Ronald Williams [RuHi86], David Parker [Park85], and Yann Le Cun [LeCu85]. The algorithm was popularized by its inclusion in the book *Parallel Distributed Processing* [RuMc86], which described the work of the Parallel Distributed Processing Group led by psychologists David Rumelhart and James McClelland. The publication of this book spurred a torrent of research in neural networks. The multilayer perceptron, trained by the backpropagation algorithm, is currently the most widely used neural network.

In this chapter we will first investigate the capabilities of multilayer networks and then present the backpropagation algorithm.

Multilayer Perceptrons

We first introduced the notation for multilayer networks in Chapter 2. For ease of reference we have reproduced the diagram of the three-layer perceptron in Figure 11.1. Note that we have simply cascaded three perceptron networks. The output of the first network is the input to the second network, and the output of the second network is the input to the third network. Each layer may have a different number of neurons, and even a different transfer function. Recall from Chapter 2 that we are using superscripts to identify the layer number. Thus, the weight matrix for the first layer is written as $\mathbf{W}^1$ and the weight matrix for the second layer is written $\mathbf{W}^2$.

To identify the structure of a multilayer network, we will sometimes use the following shorthand notation, where the number of inputs is followed by the number of neurons in each layer:

$$R - S^1 - S^2 - S^3 . \tag{11.1}$$

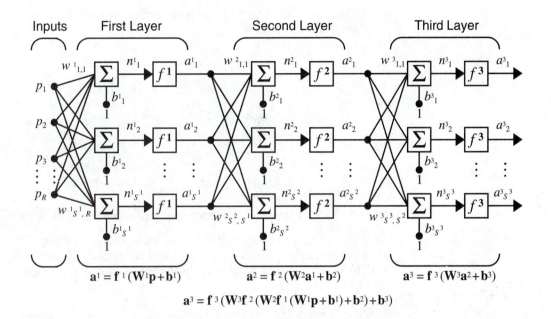

$$a^1 = f^1(W^1p + b^1) \qquad a^2 = f^2(W^2a^1 + b^2) \qquad a^3 = f^3(W^3a^2 + b^3)$$

$$a^3 = f^3(W^3f^2(W^2f^1(W^1p + b^1) + b^2) + b^3)$$

Figure 11.1 Three-Layer Network

Let's now investigate the capabilities of these multilayer perceptron networks. First we will look at the use of multilayer networks for pattern classification, and then we will discuss their application to function approximation.

Pattern Classification

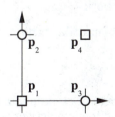

To illustrate the capabilities of the multilayer perceptron for pattern classification, consider the classic exclusive-or (XOR) problem. The input/target pairs for the XOR gate are

$$\left\{ p_1 = \begin{bmatrix} 0 \\ 0 \end{bmatrix}, t_1 = 0 \right\} \left\{ p_2 = \begin{bmatrix} 0 \\ 1 \end{bmatrix}, t_2 = 1 \right\} \left\{ p_3 = \begin{bmatrix} 1 \\ 0 \end{bmatrix}, t_3 = 1 \right\} \left\{ p_4 = \begin{bmatrix} 1 \\ 1 \end{bmatrix}, t_4 = 0 \right\}.$$

This problem, which is illustrated graphically in the figure to the left, was used by Minsky and Papert in 1969 to demonstrate the limitations of the single-layer perceptron. Because the two categories are not linearly separable, a single-layer perceptron cannot perform the classification.

A two-layer network can solve the XOR problem. In fact, there are many different multilayer solutions. One solution is to use two neurons in the first layer to create two decision boundaries. The first boundary separates p_1 from the other patterns, and the second boundary separates p_4. Then the second layer is used to combine the two boundaries together using an

11

AND operation. The decision boundaries for each first-layer neuron are shown in Figure 11.2.

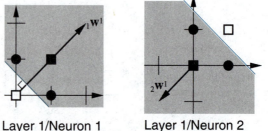

Layer 1/Neuron 1   Layer 1/Neuron 2

Figure 11.2 Decision Boundaries for XOR Network

The resulting two-layer, 2-2-1 network is shown in Figure 11.3. The overall decision regions for this network are shown in the figure in the left margin. The shaded region indicates those inputs that will produce a network output of 1.

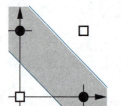

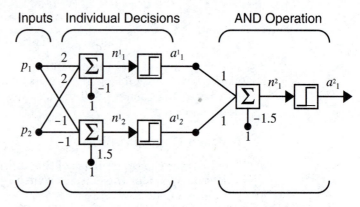

Figure 11.3 Two-Layer XOR Network

See Problems P11.1 and P11.2 for more on the use of multilayer networks for pattern classification.

Function Approximation

Up to this point in the text we have viewed neural networks mainly in the context of pattern classification. It is also instructive to view networks as function approximators. In control systems, for example, the objective is to find an appropriate feedback function that maps from measured outputs to control inputs. In adaptive filtering (Chapter 10) the objective is to find a function that maps from delayed values of an input signal to an appropriate output signal. The following example will illustrate the flexibility of the multilayer perceptron for implementing functions.

Consider the two-layer, 1-2-1 network shown in Figure 11.4. For this example the transfer function for the first layer is log-sigmoid and the transfer function for the second layer is linear. In other words,

$$f^1(n) = \frac{1}{1 + e^{-n}} \text{ and } f^2(n) = n.$$ (11.2)

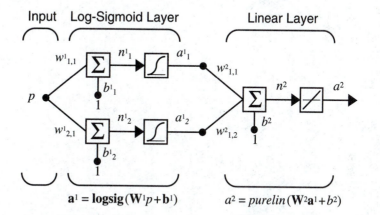

$$\mathbf{a}^1 = \mathbf{logsig}(\mathbf{W}^1 p + \mathbf{b}^1) \qquad a^2 = purelin(\mathbf{W}^2 \mathbf{a}^1 + b^2)$$

Figure 11.4 Example Function Approximation Network

Suppose that the nominal values of the weights and biases for this network are

$$w^1_{1,1} = 10, \ w^1_{2,1} = 10, \ b^1_1 = -10, \ b^1_2 = 10,$$

$$w^2_{1,1} = 1, \ w^2_{1,2} = 1, \ b^2 = 0.$$

The network response for these parameters is shown in Figure 11.5, which plots the network output a^2 as the input p is varied over the range $[-2, 2]$.

Notice that the response consists of two steps, one for each of the log-sigmoid neurons in the first layer. By adjusting the network parameters we can change the shape and location of each step, as we will see in the following discussion.

The centers of the steps occur where the net input to a neuron in the first layer is zero:

$$n^1_1 = w^1_{1,1}p + b^1_1 = 0 \implies p = -\frac{b^1_1}{w^1_{1,1}} = -\frac{-10}{10} = 1,$$ (11.3)

11

$$n_2^1 = w_{2,1}^1 p + b_2^1 = 0 \quad \Rightarrow \quad p = -\frac{b_2^1}{w_{2,1}^1} = -\frac{10}{10} = -1. \tag{11.4}$$

The steepness of each step can be adjusted by changing the network weights.

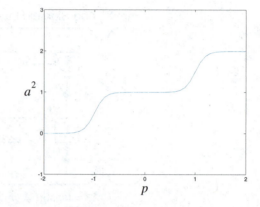

Figure 11.5 Nominal Response of Network of Figure 11.4

Figure 11.6 illustrates the effects of parameter changes on the network response. The blue curve is the nominal response. The other curves correspond to the network response when one parameter at a time is varied over the following ranges:

$$-1 \le w_{1,1}^2 \le 1 \,, \ -1 \le w_{1,2}^2 \le 1 \,, \ 0 \le b_2^1 \le 20 \,, \ -1 \le b^2 \le 1 \,. \tag{11.5}$$

Figure 11.6 (a) shows how the network biases in the first (hidden) layer can be used to locate the position of the steps. Figure 11.6 (b) illustrates how the weights determine the slope of the steps. The bias in the second (output) layer shifts the entire network response up or down, as can be seen in Figure 11.6 (d).

From this example we can see how flexible the multilayer network is. It would appear that we could use such networks to approximate almost any function, if we had a sufficient number of neurons in the hidden layer. In fact, it has been shown that two-layer networks, with sigmoid transfer functions in the hidden layer and linear transfer functions in the output layer, can approximate virtually any function of interest to any degree of accuracy, provided sufficiently many hidden units are available (see [HoSt89]).

*To experiment with the response of this two-layer network, use the Neural Network Design Demonstration Network Function (**nnd11nf**).*

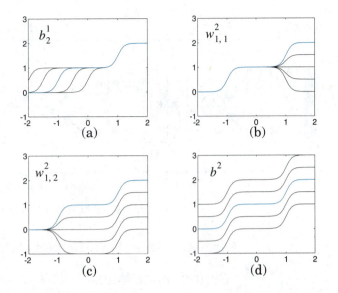

Figure 11.6 Effect of Parameter Changes on Network Response

Now that we have some idea of the power of multilayer perceptron networks for pattern recognition and function approximation, the next step is to develop an algorithm to train such networks.

The Backpropagation Algorithm

It will simplify our development of the backpropagation algorithm if we use the abbreviated notation for the multilayer network, which we introduced in Chapter 2. The three-layer network in abbreviated notation is shown in Figure 11.7.

As we discussed earlier, for multilayer networks the output of one layer becomes the input to the following layer. The equations that describe this operation are

$$\mathbf{a}^{m+1} = \mathbf{f}^{m+1}(\mathbf{W}^{m+1}\mathbf{a}^m + \mathbf{b}^{m+1}) \text{ for } m = 0, 2, \ldots, M-1, \qquad (11.6)$$

where M is the number of layers in the network. The neurons in the first layer receive external inputs:

$$\mathbf{a}^0 = \mathbf{p}, \qquad (11.7)$$

which provides the starting point for Eq. (11.6). The outputs of the neurons in the last layer are considered the network outputs:

$$\mathbf{a} = \mathbf{a}^M. \qquad (11.8)$$

11

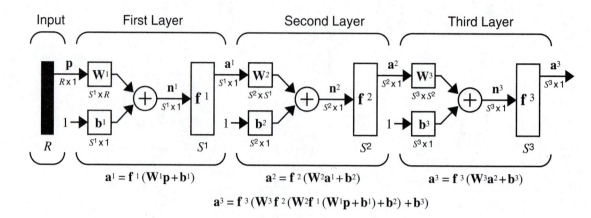

Figure 11.7 Three-Layer Network, Abbreviated Notation

Performance Index

The backpropagation algorithm for multilayer networks is a generalization of the LMS algorithm of Chapter 10, and both algorithms use the same performance index: *mean square error*. The algorithm is provided with a set of examples of proper network behavior:

$$\{\mathbf{p}_1, \mathbf{t}_1\}, \{\mathbf{p}_2, \mathbf{t}_2\}, \dots, \{\mathbf{p}_Q, \mathbf{t}_Q\}, \tag{11.9}$$

where $\mathbf{p}_q$ is an input to the network, and $\mathbf{t}_q$ is the corresponding target output. As each input is applied to the network, the network output is compared to the target. The algorithm should adjust the network parameters in order to minimize the mean square error:

$$F(\mathbf{x}) = E[e^2] = E[(t-a)^2]. \tag{11.10}$$

where $\mathbf{x}$ is the vector of network weights and biases (as in Chapter 10). If the network has multiple outputs this generalizes to

$$F(\mathbf{x}) = E[\mathbf{e}^T\mathbf{e}] = E[(\mathbf{t}-\mathbf{a})^T(\mathbf{t}-\mathbf{a})]. \tag{11.11}$$

As with the LMS algorithm, we will approximate the mean square error by

$$\hat{F}(\mathbf{x}) = (\mathbf{t}(k) - \mathbf{a}(k))^T(\mathbf{t}(k) - \mathbf{a}(k)) = \mathbf{e}^T(k)\mathbf{e}(k), \tag{11.12}$$

where the expectation of the squared error has been replaced by the squared error at iteration k.

The steepest descent algorithm for the approximate mean square error is

$$w^m_{i,j}(k+1) = w^m_{i,j}(k) - \alpha \frac{\partial \hat{F}}{\partial w^m_{i,j}}, \tag{11.13}$$

$$b^m_i(k+1) = b^m_i(k) - \alpha \frac{\partial \hat{F}}{\partial b^m_i}, \tag{11.14}$$

where α is the learning rate.

So far, this development is identical to that for the LMS algorithm. Now we come to the difficult part – the computation of the partial derivatives.

Chain Rule

For a single-layer linear network (the ADALINE) these partial derivatives are conveniently computed using Eq. (10.33) and Eq. (10.34). For the multilayer network the error is not an explicit function of the weights in the hidden layers, therefore these derivatives are not computed so easily.

Because the error is an indirect function of the weights in the hidden layers, we will use the chain rule of calculus to calculate the derivatives. To review the chain rule, suppose that we have a function f that is an explicit function only of the variable n. We want to take the derivative of f with respect to a third variable w. The chain rule is then:

$$\frac{df(n(w))}{dw} = \frac{df(n)}{dn} \times \frac{dn(w)}{dw}. \tag{11.15}$$

For example, if

$$f(n) = e^n \text{ and } n = 2w, \text{ so that } f(n(w)) = e^{2w}, \tag{11.16}$$

then

$$\frac{df(n(w))}{dw} = \frac{df(n)}{dn} \times \frac{dn(w)}{dw} = (e^n)(2). \tag{11.17}$$

We will use this concept to find the derivatives in Eq. (11.13) and Eq. (11.14):

$$\frac{\partial \hat{F}}{\partial w^m_{i,j}} = \frac{\partial \hat{F}}{\partial n^m_i} \times \frac{\partial n^m_i}{\partial w^m_{i,j}}, \tag{11.18}$$

$$\frac{\partial \hat{F}}{\partial b^m_i} = \frac{\partial \hat{F}}{\partial n^m_i} \times \frac{\partial n^m_i}{\partial b^m_i}. \tag{11.19}$$

11

The second term in each of these equations can be easily computed, since the net input to layer m is an explicit function of the weights and bias in that layer:

$$n_i^m = \sum_{j=1}^{s^{m-1}} w_{i,j}^m a_j^{m-1} + b_i^m .$$ (11.20)

Therefore

$$\frac{\partial n_i^m}{\partial w_{i,j}^m} = a_j^{m-1} , \quad \frac{\partial n_i^m}{\partial b_i^m} = 1 .$$ (11.21)

If we now define

$$s_i^m \equiv \frac{\partial \hat{F}}{\partial n_i^m} ,$$ (11.22)

(the *sensitivity* of $\hat{F}$ to changes in the ith element of the net input at layer m), then Eq. (11.18) and Eq. (11.19) can be simplified to

$$\frac{\partial \hat{F}}{\partial w_{i,j}^m} = s_i^m a_j^{m-1} ,$$ (11.23)

$$\frac{\partial \hat{F}}{\partial b_i^m} = s_i^m .$$ (11.24)

We can now express the approximate steepest descent algorithm as

$$w_{i,j}^m (k+1) = w_{i,j}^m (k) - \alpha s_i^m a_j^{m-1} ,$$ (11.25)

$$b_i^m (k+1) = b_i^m (k) - \alpha s_i^m .$$ (11.26)

In matrix form this becomes:

$$\mathbf{W}^m (k+1) = \mathbf{W}^m (k) - \alpha \mathbf{s}^m (\mathbf{a}^{m-1})^T ,$$ (11.27)

$$\mathbf{b}^m (k+1) = \mathbf{b}^m (k) - \alpha \mathbf{s}^m ,$$ (11.28)

where

$$\mathbf{s}^m \equiv \frac{\partial \hat{F}}{\partial \mathbf{n}^m} = \begin{bmatrix} \dfrac{\partial \hat{F}}{\partial n_1^m} \\[2ex] \dfrac{\partial \hat{F}}{\partial n_2^m} \\[1ex] \vdots \\[1ex] \dfrac{\partial \hat{F}}{\partial n_{S^m}^m} \end{bmatrix}. \tag{11.29}$$

(Note the close relationship between this algorithm and the LMS algorithm of Eq. (10.33) and Eq. (10.34)).

Backpropagating the Sensitivities

It now remains for us to compute the sensitivities $\mathbf{s}^m$, which requires another application of the chain rule. It is this process that gives us the term *backpropagation*, because it describes a recurrence relationship in which the sensitivity at layer m is computed from the sensitivity at layer $m+1$.

To derive the recurrence relationship for the sensitivities, we will use the following Jacobian matrix:

$$\frac{\partial \mathbf{n}^{m+1}}{\partial \mathbf{n}^m} \equiv \begin{bmatrix} \dfrac{\partial n_1^{m+1}}{\partial n_1^m} & \dfrac{\partial n_1^{m+1}}{\partial n_2^m} & \cdots & \dfrac{\partial n_1^{m+1}}{\partial n_{S^m}^m} \\[2ex] \dfrac{\partial n_2^{m+1}}{\partial n_1^m} & \dfrac{\partial n_2^{m+1}}{\partial n_2^m} & \cdots & \dfrac{\partial n_2^{m+1}}{\partial n_{S^m}^m} \\[1ex] \vdots & \vdots & & \vdots \\[1ex] \dfrac{\partial n_{S^{m+1}}^{m+1}}{\partial n_1^m} & \dfrac{\partial n_{S^{m+1}}^{m+1}}{\partial n_2^m} & \cdots & \dfrac{\partial n_{S^{m+1}}^{m+1}}{\partial n_{S^m}^m} \end{bmatrix}. \tag{11.30}$$

Next we want to find an expression for this matrix. Consider the i,j element of the matrix:

11

$$\frac{\partial n_i^{m+1}}{\partial n_j^m} = \frac{\partial \left(\sum_{l=1}^{S^m} w_{i,l}^{m+1} a_l^m + b_i^{m+1} \right)}{\partial n_j^m} = w_{i,j}^{m+1} \frac{\partial a_j^m}{\partial n_j^m} \tag{11.31}$$

$$= w_{i,j}^{m+1} \frac{\partial f^m(n_j^m)}{\partial n_j^m} = w_{i,j}^{m+1} \dot{f}^m(n_j^m) \ ,$$

where

$$\dot{f}^m(n_j^m) = \frac{\partial f^m(n_j^m)}{\partial n_j^m} \ . \tag{11.32}$$

Therefore the Jacobian matrix can be written

$$\frac{\partial \mathbf{n}^{m+1}}{\partial \mathbf{n}^m} = \mathbf{W}^{m+1} \dot{\mathbf{F}}^m(\mathbf{n}^m) \ , \tag{11.33}$$

where

$$\dot{\mathbf{F}}^m(\mathbf{n}^m) = \begin{bmatrix} \dot{f}^m(n_1^m) & 0 & \cdots & 0 \\ 0 & \dot{f}^m(n_2^m) & \cdots & 0 \\ \vdots & \vdots & & \vdots \\ 0 & 0 & & \dot{f}^m(n_{S^m}^m) \end{bmatrix} . \tag{11.34}$$

We can now write out the recurrence relation for the sensitivity by using the chain rule in matrix form:

$$\mathbf{s}^m = \frac{\partial \hat{F}}{\partial \mathbf{n}^m} = \left(\frac{\partial \mathbf{n}^{m+1}}{\partial \mathbf{n}^m} \right)^T \frac{\partial \hat{F}}{\partial \mathbf{n}^{m+1}} = \dot{\mathbf{F}}^m(\mathbf{n}^m)(\mathbf{W}^{m+1})^T \frac{\partial \hat{F}}{\partial \mathbf{n}^{m+1}}$$
$$\tag{11.35}$$
$$= \dot{\mathbf{F}}^m(\mathbf{n}^m)(\mathbf{W}^{m+1})^T \mathbf{s}^{m+1} \ .$$

Now we can see where the backpropagation algorithm derives its name. The sensitivities are propagated backward through the network from the last layer to the first layer:

$$\mathbf{s}^M \rightarrow \mathbf{s}^{M-1} \rightarrow \cdots \rightarrow \mathbf{s}^2 \rightarrow \mathbf{s}^1 \ . \tag{11.36}$$

At this point it is worth emphasizing that the backpropagation algorithm uses the same approximate steepest descent technique that we used in the LMS algorithm. The only complication is that in order to compute the gradient we need to first backpropagate the sensitivities. The beauty of backpropagation is that we have a very efficient implementation of the chain rule.

We still have one more step to make in order to complete the backpropagation algorithm. We need the starting point, s^M, for the recurrence relation of Eq. (11.35). This is obtained at the final layer:

$$s_i^M = \frac{\partial \hat{F}}{\partial n_i^M} = \frac{\partial (\mathbf{t} - \mathbf{a})^T (\mathbf{t} - \mathbf{a})}{\partial n_i^M} = \frac{\partial \sum_{j=1}^{s^M} (t_j - a_j)^2}{\partial n_i^M} = -2(t_i - a_i) \frac{\partial a_i}{\partial n_i^M}. \quad (11.37)$$

Now, since

$$\frac{\partial a_i}{\partial n_i^M} = \frac{\partial a_i^M}{\partial n_i^M} = \frac{\partial f^M (n_j^M)}{\partial n_i^M} = \dot{f}^M (n_j^M), \quad (11.38)$$

we can write

$$s_i^M = -2(t_i - a_i) \dot{f}^M (n_j^M). \quad (11.39)$$

This can be expressed in matrix form as

$$\mathbf{s}^M = -2\dot{\mathbf{F}}^M (\mathbf{n}^M) (\mathbf{t} - \mathbf{a}). \quad (11.40)$$

Summary

Let's summarize the backpropagation algorithm. The first step is to propagate the input forward through the network:

$$\mathbf{a}^0 = \mathbf{p}, \quad (11.41)$$

$$\mathbf{a}^{m+1} = \mathbf{f}^{m+1} (\mathbf{W}^{m+1} \mathbf{a}^m + \mathbf{b}^{m+1}) \text{ for } m = 0, 2, \dots, M-1, \quad (11.42)$$

$$\mathbf{a} = \mathbf{a}^M. \quad (11.43)$$

The next step is to propagate the sensitivities backward through the network:

$$\mathbf{s}^M = -2\dot{\mathbf{F}}^M (\mathbf{n}^M) (\mathbf{t} - \mathbf{a}), \quad (11.44)$$

11

$$\mathbf{s}^{m} = \dot{\mathbf{F}}^{m}(\mathbf{n}^{m}) (\mathbf{W}^{m+1})^{T} \mathbf{s}^{m+1}, \text{ for } m = M-1, \dots, 2, 1. \tag{11.45}$$

Finally, the weights and biases are updated using the approximate steepest descent rule:

$$\mathbf{W}^{m}(k+1) = \mathbf{W}^{m}(k) - \alpha \mathbf{s}^{m}(\mathbf{a}^{m-1})^{T}, \tag{11.46}$$

$$\mathbf{b}^{m}(k+1) = \mathbf{b}^{m}(k) - \alpha \mathbf{s}^{m}. \tag{11.47}$$

Example

To illustrate the backpropagation algorithm, let's choose a network and apply it to a particular problem. To begin, we will use the 1-2-1 network that we discussed earlier in this chapter. For convenience we have reproduced the network in Figure 11.8.

Next we want to define a problem for the network to solve. Suppose that we want to use the network to approximate the function

$$g(p) = 1 + \sin\left(\frac{\pi}{4}p\right) \text{ for } -2 \le p \le 2. \tag{11.48}$$

To obtain our training set we will evaluate this function at several values of p.

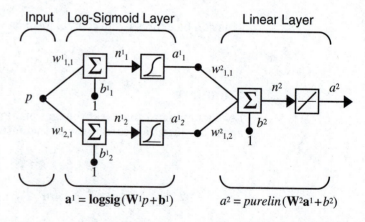

$$\mathbf{a}^{1} = \text{logsig}(\mathbf{W}^{1}p + \mathbf{b}^{1}) \qquad \mathbf{a}^{2} = purelin(\mathbf{W}^{2}\mathbf{a}^{1} + \mathbf{b}^{2})$$

Figure 11.8 Example Function Approximation Network

Before we begin the backpropagation algorithm we need to choose some initial values for the network weights and biases. Generally these are chosen to be small random values. In the next chapter we will discuss some reasons for this. For now let's choose the values

$$\mathbf{W}^1(0) = \begin{bmatrix} -0.27 \\ -0.41 \end{bmatrix}, \ \mathbf{b}^1(0) = \begin{bmatrix} -0.48 \\ -0.13 \end{bmatrix}, \ \mathbf{W}^2(0) = \begin{bmatrix} 0.09 & -0.17 \end{bmatrix}, \ \mathbf{b}^2(0) = \begin{bmatrix} 0.48 \end{bmatrix}.$$

The response of the network for these initial values is illustrated in Figure 11.9, along with the sine function we wish to approximate.

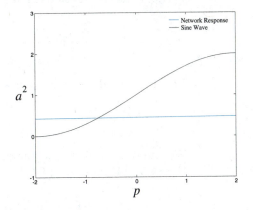

Figure 11.9 Initial Network Response

Now we are ready to start the algorithm. For our initial input we will choose $p = 1$:

$$a^0 = p = 1.$$

The output of the first layer is then

$$\mathbf{a}^1 = \mathbf{f}^1(\mathbf{W}^1\mathbf{a}^0 + \mathbf{b}^1) = \mathbf{logsig}\left(\begin{bmatrix} -0.27 \\ -0.41 \end{bmatrix} \begin{bmatrix} 1 \end{bmatrix} + \begin{bmatrix} -0.48 \\ -0.13 \end{bmatrix} \right) = \mathbf{logsig}\left(\begin{bmatrix} -0.75 \\ -0.54 \end{bmatrix} \right)$$

$$= \begin{bmatrix} \dfrac{1}{1 + e^{0.75}} \\ \dfrac{1}{1 + e^{0.54}} \end{bmatrix} = \begin{bmatrix} 0.321 \\ 0.368 \end{bmatrix}.$$

The second layer output is

$$a^2 = f^2(\mathbf{W}^2\mathbf{a}^1 + \mathbf{b}^2) = purelin\left(\begin{bmatrix} 0.09 & -0.17 \end{bmatrix} \begin{bmatrix} 0.321 \\ 0.368 \end{bmatrix} + \begin{bmatrix} 0.48 \end{bmatrix} \right) = \begin{bmatrix} 0.446 \end{bmatrix}.$$

The error would then be

11

$$e = t - a = \left\{1 + \sin\left(\frac{\pi}{4}p\right)\right\} - a^2 = \left\{1 + \sin\left(\frac{\pi}{4}1\right)\right\} - 0.446 = 1.261 .$$

The next stage of the algorithm is to backpropagate the sensitivities. Before we begin the backpropagation, recall that we will need the derivatives of the transfer functions, $\dot{f}^1(n)$ and $\dot{f}^2(n)$. For the first layer

$$\dot{f}^1(n) = \frac{d}{dn}\left(\frac{1}{1 + e^{-n}}\right) = \frac{e^{-n}}{(1 + e^{-n})^2} = \left(1 - \frac{1}{1 + e^{-n}}\right)\left(\frac{1}{1 + e^{-n}}\right) = (1 - a^1)\,(a^1) .$$

For the second layer we have

$$\dot{f}^2(n) = \frac{d}{dn}(n) = 1 .$$

We can now perform the backpropagation. The starting point is found at the second layer, using Eq. (11.44):

$$\mathbf{s}^2 = -2\dot{\mathbf{F}}^2(\mathbf{n}^2)\,(\mathbf{t} - \mathbf{a}) = -2\left[\dot{f}^2(n^2)\right](1.261) = -2\left[1\right](1.261) = -2.522 .$$

The first layer sensitivity is then computed by backpropagating the sensitivity from the second layer, using Eq. (11.45):

$$\mathbf{s}^1 = \dot{\mathbf{F}}^1(\mathbf{n}^1)\,(\mathbf{W}^2)^T\mathbf{s}^2 = \begin{bmatrix} (1 - a_1^1)\,(a_1^1) & 0 \\ 0 & (1 - a_2^1)\,(a_2^1) \end{bmatrix}\begin{bmatrix} 0.09 \\ -0.17 \end{bmatrix}\begin{bmatrix} -2.522 \end{bmatrix}$$

$$= \begin{bmatrix} (1 - 0.321)\,(0.321) & 0 \\ 0 & (1 - 0.368)\,(0.368) \end{bmatrix}\begin{bmatrix} 0.09 \\ -0.17 \end{bmatrix}\begin{bmatrix} -2.522 \end{bmatrix}$$

$$= \begin{bmatrix} 0.218 & 0 \\ 0 & 0.233 \end{bmatrix}\begin{bmatrix} -0.227 \\ 0.429 \end{bmatrix} = \begin{bmatrix} -0.0495 \\ 0.0997 \end{bmatrix} .$$

The final stage of the algorithm is to update the weights. For simplicity, we will use a learning rate $\alpha = 0.1$. (In Chapter 12 the choice of learning rate will be discussed in more detail.) From Eq. (11.46) and Eq. (11.47) we have

$$\mathbf{W}^2(1) = \mathbf{W}^2(0) - \alpha\mathbf{s}^2(\mathbf{a}^1)^T = \begin{bmatrix} 0.09 & -0.17 \end{bmatrix} - 0.1\begin{bmatrix} -2.522 \end{bmatrix}\begin{bmatrix} 0.321 & 0.368 \end{bmatrix}$$

$$= \begin{bmatrix} 0.171 & -0.0772 \end{bmatrix} ,$$

$$\mathbf{b}^2(1) = \mathbf{b}^2(0) - \alpha\mathbf{s}^2 = \begin{bmatrix} 0.48 \end{bmatrix} - 0.1\begin{bmatrix} -2.522 \end{bmatrix} = \begin{bmatrix} 0.732 \end{bmatrix},$$

$$\mathbf{W}^1(1) = \mathbf{W}^1(0) - \alpha\mathbf{s}^1(\mathbf{a}^0)^T = \begin{bmatrix} -0.27 \\ -0.41 \end{bmatrix} - 0.1\begin{bmatrix} -0.0495 \\ 0.0997 \end{bmatrix}\begin{bmatrix} 1 \end{bmatrix} = \begin{bmatrix} -0.265 \\ -0.420 \end{bmatrix},$$

$$\mathbf{b}^1(1) = \mathbf{b}^1(0) - \alpha\mathbf{s}^1 = \begin{bmatrix} -0.48 \\ -0.13 \end{bmatrix} - 0.1\begin{bmatrix} -0.0495 \\ 0.0997 \end{bmatrix} = \begin{bmatrix} -0.475 \\ -0.140 \end{bmatrix}.$$

This completes the first iteration of the backpropagation algorithm. We next proceed to choose another input p and perform another iteration of the algorithm. We continue to iterate until the difference between the network response and the target function reaches some acceptable level. We will discuss convergence criteria in more detail in Chapter 12.

To experiment with the backpropagation calculation for this two-layer network, use the Neural Network Design Demonstration Backpropagation Calculation *(nnd11bc).*

Using Backpropagation

In this section we will present some issues relating to the practical implementation of backpropagation. We will discuss the choice of network architecture, and problems with network convergence and generalization. (We will discuss implementation issues again in Chapter 12, which investigates procedures for improving the algorithm.)

Choice of Network Architecture

As we discussed earlier in this chapter, multilayer networks can be used to approximate almost any function, if we have enough neurons in the hidden layers. However, we cannot say, in general, how many layers or how many neurons are necessary for adequate performance. In this section we want to use a few examples to provide some insight into this problem.

For our first example let's assume that we want to approximate the following functions:

$$g(p) = 1 + \sin\left(\frac{i\pi}{4}p\right) \text{ for } -2 \le p \le 2, \tag{11.49}$$

where i takes on the values 1, 2, 4 and 8. As i is increased, the function becomes more complex, because we will have more periods of the sine wave over the interval $-2 \le p \le 2$. It will be more difficult for a neural network with a fixed number of neurons in the hidden layers to approximate $g(p)$ as i is increased.

For this first example we will use a 1-3-1 network, where the transfer function for the first layer is log-sigmoid and the transfer function for the second layer is linear. Recall from our example on page 11-5 that this type of two-layer network can produce a response that is a sum of three log-sigmoid functions (or as many log-sigmoids as there are neurons in the hidden layer). Clearly there is a limit to how complex a function this network can implement. Figure 11.10 illustrates the response of the network after it has been trained to approximate $g(p)$ for $i = 1, 2, 4, 8$. The final network responses are shown by the blue lines.

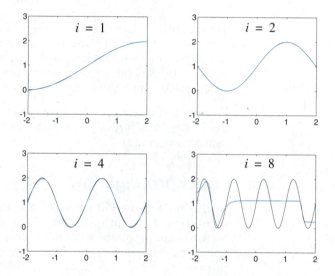

Figure 11.10 Function Approximation Using a 1-3-1 Network

We can see that for $i = 4$ the 1-3-1 network reaches its maximum capability. When $i > 4$ the network is not capable of producing an accurate approximation of $g(p)$. In the bottom right graph of Figure 11.10 we can see how the 1-3-1 network attempts to approximate $g(p)$ for $i = 8$. The mean square error between the network response and $g(p)$ is minimized, but the network response is only able to match a small part of the function.

In the next example we will approach the problem from a slightly different perspective. This time we will pick one function $g(p)$ and then use larger and larger networks until we are able to accurately represent the function. For $g(p)$ we will use

$$g(p) = 1 + \sin\left(\frac{6\pi}{4}p\right) \text{ for } -2 \le p \le 2. \tag{11.50}$$

To approximate this function we will use two-layer networks, where the transfer function for the first layer is log-sigmoid and the transfer function for the second layer is linear ($1\text{-}S^1\text{-}1$ networks). As we discussed earlier in this chapter, the response of this network is a superposition of S^1 sigmoid functions.

Figure 11.11 illustrates the network response as the number of neurons in the first layer (hidden layer) is increased. Unless there are at least five neurons in the hidden layer the network cannot accurately represent $g(p)$.

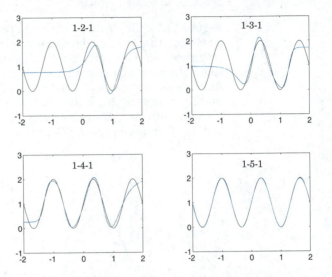

Figure 11.11 Effect of Increasing the Number of Hidden Neurons

To summarize these results, a 1-S^1-1 network, with sigmoid neurons in the hidden layer and linear neurons in the output layer, can produce a response that is a superposition of S^1 sigmoid functions. If we want to approximate a function that has a large number of inflection points, we will need to have a large number of neurons in the hidden layer.

Use the Neural Network Design Demonstration Function Approximation (**nnd11fa**) *to develop more insight into the capability of a two-layer network.*

Convergence

In the previous section we presented some examples in which the network response did not give an accurate approximation to the desired function, even though the backpropagation algorithm produced network parameters that minimized mean square error. This occurred because the capabilities of the network were inherently limited by the number of hidden neurons it contained. In this section we will provide an example in which the network is capable of approximating the function, but the learning algorithm does not produce network parameters that produce an accurate approximation. In the next chapter we will discuss this problem in more detail and explain why it occurs. For now we simply want to illustrate the problem.

11

The function that we want the network to approximate is

$$g(p) = 1 + \sin(\pi p) \quad \text{for } -2 \le p \le 2. \tag{11.51}$$

To approximate this function we will use a 1-3-1 network, where the transfer function for the first layer is log-sigmoid and the transfer function for the second layer is linear.

Figure 11.12 illustrates a case where the learning algorithm converges to a solution that minimizes mean square error. The thin blue lines represent intermediate iterations, and the thick blue line represents the final solution, when the algorithm has converged. (The numbers next to each curve indicate the sequence of iterations, where 0 represents the initial condition and 5 represents the final solution. The numbers do not correspond to the iteration number. There were many iterations for which no curve is represented. The numbers simply indicate an ordering.)

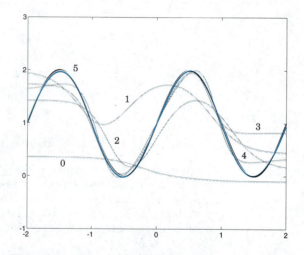

Figure 11.12 Convergence to a Global Minimum

Figure 11.13 illustrates a case where the learning algorithm converges to a solution that does not minimize mean square error. The thick blue line (marked with a 5) represents the network response at the final iteration. The gradient of the mean square error is zero at the final iteration, therefore we have a local minima, but we know that a better solution exists, as evidenced by Figure 11.12. The only difference between this result and the result shown in Figure 11.12 is the initial condition. From one initial condition the algorithm converged to a global minimum point, while from another initial condition the algorithm converged to a local minimum point.

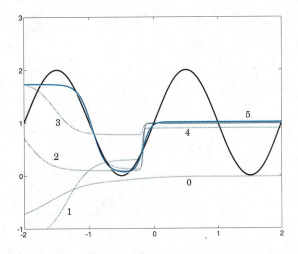

Figure 11.13 Convergence to a Local Minimum

Note that this result could not have occurred with the LMS algorithm. The mean square error performance index for the ADALINE network is a quadratic function with a single minimum point (under most conditions). Therefore the LMS algorithm is guaranteed to converge to the global minimum as long as the learning rate is small enough. The mean square error for the multilayer network is generally much more complex and has many local minima (as we will see in the next chapter). When the backpropagation algorithm converges we cannot be sure that we have an optimum solution. It is best to try several different initial conditions in order to ensure that an optimum solution has been obtained.

Generalization

In most cases the multilayer network is trained with a finite number of examples of proper network behavior:

$$\{\mathbf{p}_1, \mathbf{t}_1\}, \{\mathbf{p}_2, \mathbf{t}_2\}, \dots, \{\mathbf{p}_Q, \mathbf{t}_Q\} . \tag{11.52}$$

This training set is normally representative of a much larger class of possible input/output pairs. It is important that the network successfully *generalize* what it has learned to the total population.

For example, suppose that the training set is obtained by sampling the following function:

$$g(p) = 1 + \sin\left(\frac{\pi}{4}p\right), \tag{11.53}$$

at the points $p = -2, -1.6, -1.2, \dots, 1.6, 2$. (There are a total of 11 input/target pairs.) In Figure 11.14 we see the response of a 1-2-1 network that has

11

been trained on this data. The black line represents $g(p)$, the blue line represents the network response, and the '+' symbols indicate the training set.

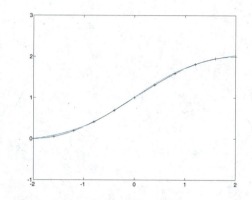

Figure 11.14 1-2-1 Network Approximation of $g(p)$

We can see that the network response is an accurate representation of $g(p)$. If we were to find the response of the network at a value of p that was not contained in the training set (e.g., $p = -0.2$), the network would still produce an output close to $g(p)$. This network generalizes well.

Now consider Figure 11.15, which shows the response of a 1-9-1 network that has been trained on the same data set. Note that the network response accurately models $g(p)$ at all of the training points. However, if we compute the network response at a value of p not contained in the training set (e.g., $p = -0.2$) the network might produce an output far from the true response $g(p)$. This network does not generalize well.

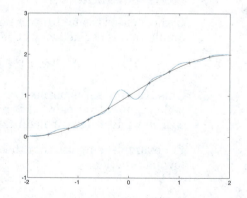

Figure 11.15 1-9-1 Network Approximation of $g(p)$

The 1-9-1 network has too much flexibility for this problem; it has a total of 28 adjustable parameters (18 weights and 10 biases), and yet there are only 11 data points in the training set. The 1-2-1 network has only 7 parameters and is therefore much more restricted in the types of functions that it can implement.

For a network to be able to generalize, it should have fewer parameters than there are data points in the training set. In neural networks, as in all modeling problems, we want to use the simplest network that can adequately represent the training set. Don't use a bigger network when a smaller network will work (a concept often referred to as Ockham's Razor).

An alternative to using the simplest network is to stop the training before the network overfits. A reference to this procedure and other techniques to improve generalization are given in Chapter 19.

To experiment with generalization in neural networks, use the Neural Network Design Demonstration Generalization (**nnd11gn**).

Summary of Results

Multilayer Network

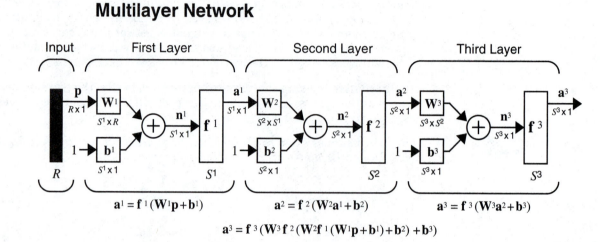

$$a^1 = f^1(W^1p + b^1) \qquad a^2 = f^2(W^2a^1 + b^2) \qquad a^3 = f^3(W^3a^2 + b^3)$$

$$a^3 = f^3(W^3 f^2(W^2 f^1(W^1p + b^1) + b^2) + b^3)$$

Backpropagation Algorithm

Performance Index

$$F(\mathbf{x}) = E[\mathbf{e}^T \mathbf{e}] = E[(\mathbf{t} - \mathbf{a})^T (\mathbf{t} - \mathbf{a})]$$

Approximate Performance Index

$$\hat{F}(\mathbf{x}) = \mathbf{e}^T(k)\mathbf{e}(k) = (\mathbf{t}(k) - \mathbf{a}(k))^T (\mathbf{t}(k) - \mathbf{a}(k))$$

Sensitivity

$$\mathbf{s}^m \equiv \frac{\partial \hat{F}}{\partial \mathbf{n}^m} = \begin{bmatrix} \dfrac{\partial \hat{F}}{\partial n_1^m} \\[2mm] \dfrac{\partial \hat{F}}{\partial n_2^m} \\[1mm] \vdots \\[1mm] \dfrac{\partial \hat{F}}{\partial n_{S^m}^m} \end{bmatrix}$$

Forward Propagation

$$\mathbf{a}^0 = \mathbf{p},$$

$$\mathbf{a}^{m+1} = \mathbf{f}^{m+1}(\mathbf{W}^{m+1}\mathbf{a}^m + \mathbf{b}^{m+1}) \text{ for } m = 0, 2, \ldots, M-1,$$

$$\mathbf{a} = \mathbf{a}^M.$$

Backward Propagation

$$\mathbf{s}^M = -2\dot{\mathbf{F}}^M(\mathbf{n}^M)(\mathbf{t} - \mathbf{a}),$$

$$\mathbf{s}^m = \dot{\mathbf{F}}^m(\mathbf{n}^m)(\mathbf{W}^{m+1})^T\mathbf{s}^{m+1}, \text{ for } m = M-1, \ldots, 2, 1,$$

where

$$\dot{\mathbf{F}}^m(\mathbf{n}^m) = \begin{bmatrix} \dot{f}^m(n_1^m) & 0 & \cdots & 0 \\ 0 & \dot{f}^m(n_2^m) & \cdots & 0 \\ \vdots & \vdots & & \vdots \\ 0 & 0 & & \dot{f}^m(n_{S^m}^m) \end{bmatrix},$$

$$\dot{f}^m(n_j^m) = \frac{\partial f^m(n_j^m)}{\partial n_j^m}.$$

Weight Update (Approximate Steepest Descent)

$$\mathbf{W}^m(k+1) = \mathbf{W}^m(k) - \alpha\mathbf{s}^m(\mathbf{a}^{m-1})^T,$$

$$\mathbf{b}^m(k+1) = \mathbf{b}^m(k) - \alpha\mathbf{s}^m.$$

11

Solved Problems

P11.1 **Consider the two classes of patterns that are shown in Figure P11.1. Class I represents vertical lines and Class II represents horizontal lines.**

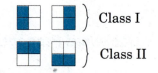

Figure P11.1 Pattern Classes for Problem P11.1

    i. Are these categories linearly separable?

    ii. Design a multilayer network to distinguish these categories.

i. Let's begin by converting the patterns to vectors by scanning each 2X2 grid one column at a time. Each white square will be represented by a "–1" and each blue square by a "1". The vertical lines (Class I patterns) then become

$$\mathbf{p}_1 = \begin{bmatrix} 1 \\ 1 \\ -1 \\ -1 \end{bmatrix} \text{ and } \mathbf{p}_2 = \begin{bmatrix} -1 \\ -1 \\ 1 \\ 1 \end{bmatrix},$$

and the horizontal lines (Class II patterns) become

$$\mathbf{p}_3 = \begin{bmatrix} 1 \\ -1 \\ 1 \\ -1 \end{bmatrix} \text{ and } \mathbf{p}_4 = \begin{bmatrix} -1 \\ 1 \\ -1 \\ 1 \end{bmatrix}.$$

In order for these categories to be linearly separable we must be able to place a hyperplane between the two categories. This means there must be a weight matrix $\mathbf{W}$ and a bias b such that

$$\mathbf{W}\mathbf{p}_1 + b > 0, \ \mathbf{W}\mathbf{p}_2 + b > 0, \ \mathbf{W}\mathbf{p}_3 + b < 0, \ \mathbf{W}\mathbf{p}_4 + b < 0.$$

These conditions can be converted to

$$\begin{bmatrix} w_{1,1} & w_{1,2} & w_{1,3} & w_{1,4} \end{bmatrix} \begin{bmatrix} 1 \\ 1 \\ -1 \\ -1 \end{bmatrix} = \begin{bmatrix} w_{1,1} + w_{1,2} - w_{1,3} - w_{1,4} \end{bmatrix} > 0,$$

$$\begin{bmatrix} -w_{1,1} - w_{1,2} + w_{1,3} + w_{1,4} \end{bmatrix} > 0,$$

$$\begin{bmatrix} w_{1,1} - w_{1,2} + w_{1,3} - w_{1,4} \end{bmatrix} < 0,$$

$$\begin{bmatrix} -w_{1,1} + w_{1,2} - w_{1,3} + w_{1,4} \end{bmatrix} < 0.$$

The first two conditions reduce to

$$w_{1,1} + w_{1,2} > w_{1,3} + w_{1,4} \text{ and } w_{1,3} + w_{1,4} > w_{1,1} + w_{1,2},$$

which are contradictory. The final two conditions reduce to

$$w_{1,1} + w_{1,3} > w_{1,2} + w_{1,4} \text{ and } w_{1,2} + w_{1,4} > w_{1,1} + w_{1,3},$$

which are also contradictory. Therefore there is no hyperplane that can separate these two categories.

ii. There are many different multilayer networks that could solve this problem. We will design a network by first noting that for the Class I vectors either the first two elements or the last two elements will be "1". The Class II vectors have alternating "1" and "–1" patterns. This leads to the network shown in Figure P11.2.

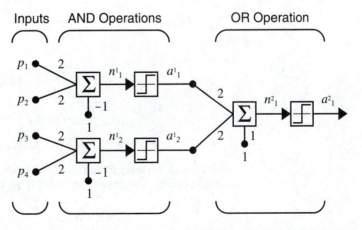

Figure P11.2 Network to Categorize Horizontal and Vertical Lines

The first neuron in the first layer tests the first two elements of the input vector. If they are both "1" it outputs a "1", otherwise it outputs a "-1". The second neuron in the first layer tests the last two elements of the input vector in the same way. Both of the neurons in the first layer perform AND operations. The second layer of the network tests whether either of the outputs of the first layer are "1". It performs an OR operation. In this way, the network will output a "1" if either the first two elements or the last two elements of the input vector are both "1".

P11.2 **Figure P11.3 illustrates a classification problem, where Class I vectors are represented by light circles, and Class II vectors are represented by dark circles. These categories are not linearly separable. Design a multilayer network to correctly classify these categories.**

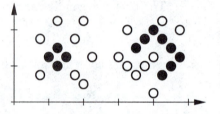

Figure P11.3 Classification Problem

We will solve this problem with a procedure that can be used for arbitrary classification problems. It requires a three-layer network, with hard-limiting neurons in each layer. In the first layer we create a set of linear decision boundaries that separate every Class I vector from every Class II vector. For this problem we used 11 such boundaries. They are shown in Figure P11.4.

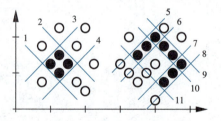

Figure P11.4 First Layer Decision Boundaries

Each row of the weight matrix in the first layer corresponds to one decision boundary. The weight matrix and bias vector for the first layer are

$$(\mathbf{W}^1)^T = \begin{bmatrix} 1 & -1 & 1 & -1 & 1 & -1 & 1 & -1 & -1 & 1 & 1 \\ 1 & -1 & -1 & 1 & -1 & 1 & -1 & 1 & -1 & 1 & 1 \end{bmatrix},$$

$$(\mathbf{b}^1)^T = \begin{bmatrix} -2 & 3 & 0.5 & 0.5 & -1.75 & 2.25 & -3.25 & 3.75 & 6.25 & -5.75 & -4.75 \end{bmatrix}.$$

(Review Chapters 3, 4 and 10 for procedures for calculating the appropriate weight matrix and bias for a given decision boundary.) Now we can combine the outputs of the 11 first layer neurons into groups with a second layer of AND neurons, such as those we used in the first layer of the network in Problem P11.1. The second layer weight matrix and bias are

$$\mathbf{W}^2 = \begin{bmatrix} 1 & 1 & 1 & 1 & 0 & 0 & 0 & 0 & 0 & 0 & 0 \\ 0 & 0 & 0 & 0 & 1 & 1 & 0 & 0 & 1 & 0 & 1 \\ 0 & 0 & 0 & 0 & 1 & 0 & 0 & 1 & 1 & 1 & 0 \\ 0 & 0 & 0 & 0 & 0 & 0 & 1 & 1 & 1 & 0 & 1 \end{bmatrix}, \mathbf{b}^T = \begin{bmatrix} -3 \\ -3 \\ -3 \\ -3 \end{bmatrix}.$$

The four decision boundaries for the second layer are shown in Figure P11.5. For example, the neuron 2 decision boundary is obtained by combining the boundaries 5, 6, 9 and 11 from layer 1. This can be seen by looking at row 2 of $\mathbf{W}^2$.

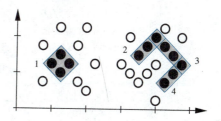

Figure P11.5 Second Layer Decision Regions

In the third layer of the network we will combine together the four decision regions of the second layer into one decision region using an OR operation, just as in the last layer of the network in Problem P11.1. The weight matrix and bias for the third layer are

$$\mathbf{W}^3 = \begin{bmatrix} 1 & 1 & 1 & 1 \end{bmatrix}, \mathbf{b}^3 = \begin{bmatrix} 3 \end{bmatrix}.$$

The complete network is shown in Figure P11.6.

The procedure that we used to develop this network can be used to solve classification problems with arbitrary decision boundaries as long as we have enough neurons in the hidden layers. The idea is to use the first layer to create a number of linear boundaries, which can be combined by using AND neurons in the second layer and OR neurons in the third layer. The decision regions of the second layer are convex, but the final decision boundaries created by the third layer can have arbitrary shapes.

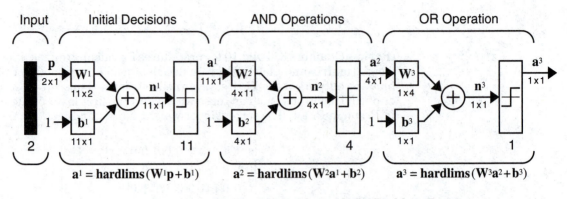

Figure P11.6 Network for Problem P11.2

The final network decision regions are given in Figure P11.7. Any vector in the shaded areas will produce a network output of 1, which corresponds to Class II. All other vectors will produce a network output of –1, which corresponds to Class I.

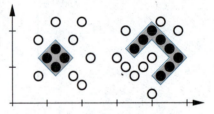

Figure P11.7 Final Decision Regions

P11.3 Show that a multilayer network with linear transfer functions is equivalent to a single-layer linear network.

For a multilayer linear network the forward equations would be

$$\mathbf{a}^1 = \mathbf{W}^1\mathbf{p} + \mathbf{b}^1$$

$$\mathbf{a}^2 = \mathbf{W}^2\mathbf{a}^1 + \mathbf{b}^2 = \mathbf{W}^2\mathbf{W}^1\mathbf{p} + [\mathbf{W}^2\mathbf{b}^1 + \mathbf{b}^2] \, ,$$

$$\mathbf{a}^3 = \mathbf{W}^3\mathbf{a}^2 + \mathbf{b}^3 = \mathbf{W}^3\mathbf{W}^2\mathbf{W}^1\mathbf{p} + [\mathbf{W}^3\mathbf{W}^2\mathbf{b}^1 + \mathbf{W}^3\mathbf{b}^2 + \mathbf{b}^3] \, .$$

If we continue this process we can see that for an M-layer linear network, the equivalent single-layer linear network would have the following weight matrix and bias vector

$$\mathbf{W} = \mathbf{W}^M\mathbf{W}^{M-1}\ldots\mathbf{W}^2\mathbf{W}^1 \, ,$$

$$\mathbf{b} = [\mathbf{W}^M \mathbf{W}^{M-1} \dots \mathbf{W}^2] \mathbf{b}^1 + [\mathbf{W}^M \mathbf{W}^{M-1} \dots \mathbf{W}^3] \mathbf{b}^2 + \cdots + \mathbf{b}^M.$$

P11.4 **The purpose of this problem is to illustrate the use of the chain rule. Consider the following dynamic system:**

$$y(k+1) = f(y(k)).$$

We want to choose the initial condition $y(0)$ so that at some final time $k = K$ the system output $y(K)$ will be as close as possible to some target output t. We will minimize the performance index

$$F(y(0)) = (t - y(K))^2$$

using steepest descent, so we need the gradient

$$\frac{\partial}{\partial y(0)} F(y(0)).$$

Find a procedure for computing this using the chain rule.

The gradient is

$$\frac{\partial}{\partial y(0)} F(y(0)) = \frac{\partial (t - y(K))^2}{\partial y(0)} = 2(t - y(K)) \left[-\frac{\partial}{\partial y(0)} y(K) \right].$$

The key term is

$$\left[\frac{\partial}{\partial y(0)} y(K) \right],$$

which cannot be computed directly, since $y(K)$ is not an explicit function of $y(0)$. Let's define an intermediate term

$$r(k) \equiv \frac{\partial}{\partial y(0)} y(k).$$

Then we can use the chain rule:

$$r(k+1) = \frac{\partial}{\partial y(0)} y(k+1) = \frac{\partial y(k+1)}{\partial y(k)} \times \frac{\partial y(k)}{\partial y(0)} = \frac{\partial y(k+1)}{\partial y(k)} \times r(k).$$

From the system dynamics we know

$$\frac{\partial y(k+1)}{\partial y(k)} = \frac{\partial f(y(k))}{\partial y(k)} = \dot{f}(y(k)).$$

Therefore the recursive equation for the computation of $r(k)$ is

11

$$r(k+1) = \dot{f}(y(k)) r(k).$$

This is initialized at $k = 0$:

$$r(0) = \frac{\partial y(0)}{\partial y(0)} = 1.$$

The total procedure for computing the gradient is then

$$r(0) = 1,$$

$$r(k+1) = \dot{f}(y(k)) r(k), \text{ for } k = 0, 1, \ldots, K-1,$$

$$\frac{\partial}{\partial y(0)} F(y(0)) = 2(t - y(K)) [-r(K)].$$

P11.5 **Consider the two-layer network shown in Figure P11.8. The initial weights and biases are set to**

$$w^1 = 1, b^1 = 1, w^2 = -2, b^2 = 1.$$

An input/target pair is given to be

$$((p = 1), (t = 1)).$$

   i. **Find the squared error** $(e)^2$ **as an explicit function of all weights and biases.**

  ii. **Using part (i) find** $\partial(e)^2/\partial w^1$ **at the initial weights and biases.**

 iii. **Repeat part (ii) using backpropagation and compare results.**

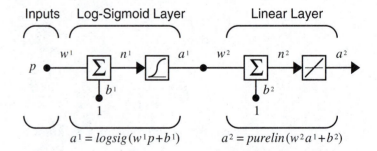

Figure P11.8 Two-Layer Network for Problem P11.5

i. The squared error is given by

$$(e)^2 = (t - a^2)^2 = \left(t - \{w^2 \frac{1}{(1 + \exp(-(w^1 p + b^1)))} + b^2\}\right)^2.$$

ii. The derivative is

$$\frac{\partial(e)^2}{\partial w^1} = 2e \frac{\partial e}{\partial w^1} = 2e \left\{ -w^2 \frac{1}{(1 + \exp(-(w^1 p + b^1)))^2} \exp(-(w^1 p + b^1))(-p) \right\}$$

To evaluate this at the initial weights and biases we find

$$a^1 = \frac{1}{(1 + \exp(-(w^1 p + b^1)))} = \frac{1}{(1 + \exp(-(1(1) + 1)))} = 1.1565$$

$$a^2 = w^2 a^1 + b^2 = (-2)1.1565 + 1 = -1.313$$

$$e = (t - a^2) = (1 - (-1.313)) = 2.313$$

$$\frac{\partial(e)^2}{\partial w^1} = 2e \left\{ -w^2 \frac{1}{(1 + \exp(-(w^1 p + b^1)))^2} \exp(-(w^1 p + b^1))(-p) \right\}$$

$$= 2(2.313) \{ -(-2) \frac{1}{(1 + \exp(-(1(1) + 1)))^2} \exp(-(1(1) + 1))(-1) \}$$

$$= 4.626 \left(-0.2707 \frac{1}{(0.8647)^2} \right) = -1.6748 .$$

iii. To backpropagate the sensitivities we use Eq. (11.44) and Eq. (11.45):

$$s^2 = -2\dot{F}^2(n^2)(t - a) = -2(1)(1 - (-1.313)) = -4.626,$$

$$s^1 = \dot{F}^1(n^1)(W^2)^T s^2 = [a^1(1 - a^1)](-2)s^2$$

$$= [1.1565(1 - 1.1565)](-2)(-4.626) = -1.6748 .$$

From Eq. (11.23) we can compute $\partial(e)^2 / \partial w^1$:

$$\frac{\partial(e)^2}{\partial w^1} = s^1 a^0 = s^1 p = (-1.6748)(1) = -1.6748 .$$

This agrees with our result from part (ii).

11

P11.6 **Earlier in this chapter we showed that if the neuron transfer function is log-sigmoid,**

$$a = f(n) = \frac{1}{1 + e^{-n}},$$

then the derivative can be conveniently computed by

$$\dot{f}(n) = a(1-a).$$

Find a convenient way to compute the derivative for the hyperbolic tangent sigmoid:

$$a = f(n) = tansig(n) = \frac{e^n - e^{-n}}{e^n + e^{-n}}.$$

Computing the derivative directly we find

$$\dot{f}(n) = \frac{df(n)}{dn} = \frac{d}{dn}\left(\frac{e^n - e^{-n}}{e^n + e^{-n}}\right) = -\frac{e^n - e^{-n}}{(e^n + e^{-n})^2}(e^n - e^{-n}) + \frac{e^n + e^{-n}}{e^n + e^{-n}}$$

$$= 1 - \frac{(e^n - e^{-n})^2}{(e^n + e^{-n})^2} = 1 - (a)^2.$$

P11.7 **For the network shown in Figure P11.9 the initial weights and biases are chosen to be**

$$w^1(0) = -1, \; b^1(0) = 1, \; w^2(0) = -2, \; b^2(0) = 1.$$

An input/target pair is given to be

$$((p = -1),(t = 1)).$$

Perform one iteration of backpropagation with $\alpha = 1$.

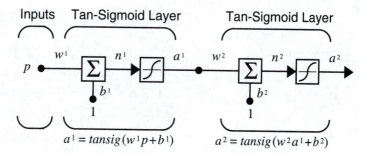

Figure P11.9 Two-Layer Tan-Sigmoid Network

The first step is to propagate the input through the network.

$$n^1 = w^1 p + b^1 = (-1)(-1) + 1 = 2$$

$$a^1 = tansig(n^1) = \frac{\exp(n^1) - \exp(-n^1)}{\exp(n^1) + \exp(-n^1)} = \frac{\exp(2) - \exp(-2)}{\exp(2) + \exp(-2)} = 0.964$$

$$n^2 = w^2 a^1 + b^2 = (-2)(0.964) + 1 = -0.928$$

$$a^2 = tansig(n^2) = \frac{\exp(n^2) - \exp(-n^2)}{\exp(n^2) + \exp(-n^2)} = \frac{\exp(-0.928) - \exp(0.928)}{\exp(-0.928) + \exp(0.928)}$$

$$= -0.7297$$

$$e = (t - a^2) = (1 - (-0.7297)) = 1.7297$$

Now we backpropagate the sensitivities using Eq. (11.44) and Eq. (11.45).

$$\mathbf{s}^2 = -2\dot{\mathbf{F}}^2(\mathbf{n}^2)(\mathbf{t} - \mathbf{a}) = -2[1 - (a^2)^2](e) = -2[1 - (-0.7297)^2]1.7297$$

$$= -1.6175$$

$$\mathbf{s}^1 = \dot{\mathbf{F}}^1(\mathbf{n}^1)(\mathbf{W}^2)^T \mathbf{s}^2 = [1 - (a^1)^2]w^2 \mathbf{s}^2 = [1 - (0.964)^2](-2)(-1.6175)$$

$$= 0.2285$$

Finally, the weights and biases are updated using Eq. (11.46) and Eq. (11.47):

11

$$w^2(1) = w^2(0) - \alpha s^2 (a^1)^T = (-2) - 1(-1.6175)(0.964) = -0.4407,$$

$$w^1(1) = w^1(0) - \alpha s^1 (a^0)^T = (-1) - 1(0.2285)(-1) = -0.7715,$$

$$b^2(1) = b^2(0) - \alpha s^2 = 1 - 1(-1.6175) = 2.6175,$$

$$b^1(1) = b^1(0) - \alpha s^1 = 1 - 1(0.2285) = 0.7715.$$

P11.8 **In Figure P11.10 we have a network that is a slight modification to the standard two-layer feedforward network. It has a connection from the input directly to the second layer. Derive the backpropagation algorithm for this network.**

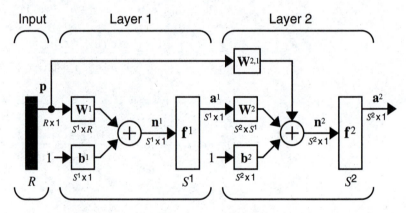

Figure P11.10 Network with Bypass Connection

We begin with the forward equations:

$$\mathbf{n}^1 = \mathbf{W}^1\mathbf{p} + \mathbf{b}^1,$$

$$\mathbf{a}^1 = \mathbf{f}^1(\mathbf{n}^1) = \mathbf{f}^1(\mathbf{W}^1\mathbf{p} + \mathbf{b}^1),$$

$$\mathbf{n}^2 = \mathbf{W}^2\mathbf{a}^1 + \mathbf{W}^{2,1}\mathbf{p} + \mathbf{b}^2,$$

$$\mathbf{a}^2 = \mathbf{f}^2(\mathbf{n}^2) = \mathbf{f}^2(\mathbf{W}^2\mathbf{a}^1 + \mathbf{W}^{2,1}\mathbf{p} + \mathbf{b}^2).$$

The backpropagation equations for the sensitivities will not change from those for a standard two-layer network. The sensitivities are the derivatives of the squared error with respect to the net inputs; these derivatives don't change, since we are simply adding a term to the net input.

Next we need the elements of the gradient for the weight update equations. For the standard weights and biases we have

$$\frac{\partial \hat{F}}{\partial w_{i,j}^m} = \frac{\partial \hat{F}}{\partial n_i^m} \times \frac{\partial n_i^m}{\partial w_{i,j}^m} = s_i^m a_j^{m-1},$$

$$\frac{\partial \hat{F}}{\partial b_i^m} = \frac{\partial \hat{F}}{\partial n_i^m} \times \frac{\partial n_i^m}{\partial b_i^m} = s_i^m.$$

Therefore the update equations for $\mathbf{W}^1$, $\mathbf{b}^1$, $\mathbf{W}^2$ and $\mathbf{b}^2$ do not change. We do need an additional equation for $\mathbf{W}^{2,1}$:

$$\frac{\partial \hat{F}}{\partial w_{i,j}^{2,1}} = \frac{\partial \hat{F}}{\partial n_i^2} \times \frac{\partial n_i^2}{\partial w_{i,j}^{2,1}} = s_i^2 \times \frac{\partial n_i^2}{\partial w_{i,j}^{2,1}}.$$

To find the derivative on the right-hand side of this equation note that

$$n_i^2 = \sum_{j=1}^{s^1} w_{i,j}^2 a_j^1 + \sum_{j=1}^{R} w_{i,j}^{2,1} p_j + b_i^2.$$

Therefore

$$\frac{\partial n_i^2}{\partial w_{i,j}^{2,1}} = p_j \text{ and } \frac{\partial \hat{F}}{\partial w_{i,j}^{2,1}} = s_i^2 p_j.$$

The update equations can thus be written in matrix form as:

$$\mathbf{W}^m(k+1) = \mathbf{W}^m(k) - \alpha \mathbf{s}^m (\mathbf{a}^{m-1})^T, \ m = 1, 2,$$

$$\mathbf{b}^m(k+1) = \mathbf{b}^m(k) - \alpha \mathbf{s}^m, \ m = 1, 2.$$

$$\mathbf{W}^{2,1}(k+1) = \mathbf{W}^{2,1}(k) - \alpha \mathbf{s}^2 (\mathbf{a}^0)^T = \mathbf{W}^{2,1}(k) - \alpha \mathbf{s}^2 (\mathbf{p})^T.$$

The main point of this problem is that the backpropagation concept can be used on networks more general than the standard multilayer feedforward network.

P11.9 **Find an algorithm, based on the backpropagation concept, that can be used to update the weights w_1 and w_2 in the recurrent network shown in Figure P11.11.**

11

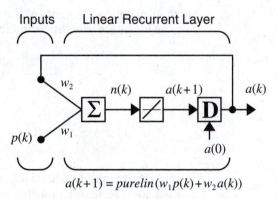

$$a(k+1) = purelin(w_1 p(k) + w_2 a(k))$$

Figure P11.11 Linear Recurrent Network

The first step is to define our performance index. As with the multilayer networks, we will use squared error:

$$\hat{F}(\mathbf{x}) = (t(k) - a(k))^2 = (e(k))^2.$$

For our weight updates we will use the steepest descent algorithm:

$$\Delta w_i = -\alpha \frac{\partial}{\partial w_i} \hat{F}(\mathbf{x}).$$

These derivatives can be computed as follows:

$$\frac{\partial}{\partial w_i} \hat{F}(\mathbf{x}) = \frac{\partial}{\partial w_i} (t(k) - a(k))^2 = 2(t(k) - a(k)) \left\{ -\frac{\partial a(k)}{\partial w_i} \right\}.$$

Therefore, the key terms we need to compute are

$$\frac{\partial a(k)}{\partial w_i}.$$

To compute these terms we first need to write out the network equation:

$$a(k+1) = purelin(w_1 p(k) + w_2 a(k)) = w_1 p(k) + w_2 a(k).$$

Next we take the derivative of both sides of this equation with respect to the network weights:

$$\frac{\partial a(k+1)}{\partial w_1} = p(k) + w_2 \frac{\partial a(k)}{\partial w_1},$$

$$\frac{\partial a(k+1)}{\partial w_2} = a(k) + w_2 \frac{\partial a(k)}{\partial w_2}.$$

(Note that we had to take account of the fact that $a(k)$ is itself a function of w_1 and w_2.) These two recursive equations are then used to compute the derivatives needed for the steepest descent weight update. The equations are initialized with

$$\frac{\partial a(0)}{\partial w_1} = 0, \ \frac{\partial a(0)}{\partial w_2} = 0,$$

since the initial condition is not a function of the weight.

To illustrate the process, let's say that $a(0) = 0$. The first network update would be

$$a(1) = w_1 p(0) + w_2 a(0) = w_1 p(0).$$

The first derivatives would be computed:

$$\frac{\partial a(1)}{\partial w_1} = p(0) + w_2 \frac{\partial a(0)}{\partial w_1} = p(0), \ \frac{\partial a(1)}{\partial w_2} = a(0) + w_2 \frac{\partial a(0)}{\partial w_2} = 0.$$

The first weight updates would be

$$\Delta w_i = -\alpha \frac{\partial}{\partial w_i} \hat{F}(\mathbf{x}) = -\alpha \left[2(t(1) - a(1)) \{ -\frac{\partial a(1)}{\partial w_i} \} \right]$$

$$\Delta w_1 = -2\alpha (t(1) - a(1)) \{ -p(0) \}$$

$$\Delta w_2 = -2\alpha (t(1) - a(1)) \{ 0 \} = 0.$$

This algorithm is a type of *dynamic backpropagation*, in which the gradient is computed by means of a difference equation.

P11.10 **Show that backpropagation reduces to the LMS algorithm for a single-layer linear network (ADALINE).**

The sensitivity calculation for a single-layer linear network would be:

$$\mathbf{s}^1 = -2\dot{\mathbf{F}}^1(\mathbf{n}^1)(\mathbf{t} - \mathbf{a}) = -2\mathbf{I}(\mathbf{t} - \mathbf{a}) = -2\mathbf{e},$$

The weight update (Eq. (11.46) and Eq. (11.47)) would be

$$\mathbf{W}^1(k+1) = \mathbf{W}^1(k) - \alpha \mathbf{s}^1 (\mathbf{a}^0)^T = \mathbf{W}^1(k) - \alpha(-2\mathbf{e})\mathbf{p}^T = \mathbf{W}^1(k) + 2\alpha\mathbf{e}\mathbf{p}^T$$

$$\mathbf{b}^1(k+1) = \mathbf{b}^1(k) - \alpha \mathbf{s}^1 = \mathbf{b}^1(k) - \alpha(-2\mathbf{e}) = \mathbf{b}^1(k) + 2\alpha\mathbf{e}.$$

This is identical to the LMS algorithm of Chapter 10.

11

Epilogue

In this chapter we have presented the multilayer perceptron network and the backpropagation learning rule. The multilayer network is a powerful extension of the single-layer perceptron network. Whereas the single-layer network is only able to classify linearly separable patterns, the multilayer network can be used for arbitrary classification problems. In addition, multilayer networks can be used as universal function approximators. It has been shown that a two-layer network, with sigmoid-type transfer functions in the hidden layer, can approximate any practical function, given enough neurons in the hidden layer.

The backpropagation algorithm is an extension of the LMS algorithm that can be used to train multilayer networks. Both LMS and backpropagation are approximate steepest descent algorithms that minimize squared error. The only difference between them is in the way in which the gradient is calculated. The backpropagation algorithm uses the chain rule in order to compute the derivatives of the squared error with respect to the weights and biases in the hidden layers. It is called backpropagation because the derivatives are computed first at the last layer of the network, and then propagated backward through the network, using the chain rule, to compute the derivatives in the hidden layers.

One of the major problems with backpropagation has been the long training times. It is not feasible to use the basic backpropagation algorithm on practical problems, because it can take weeks to train a network, even on a large computer. Since backpropagation was first popularized, there has been considerable work on methods to accelerate the convergence of the algorithm. In Chapter 12 we will discuss the reasons for the slow convergence of backpropagation and will present several techniques for improving the performance of the algorithm.

Further Reading

[HoSt89] K. M. Hornik, M. Stinchcombe and H. White, "Multilayer feedforward networks are universal approximators," *Neural Networks*, vol. 2, no. 5, pp. 359–366, 1989.

This paper proves that multilayer feedforward networks with arbitrary squashing functions can approximate any Borel integrable function from one finite dimensional space to another finite dimensional space.

[LeCu85] Y. Le Cun, "Une procedure d'apprentissage pour reseau a seuil assymetrique," *Cognitiva*, vol. 85, pp. 599–604, 1985.

Yann Le Cun discovered the backpropagation algorithm at about the same time as Parker and Rumelhart, Hinton and Williams. This paper describes his algorithm.

[Park85] D. B. Parker, "Learning-logic: Casting the cortex of the human brain in silicon," Technical Report TR-47, Center for Computational Research in Economics and Management Science, MIT, Cambridge, MA, 1985.

David Parker independently derived the backpropagation algorithm at about the same time as Le Cun and Rumelhart, Hinton and Williams. This report describes his algorithm.

[RuHi86] D. E. Rumelhart, G. E. Hinton and R. J. Williams, "Learning representations by back-propagating errors," *Nature*, vol. 323, pp. 533–536, 1986.

This paper contains the most widely publicized description of the backpropagation algorithm.

[RuMc86] D. E. Rumelhart and J. L. McClelland, eds., *Parallel Distributed Processing: Explorations in the Microstructure of Cognition*, vol. 1, Cambridge, MA: MIT Press, 1986.

This book was one of the two key influences in the resurgence of interest in the neural networks field during the 1980s. Among other topics, it presents the backpropagation algorithm for training multilayer neural networks.

[Werbo74] P. J. Werbos, "Beyond regression: New tools for prediction and analysis in the behavioral sciences," Ph.D. Thesis, Harvard University, Cambridge, MA, 1974.

This Ph.D. thesis contains what appears to be the first description of the backpropagation algorithm (although that

11

name is not used). The algorithm is described here in the context of general networks, with neural networks as a special case. Backpropagation did not become widely known until it was rediscovered in the mid 1980s by Rumelhart, Hinton and Williams [RuHi86], David Parker [Park85] and Yann Le Cun [LeCu85].

Exercises

E11.1 Design a multilayer network to perform the classification illustrated in Figure E11.1. The network should output a 1 whenever the input vector is in the shaded region (or on the boundary) and a –1 otherwise.

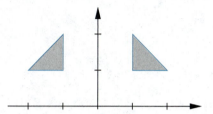

Figure E11.1 Pattern Classification Regions

E11.2 Find a single-layer network that has the same input/output characteristic as the network in Figure E11.2.

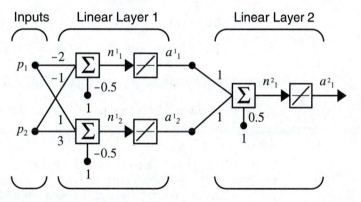

Figure E11.2 Two-Layer Linear Network

E11.3 Choose the weights and biases for the 1-2-1 network shown in Figure 11.4 so that the network response passes through the points indicated by the blue circles in Figure E11.3.

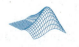

Use the Neural Network Design Demonstration Two-Layer Network Function (**nnd11nf**) *to check your result.*

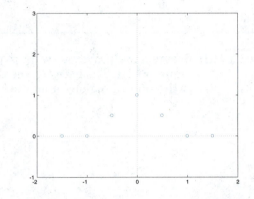

Figure E11.3 Function Approximation Exercise

E11.4 Use the chain rule to find the derivative $\partial f / \partial w$ in the following cases:

    i. $f(n) = \sin(n)$, $n(w) = w^2$.

    ii. $f(n) = \tanh(n)$, $n(w) = 5w$.

    iii. $f(n) = \exp(n)$, $n(w) = \cos(w)$.

    iv. $f(n) = \text{logsig}(n)$, $n(w) = \exp(w)$.

E11.5 Repeat Problem P11.4 using the "backward" method described below.

In Problem P11.4. we had the dynamic system

$$y(k+1) = f(y(k)).$$

We had to choose the initial condition $y(0)$ so that at some final time $k = K$ the system output $y(K)$ would be as close as possible to some target output t. We minimized the performance index

$$F(y(0)) = (t - y(K))^2 = e^2(K)$$

using steepest descent, so we needed the gradient

$$\frac{\partial}{\partial y(0)} F(y(0)).$$

We developed a procedure for computing this gradient using the chain rule. The procedure involved a recursive equation for the term

$$r(k) \equiv \frac{\partial}{\partial y(0)} y(k),$$

which evolved forward in time. The gradient can also be computed in a different way by evolving the term

$$q(k) \equiv \frac{\partial}{\partial y(k)} e^2(K)$$

backward through time.

E11.6 Consider again the backpropagation example that begins on page 11-14.

   i. Find the squared error $(e)^2$ as an explicit function of all weights and biases.

   ii. Using part (i), find $\partial(e)^2 / \partial w_{1,1}^1$ at the initial weights and biases.

   iii. Compare the results of part (ii) with the backpropagation results described in the text.

E11.7 For the network shown in Figure E11.4 the initial weights and biases are chosen to be

$$w^1(0) = 1, \, b^1(0) = -2, \, w^2(0) = 1, \, b^2(0) = 1.$$

The network transfer functions are

$$f^1(n) = (n)^2, \, f^2(n) = \frac{1}{n},$$

and an input/target pair is given to be

$$((p = 1), (t = 1)).$$

Perform one iteration of backpropagation with $\alpha = 1$.

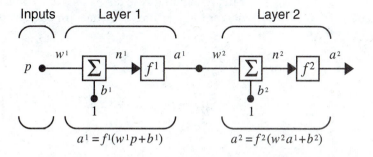

Figure E11.4 Two-Layer Network for Exercise E11.7

E11.8 For the network shown in Figure E11.5 the neuron transfer function is

$$f^1(n) = (n)^2,$$

and an input/target pair is given to be

$$\left(\mathbf{p} = \begin{bmatrix} 1 \\ 1 \end{bmatrix} \right), \left(\mathbf{t} = \begin{bmatrix} 8 \\ 2 \end{bmatrix} \right).$$

Perform one iteration of backpropagation with $\alpha = 1$.

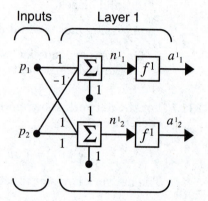

Figure E11.5 Single-Layer Network for Exercise E11.8

E11.9 The network shown in Figure E11.6 does not use our standard neuron format. The network output uses a product of network inputs:

$$a = w_1 p_1 + w_{1,2} p_1 p_2 + w_2 p_2 + b.$$

Find a learning rule for w_1, $w_{1,2}$, w_2 and b using an approximate steepest descent algorithm, as is used in backpropagation.

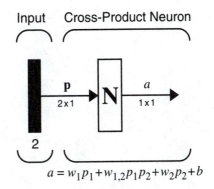

Figure E11.6 Cross-Product Network

E11.10 In Figure E11.7 we have a two-layer network that has an additional connection from the input directly to the second layer. Derive the backpropagation algorithm for this network.

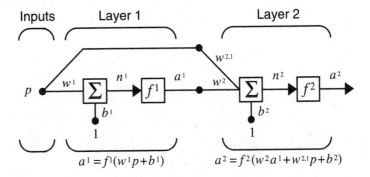

Figure E11.7 Two-Layer Network with Bypass Connection

E11.11 Write a MATLAB program to implement the backpropagation algorithm for the 1-2-1 network shown in Figure 11.4. Choose the initial weights and biases to be random numbers uniformly distributed between –0.5 and 0.5 (using the MATLAB function **rand**), and train the network to approximate the function

$$g(p) = 1 + \sin\left(\frac{\pi}{8}p\right) \text{ for } -2 \leq p \leq 2.$$

Try several different values for the learning rate α, and use several different initial conditions. Discuss the convergence properties of the algorithm.

12 Variations on Backpropagation

Objectives

The backpropagation algorithm introduced in Chapter 11 was a major breakthrough in neural network research. However, the basic algorithm is too slow for most practical applications. In this chapter we present several variations of backpropagation that provide significant speedup and make the algorithm more practical.

We will begin by using a function approximation example to illustrate why the backpropagation algorithm is slow in converging. Then we will present several modifications to the algorithm. Recall that backpropagation is an approximate steepest descent algorithm. In Chapter 9 we saw that steepest descent is the simplest, and often the slowest, minimization method. The conjugate gradient algorithm and Newton's method generally provide faster convergence. In this chapter we will explain how these faster procedures can be used to speed up the convergence of backpropagation.

Theory and Examples

When the basic backpropagation algorithm is applied to a practical problem the training may take days or weeks of computer time. This has encouraged considerable research on methods to accelerate the convergence of the algorithm.

The research on faster algorithms falls roughly into two categories. The first category involves the development of heuristic techniques, which arise out of a study of the distinctive performance of the standard backpropagation algorithm. These heuristic techniques include such ideas as varying the learning rate, using momentum and rescaling variables (e.g., [VoMa88], [Jacob88], [Toll90] and [RiIr90]). In this chapter we will discuss the use of momentum and variable learning rates.

Another category of research has focused on standard numerical optimization techniques (e.g., [Shan90], [Barn92], [Batt92] and [Char92]). As we have discussed in Chapters 10 and 11, training feedforward neural networks to minimize squared error is simply a numerical optimization problem. Because numerical optimization has been an important research subject for 30 or 40 years (see Chapter 9), it seems reasonable to look for fast training algorithms in the large number of existing numerical optimization techniques. There is no need to "reinvent the wheel" unless absolutely necessary. In this chapter we will present two existing numerical optimization techniques that have been very successfully applied to the training of multilayer perceptrons: the conjugate gradient algorithm and the Levenberg-Marquardt algorithm (a variation of Newton's method).

SDBP We should emphasize that all of the algorithms that we will describe in this chapter use the backpropagation procedure, in which derivatives are processed from the last layer of the network to the first. For this reason they could all be called "backpropagation" algorithms. The differences between the algorithms occur in the way in which the resulting derivatives are used to update the weights. In some ways it is unfortunate that the algorithm we usually refer to as backpropagation is in fact a steepest descent algorithm. In order to clarify our discussion, for the remainder of this chapter we will refer to the basic backpropagation algorithm as steepest descent backpropagation (*SDBP*).

In the next section we will use a simple example to explain why SDBP has problems with convergence. Then, in the following sections, we will present various procedures to improve the convergence of the algorithm.

Drawbacks of Backpropagation

Recall from Chapter 10 that the LMS algorithm is guaranteed to converge to a solution that minimizes the mean squared error, so long as the learning rate is not too large. This is true because the mean squared error for a single-layer linear network is a quadratic function. The quadratic function has only a single stationary point. In addition, the Hessian matrix of a quadratic function is constant, therefore the curvature of the function in a given direction does not change, and the function contours are elliptical.

SDBP is a generalization of the LMS algorithm. Like LMS, it is also an approximate steepest descent algorithm for minimizing the mean squared error. In fact, SDBP is equivalent to the LMS algorithm when used on a single-layer linear network. (See Problem P11.10.) When applied to multilayer networks, however, the characteristics of SDBP are quite different. This has to do with the differences between the mean squared error performance surfaces of single-layer linear networks and multilayer nonlinear networks. While the performance surface for a single-layer linear network has a single minimum point and constant curvature, the performance surface for a multilayer network may have many local minimum points, and the curvature can vary widely in different regions of the parameter space. This will become clear in the example that follows.

Performance Surface Example

To investigate the mean squared error performance surface for multilayer networks we will employ a simple function approximation example. We will use the 1-2-1 network shown in Figure 12.1, with log-sigmoid transfer functions in both layers.

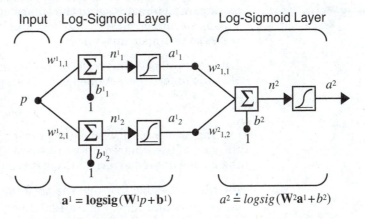

Figure 12.1 1-2-1 Function Approximation Network

In order to simplify our analysis, we will give the network a problem for which we know the optimal solution. The function we will approximate is the response of the same 1-2-1 network, with the following values for the weights and biases:

$$w_{1,1}^1 = 10 \,, \; w_{2,1}^1 = 10 \,, \; b_1^1 = -5 \,, \; b_2^1 = 5 \,, \tag{12.1}$$

$$w_{1,1}^2 = 1 \,, \; w_{1,2}^2 = 1 \,, \; b^2 = -1 \,. \tag{12.2}$$

The network response for these parameters is shown in Figure 12.2, which plots the network output a^2 as the input p is varied over the range $[-2, 2]$.

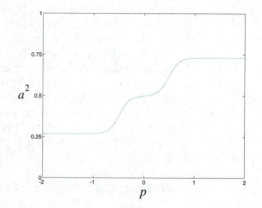

Figure 12.2 Nominal Function

We want to train the network of Figure 12.1 to approximate the function displayed in Figure 12.2. The approximation will be exact when the network parameters are set to the values given in Eq. (12.1) and Eq. (12.2). This is, of course, a very contrived problem, but it is simple and it illustrates some important concepts.

Let's now consider the performance index for our problem. We will assume that the function is sampled at the values

$$p = -2, -1.9, -1.8, \ldots, 1.9, 2 \,, \tag{12.3}$$

and that each occurs with equal probability. The performance index will be the sum of the squared errors at these 41 points. (We won't bother to find the mean squared error, which just requires dividing by 41.)

In order to be able to graph the performance index, we will vary only two parameters at a time. Figure 12.3 illustrates the squared error when only $w_{1,1}^1$ and $w_{1,1}^2$ are being adjusted, while the other parameters are set to their optimal values given in Eq. (12.1) and Eq. (12.2). Note that the minimum error will be zero, and it will occur when $w_{1,1}^1 = 10$ and $w_{1,1}^2 = 1$, as indicated by the open blue circle in the figure.

There are several features to notice about this error surface. First, it is clearly not a quadratic function. The curvature varies drastically over the parameter space. For this reason it will be difficult to choose an appropriate learning rate for the steepest descent algorithm. In some regions the surface is very flat, which would allow a large learning rate, while in other regions the curvature is high, which would require a small learning rate. (Refer to discussions in Chapters 9 and 10 on the choice of learning rate for the steepest descent algorithm.)

It should be noted that the flat regions of the performance surface should not be unexpected, given the sigmoid transfer functions used by the network. The sigmoid is very flat for large inputs.

A second feature of this error surface is the existence of more than one local minimum point. The global minimum point is located at $w_{1,1}^1 = 10$ and $w_{1,1}^2 = 1$, along the valley that runs parallel to the $w_{1,1}^1$ axis. However, there is also a local minimum, which is located in the valley that runs parallel to the $w_{1,1}^2$ axis. (This local minimum is actually off the graph at $w_{1,1}^1 = 0.88$, $w_{1,1}^2 = 38.6$.) In the next section we will investigate the performance of backpropagation on this surface.

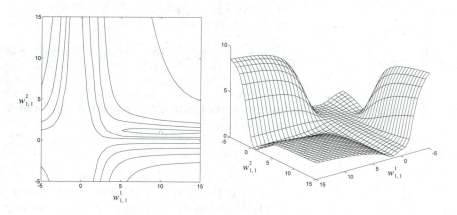

Figure 12.3 Squared Error Surface Versus $w_{1,1}^1$ and $w_{1,1}^2$

Figure 12.4 illustrates the squared error when $w_{1,1}^1$ and b_1^1 are being adjusted, while the other parameters are set to their optimal values. Note that the minimum error will be zero, and it will occur when $w_{1,1}^1 = 10$ and $b_1^1 = -5$, as indicated by the open blue circle in the figure.

Again we find that the surface has a very contorted shape, steep in some regions and very flat in others. Surely the standard steepest descent algorithm will have some trouble with this surface. For example, if we have an initial guess of $w_{1,1}^1 = 0$, $b_1^1 = -10$, the gradient will be very close to zero, and the steepest descent algorithm would effectively stop, even though it is not close to a local minimum point.

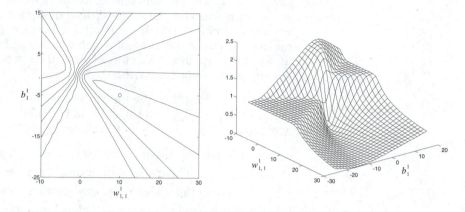

Figure 12.4 Squared Error Surface Versus $w^1_{1,1}$ and b^1_1

Figure 12.5 illustrates the squared error when b^1_1 and b^2_1 are being adjusted, while the other parameters are set to their optimal values. The minimum error is located at $b^1_1 = -5$ and $b^2_1 = 5$, as indicated by the open blue circle in the figure.

This surface illustrates an important property of multilayer networks: they have a symmetry to them. Here we see that there are two local minimum points and they both have the same value of squared error. The second solution corresponds to the same network being turned upside down (i.e., the top neuron in the first layer is exchanged with the bottom neuron). It is because of this characteristic of neural networks that we do not set the initial weights and biases to zero. The symmetry causes zero to be a saddle point of the performance surface.

This brief study of the performance surfaces for multilayer networks gives us some hints as to how to set the initial guess for the SDBP algorithm. First, we do not want to set the initial parameters to zero. This is because the origin of the parameter space tends to be a saddle point for the performance surface. Second, we do not want to set the initial parameters to large values. This is because the performance surface tends to have very flat regions as we move far away from the optimum point.

Typically we choose the initial weights and biases to be small random values. In this way we stay away from a possible saddle point at the origin without moving out to the very flat regions of the performance surface. (Another procedure for choosing the initial parameters is described in [NgWi90].) As we will see in the next section, it is also useful to try several different initial guesses, in order to be sure that the algorithm converges to a global minimum point.

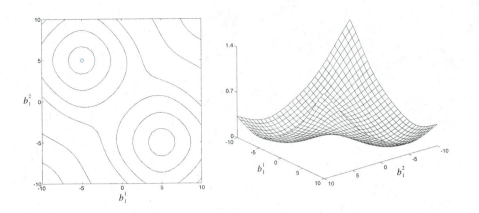

Figure 12.5 Squared Error Surface Versus b_1^1 and b_1^2

Convergence Example

Now that we have examined the performance surface, let's investigate the performance of SDBP. For this section we will use a variation of the standard algorithm, called *batching*, in which the parameters are updated only after the entire training set has been presented. The gradients calculated at each training example are averaged together to produce a more accurate estimate of the gradient. (If the training set is complete, i.e., covers all possible input/output pairs, then the gradient estimate will be exact.)

Batching

In Figure 12.6 we see two trajectories of SDBP (batch mode) when only two parameters, $w_{1,1}^1$ and $w_{1,1}^2$ are adjusted. For the initial condition labeled "a" the algorithm does eventually converge to the optimal solution, but the convergence is slow. The reason for the slow convergence is the change in curvature of the surface over the path of the trajectory. After an initial moderate slope, the trajectory passes over a very flat surface, until it falls into a very gently sloping valley. If we were to increase the learning rate, the algorithm would converge faster while passing over the initial flat surface, but would become unstable when falling into the valley, as we will see in a moment.

Trajectory "b" illustrates how the algorithm can converge to a local minimum point. The trajectory is trapped in a valley and diverges from the optimal solution. If allowed to continue the trajectory converges to $w_{1,1}^1 = 0.88$, $w_{1,1}^2 = 38.6$. The existence of multiple local minimum points is typical of the performance surface of multilayer networks. For this reason it is best to try several different initial guesses in order to ensure that a global minimum has been obtained. (Some of the local minimum points may have the same value of squared error, as we saw in Figure 12.5, so we would not expect the algorithm to converge to the same parameter values for each initial guess. We just want to be sure that the same minimum error is obtained.)

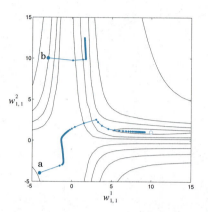

Figure 12.6 Two SDBP (Batch Mode) Trajectories

The progress of the algorithm can also be seen in Figure 12.7, which shows the squared error versus the iteration number. The curve on the left corresponds to trajectory "a" and the curve on the right corresponds to trajectory "b." These curves are typical of SDBP, with long periods of little progress and then short periods of rapid advance.

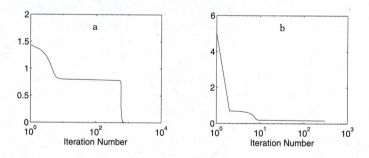

Figure 12.7 Squared Error Convergence Patterns

We can see that the flat sections in Figure 12.7 correspond to times when the algorithm is traversing a flat section of the performance surface, as shown in Figure 12.6. During these periods we would like to increase the learning rate, in order to speed up convergence. However, if we increase the learning rate the algorithm will become unstable when it reaches steeper portions of the performance surface.

This effect is illustrated in Figure 12.8. The trajectory shown here corresponds to trajectory "a" in Figure 12.6, except that a larger learning rate was used. The algorithm converges faster at first, but when the trajectory reaches the narrow valley that contains the minimum point the algorithm begins to diverge. This suggests that it would be useful to vary the learning rate. We could increase the learning rate on flat surfaces and then decrease the learning rate as the slope increased. The question is: "How will the algorithm know when it is on a flat surface?" We will discuss this in a later section.

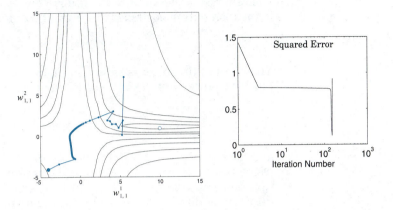

Figure 12.8 Trajectory with Learning Rate Too Large

Another way to improve convergence would be to smooth out the trajectory. Note in Figure 12.8 that when the algorithm begins to diverge it is oscillating back and forth across a narrow valley. If we could filter the trajectory, by averaging the updates to the parameters, this might smooth out the oscillations and produce a stable trajectory. We will discuss this procedure in the next section.

 To experiment with this backpropagation example, use the Neural Network Design Demonstration Steepest Descent Backpropagation *(*nnd12sdbp*).*

Heuristic Modifications of Backpropagation

Now that we have investigated some of the drawbacks of backpropagation (steepest descent), let's consider some procedures for improving the algorithm. In this section we will discuss two heuristic methods. In a later section we will present two methods based on standard numerical optimization algorithms.

Momentum

The first method we will discuss is the use of momentum. This is a modification based on our observation in the last section that convergence might be improved if we could smooth out the oscillations in the trajectory. We can do this with a low-pass filter.

Before we apply momentum to a neural network application, let's investigate a simple example to illustrate the smoothing effect. Consider the following first-order filter:

$$y(k) = \gamma y(k-1) + (1-\gamma)w(k), \tag{12.4}$$

where $w(k)$ is the input to the filter, $y(k)$ is the output of the filter and γ is the momentum coefficient that must satisfy

$$0 \le \gamma < 1. \tag{12.5}$$

The effect of this filter is shown in Figure 12.9. For these examples the input to the filter was taken to be the sine wave:

$$w(k) = 1 + \sin\left(\frac{2\pi k}{16}\right), \tag{12.6}$$

and the momentum coefficient was set to $\gamma = 0.9$ (left graph) and $\gamma = 0.98$ (right graph). Here we can see that the oscillation of the filter output is less than the oscillation in the filter input (as we would expect for a low-pass filter). In addition, as γ is increased the oscillation in the filter output is reduced. Notice also that the average filter output is the same as the average filter input, although as γ is increased the filter output is slower to respond.

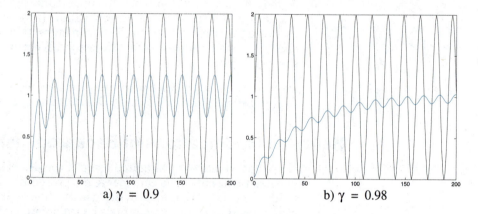

a) $\gamma = 0.9$ b) $\gamma = 0.98$

Figure 12.9 Smoothing Effect of Momentum

To summarize, the filter tends to reduce the amount of oscillation, while still tracking the average value. Now let's see how this works on the neural network problem. First, recall that the parameter updates for SDBP (Eq. (11.46) and Eq. (11.47)) are

$$\Delta \mathbf{W}^m(k) = -\alpha \mathbf{s}^m (\mathbf{a}^{m-1})^T, \tag{12.7}$$

$$\Delta \mathbf{b}^m(k) = -\alpha \mathbf{s}^m. \tag{12.8}$$

Momentum

MOBP

When the *momentum* filter is added to the parameter changes, we obtain the following equations for the momentum modification to backpropagation (*MOBP*):

$$\Delta\mathbf{W}^m(k) = \gamma\Delta\mathbf{W}^m(k-1) - (1-\gamma)\,\alpha\mathbf{s}^m(\mathbf{a}^{m-1})^T,\qquad (12.9)$$

$$\Delta\mathbf{b}^m(k) = \gamma\Delta\mathbf{b}^m(k-1) - (1-\gamma)\,\alpha\mathbf{s}^m.\qquad (12.10)$$

If we now apply these modified equations to the example in the preceding section, we obtain the results shown in Figure 12.10. (For this example we have used a batching form of MOBP, in which the parameters are updated only after the entire training set has been presented. The gradients calculated at each training example are averaged together to produce a more accurate estimate of the gradient.) This trajectory corresponds to the same initial condition and learning rate shown in Figure 12.8, but with a momentum coefficient of $\gamma = 0.8$. We can see that the algorithm is now stable. By the use of momentum we have been able to use a larger learning rate, while maintaining the stability of the algorithm. Another feature of momentum is that it tends to accelerate convergence when the trajectory is moving in a consistent direction.

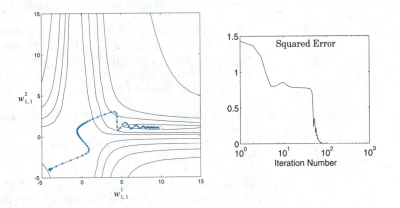

Figure 12.10 Trajectory with Momentum

If you look carefully at the trajectory in Figure 12.10, you can see why the procedure is given the name *momentum*. It tends to make the trajectory continue in the same direction. The larger the value of γ, the more "momentum" the trajectory has.

To experiment with momentum, use the Neural Network Design Demonstration Momentum Backpropagation (**nnd12mobp**)*.*

Variable Learning Rate

We suggested earlier in this chapter that we might be able to speed up convergence if we increase the learning rate on flat surfaces and then decrease the learning rate when the slope increases. In this section we want to explore this concept.

Recall that the mean squared error performance surface for single-layer linear networks is always a quadratic function, and the Hessian matrix is therefore constant. The maximum stable learning rate for the steepest descent algorithm is two divided by the maximum eigenvalue of the Hessian matrix. (See Eq. (9.25).)

As we have seen, the error surface for the multilayer network is not a quadratic function. The shape of the surface can be very different in different regions of the parameter space. Perhaps we can speed up convergence by adjusting the learning rate during the course of training. The trick will be to determine when to change the learning rate and by how much.

There are many different approaches for varying the learning rate. We will describe a very straightforward batching procedure [VoMa88], where the learning rate is varied according to the performance of the algorithm. The rules of the *variable learning rate* backpropagation algorithm (*VLBP*) are:

Variable Learning Rate
VLBP

1. If the squared error (over the entire training set) increases by more than some set percentage ζ (typically one to five percent) after a weight update, then the weight update is discarded, the learning rate is multiplied by some factor $0 < \rho < 1$, and the momentum coefficient γ (if it is used) is set to zero.

2. If the squared error decreases after a weight update, then the weight update is accepted and the learning rate is multiplied by some factor $\eta > 1$. If γ has been previously set to zero, it is reset to its original value.

3. If the squared error increases by less than ζ, then the weight update is accepted but the learning rate and the momentum coefficient are unchanged.

(See Problem P12.3 for a numerical example of VLBP.)

To illustrate VLBP, let's apply it to the function approximation problem of the previous section. Figure 12.11 displays the trajectory for the algorithm using the same initial guess, initial learning rate and momentum coefficient as was used in Figure 12.10. The new parameters were assigned the values

$$\eta = 1.05, \ \rho = 0.7 \text{ and } \zeta = 4\%. \tag{12.11}$$

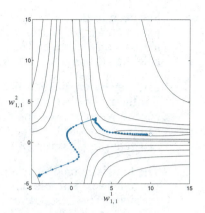

Figure 12.11 Variable Learning Rate Trajectory

Notice how the learning rate, and therefore the step size, tends to increase when the trajectory is traveling in a straight line with constantly decreasing error. This effect can also be seen in Figure 12.12, which shows the squared error and the learning rate versus iteration number.

When the trajectory reaches a narrow valley, the learning rate is rapidly decreased. Otherwise the trajectory would have become oscillatory, and the error would have increased dramatically. For each potential step where the error would have increased by more than 4% the learning rate is reduced and the momentum is eliminated, which allows the trajectory to make the quick turn to follow the valley toward the minimum point. The learning rate then increases again, which accelerates the convergence. The learning rate is reduced again when the trajectory overshoots the minimum point when the algorithm has almost converged. This process is typical of a VLBP trajectory.

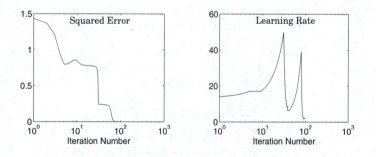

Figure 12.12 Convergence Characteristics of Variable Learning Rate

There are many variations on this variable learning rate algorithm. Jacobs [Jaco88] proposed the *delta-bar-delta* learning rule, in which each network parameter (weight or bias) has its own learning rate. The algorithm increases the learning rate for a network parameter if the parameter change has been in the same direction for several iterations. If the direction of the parameter change alternates, then the learning rate is reduced. The *SuperSAB* algorithm of Tollenaere [Toll90] is similar to the delta-bar-delta rule, but it has more complex rules for adjusting the learning rates.

Another heuristic modification to SDBP is the Quickprop algorithm of Fahlman [Fahl88]. It assumes that the error surface is parabolic and concave upward around the minimum point and that the effect of each weight can be considered independently. (References to other SDBP modifications are given in Chapter 19.)

The heuristic modifications to SDBP can often provide much faster convergence for some problems. However, there are two main drawbacks to these methods. The first is that the modifications require that several parameters be set (e.g., ζ, ρ and γ), while the only parameter required for SDBP is the learning rate. Some of the more complex heuristic modifications can have five or six parameters to be selected. Often the performance of the algorithm is sensitive to changes in these parameters. The choice of parameters is also problem dependent. The second drawback to these modifications to SDBP is that they can sometimes fail to converge on problems for which SDBP will eventually find a solution. Both of these drawbacks tend to occur more often when using the more complex algorithms.

To experiment with VLBP, use the Neural Network Design Demonstration Variable Learning Rate Backpropagation (`nnd12vlbp`*).*

Numerical Optimization Techniques

Now that we have investigated some of the heuristic modifications to SDBP, let's consider those methods that are based on standard numerical optimization techniques. We will investigate two techniques: conjugate gradient and Levenberg-Marquardt. The conjugate gradient algorithm for quadratic functions was presented in Chapter 9. We need to add two procedures to this algorithm in order to apply it to more general functions.

The second numerical optimization method we will discuss in this chapter is the Levenberg-Marquardt algorithm, which is a modification to Newton's method that is well-suited to neural network training.

Conjugate Gradient

In Chapter 9 we presented three numerical optimization techniques: steepest descent, conjugate gradient and Newton's method. Steepest descent is the simplest algorithm, but is often slow in converging. Newton's method is much faster, but requires that the Hessian matrix and its inverse be calculated. The conjugate gradient algorithm is something of a compromise; it does not require the calculation of second derivatives, and yet it still has the quadratic convergence property. (It converges to the minimum of a quadratic function in a finite number of iterations.) In this section we will describe how the conjugate gradient algorithm can be used to train multilayer networks. We will call this algorithm *conjugate gradient back-propagation (CGBP)*.

CGBP

Let's begin by reviewing the conjugate gradient algorithm. For ease of reference, we will repeat the algorithm steps from Chapter 9 (page 9-18):

1. Select the first search direction $\mathbf{p}_0$ to be the negative of the gradient, as in Eq. (9.59):

$$\mathbf{p}_0 = -\mathbf{g}_0,\tag{12.12}$$

where

$$\mathbf{g}_k \equiv \nabla F(\mathbf{x})\big|_{\mathbf{x} = \mathbf{x}_k}.\tag{12.13}$$

2. Take a step according to Eq. (9.57), selecting the learning rate α_k to minimize the function along the search direction:

$$\mathbf{x}_{k+1} = \mathbf{x}_k + \alpha_k \mathbf{p}_k.\tag{12.14}$$

3. Select the next search direction according to Eq. (9.60), using Eq. (9.61), Eq. (9.62), or Eq. (9.63) to calculate β_k:

$$\mathbf{p}_k = -\mathbf{g}_k + \beta_k \mathbf{p}_{k-1},\tag{12.15}$$

with

$$\beta_k = \frac{\Delta \mathbf{g}_{k-1}^T \mathbf{g}_k}{\Delta \mathbf{g}_{k-1}^T \mathbf{p}_{k-1}} \text{ or } \beta_k = \frac{\mathbf{g}_k^T \mathbf{g}_k}{\mathbf{g}_{k-1}^T \mathbf{g}_{k-1}} \text{ or } \beta_k = \frac{\Delta \mathbf{g}_{k-1}^T \mathbf{g}_k}{\mathbf{g}_{k-1}^T \mathbf{g}_{k-1}}.\tag{12.16}$$

4. If the algorithm has not converged, continue from step 2.

This conjugate gradient algorithm cannot be applied directly to the neural network training task, because the performance index is not quadratic. This affects the algorithm in two ways. First, we will not be able to use Eq. (9.31) to minimize the function along a line, as required in step 2. Second, the exact minimum will not normally be reached in a finite number of steps, and therefore the algorithm will need to be reset after some set number of iterations.

Let's address the linear search first. We need to have a general procedure for locating the minimum of a function in a specified direction. This will involve two steps: interval location and interval reduction. The purpose of the interval location step is to find some initial interval that contains a local minimum. The interval reduction step then reduces the size of the initial interval until the minimum is located to the desired accuracy.

Interval Location

We will use a function comparison method [Scal85] to perform the *interval location* step. This procedure is illustrated in Figure 12.13. We begin by evaluating the performance index at an initial point, represented by a_1 in the figure. This point corresponds to the current values of the network weights and biases. In other words, we are evaluating

$$F(\mathbf{x}_0) . \tag{12.17}$$

The next step is to evaluate the function at a second point, represented by b_1 in the figure, which is a distance ε from the initial point, along the first search direction $\mathbf{p}_0$. In other words, we are evaluating

$$F(\mathbf{x}_0 + \varepsilon \mathbf{p}_0) . \tag{12.18}$$

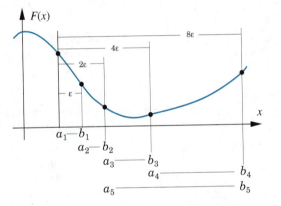

Figure 12.13 Interval Location

We then continue to evaluate the performance index at new points b_i, successively doubling the distance between points. This process stops when the function increases between two consecutive evaluations. In Figure 12.13 this is represented by b_3 to b_4. At this point we know that the minimum is bracketed by the two points a_5 and b_5. We cannot narrow the interval any further, because the minimum may occur either in the interval $[a_4, b_4]$ or in the interval $[a_3, b_3]$. These two possibilities are illustrated in Figure 12.14 (a).

Interval Reduction

Now that we have located an interval containing the minimum, the next step in the linear search is *interval reduction*. This will involve evaluating the function at points inside the interval $[a_5, b_5]$, which was selected in the interval location step. From Figure 12.14 we can see that we will need to evaluate the function at two internal points (at least) in order to reduce the size of the interval of uncertainty. Figure 12.14 (a) shows that one internal function evaluation does not provide us with any information on the location of the minimum. However, if we evaluate the function at two points c and d, as in Figure 12.14 (b), we can reduce the interval of uncertainty. If

$F(c) > F(d)$, as shown in Figure 12.14 (b), then the minimum must occur in the interval $[c, b]$. Conversely, if $F(c) < F(d)$, then the minimum must occur in the interval $[a, d]$. (Note that we are assuming that there is a single minimum located in the initial interval. More about that later.)

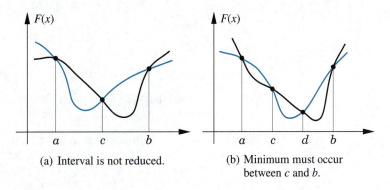

(a) Interval is not reduced.   (b) Minimum must occur between c and b.

Figure 12.14 Reducing the Size of the Interval of Uncertainty

The procedure described above suggests a method for reducing the size of the interval of uncertainty. We now need to decide how to determine the locations of the internal points c and d. There are several ways to do this (see [Scal85]). We will use a method called the *Golden Section search*, which is designed to reduce the number of function evaluations required. At each iteration one new function evaluation is required. For example, in the case illustrated in Figure 12.14 (b) point a would be discarded and point c would become an outside point. Then a new point c would be placed between the original points c and d. The trick is to place the new point so that the interval of uncertainty will be reduced as quickly as possible.

Golden Section Search

The algorithm for the Golden Section search is as follows [Scal85]:

$$\tau = 0.618$$

Set $c_1 = a_1 + (1 - \tau)(b_1 - a_1)$, $F_c = F(c_1)$.

$d_1 = b_1 - (1 - \tau)(b_1 - a_1)$, $F_d = F(d_1)$.

For $k = 1, 2, \ldots$ repeat

If $F_c < F_d$ then

Set $a_{k+1} = a_k$; $b_{k+1} = d_k$; $d_{k+1} = c_k$

$c_{k+1} = a_{k+1} + (1 - \tau)(b_{k+1} - a_{k+1})$

$F_d = F_c$; $F_c = F(c_{k+1})$

else

$$\text{Set} \quad a_{k+1} = c_k ; \, b_{k+1} = b_k ; \, c_{k+1} = d_k$$

$$d_{k+1} = b_{k+1} - (1-\tau) \, (b_{k+1} - a_{k+1})$$

$$F_c = F_d ; \, F_d = F(d_{k+1})$$

    end

    end until $b_{k+1} - a_{k+1} < tol$

Where *tol* is the accuracy tolerance set by the user.

(See Problem P12.4 for a numerical example of the interval location and interval reduction procedures.)

There is one more modification to the conjugate gradient algorithm that needs to be made before we apply it to neural network training. For quadratic functions the algorithm will converge to the minimum in at most n iterations, where n is the number of parameters being optimized. The mean squared error performance index for multilayer networks is not quadratic, therefore the algorithm would not normally converge in n iterations. The development of the conjugate gradient algorithm does not indicate what search direction to use once a cycle of n iterations has been completed. There have been many procedures suggested, but the simplest method is to reset the search direction to the steepest descent direction (negative of the gradient) after n iterations [Scal85]. We will use this method.

Let's now apply the conjugate gradient algorithm to the function approximation example that we have been using to demonstrate the other neural network training algorithms. We will use the backpropagation algorithm to compute the gradient (using Eq. (11.23) and Eq. (11.24)) and the conjugate gradient algorithm to determine the weight updates. This is a batch mode algorithm, as the gradient is computed after the entire training set has been presented to the network.

Figure 12.15 shows the intermediate steps of the CGBP algorithm for the first three iterations. The interval location process is illustrated by the open blue circles; each one represents one evaluation of the function. The final interval is indicated by the larger open black circles. The black dots in Figure 12.15 indicate the location of the new interior points during the Golden Section search, one for each iteration of the procedure. The final point is indicated by a blue dot.

Figure 12.16 shows the total trajectory to convergence. Notice that the CGBP algorithm converges in many fewer iterations than the other algorithms that we have tested. This is a little deceiving, since each iteration of CGBP requires more computations than the other methods; there are many function evaluations involved in each iteration of CGBP. Even so, CGBP has been shown to be one of the fastest batch training algorithms for multilayer networks [Char92].

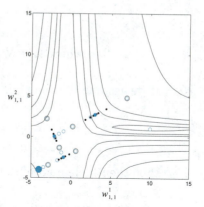

Figure 12.15 Intermediate Steps of CGBP

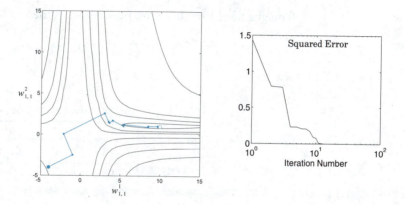

Figure 12.16 Conjugate Gradient Trajectory

To experiment with CGBP, use the Neural Network Design Demonstrations Conjugate Gradient Line Search (nnd12cgls) and Conjugate Gradient Backpropagation (nnd12cgbp).

Levenberg-Marquardt Algorithm

The Levenberg-Marquardt algorithm is a variation of Newton's method that was designed for minimizing functions that are sums of squares of other nonlinear functions. This is very well suited to neural network training where the performance index is the mean squared error.

Basic Algorithm

Let's begin by considering the form of Newton's method where the performance index is a sum of squares. Recall from Chapter 9 that Newton's method for optimizing a performance index $F(\mathbf{x})$ is

$$\mathbf{x}_{k+1} = \mathbf{x}_k - \mathbf{A}_k^{-1}\mathbf{g}_k,$$ (12.19)

where $\mathbf{A}_k \equiv \nabla^2 F(\mathbf{x})\big|_{\mathbf{x}=\mathbf{x}_k}$ and $\mathbf{g}_k \equiv \nabla F(\mathbf{x})\big|_{\mathbf{x}=\mathbf{x}_k}$.

If we assume that $F(\mathbf{x})$ is a sum of squares function:

$$F(\mathbf{x}) = \sum_{i=1}^{N} v_i^2(\mathbf{x}) = \mathbf{v}^T(\mathbf{x})\mathbf{v}(\mathbf{x}),$$ (12.20)

then the jth element of the gradient would be

$$[\nabla F(\mathbf{x})]_j = \frac{\partial F(\mathbf{x})}{\partial x_j} = 2\sum_{i=1}^{N} v_i(\mathbf{x})\frac{\partial v_i(\mathbf{x})}{\partial x_j}.$$ (12.21)

The gradient can therefore be written in matrix form:

$$\nabla F(\mathbf{x}) = 2\mathbf{J}^T(\mathbf{x})\mathbf{v}(\mathbf{x}),$$ (12.22)

where

$$\mathbf{J}(\mathbf{x}) = \begin{bmatrix} \dfrac{\partial v_1(\mathbf{x})}{\partial x_1} & \dfrac{\partial v_1(\mathbf{x})}{\partial x_2} & \cdots & \dfrac{\partial v_1(\mathbf{x})}{\partial x_n} \\[2ex] \dfrac{\partial v_2(\mathbf{x})}{\partial x_1} & \dfrac{\partial v_2(\mathbf{x})}{\partial x_2} & \cdots & \dfrac{\partial v_2(\mathbf{x})}{\partial x_n} \\[1ex] \vdots & \vdots & & \vdots \\[1ex] \dfrac{\partial v_N(\mathbf{x})}{\partial x_1} & \dfrac{\partial v_N(\mathbf{x})}{\partial x_2} & \cdots & \dfrac{\partial v_N(\mathbf{x})}{\partial x_n} \end{bmatrix}.$$ (12.23)

Jacobian Matrix is the *Jacobian matrix*.

Next we want to find the Hessian matrix. The k, j element of the Hessian matrix would be

$$[\nabla^2 F(\mathbf{x})]_{k,j} = \frac{\partial^2 F(\mathbf{x})}{\partial x_k \partial x_j} = 2\sum_{i=1}^{N}\left\{\frac{\partial v_i(\mathbf{x})}{\partial x_k}\frac{\partial v_i(\mathbf{x})}{\partial x_j} + v_i(\mathbf{x})\frac{\partial^2 v_i(\mathbf{x})}{\partial x_k \partial x_j}\right\}.$$ (12.24)

The Hessian matrix can then be expressed in matrix form:

$$\nabla^2 F(\mathbf{x}) = 2\mathbf{J}^T(\mathbf{x})\mathbf{J}(\mathbf{x}) + 2\mathbf{S}(\mathbf{x}),$$ (12.25)

where

$$\mathbf{S}(\mathbf{x}) = \sum_{i=1}^{N} v_i(\mathbf{x}) \nabla^2 v_i(\mathbf{x}) . \qquad (12.26)$$

If we assume that $\mathbf{S}(\mathbf{x})$ is small, we can approximate the Hessian matrix as

$$\nabla^2 F(\mathbf{x}) \cong 2\mathbf{J}^T(\mathbf{x})\mathbf{J}(\mathbf{x}) . \qquad (12.27)$$

Gauss-Newton

If we then substitute Eq. (12.27) and Eq. (12.22) into Eq. (12.19), we obtain the *Gauss-Newton* method:

$$\mathbf{x}_{k+1} = \mathbf{x}_k - [2\mathbf{J}^T(\mathbf{x}_k)\mathbf{J}(\mathbf{x}_k)]^{-1} 2\mathbf{J}^T(\mathbf{x}_k)\mathbf{v}(\mathbf{x}_k)$$
$$\qquad (12.28)$$
$$= \mathbf{x}_k - [\mathbf{J}^T(\mathbf{x}_k)\mathbf{J}(\mathbf{x}_k)]^{-1}\mathbf{J}^T(\mathbf{x}_k)\mathbf{v}(\mathbf{x}_k) .$$

Note that the advantage of Gauss-Newton over the standard Newton's method is that it does not require calculation of second derivatives.

One problem with the Gauss-Newton method is that the matrix $\mathbf{H} = \mathbf{J}^T\mathbf{J}$ may not be invertible. This can be overcome by using the following modification to the approximate Hessian matrix:

$$\mathbf{G} = \mathbf{H} + \mu\mathbf{I} . \qquad (12.29)$$

To see how this matrix can be made invertible, suppose that the eigenvalues and eigenvectors of $\mathbf{H}$ are $\{\lambda_1, \lambda_2, \dots, \lambda_n\}$ and $\{\mathbf{z}_1, \mathbf{z}_2, \dots, \mathbf{z}_n\}$. Then

$$\mathbf{G}\mathbf{z}_i = [\mathbf{H} + \mu\mathbf{I}]\mathbf{z}_i = \mathbf{H}\mathbf{z}_i + \mu\mathbf{z}_i = \lambda_i\mathbf{z}_i + \mu\mathbf{z}_i = (\lambda_i + \mu)\mathbf{z}_i . \qquad (12.30)$$

Therefore the eigenvectors of $\mathbf{G}$ are the same as the eigenvectors of $\mathbf{H}$, and the eigenvalues of $\mathbf{G}$ are $(\lambda_i + \mu)$. $\mathbf{G}$ can be made positive definite by increasing μ until $(\lambda_i + \mu) > 0$ for all i, and therefore the matrix will be invertible.

Levenberg-Marquardt

This leads to the *Levenberg-Marquardt* algorithm [Scal85]:

$$\mathbf{x}_{k+1} = \mathbf{x}_k - [\mathbf{J}^T(\mathbf{x}_k)\mathbf{J}(\mathbf{x}_k) + \mu_k\mathbf{I}]^{-1}\mathbf{J}^T(\mathbf{x}_k)\mathbf{v}(\mathbf{x}_k) . \qquad (12.31)$$

or

$$\Delta\mathbf{x}_k = -[\mathbf{J}^T(\mathbf{x}_k)\mathbf{J}(\mathbf{x}_k) + \mu_k\mathbf{I}]^{-1}\mathbf{J}^T(\mathbf{x}_k)\mathbf{v}(\mathbf{x}_k) . \qquad (12.32)$$

This algorithm has the very useful feature that as μ_k is increased it approaches the steepest descent algorithm with small learning rate:

$$\mathbf{x}_{k+1} \cong \mathbf{x}_k - \frac{1}{\mu_k}\mathbf{J}^T(\mathbf{x}_k)\mathbf{v}(\mathbf{x}_k) = \mathbf{x}_k - \frac{1}{2\mu_k}\nabla F(\mathbf{x}) \text{ , for large } \mu_k, \quad (12.33)$$

while as μ_k is decreased to zero the algorithm becomes Gauss-Newton.

The algorithm begins with μ_k set to some small value (e.g., $\mu_k = 0.01$). If a step does not yield a smaller value for $F(\mathbf{x})$, then the step is repeated with μ_k multiplied by some factor $\vartheta > 1$ (e.g., $\vartheta = 10$). Eventually $F(\mathbf{x})$ should decrease, since we would be taking a small step in the direction of steepest descent. If a step does produce a smaller value for $F(\mathbf{x})$, then μ_k is divided by ϑ for the next step, so that the algorithm will approach Gauss-Newton, which should provide faster convergence. The algorithm provides a nice compromise between the speed of Newton's method and the guaranteed convergence of steepest descent.

Now let's see how we can apply the Levenberg-Marquardt algorithm to the multilayer network training problem. The performance index for multilayer network training is the mean squared error (see Eq. (11.11)). If each target occurs with equal probability, the mean squared error is proportional to the sum of squared errors over the Q targets in the training set:

$$
\begin{aligned}
F(\mathbf{x}) &= \sum_{q=1}^{Q}(\mathbf{t}_q - \mathbf{a}_q)^T(\mathbf{t}_q - \mathbf{a}_q) \\
&= \sum_{q=1}^{Q}\mathbf{e}_q^T\mathbf{e}_q = \sum_{q=1}^{Q}\sum_{j=1}^{S^M}(e_{j,q})^2 = \sum_{i=1}^{N}(v_i)^2 ,
\end{aligned}
\quad (12.34)
$$

where $e_{j,q}$ is the jth element of the error for the qth input/target pair.

Eq. (12.34) is equivalent to the performance index, Eq. (12.20), for which Levenberg-Marquardt was designed. Therefore it should be a straightforward matter to adapt the algorithm for network training. It turns out that this is true in concept, but it does require some care in working out the details.

Jacobian Calculation

The key step in the Levenberg-Marquardt algorithm is the computation of the Jacobian matrix. To perform this computation we will use a variation of the backpropagation algorithm. Recall that in the standard backpropagation procedure we compute the derivatives of the squared errors, with respect to the weights and biases of the network. To create the Jacobian matrix we need to compute the derivatives of the errors, instead of the derivatives of the squared errors.

It is a simple matter conceptually to modify the backpropagation algorithm to compute the elements of the Jacobian matrix. Unfortunately, although the basic concept is simple, the details of the implementation can be a little tricky. For that reason you may want to skim through the rest of this section on your first reading, in order to obtain an overview of the general flow of the presentation, and return later to pick up the details. It may also be helpful to review the development of the backpropagation algorithm in Chapter 11 before proceeding.

Before we present the procedure for computing the Jacobian, let's take a closer look at its form (Eq. (12.23)). Note that the error vector is

$$\mathbf{v}^T = \begin{bmatrix} v_1 & v_2 & \cdots & v_N \end{bmatrix} = \begin{bmatrix} e_{1,1} & e_{2,1} & \cdots & e_{S^M,1} & e_{1,2} & \cdots & e_{S^M,Q} \end{bmatrix}, \quad (12.35)$$

the parameter vector is

$$\mathbf{x}^T = \begin{bmatrix} x_1 & x_2 & \cdots & x_n \end{bmatrix} = \begin{bmatrix} w_{1,1}^1 & w_{1,2}^1 & \cdots & w_{S^1,R}^1 & b_1^1 & \cdots & b_{S^1}^1 & w_{1,1}^2 & \cdots & b_{S^M}^M \end{bmatrix}, \quad (12.36)$$

$N = Q \times S^M$ and $n = S^1(R+1) + S^2(S^1+1) + \cdots + S^M(S^{M-1}+1)$.

Therefore, if we make these substitutions into Eq. (12.23), the Jacobian matrix for multilayer network training can be written

$$\mathbf{J}(\mathbf{x}) = \begin{bmatrix} \dfrac{\partial e_{1,1}}{\partial w_{1,1}^1} & \dfrac{\partial e_{1,1}}{\partial w_{1,2}^1} & \cdots & \dfrac{\partial e_{1,1}}{\partial w_{S^1,R}^1} & \dfrac{\partial e_{1,1}}{\partial b_1^1} & \cdots \\[2ex] \dfrac{\partial e_{2,1}}{\partial w_{1,1}^1} & \dfrac{\partial e_{2,1}}{\partial w_{1,2}^1} & \cdots & \dfrac{\partial e_{2,1}}{\partial w_{S^1,R}^1} & \dfrac{\partial e_{2,1}}{\partial b_1^1} & \cdots \\[2ex] \vdots & \vdots & & \vdots & \vdots & \\[2ex] \dfrac{\partial e_{S^M,1}}{\partial w_{1,1}^1} & \dfrac{\partial e_{S^M,1}}{\partial w_{1,2}^1} & \cdots & \dfrac{\partial e_{S^M,1}}{\partial w_{S^1,R}^1} & \dfrac{\partial e_{S^M,1}}{\partial b_1^1} & \cdots \\[2ex] \dfrac{\partial e_{1,2}}{\partial w_{1,1}^1} & \dfrac{\partial e_{1,2}}{\partial w_{1,2}^1} & \cdots & \dfrac{\partial e_{1,2}}{\partial w_{S^1,R}^1} & \dfrac{\partial e_{1,2}}{\partial b_1^1} & \cdots \\[2ex] \vdots & \vdots & & \vdots & \vdots & \end{bmatrix}. \quad (12.37)$$

The terms in this Jacobian matrix can be computed by a simple modification to the backpropagation algorithm.

Standard backpropagation calculates terms like

$$\frac{\partial \hat{F}(\mathbf{x})}{\partial x_l} = \frac{\partial \mathbf{e}_q^T \mathbf{e}_q}{\partial x_l}. \quad (12.38)$$

For the elements of the Jacobian matrix that are needed for the Levenberg-Marquardt algorithm we need to calculate terms like

$$[\mathbf{J}]_{h, l} = \frac{\partial v_h}{\partial x_l} = \frac{\partial e_{k, q}}{\partial x_l} . \tag{12.39}$$

Recall from Eq. (11.18) in our derivation of backpropagation that

$$\frac{\partial \hat{F}}{\partial w_{i, j}^m} = \frac{\partial \hat{F}}{\partial n_i^m} \times \frac{\partial n_i^m}{\partial w_{i, j}^m} , \tag{12.40}$$

where the first term on the right-hand side was defined as the sensitivity:

$$s_i^m \equiv \frac{\partial \hat{F}}{\partial n_i^m} . \tag{12.41}$$

The backpropagation process computed the sensitivities through a recurrence relationship from the last layer backward to the first layer. We can use the same concept to compute the terms needed for the Jacobian matrix (Eq. (12.37)) if we define a new *Marquardt sensitivity*:

Marquardt Sensitivity

$$\tilde{s}_{i, h}^m \equiv \frac{\partial v_h}{\partial n_{i, q}^m} = \frac{\partial e_{k, q}}{\partial n_{i, q}^m} , \tag{12.42}$$

where, from Eq. (12.35), $h = (q-1) S^M + k$.

Now we can compute elements of the Jacobian by

$$[\mathbf{J}]_{h, l} = \frac{\partial v_h}{\partial x_l} = \frac{\partial e_{k, q}}{\partial w_{i, j}^m} = \frac{\partial e_{k, q}}{\partial n_{i, q}^m} \times \frac{\partial n_{i, q}^m}{\partial w_{i, j}^m} = \tilde{s}_{i, h}^m \times \frac{\partial n_{i, q}^m}{\partial w_{i, j}^m} = \tilde{s}_{i, h}^m \times a_{j, q}^{m-1} , \tag{12.43}$$

or if x_l is a bias,

$$[\mathbf{J}]_{h, l} = \frac{\partial v_h}{\partial x_l} = \frac{\partial e_{k, q}}{\partial b_i^m} = \frac{\partial e_{k, q}}{\partial n_{i, q}^m} \times \frac{\partial n_{i, q}^m}{\partial b_i^m} = \tilde{s}_{i, h}^m \times \frac{\partial n_{i, q}^m}{\partial b_i^m} = \tilde{s}_{i, h}^m . \tag{12.44}$$

The Marquardt sensitivities can be computed through the same recurrence relations as the standard sensitivities (Eq. (11.35)) with one modification at the final layer, which for standard backpropagation is computed with Eq. (11.40). For the Marquardt sensitivities at the final layer we have

$$\tilde{s}_{i,h}^{M} = \frac{\partial v_h}{\partial n_{i,q}^{M}} = \frac{\partial e_{k,q}}{\partial n_{i,q}^{M}} = \frac{\partial (t_{k,q} - a_{k,q}^{M})}{\partial n_{i,q}^{M}} = -\frac{\partial a_{k,q}^{M}}{\partial n_{i,q}^{M}}$$

$$= \begin{cases} -\dot{f}^{M}(n_{i,q}^{M}) & \text{for } i = k \\ 0 & \text{for } i \neq k \end{cases}. \tag{12.45}$$

Therefore when the input $\mathbf{p}_q$ has been applied to the network and the corresponding network output $\mathbf{a}_q^{M}$ has been computed, the Levenberg-Marquardt backpropagation is initialized with

$$\tilde{\mathbf{S}}_q^{M} = -\dot{\mathbf{F}}^{M}(\mathbf{n}_q^{M}), \tag{12.46}$$

where $\dot{\mathbf{F}}^{M}(\mathbf{n}^{M})$ is defined in Eq. (11.34). Each column of the matrix $\tilde{\mathbf{S}}_q^{M}$ must be backpropagated through the network using Eq. (11.35) to produce one row of the Jacobian matrix. The columns can also be backpropagated together using

$$\tilde{\mathbf{S}}_q^{m} = \dot{\mathbf{F}}^{m}(\mathbf{n}_q^{m})(\mathbf{W}^{m+1})^{T}\tilde{\mathbf{S}}_q^{m+1}. \tag{12.47}$$

The total Marquardt sensitivity matrices for each layer are then created by augmenting the matrices computed for each input:

$$\tilde{\mathbf{S}}^{m} = \left[\tilde{\mathbf{S}}_1^{m} \mid \tilde{\mathbf{S}}_2^{m} \mid \cdots \mid \tilde{\mathbf{S}}_Q^{m}\right]. \tag{12.48}$$

Note that for each input that is presented to the network we will backpropagate S^{M} sensitivity vectors. This is because we are computing the derivatives of each individual error, rather than the derivative of the sum of squares of the errors. For every input applied to the network there will be S^{M} errors (one for each element of the network output). For each error there will be one row of the Jacobian matrix.

After the sensitivities have been backpropagated, the Jacobian matrix is computed using Eq. (12.43) and Eq. (12.44). See Problem P12.5 for a numerical illustration of the Jacobian computation.

The iterations of the Levenberg-Marquardt backpropagation algorithm LMBP (*LMBP*) can be summarized as follows:

1. Present all inputs to the network and compute the corresponding network outputs (using Eq. (11.41) and Eq. (11.42)) and the errors $\mathbf{e}_q = \mathbf{t}_q - \mathbf{a}_q^{M}$. Compute the sum of squared errors over all inputs, $F(\mathbf{x})$,

using Eq. (12.34).

2. Compute the Jacobian matrix, Eq. (12.37). Calculate the sensitivities with the recurrence relations Eq. (12.47), after initializing with Eq. (12.46). Augment the individual matrices into the Marquardt sensitivities using Eq. (12.48). Compute the elements of the Jacobian matrix with Eq. (12.43) and Eq. (12.44).

3. Solve Eq. (12.32) to obtain $\Delta\mathbf{x}_k$.

4. Recompute the sum of squared errors using $\mathbf{x}_k + \Delta\mathbf{x}_k$. If this new sum of squares is smaller than that computed in step 1, then divide μ by ϑ, let $\mathbf{x}_{k+1} = \mathbf{x}_k + \Delta\mathbf{x}_k$ and go back to step 1. If the sum of squares is not reduced, then multiply μ by ϑ and go back to step 3.

The algorithm is assumed to have converged when the norm of the gradient, Eq. (12.22), is less than some predetermined value, or when the sum of squares has been reduced to some error goal.

To illustrate LMBP, let's apply it to the function approximation problem introduced at the beginning of this chapter. We will begin by looking at the basic Levenberg-Marquardt step. Figure 12.17 illustrates the possible steps the LMBP algorithm could take on the first iteration.

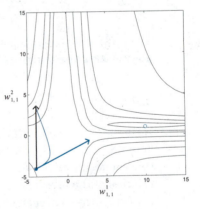

Figure 12.17 Levenberg-Marquardt Step

The black arrow represents the direction taken for small μ_k, which corresponds to the Gauss-Newton direction. The blue arrow represents the direction taken for large μ_k, which corresponds to the steepest descent direction. (This was the initial direction taken by all of the previous algorithms discussed.) The blue curve represents the Levenberg-Marquardt step for all intermediate values of μ_k. Note that as μ_k is increased the algorithm moves toward a small step in the direction of steepest descent. This guarantees that the algorithm will always be able to reduce the sum of squares at each iteration.

Figure 12.18 shows the path of the LMBP trajectory to convergence, with $\mu_0 = 0.01$ and $\vartheta = 5$. Note that the algorithm converges in fewer iterations than any of the methods we have discussed so far. Of course this algorithm also requires more computation per iteration than any of the other algorithms, since it involves a matrix inversion. Even given the large number of computations, however, the LMBP algorithm appears to be the fastest neural network training algorithm for moderate numbers of network parameters [HaMe94].

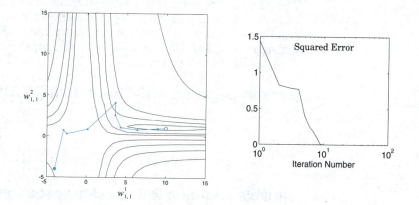

Figure 12.18 LMBP Trajectory

*To experiment with the LMBP algorithm, use the Neural Network Design Demonstrations Marquardt Step (**nnd12ms**) and Marquardt Backpropagation (**nnd12m**).*

The key drawback of the LMBP algorithm is the storage requirement. The algorithm must store the approximate Hessian matrix $\mathbf{J}^T\mathbf{J}$. This is an $n \times n$ matrix, where n is the number of parameters (weights and biases) in the network. Recall that the other methods discussed need only store the gradient, which is an n-dimensional vector. When the number of parameters is very large, it may be impractical to use the Levenberg-Marquardt algorithm. (What constitutes "very large" depends on the available memory on your computer, but typically a few thousand parameters is an upper limit.)

Summary of Results

Heuristic Variations of Backpropagation

Batching

The parameters are updated only after the entire training set has been presented. The gradients calculated for each training example are averaged together to produce a more accurate estimate of the gradient. (If the training set is complete, i.e., covers all possible input/output pairs, then the gradient estimate will be exact.)

Backpropagation with Momentum (MOBP)

$$\Delta \mathbf{W}^m(k) = \gamma \Delta \mathbf{W}^m(k-1) - (1-\gamma)\alpha \mathbf{s}^m (\mathbf{a}^{m-1})^T$$

$$\Delta \mathbf{b}^m(k) = \gamma \Delta \mathbf{b}^m(k-1) - (1-\gamma)\alpha \mathbf{s}^m$$

Variable Learning Rate Backpropagation (VLBP)

1. If the squared error (over the entire training set) increases by more than some set percentage ζ (typically one to five percent) after a weight update, then the weight update is discarded, the learning rate is multiplied by some factor $\rho < 1$, and the momentum coefficient γ (if it is used) is set to zero.

2. If the squared error decreases after a weight update, then the weight update is accepted and the learning rate is multiplied by some factor $\eta > 1$. If γ has been previously set to zero, it is reset to its original value.

3. If the squared error increases by less than ζ, then the weight update is accepted but the learning rate and the momentum coefficient are unchanged.

Numerical Optimization Techniques

Conjugate Gradient

Interval Location

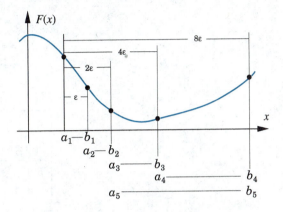

Interval Reduction (Golden Section Search)

$\tau = 0.618$

Set $\quad c_1 = a_1 + (1 - \tau)(b_1 - a_1)$, $F_c = F(c_1)$.

$\quad\quad d_1 = b_1 - (1 - \tau)(b_1 - a_1)$, $F_d = F(d_1)$.

For $k = 1, 2, \ldots$ repeat

$\quad$ If $F_c < F_d$ then

$\quad\quad\quad$ Set $\quad a_{k+1} = a_k$; $b_{k+1} = d_k$; $d_{k+1} = c_k$

$\quad\quad\quad\quad\quad\quad c_{k+1} = a_{k+1} + (1 - \tau)(b_{k+1} - a_{k+1})$

$\quad\quad\quad\quad\quad\quad F_d = F_c$; $F_c = F(c_{k+1})$

$\quad$ else

$\quad\quad\quad$ Set $\quad a_{k+1} = c_k$; $b_{k+1} = b_k$; $c_{k+1} = d_k$

$\quad\quad\quad\quad\quad\quad d_{k+1} = b_{k+1} - (1 - \tau)(b_{k+1} - a_{k+1})$

$\quad\quad\quad\quad\quad\quad F_c = F_d$; $F_d = F(d_{k+1})$

$\quad$ end

$\quad$ end until $b_{k+1} - a_{k+1} < tol$

Levenberg-Marquardt Backpropagation (LMBP)

$$\Delta \mathbf{x}_k = -[\mathbf{J}^T(\mathbf{x}_k)\mathbf{J}(\mathbf{x}_k) + \mu_k \mathbf{I}]^{-1}\mathbf{J}^T(\mathbf{x}_k)\mathbf{v}(\mathbf{x}_k)$$

$$\mathbf{v}^T = \begin{bmatrix} v_1 & v_2 & \dots & v_N \end{bmatrix} = \begin{bmatrix} e_{1,1} & e_{2,1} & \dots & e_{S^M,1} & e_{1,2} & \dots & e_{S^M,Q} \end{bmatrix}$$

$$\mathbf{x}^T = \begin{bmatrix} x_1 & x_2 & \dots & x_n \end{bmatrix} = \begin{bmatrix} w_{1,1}^1 & w_{1,2}^1 & \dots & w_{S^1,R}^1 & b_1^1 & \dots & b_{S^1}^1 & w_{1,1}^2 & \dots & b_{S^M}^M \end{bmatrix}$$

$$N = Q \times S^M \text{ and } n = S^1(R+1) + S^2(S^1+1) + \dots + S^M(S^{M-1}+1)$$

$$\mathbf{J}(\mathbf{x}) = \begin{bmatrix} \dfrac{\partial e_{1,1}}{\partial w_{1,1}^1} & \dfrac{\partial e_{1,1}}{\partial w_{1,2}^1} & \cdots & \dfrac{\partial e_{1,1}}{\partial w_{S^1,R}^1} & \dfrac{\partial e_{1,1}}{\partial b_1^1} & \cdots \\[2ex] \dfrac{\partial e_{2,1}}{\partial w_{1,1}^1} & \dfrac{\partial e_{2,1}}{\partial w_{1,2}^1} & \cdots & \dfrac{\partial e_{2,1}}{\partial w_{S^1,R}^1} & \dfrac{\partial e_{2,1}}{\partial b_1^1} & \cdots \\[2ex] \vdots & \vdots & & \vdots & \vdots & \\[1ex] \dfrac{\partial e_{S^M,1}}{\partial w_{1,1}^1} & \dfrac{\partial e_{S^M,1}}{\partial w_{1,2}^1} & \cdots & \dfrac{\partial e_{S^M,1}}{\partial w_{S^1,R}^1} & \dfrac{\partial e_{S^M,1}}{\partial b_1^1} & \cdots \\[2ex] \dfrac{\partial e_{1,2}}{\partial w_{1,1}^1} & \dfrac{\partial e_{1,2}}{\partial w_{1,2}^1} & \cdots & \dfrac{\partial e_{1,2}}{\partial w_{S^1,R}^1} & \dfrac{\partial e_{1,2}}{\partial b_1^1} & \cdots \\[2ex] \vdots & \vdots & & \vdots & \vdots & \end{bmatrix}$$

$$[\mathbf{J}]_{h,l} = \frac{\partial v_h}{\partial x_l} = \frac{\partial e_{k,q}}{\partial w_{i,j}^m} = \frac{\partial e_{k,q}}{\partial n_{i,q}^m} \times \frac{\partial n_{i,q}^m}{\partial w_{i,j}^m} = \tilde{s}_{i,h}^m \times \frac{\partial n_{i,q}^m}{\partial w_{i,j}^m} = \tilde{s}_{i,h}^m \times a_{j,q}^{m-1} \text{ for weight } x_l$$

$$[\mathbf{J}]_{h,l} = \frac{\partial v_h}{\partial x_l} = \frac{\partial e_{k,q}}{\partial b_i^m} = \frac{\partial e_{k,q}}{\partial n_{i,q}^m} \times \frac{\partial n_{i,q}^m}{\partial b_i^m} = \tilde{s}_{i,h}^m \times \frac{\partial n_{i,q}^m}{\partial b_i^m} = \tilde{s}_{i,h}^m \text{ for bias } x_l$$

$$\tilde{s}_{i,h}^m \equiv \frac{\partial v_h}{\partial n_{i,q}^m} = \frac{\partial e_{k,q}}{\partial n_{i,q}^m} \text{ (Marquardt Sensitivity) where } h = (q-1)S^M + k$$

$$\tilde{\mathbf{S}}_q^M = -\dot{\mathbf{F}}^M(\mathbf{n}_q^M)$$

$$\tilde{\mathbf{S}}_q^m = \dot{\mathbf{F}}^m(\mathbf{n}_q^m)(\mathbf{W}^{m+1})^T \tilde{\mathbf{S}}_q^{m+1}$$

$$\tilde{\mathbf{S}}^m = \begin{bmatrix} \tilde{\mathbf{S}}_1^m & | & \tilde{\mathbf{S}}_2^m & | & \cdots & | & \tilde{\mathbf{S}}_Q^m \end{bmatrix}$$

Levenberg-Marquardt Iterations

1. Present all inputs to the network and compute the corresponding network outputs (using Eq. (11.41) and Eq. (11.42)) and the errors $\mathbf{e}_q = \mathbf{t}_q - \mathbf{a}_q^M$. Compute the sum of squared errors over all inputs, $F(\mathbf{x})$, using Eq. (12.34).

2. Compute the Jacobian matrix, Eq. (12.37). Calculate the sensitivities with the recurrence relations Eq. (12.47), after initializing with Eq. (12.46). Augment the individual matrices into the Marquardt sensitivities using Eq. (12.48). Compute the elements of the Jacobian matrix with Eq. (12.43) and Eq. (12.44).

3. Solve Eq. (12.32) to obtain $\Delta\mathbf{x}_k$.

4. Recompute the sum of squared errors using $\mathbf{x}_k + \Delta\mathbf{x}_k$. If this new sum of squares is smaller than that computed in step 1, then divide μ by ϑ, let $\mathbf{x}_{k+1} = \mathbf{x}_k + \Delta\mathbf{x}_k$ and go back to step 1. If the sum of squares is not reduced, then multiply μ by ϑ and go back to step 3.

Solved Problems

P12.1 **We want to train the network shown in Figure P12.1 on the training set**

$$\{ (\mathbf{p}_1 = \begin{bmatrix} -3 \end{bmatrix}), (\mathbf{t}_1 = \begin{bmatrix} 0.5 \end{bmatrix})\} , \{ (\mathbf{p}_2 = \begin{bmatrix} 2 \end{bmatrix}), (\mathbf{t}_2 = \begin{bmatrix} 1 \end{bmatrix})\} ,$$

starting from the initial guess

$$w(0) = 0.4, \, b(0) = 0.15.$$

Demonstrate the effect of batching by computing the direction of the initial step for SDBP with and without batching.

Input   Log-Sigmoid Layer

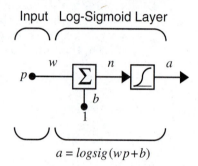

$$a = logsig(wp+b)$$

Figure P12.1 Network for Problem P12.1

Let's begin by computing the direction of the initial step if batching is not used. In this case the first step is computed from the first input/target pair. The forward and backpropagation steps are

$$a = logsig(wp + b) = \frac{1}{1 + \exp(-(0.4(-3) + 0.15))} = 0.2592$$

$$e = t - a = 0.5 - 0.2592 = 0.2408$$

$$s = -2\dot{f}(n)e = -2a(1-a)e = -2(0.2592)(1-0.2592)0.2408 = -0.0925.$$

The direction of the initial step is the negative of the gradient. For the weight this will be

$$-sp = -(-0.0925)(-3) = -0.2774.$$

For the bias we have

$$-s = -(-0.0925) = 0.0925.$$

Therefore the direction of the initial step in the (w, b) plane would be

$$\begin{bmatrix} -0.2774 \\ 0.0925 \end{bmatrix}.$$

Now let's consider the initial direction for the batch mode algorithm. In this case the gradient is found by adding together the individual gradients found from the two sets of input/target pairs. For this we need to apply the second input to the network and perform the forward and backpropagation steps:

$$a = logsig\,(wp + b) = \frac{1}{1 + \exp\,(-(0.4\,(2) + 0.15))} = 0.7211$$

$$e = t - a = 1 - 0.7211 = 0.2789$$

$$s = -2\dot{f}\,(n)\,e = -2a\,(1 - a)\,e = -2\,(0.7211)\,(1 - 0.7211)\,0.2789 = -0.1122\,.$$

The direction of the step is the negative of the gradient. For the weight this will be

$$-sp = -(-0.1122)\,(2) = 0.2243\,.$$

For the bias we have

$$-s = -(-0.1122) = 0.1122\,.$$

The partial gradient for the second input/target pair is therefore

$$\begin{bmatrix} 0.2243 \\ 0.1122 \end{bmatrix}.$$

If we now add the results from the two input/target pairs we find the direction of the first step of the batch mode SDBP to be

$$\frac{1}{2}\left(\begin{bmatrix} -0.2774 \\ 0.0925 \end{bmatrix} + \begin{bmatrix} 0.2243 \\ 0.1122 \end{bmatrix} \right) = \frac{1}{2}\begin{bmatrix} -0.0531 \\ 0.2047 \end{bmatrix} = \begin{bmatrix} -0.0265 \\ 0.1023 \end{bmatrix}.$$

The results are illustrated in Figure P12.2. The blue circle indicates the initial guess. The two blue arrows represent the directions of the partial gradients for each of the two input/target pairs, and the black arrow represents the direction of the total gradient. The function that is plotted is the sum of squared errors for the entire training set. Note that the individual partial gradients can point in quite different directions than the true gradient. However, on the average, over several iterations, the path will generally follow the steepest descent trajectory.

The relative effectiveness of the batch mode over the incremental approach depends very much on the particular problem. The incremental approach requires less storage, and, if the inputs are presented randomly to the network, the trajectory is stochastic, which makes the algorithm somewhat less likely to be trapped in a local minimum. It may also take longer to converge than the batch mode algorithm.

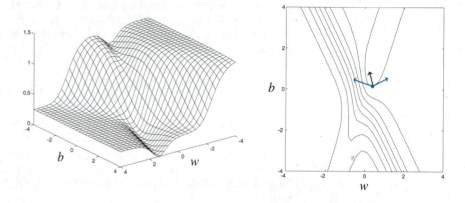

Figure P12.2 Effect of Batching in Problem P12.1

P12.2 **In Chapter 9 we proved that the steepest descent algorithm, when applied to a quadratic function, would be stable if the learning rate was less than 2 divided by the maximum eigenvalue of the Hessian matrix. Show that if a momentum term is added to the steepest descent algorithm there will always be a momentum coefficient that will make the algorithm stable, regardless of the learning rate. Follow the format of the proof on page 9-6.**

The standard steepest descent algorithm is

$$\Delta \mathbf{x}_k = -\alpha \nabla F(\mathbf{x}_k) = -\alpha \mathbf{g}_k,$$

If we add momentum this becomes

$$\Delta \mathbf{x}_k = \gamma \Delta \mathbf{x}_{k-1} - (1 - \gamma) \alpha \mathbf{g}_k.$$

Recall from Chapter 8 that the quadratic function has the form

$$F(\mathbf{x}) = \frac{1}{2} \mathbf{x}^T \mathbf{A} \mathbf{x} + \mathbf{d}^T \mathbf{x} + c,$$

and the gradient of the quadratic function is

$$\nabla F(\mathbf{x}) = \mathbf{A} \mathbf{x} + \mathbf{d}.$$

If we now insert this expression into our expression for the steepest descent algorithm with momentum we obtain

$$\Delta \mathbf{x}_k = \gamma \Delta \mathbf{x}_{k-1} - (1 - \gamma) \alpha (\mathbf{A}\mathbf{x}_k + \mathbf{d}) .$$

Using the definition $\Delta \mathbf{x}_k = \mathbf{x}_{k+1} - \mathbf{x}_k$ this can be rewritten

$$\mathbf{x}_{k+1} - \mathbf{x}_k = \gamma (\mathbf{x}_k - \mathbf{x}_{k-1}) - (1 - \gamma) \alpha (\mathbf{A}\mathbf{x}_k + \mathbf{d})$$

or

$$\mathbf{x}_{k+1} = [(1 + \gamma) \mathbf{I} - (1 - \gamma) \alpha \mathbf{A}] \mathbf{x}_k - \gamma \mathbf{x}_{k-1} - (1 - \gamma) \alpha \mathbf{d} .$$

Now define a new vector

$$\tilde{\mathbf{x}}_k = \begin{bmatrix} \mathbf{x}_{k-1} \\ \mathbf{x}_k \end{bmatrix}.$$

The momentum variation of steepest descent can then be written

$$\tilde{\mathbf{x}}_{k+1} = \begin{bmatrix} \mathbf{0} & \mathbf{I} \\ -\gamma \mathbf{I} & [(1 + \gamma) \mathbf{I} - (1 - \gamma) \alpha \mathbf{A}] \end{bmatrix} \tilde{\mathbf{x}}_k + \begin{bmatrix} \mathbf{0} \\ -(1 - \gamma) \alpha \mathbf{d} \end{bmatrix} = \mathbf{W} \tilde{\mathbf{x}}_k + \mathbf{v} .$$

This is a linear dynamic system that will be stable if the eigenvalues of $\mathbf{W}$ are less than one in magnitude. We will find the eigenvalues of $\mathbf{W}$ in stages. First, rewrite $\mathbf{W}$ as

$$\mathbf{W} = \begin{bmatrix} \mathbf{0} & \mathbf{I} \\ -\gamma \mathbf{I} & \mathbf{T} \end{bmatrix} \text{ where } \mathbf{T} = [(1 + \gamma) \mathbf{I} - (1 - \gamma) \alpha \mathbf{A}] .$$

The eigenvalues and eigenvectors of $\mathbf{W}$ should satisfy

$$\mathbf{W}\mathbf{z}^w = \lambda^w \mathbf{z}^w, \text{ or } \begin{bmatrix} \mathbf{0} & \mathbf{I} \\ -\gamma \mathbf{I} & \mathbf{T} \end{bmatrix} \begin{bmatrix} \mathbf{z}_1^w \\ \mathbf{z}_2^w \end{bmatrix} = \lambda^w \begin{bmatrix} \mathbf{z}_1^w \\ \mathbf{z}_2^w \end{bmatrix}.$$

This means that

$$\mathbf{z}_2^w = \lambda^w \mathbf{z}_1^w \text{ and } -\gamma \mathbf{z}_1^w + \mathbf{T}\mathbf{z}_2^w = \lambda^w \mathbf{z}_2^w .$$

At this point we will choose $\mathbf{z}_2^w$ to be an eigenvector of the matrix $\mathbf{T}$, with corresponding eigenvalue λ^t. (If this choice is not appropriate it will lead to a contradiction.) Therefore the previous equations become

$$\mathbf{z}_2^w = \lambda^w \mathbf{z}_1^w \text{ and } -\gamma \mathbf{z}_1^w + \lambda^t \mathbf{z}_2^w = \lambda^w \mathbf{z}_2^w.$$

If we substitute the first equation into the second equation we find

$$-\frac{\gamma}{\lambda^w}\mathbf{z}_2^w + \lambda^t \mathbf{z}_2^w = \lambda^w \mathbf{z}_2^w \text{ or } [(\lambda^w)^2 - \lambda^t(\lambda^w) + \gamma]\mathbf{z}_2^w = 0.$$

Therefore for each eigenvalue λ^t of $\mathbf{T}$ there will be two eigenvalues λ^w of $\mathbf{W}$ that are roots of the quadratic equation

$$(\lambda^w)^2 - \lambda^t(\lambda^w) + \gamma = 0.$$

From the quadratic formula we have

$$\lambda^w = \frac{\lambda^t \pm \sqrt{(\lambda^t)^2 - 4\gamma}}{2}.$$

For the algorithm to be stable the magnitude of each eigenvalue must be less than 1. We will show that there always exists some range of γ for which this is true.

Note that if the eigenvalues λ^w are complex then their magnitude will be $\sqrt{\gamma}$:

$$|\lambda^w| = \sqrt{\frac{(\lambda^t)^2}{4} + \frac{4\gamma - (\lambda^t)^2}{4}} = \sqrt{\gamma}.$$

(This is true only for real λ^t. We will show later that λ^t is real.) Since γ is between 0 and 1, the magnitude of the eigenvalue must be less than 1. It remains to show that there exists some range of γ for which all of the eigenvalues are complex.

In order for λ^w to be complex we must have

$$(\lambda^t)^2 - 4\gamma < 0 \text{ or } |\lambda^t| < 2\sqrt{\gamma}.$$

Let's now consider the eigenvalues λ^t of $\mathbf{T}$. These eigenvalues can be expressed in terms of the eigenvalues of $\mathbf{A}$. Let $\{\lambda_1, \lambda_2, \ldots, \lambda_n\}$ and $\{\mathbf{z}_1, \mathbf{z}_2, \ldots, \mathbf{z}_n\}$ be the eigenvalues and eigenvectors of the Hessian matrix. Then

$$\mathbf{T}\mathbf{z}_i = [(1+\gamma)\mathbf{I} - (1-\gamma)\alpha\mathbf{A}]\mathbf{z}_i = (1+\gamma)\mathbf{z}_i - (1-\gamma)\alpha\mathbf{A}\mathbf{z}_i$$

$$= (1+\gamma)\mathbf{z}_i - (1-\gamma)\alpha\lambda_i\mathbf{z}_i = \{(1+\gamma) - (1-\gamma)\alpha\lambda_i\}\mathbf{z}_i = \lambda_i^t\mathbf{z}_i.$$

Therefore the eigenvectors of $\mathbf{T}$ are the same as the eigenvectors of $\mathbf{A}$, and the eigenvalues of $\mathbf{T}$ are

$$\lambda_i^t = \{ (1 + \gamma) - (1 - \gamma) \alpha \lambda_i \} .$$

(Note that λ_i^t is real, since γ, α and λ_i for symmetric $\mathbf{A}$ are real.) Therefore, in order for λ^w to be complex we must have

$$\left| \lambda^t \right| < 2\sqrt{\gamma} \text{ or } \left| (1 + \gamma) - (1 - \gamma) \alpha \lambda_i \right| < 2\sqrt{\gamma}.$$

For $\gamma = 1$ both sides of the inequality will equal 2. The function on the right of the inequality, as a function of γ, has a slope of 1 at $\gamma = 1$. The function on the left of the inequality has a slope of $1 - \alpha \lambda_i$. Since the eigenvalues of the Hessian will be positive real numbers if the function has a strong minimum, and the learning rate is a positive number, this slope must be less than 1. This shows that the inequality will always hold for γ close enough to 1.

To summarize the results, we have shown that if a momentum term is added to the steepest descent algorithm on a quadratic function, then there will always be a momentum coefficient that will make the algorithm stable, regardless of the learning rate. In addition we have shown that if γ is close enough to 1, then the magnitudes of the eigenvalues of $\mathbf{W}$ will be $\sqrt{\gamma}$. It can be shown (see [Brog91]) that the magnitudes of the eigenvalues determine how fast the algorithm will converge. The smaller the magnitude, the faster the convergence. As the magnitude approaches 1, the convergence time increases.

We can demonstrate these results using the example on page 9-7. There we showed that the steepest descent algorithm, when applied to the function $F(\mathbf{x}) = x_1^2 + 25x_2^2$, was unstable for a learning rate $\alpha \geq 0.4$. In Figure P12.3 we see the steepest descent trajectory (with momentum) with $\alpha = 0.041$ and $\gamma = 0.2$. Compare this trajectory with Figure 9.3, which uses the same learning rate but no momentum.

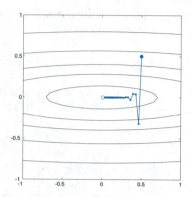

Figure P12.3 Trajectory for $\alpha = 0.041$ and $\gamma = 0.2$

P12.3 **Execute three iterations of the variable learning rate algorithm on the following function (from the Chapter 9 example on page 9-7):**

$$F(\mathbf{x}) = x_1^2 + 25x_2^2,$$

starting from the initial guess

$$\mathbf{x}_0 = \begin{bmatrix} 0.5 \\ 0.5 \end{bmatrix},$$

and use the following values for the algorithm parameters:

$$\alpha = 0.05, \ \gamma = 0.2, \ \eta = 1.5, \ \rho = 0.5, \ \zeta = 5\%.$$

The first step is to evaluate the function at the initial guess:

$$F(\mathbf{x}_0) = \frac{1}{2}\mathbf{x}_0^T \begin{bmatrix} 2 & 0 \\ 0 & 50 \end{bmatrix} \mathbf{x}_0 = \frac{1}{2}\begin{bmatrix} 0.5 & 0.5 \end{bmatrix} \begin{bmatrix} 2 & 0 \\ 0 & 50 \end{bmatrix} \begin{bmatrix} 0.5 \\ 0.5 \end{bmatrix} = 6.5.$$

The next step is to find the gradient:

$$\nabla F(\mathbf{x}) = \begin{bmatrix} \dfrac{\partial}{\partial x_1}F(\mathbf{x}) \\ \dfrac{\partial}{\partial x_2}F(\mathbf{x}) \end{bmatrix} = \begin{bmatrix} 2x_1 \\ 50x_2 \end{bmatrix}.$$

If we evaluate the gradient at the initial guess we find:

$$\mathbf{g}_0 = \nabla F(\mathbf{x}) \Big|_{\mathbf{x} = \mathbf{x}_0} = \begin{bmatrix} 1 \\ 25 \end{bmatrix}.$$

With the initial learning rate of $\alpha = 0.05$, the tentative first step of the algorithm is

$$\Delta \mathbf{x}_0 = \gamma \Delta \mathbf{x}_{-1} - (1 - \gamma) \alpha \mathbf{g}_0 = 0.2 \begin{bmatrix} 0 \\ 0 \end{bmatrix} - 0.8 (0.05) \begin{bmatrix} 1 \\ 25 \end{bmatrix} = \begin{bmatrix} -0.04 \\ -1 \end{bmatrix}$$

$$\mathbf{x}_1^t = \mathbf{x}_0 + \Delta \mathbf{x}_0 = \begin{bmatrix} 0.5 \\ 0.5 \end{bmatrix} + \begin{bmatrix} -0.04 \\ -1 \end{bmatrix} = \begin{bmatrix} 0.46 \\ -0.5 \end{bmatrix}.$$

To verify that this is a valid step we must test the value of the function at this new point:

$$F(\mathbf{x}_1^t) = \frac{1}{2} (\mathbf{x}_1^t)^T \begin{bmatrix} 2 & 0 \\ 0 & 50 \end{bmatrix} \mathbf{x}_1^t = \frac{1}{2} \begin{bmatrix} 0.46 & -0.5 \end{bmatrix} \begin{bmatrix} 2 & 0 \\ 0 & 50 \end{bmatrix} \begin{bmatrix} 0.46 \\ -0.5 \end{bmatrix} = 6.4616.$$

This is less than $F(\mathbf{x}_0)$. Therefore this tentative step is accepted and the learning rate is increased:

$$\mathbf{x}_1 = \mathbf{x}_1^t = \begin{bmatrix} 0.46 \\ -0.5 \end{bmatrix}, \ F(\mathbf{x}_1) = 6.4616 \text{ and } \alpha = \eta \alpha = 1.5 (0.05) = 0.075.$$

The tentative second step of the algorithm is

$$\Delta \mathbf{x}_1 = \gamma \Delta \mathbf{x}_0 - (1 - \gamma) \alpha \mathbf{g}_1 = 0.2 \begin{bmatrix} -0.04 \\ -1 \end{bmatrix} - 0.8 (0.075) \begin{bmatrix} 0.92 \\ -25 \end{bmatrix} = \begin{bmatrix} -0.0632 \\ 1.3 \end{bmatrix}$$

$$\mathbf{x}_2^t = \mathbf{x}_1 + \Delta \mathbf{x}_1 = \begin{bmatrix} 0.46 \\ -0.5 \end{bmatrix} + \begin{bmatrix} -0.0632 \\ 1.3 \end{bmatrix} = \begin{bmatrix} 0.3968 \\ 0.8 \end{bmatrix}.$$

We evaluate the function at this point:

$$F(\mathbf{x}_2^t) = \frac{1}{2} (\mathbf{x}_2^t)^T \begin{bmatrix} 2 & 0 \\ 0 & 50 \end{bmatrix} \mathbf{x}_2^t = \frac{1}{2} \begin{bmatrix} 0.3968 & 0.8 \end{bmatrix} \begin{bmatrix} 2 & 0 \\ 0 & 50 \end{bmatrix} \begin{bmatrix} 0.3968 \\ 0.8 \end{bmatrix} = 16.157.$$

Since this is more than 5% larger than $F(\mathbf{x}_1)$, we reject this step, reduce the learning rate and set the momentum coefficient to zero.

$$\mathbf{x}_2 = \mathbf{x}_1, \ F(\mathbf{x}_2) = F(\mathbf{x}_1) = 6.4616, \ \alpha = \rho \alpha = 0.5 (0.075) = 0.0375, \ \gamma = 0$$

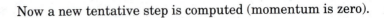

Now a new tentative step is computed (momentum is zero).

$$\Delta \mathbf{x}_2 = -\alpha \mathbf{g}_2 = -(0.0375)\begin{bmatrix} 0.92 \\ -25 \end{bmatrix} = \begin{bmatrix} -0.0345 \\ 0.9375 \end{bmatrix}$$

$$\mathbf{x}_3^t = \mathbf{x}_2 + \Delta \mathbf{x}_2 = \begin{bmatrix} 0.46 \\ -0.5 \end{bmatrix} + \begin{bmatrix} -0.0345 \\ 0.9375 \end{bmatrix} = \begin{bmatrix} 0.4255 \\ 0.4375 \end{bmatrix}$$

$$F(\mathbf{x}_3^t) = \frac{1}{2}(\mathbf{x}_3^t)^T \begin{bmatrix} 2 & 0 \\ 0 & 50 \end{bmatrix} \mathbf{x}_3^t = \frac{1}{2}\begin{bmatrix} 0.4255 & 0.4375 \end{bmatrix}\begin{bmatrix} 2 & 0 \\ 0 & 50 \end{bmatrix}\begin{bmatrix} 0.4255 \\ 0.4375 \end{bmatrix} = 4.966$$

This is less than $F(\mathbf{x}_2)$. Therefore this step is accepted, the momentum is reset to its original value, and the learning rate is increased.

$$\mathbf{x}_3 = \mathbf{x}_3^t, \ \gamma = 0.2, \ \alpha = \eta\alpha = 1.5(0.0375) = 0.05625$$

This completes the third iteration.

P12.4 **Recall the example from Chapter 9 that we used to demonstrate the conjugate gradient algorithm (page 9-18):**

$$F(\mathbf{x}) = \frac{1}{2}\mathbf{x}^T \begin{bmatrix} 2 & 1 \\ 1 & 2 \end{bmatrix}\mathbf{x},$$

with initial guess

$$\mathbf{x}_0 = \begin{bmatrix} 0.8 \\ -0.25 \end{bmatrix}.$$

Perform one iteration of the conjugate gradient algorithm. For the linear minimization use interval location by function evaluation and interval reduction by the Golden Section search.

The gradient of this function is

$$\nabla F(\mathbf{x}) = \begin{bmatrix} 2x_1 + x_2 \\ x_1 + 2x_2 \end{bmatrix}.$$

As with steepest descent, the first search direction for the conjugate gradient algorithm is the negative of the gradient:

$$\mathbf{p}_0 = -\mathbf{g}_0 = -\nabla F(\mathbf{x})^T \Big|_{\mathbf{x} = \mathbf{x}_0} = \begin{bmatrix} -1.35 \\ -0.3 \end{bmatrix}.$$

For the first iteration we need to minimize $F(\mathbf{x})$ along the line

$$\mathbf{x}_1 = \mathbf{x}_0 + \alpha_0 \mathbf{p}_0 = \begin{bmatrix} 0.8 \\ -0.25 \end{bmatrix} + \alpha_0 \begin{bmatrix} -1.35 \\ -0.3 \end{bmatrix}.$$

The first step is interval location. Assume that the initial step size is $\varepsilon = 0.075$. Then the interval location would proceed as follows:

$$F(a_1) = F\left(\begin{bmatrix} 0.8 \\ -0.25 \end{bmatrix} \right) = 0.565,$$

$$b_1 = \varepsilon = 0.075, \ F(b_1) = F\left(\begin{bmatrix} 0.8 \\ -0.25 \end{bmatrix} + 0.075 \begin{bmatrix} -1.35 \\ -0.3 \end{bmatrix} \right) = 0.3721$$

$$b_2 = 2\varepsilon = 0.15, \ F(b_2) = F\left(\begin{bmatrix} 0.8 \\ -0.25 \end{bmatrix} + 0.15 \begin{bmatrix} -1.35 \\ -0.3 \end{bmatrix} \right) = 0.2678$$

$$b_3 = 4\varepsilon = 0.3, \ F(b_3) = F\left(\begin{bmatrix} 0.8 \\ -0.25 \end{bmatrix} + 0.3 \begin{bmatrix} -1.35 \\ -0.3 \end{bmatrix} \right) = 0.1373$$

$$b_4 = 8\varepsilon = 0.6, \ F(b_4) = F\left(\begin{bmatrix} 0.8 \\ -0.25 \end{bmatrix} + 0.6 \begin{bmatrix} -1.35 \\ -0.3 \end{bmatrix} \right) = 0.1893.$$

Since the function increases between two consecutive evaluations we know that the minimum must occur in the interval [0.15, 0.6]. This process is illustrated by the open blue circles in Figure P12.4, and the final interval is indicated by the large open black circles.

The next step in the linear minimization is interval reduction using the Golden Section search. This proceeds as follows:

$$c_1 = a_1 + (1 - \tau)(b_1 - a_1) = 0.15 + (0.382)(0.6 - 0.15) = 0.3219,$$

$$d_1 = b_1 - (1 - \tau)(b_1 - a_1) = 0.6 - (0.382)(0.6 - 0.15) = 0.4281,$$

$$F_a = 0.2678, \ F_b = 0.1893, \ F_c = 0.1270, \ F_d = 0.1085.$$

Since $F_c > F_d$, we have

$$a_2 = c_1 = 0.3219, \, b_2 = b_1 = 0.6, \, c_2 = d_1 = 0.4281$$

$$d_2 = b_2 - (1 - \tau)(b_2 - a_2) = 0.6 - (0.382)(0.6 - 0.3219) = 0.4938,$$

$$F_a = F_c = 0.1270, \, F_c = F_d = 0.1085, \, F_d = F(d_2) = 0.1232.$$

This time $F_c < F_d$, therefore

$$a_3 = a_2 = 0.3219, \, b_3 = d_2 = 0.4938, \, d_3 = c_2 = 0.4281,$$

$$c_3 = a_3 + (1 - \tau)(b_3 - a_3) = 0.3219 + (0.382)(0.4938 - 0.3219) = 0.3876,$$

$$F_b = F_d = 0.1232, \, F_d = F_c = 0.1085, \, F_c = F(c_3) = 0.1094.$$

This routine continues until $b_{k+1} - a_{k+1} < tol$. The black dots in Figure P12.4 indicate the location of the new interior points, one for each iteration of the procedure. The final point is indicated by a blue dot. Compare this result with the first iteration shown in Figure 9.10.

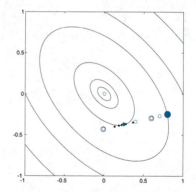

Figure P12.4 Linear Minimization Example

P12.5 **To illustrate the computation of the Jacobian matrix for the Levenberg-Marquardt method, consider using the network of Figure P12.5 for function approximation. The network transfer functions are chosen to be**

$$f^1(n) = (n)^2, \, f^2(n) = n.$$

Therefore their derivatives are

$$\dot{f}^1(n) = 2n, \, \dot{f}^2(n) = 1.$$

Assume that the training set consists of

$$\{\,(\mathbf{p}_1 = \begin{bmatrix}1\end{bmatrix}),\,(\mathbf{t}_1 = \begin{bmatrix}1\end{bmatrix})\}\,,\,\{\,(\mathbf{p}_2 = \begin{bmatrix}2\end{bmatrix}),\,(\mathbf{t}_2 = \begin{bmatrix}2\end{bmatrix})\}\,,$$

and that the parameters are initialized to

$$\mathbf{W}^1 = \begin{bmatrix}1\end{bmatrix},\,\mathbf{b}^1 = \begin{bmatrix}0\end{bmatrix},\,\mathbf{W}^2 = \begin{bmatrix}2\end{bmatrix},\,\mathbf{b}^1 = \begin{bmatrix}1\end{bmatrix}.$$

Find the Jacobian matrix for the first step of the Levenberg-Marquardt method.

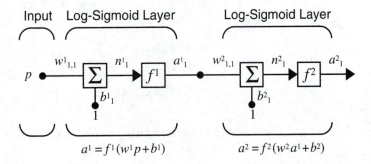

Figure P12.5 Two-Layer Network for LMBP Demonstration

The first step is to propagate the inputs through the network and compute the errors.

$$\mathbf{a}_1^0 = \mathbf{p}_1 = \begin{bmatrix}1\end{bmatrix}$$

$$\mathbf{n}_1^1 = \mathbf{W}^1\mathbf{a}_1^0 + \mathbf{b}^1 = \begin{bmatrix}1\end{bmatrix}\begin{bmatrix}1\end{bmatrix} + \begin{bmatrix}0\end{bmatrix} = \begin{bmatrix}1\end{bmatrix},\,\mathbf{a}_1^1 = \mathbf{f}^1(\mathbf{n}_1^1) = (\begin{bmatrix}1\end{bmatrix})^2 = \begin{bmatrix}1\end{bmatrix}$$

$$\mathbf{n}_1^2 = \mathbf{W}^2\mathbf{a}_1^1 + \mathbf{b}^2 = (\begin{bmatrix}2\end{bmatrix}\begin{bmatrix}1\end{bmatrix} + \begin{bmatrix}1\end{bmatrix}) = \begin{bmatrix}3\end{bmatrix},\,\mathbf{a}_1^2 = \mathbf{f}^2(\mathbf{n}_1^2) = (\begin{bmatrix}3\end{bmatrix}) = \begin{bmatrix}3\end{bmatrix}$$

$$\mathbf{e}_1 = (\mathbf{t}_1 - \mathbf{a}_1^2) = (\begin{bmatrix}1\end{bmatrix} - \begin{bmatrix}3\end{bmatrix}) = \begin{bmatrix}-2\end{bmatrix}$$

$$\mathbf{a}_2^0 = \mathbf{p}_2 = \begin{bmatrix}2\end{bmatrix}$$

$$\mathbf{n}_2^1 = \mathbf{W}^1\mathbf{a}_2^0 + \mathbf{b}^1 = \begin{bmatrix}1\end{bmatrix}\begin{bmatrix}2\end{bmatrix} + \begin{bmatrix}0\end{bmatrix} = \begin{bmatrix}2\end{bmatrix},\,\mathbf{a}_2^1 = \mathbf{f}^1(\mathbf{n}_2^1) = (\begin{bmatrix}2\end{bmatrix})^2 = \begin{bmatrix}4\end{bmatrix}$$

$$\mathbf{n}_2^2 = \mathbf{W}^2\mathbf{a}_2^1 + \mathbf{b}^2 = (\begin{bmatrix}2\end{bmatrix}\begin{bmatrix}4\end{bmatrix} + \begin{bmatrix}1\end{bmatrix}) = \begin{bmatrix}9\end{bmatrix},\,\mathbf{a}_2^2 = \mathbf{f}^2(\mathbf{n}_2^2) = (\begin{bmatrix}9\end{bmatrix}) = \begin{bmatrix}9\end{bmatrix}$$

$$\mathbf{e}_1 = (\mathbf{t}_1 - \mathbf{a}_1^2) = (\begin{bmatrix}2\end{bmatrix} - \begin{bmatrix}9\end{bmatrix}) = \begin{bmatrix}-7\end{bmatrix}$$

The next step is to initialize and backpropagate the Marquardt sensitivities using Eq. (12.46) and Eq. (12.47).

$$\tilde{\mathbf{S}}_1^2 = -\dot{\mathbf{F}}^2(\mathbf{n}_1^2) = -\begin{bmatrix}1\end{bmatrix}$$

$$\tilde{\mathbf{S}}_1^1 = \dot{\mathbf{F}}^1(\mathbf{n}_1^1)(\mathbf{W}^2)^T \tilde{\mathbf{S}}_1^2 = \begin{bmatrix}2n_{1,1}^1\end{bmatrix}\begin{bmatrix}2\end{bmatrix}\begin{bmatrix}-1\end{bmatrix} = \begin{bmatrix}2(1)\end{bmatrix}\begin{bmatrix}2\end{bmatrix}\begin{bmatrix}-1\end{bmatrix} = \begin{bmatrix}-4\end{bmatrix}$$

$$\tilde{\mathbf{S}}_2^2 = -\dot{\mathbf{F}}^2(\mathbf{n}_2^2) = -\begin{bmatrix}1\end{bmatrix}$$

$$\tilde{\mathbf{S}}_2^1 = \dot{\mathbf{F}}^1(\mathbf{n}_2^1)(\mathbf{W}^2)^T \tilde{\mathbf{S}}_2^2 = \begin{bmatrix}2n_{1,2}^2\end{bmatrix}\begin{bmatrix}2\end{bmatrix}\begin{bmatrix}-1\end{bmatrix} = \begin{bmatrix}2(2)\end{bmatrix}\begin{bmatrix}2\end{bmatrix}\begin{bmatrix}-1\end{bmatrix} = \begin{bmatrix}-8\end{bmatrix}$$

$$\tilde{\mathbf{S}}^1 = \begin{bmatrix}\tilde{\mathbf{S}}_1^1 | \tilde{\mathbf{S}}_2^1\end{bmatrix} = \begin{bmatrix}-4 & -8\end{bmatrix}, \tilde{\mathbf{S}}^2 = \begin{bmatrix}\tilde{\mathbf{S}}_1^2 | \tilde{\mathbf{S}}_2^2\end{bmatrix} = \begin{bmatrix}-1 & -1\end{bmatrix}$$

We can now compute the Jacobian matrix using Eq. (12.43), Eq. (12.44) and Eq. (12.37).

$$\mathbf{J}(\mathbf{x}) = \begin{bmatrix} \dfrac{\partial v_1}{\partial x_1} & \dfrac{\partial v_1}{\partial x_2} & \dfrac{\partial v_1}{\partial x_3} & \dfrac{\partial v_1}{\partial x_4} \\[2mm] \dfrac{\partial v_2}{\partial x_1} & \dfrac{\partial v_2}{\partial x_2} & \dfrac{\partial v_2}{\partial x_3} & \dfrac{\partial v_2}{\partial x_4} \end{bmatrix} = \begin{bmatrix} \dfrac{\partial e_{1,1}}{\partial w_{1,1}^1} & \dfrac{\partial e_{1,1}}{\partial b_1^1} & \dfrac{\partial e_{1,1}}{\partial w_{1,1}^2} & \dfrac{\partial e_{1,1}}{\partial b_1^2} \\[2mm] \dfrac{\partial e_{1,2}}{\partial w_{1,1}^1} & \dfrac{\partial e_{1,2}}{\partial b_1^1} & \dfrac{\partial e_{1,2}}{\partial w_{1,1}^2} & \dfrac{\partial e_{1,2}}{\partial b_1^2} \end{bmatrix}$$

$$[\mathbf{J}]_{1,1} = \frac{\partial v_1}{\partial x_1} = \frac{\partial e_{1,1}}{\partial w_{1,1}^1} = \frac{\partial e_{1,1}}{\partial n_{1,1}^1} \times \frac{\partial n_{1,1}^1}{\partial w_{1,1}^1} = \tilde{s}_{1,1}^1 \times \frac{\partial n_{1,1}^1}{\partial w_{1,1}^1} = \tilde{s}_{1,1}^1 \times a_{1,1}^0$$

$$= (-4)(1) = -4$$

$$[\mathbf{J}]_{1,2} = \frac{\partial v_1}{\partial x_2} = \frac{\partial e_{1,1}}{\partial b_1^1} = \frac{\partial e_{1,1}}{\partial n_{1,1}^1} \times \frac{\partial n_{1,1}^1}{\partial b_1^1} = \tilde{s}_{1,1}^1 \times \frac{\partial n_{1,1}^1}{\partial b_1^1} = \tilde{s}_{1,1}^1 = -4$$

$$[\mathbf{J}]_{1,3} = \frac{\partial v_1}{\partial x_3} = \frac{\partial e_{1,1}}{\partial n_{1,1}^2} \times \frac{\partial n_{1,1}^2}{\partial w_{1,1}^2} = \tilde{s}_{1,1}^2 \times \frac{\partial n_{1,1}^2}{\partial w_{1,1}^2} = \tilde{s}_{1,1}^2 \times a_{1,1}^1 = (-1)(1) = -1$$

$$[\mathbf{J}]_{1,4} = \frac{\partial v_1}{\partial x_4} = \frac{\partial e_{1,1}}{\partial n_{1,1}^2} \times \frac{\partial n_{1,1}^1}{\partial b_1^2} = \tilde{s}_{1,1}^2 \times \frac{\partial n_{1,1}^2}{\partial b_1^2} = \tilde{s}_{1,1}^2 = -1$$

$$[\mathbf{J}]_{2,1} = \frac{\partial v_2}{\partial x_1} = \frac{\partial e_{1,2}}{\partial n_{1,2}^1} \times \frac{\partial n_{1,2}^1}{\partial w_{1,1}^1} = \tilde{s}_{1,2}^1 \times \frac{\partial n_{1,2}^1}{\partial w_{1,1}^1} = \tilde{s}_{1,2}^1 \times a_{1,2}^0 = (-8)\,(2) = -16$$

$$[\mathbf{J}]_{2,2} = \frac{\partial v_2}{\partial x_2} = \frac{\partial e_{1,2}}{\partial b_1^1} = \frac{\partial e_{1,2}}{\partial n_{1,2}^1} \times \frac{\partial n_{1,2}^1}{\partial b_1^1} = \tilde{s}_{1,2}^1 \times \frac{\partial n_{1,2}^1}{\partial b_1^1} = \tilde{s}_{1,2}^1 = -8$$

$$[\mathbf{J}]_{2,3} = \frac{\partial v_2}{\partial x_3} = \frac{\partial e_{1,2}}{\partial n_{1,2}^2} \times \frac{\partial n_{1,2}^2}{\partial w_{1,1}^2} = \tilde{s}_{1,2}^2 \times \frac{\partial n_{1,2}^2}{\partial w_{1,1}^2} = \tilde{s}_{1,2}^2 \times a_{1,2}^1 = (-1)\,(4) = -4$$

$$[\mathbf{J}]_{2,4} = \frac{\partial v_2}{\partial x_4} = \frac{\partial e_{1,2}}{\partial b_1^2} = \frac{\partial e_{1,2}}{\partial n_{1,2}^2} \times \frac{\partial n_{1,2}^2}{\partial b_1^2} = \tilde{s}_{1,2}^2 \times \frac{\partial n_{1,2}^2}{\partial b_1^2} = \tilde{s}_{1,2}^2 = -1$$

Therefore the Jacobian matrix is

$$\mathbf{J}(\mathbf{x}) = \begin{bmatrix} -4 & -4 & -1 & -1 \\ -16 & -8 & -4 & -1 \end{bmatrix} \ .$$

Epilogue

One of the major problems with the basic backpropagation algorithm (steepest descent backpropagation — SDBP) has been the long training times. It is not feasible to use SDBP on practical problems, because it can take weeks to train a network, even on a large computer. Since backpropagation was first popularized, there has been considerable work on methods to accelerate the convergence of the algorithm. In this chapter we have discussed the reasons for the slow convergence of SDBP and have presented several techniques for improving the performance of the algorithm.

The techniques for speeding up convergence have fallen into two main categories: heuristic methods and standard numerical optimization methods. We have discussed two heuristic methods: momentum (MOBP) and variable learning rate (VLBP). MOBP is simple to implement, can be used in batch mode or incremental mode and is significantly faster than SDBP. It does require the selection of the momentum coefficient, but γ is limited to the range $[0, 1]$ and the algorithm is not extremely sensitive to this choice.

The VLBP algorithm is faster than MOBP but must be used in batch mode. For this reason it requires more storage. VLBP also requires the selection of a total of five parameters. The algorithm is reasonably robust, but the choice of the parameters can affect the convergence speed and is problem dependent.

We also presented two standard numerical optimization techniques: conjugate gradient (CGBP) and Levenberg-Marquardt (LMBP). CGBP is generally faster than VLBP. It is a batch mode algorithm, which requires a linear search at each iteration, but its storage requirements are not significantly different than VLBP. There are many variations of the conjugate gradient algorithm proposed for neural network applications. We have presented only one.

The LMBP algorithm is the fastest algorithm that we have tested for training multilayer networks of moderate size, even though it requires a matrix inversion at each iteration. It requires that two parameters be selected, but the algorithm does not appear to be sensitive to this selection. The main drawback of LMBP is the storage requirement. The $\mathbf{J}^T\mathbf{J}$ matrix, which must be inverted, is $n \times n$, where n is the total number of weights and biases in the network. If the network has more than a few thousand parameters, the LMBP algorithm becomes impractical on current machines.

There are many other variations on backpropagation that have not been discussed in this chapter. Some references to other techniques are given in Chapter 19.

Further Reading

[Barn92]   E. Barnard, "Optimization for training neural nets," *IEEE Trans. on Neural Networks*, vol. 3, no. 2, pp. 232–240, 1992.

A number of optimization algorithms that have promise for neural network training are discussed in this paper.

[Batt92]   R. Battiti, "First- and second-order methods for learning: Between steepest descent and Newton's method," *Neural Computation*, vol. 4, no. 2, pp. 141–166, 1992.

This paper is an excellent survey of the current optimization algorithms that are suitable for neural network training.

[Char92]   C. Charalambous, "Conjugate gradient algorithm for efficient training of artificial neural networks," *IEE Proceedings*, vol. 139, no. 3, pp. 301–310, 1992.

This paper explains how the conjugate gradient algorithm can be used to train multilayer networks. Comparisons are made to other training algorithms.

[Fahl88]   S. E. Fahlman, "Faster-learning variations on back-propagation: An empirical study," In D. Touretsky, G. Hinton & T. Sejnowski, eds., *Proceedings of the 1988 Connectionist Models Summer School*, San Mateo, CA: Morgan Kaufmann, pp. 38–51, 1988.

The QuickProp algorithm, which is described in this paper, is one of the more popular heuristic modifications to backpropagation. It assumes that the error curve can be approximated by a parabola, and that the effect of each weight can be considered independently. QuickProp provides significant speedup over standard backpropagation on many problems.

[HaMe94]   M. T. Hagan and M. Menhaj, "Training feedforward networks with the Marquardt algorithm," *IEEE Transactions on Neural Networks*, vol. 5, no. 6, 1994.

This paper describes the use of the Levenberg-Marquardt algorithm for training multilayer networks and compares the performance of the algorithm with variable learning rate backpropagation and conjugate gradient. The Levenberg-Marquardt algorithm is faster, but requires more storage.

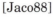

[Jaco88]   R. A. Jacobs, "Increased rates of convergence through learning rate adaptation," *Neural Networks*, vol. 1, no. 4, pp. 295–308, 1988.

This is another early paper discussing the use of variable learning rate backpropagation. The procedure described here is called the delta-bar-delta learning rule, in which each network parameter has its own learning rate that varies at each iteration.

[NgWi90]   D. Nguyen and B. Widrow, "Improving the learning speed of 2-layer neural networks by choosing initial values of the adaptive weights," *Proceedings of the IJCNN*, vol. 3, pp. 21–26, July 1990.

This paper describes a procedure for setting the initial weights and biases for the backpropagation algorithm. It uses the shape of the sigmoid transfer function and the range of the input variables to determine how large the weights should be, and then uses the biases to center the sigmoids in the operating region. The convergence of backpropagation is improved significantly by this procedure.

[RiIr90]   A. K. Rigler, J. M. Irvine and T. P. Vogl, "Rescaling of variables in back propagation learning," *Neural Networks*, vol. 3, no. 5, pp. 561–573, 1990.

This paper notes that the derivative of a sigmoid function is very small on the tails. This means that the elements of the gradient associated with the first few layers will generally be smaller that those associated with the last layer. The terms in the gradient are then scaled to equalize them.

[Scal85]   L. E. Scales, *Introduction to Non-Linear Optimization*. New York: Springer-Verlag, 1985.

Scales has written a very readable text describing the major optimization algorithms. The book emphasizes methods of optimization rather than existence theorems and proofs of convergence. Algorithms are presented with intuitive explanations, along with illustrative figures and examples. Pseudocode is presented for most algorithms.

[Shan90]   D. F. Shanno, "Recent advances in numerical techniques for large-scale optimization," *Neural Networks for Control*, Miller, Sutton and Werbos, eds., Cambridge MA: MIT Press, 1990.

This paper discusses some conjugate gradient and quasi-Newton optimization algorithms that could be used for neural network training.

[Toll90]   T. Tollenaere, "SuperSAB: Fast adaptive back propagation with good scaling properties," *Neural Networks*, vol. 3, no. 5, pp. 561–573, 1990.

This paper presents a variable learning rate backpropagation algorithm in which different learning rates are used for each weight.

[VoMa88]   T. P. Vogl, J. K. Mangis, A. K. Zigler, W. T. Zink and D. L. Alkon, "Accelerating the convergence of the backpropagation method," *Biological Cybernetics.*, vol. 59, pp. 256–264, Sept. 1988.

This was one of the first papers to introduce several heuristic techniques for accelerating the convergence of backpropagation. It included batching, momentum and variable learning rate.

Exercises

E12.1 We want to train the network shown in Figure E12.1 on the training set

$$\{ (\mathbf{p}_1 = \begin{bmatrix} -2 \end{bmatrix}), (\mathbf{t}_1 = \begin{bmatrix} 0.8 \end{bmatrix}) \}, \{ (\mathbf{p}_2 = \begin{bmatrix} 2 \end{bmatrix}), (\mathbf{t}_2 = \begin{bmatrix} 1 \end{bmatrix}) \},$$

where each pair is equally likely to occur.

Write a MATLAB M-file to create a contour plot for the mean squared error performance index.

Input   Log-Sigmoid Layer

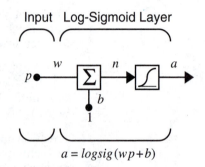

$a = logsig\,(wp+b)$

Figure E12.1 Network for Exercise E12.1

E12.2 Demonstrate the effect of batching by computing the direction of the initial step for SDBP with and without batching for the problem described in Exercise E12.1, starting from the initial guess

$$w\,(0) \ = \ 0\,,\ b\,(0) \ = \ 0.5\,.$$

E12.3 Recall the quadratic function used in Problem P9.1:

$$F\,(\mathbf{x}) \ = \ \frac{1}{2}\mathbf{x}^T \begin{bmatrix} 10 & -6 \\ -6 & 10 \end{bmatrix} \mathbf{x} + \begin{bmatrix} 4 & 4 \end{bmatrix} \mathbf{x}\,.$$

We want to use the steepest descent algorithm with momentum to minimize this function.

i. Suppose that the learning rate is $\alpha = 0.2$. Find a value for the momentum coefficient γ for which the algorithm will be stable. Use the ideas presented in Problem P12.2.

ii. Suppose that the learning rate is $\alpha = 20$. Find a value for the momentum coefficient γ for which the algorithm will be stable.

```
» 2 + 2
ans =
    4
```

iii. Write a MATLAB program to plot the trajectories of the algorithm for the α and γ values of both part (i) and part (ii) on the contour plot of $F(\mathbf{x})$, starting from the initial guess

$$\mathbf{x}_0 = \begin{bmatrix} -1 \\ -2.5 \end{bmatrix}.$$

E12.4 For the function of Exercise E12.3, perform three iterations of the variable learning rate algorithm, with initial guess

$$\mathbf{x}_0 = \begin{bmatrix} -1 \\ -2.5 \end{bmatrix}.$$

Plot the algorithm trajectory on a contour plot of $F(\mathbf{x})$. Use the algorithm parameters

$$\alpha = 0.4, \gamma = 0.1, \eta = 1.5, \rho = 0.5, \zeta = 5\%.$$

E12.5 For the function of Exercise E12.3, perform one iteration of the conjugate gradient algorithm, with initial guess

$$\mathbf{x}_0 = \begin{bmatrix} -1 \\ -2.5 \end{bmatrix}.$$

For the linear minimization use interval location by function evaluation and interval reduction by the Golden Section search. Plot the path of the search on a contour plot of $F(\mathbf{x})$.

E12.6 We want to use the network of Figure E12.2 to approximate the function

$$g(p) = 1 + \sin\left(\frac{\pi}{4}p\right) \text{ for } -2 \le p \le 2.$$

The initial network parameters are chosen to be

$$\mathbf{w}^1(0) = \begin{bmatrix} -0.27 \\ -0.41 \end{bmatrix}, \mathbf{b}^1(0) = \begin{bmatrix} -0.48 \\ -0.13 \end{bmatrix}, \mathbf{w}^2(0) = \begin{bmatrix} 0.09 & -0.17 \end{bmatrix}, \mathbf{b}^2(0) = \begin{bmatrix} 0.48 \end{bmatrix}.$$

To create the training set we sample the function $g(p)$ at the points $p = 1$ and $p = 0$. Find the Jacobian matrix for the first step of the LMBP algorithm. (Some of the information you will need has been computed in the example starting on page 11-14.)

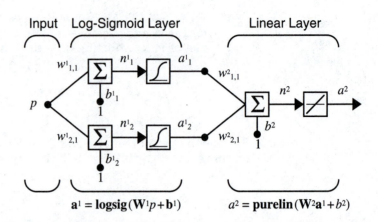

$$\mathbf{a}^1 = \mathbf{logsig}(\mathbf{W}^1 p + \mathbf{b}^1) \qquad a^2 = \mathbf{purelin}(\mathbf{W}^2 \mathbf{a}^1 + b^2)$$

Figure E12.2 Network for Exercise E12.6

E12.7 Show that for a linear network the LMBP algorithm will converge to an optimum solution in one iteration if $\mu = 0$.

E12.8 In Exercise E11.11 you wrote a MATLAB program to implement the SDBP algorithm for the 1-2-1 network shown in Figure E12.2, and trained the network to approximate the function

$$g(p) = 1 + \sin\left(\frac{\pi}{8}p\right) \text{ for } -2 \le p \le 2.$$

Repeat this exercise, modifying your program to use the training procedures discussed in this chapter: batch mode SDBP, MOBP, VLBP, CGBP and LMBP. Compare the convergence results of the various methods.

13 Associative Learning

Objectives

The neural networks we have discussed so far (in Chapters 4, 7, 10–12) have all been trained in a supervised manner. Each network required a target signal to define correct network behavior.

In contrast, this chapter introduces a collection of simple rules that allow unsupervised learning. These rules give networks the ability to learn associations between patterns that occur together frequently. Once learned, associations allow networks to perform useful tasks such as pattern recognition and recall.

Despite the simplicity of the rules in this chapter, they will form the foundation for powerful networks in Chapters 14–16.

Theory and Examples

This chapter is all about associations: how associations can be represented by a network, how a network can learn new associations.

What is an association? An association is any link between a system's input and output such that when a pattern A is presented to the system it will respond with pattern B. When two patterns are linked by an association, the input pattern is often referred to as the *stimulus*. Likewise, the output pattern is referred to as the *response*.

Stimulus
Response

Associations are so fundamental that they formed the foundation of the behaviorist school of psychology. This branch of psychology attempted to explain much of animal and human behavior by using associations and rules for learning associations. (This approach has since been largely discredited.)

One of the earliest influences on the behaviorist school of psychology was the classic experiment of Ivan Pavlov, in which he trained a dog to salivate at the sound of a bell, by ringing the bell whenever food was presented. This is an example of what is now called classical conditioning. B. F. Skinner was one of the most influential proponents of the behaviorist school. His classic experiment involved training a rat to press a bar in order to obtain a food pellet. This is an example of instrumental conditioning.

It was to provide a biological explanation for some of this behavior that led Donald Hebb to his postulate, previously quoted in Chapter 7 [Hebb49]:

"When an axon of cell A is near enough to excite a cell B and repeatedly or persistently takes part in firing it, some growth process or metabolic change takes place in one or both cells such that A's efficiency, as one of the cells firing B, is increased."

In Chapter 7 we analyzed the performance of a supervised learning rule based on Hebb's postulate. In this chapter we will discuss unsupervised forms of Hebbian learning, as well as other related associative learning rules.

A number of researchers have contributed to the development of associative learning. In particular, Tuevo Kohonen, James Anderson and Stephen Grossberg have been very influential. Anderson and Kohonen independently developed the linear associator network in the late 1960s and early 1970s ([Ande72], [Koho72]). Grossberg introduced nonlinear continuous-time associative networks during the same time period (e.g., [Gross68]). All of these researchers, in addition to many others, have continued the development of associative learning up to the present time.

In this chapter we will discuss the elemental associative learning rules. Then, in Chapters 14–16 we will present more complex networks that use associative learning as a primary component. Chapter 14 will describe Kohonen networks, and Chapters 15 and 16 will discuss Grossberg networks.

Simple Associative Network

Let's take a look at the simplest network capable of implementing an association. An example is the single-input hard limit neuron shown in Figure 13.1.

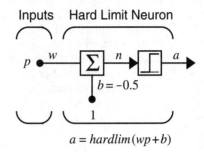

$$a = hardlim(wp+b)$$

Figure 13.1 Single-Input Hard Limit Associator

The neuron's output a is determined from its input p according to

$$a = hardlim(wp+b) = hardlim(wp-0.5). \qquad (13.1)$$

For simplicity, we will restrict the value of p to be either 0 or 1, indicating whether a stimulus is absent or present. Note that a is limited to the same values by the hard limit transfer function. It indicates the presence or absence of the network's response.

$$p = \begin{cases} 1, & \text{stimulus} \\ 0, & \text{no stimulus} \end{cases} \qquad a = \begin{cases} 1, & \text{response} \\ 0, & \text{no response} \end{cases} \qquad (13.2)$$

The presence of an association between the stimulus $p = 1$, and the response $a = 1$ is dictated by the value of w. The network will respond to the stimulus only if w is greater than $-b$ (in this case 0.5).

The learning rules discussed in this chapter are normally used in the framework of a larger network, such as the competitive networks of Chapters 14–16. In order to demonstrate the operation of the associative learning rules, without using complex networks, we will use simple networks that have two types of inputs.

Unconditioned Stimulus One set of inputs will represent the *unconditioned stimulus*. This is analogous to the food presented to the dog in Pavlov's experiment. Another set **Conditioned Stimulus** of inputs will represent the *conditioned stimulus*. This is analogous to the bell in Pavlov's experiment. Initially the dog salivates only when food is presented. This is an innate characteristic that does not have to be learned. However, when the bell is repeatedly paired with the food, the dog is conditioned to salivate at the sound of the bell, even when no food is present.

We will represent the unconditioned stimulus as $\mathbf{p}^0$ and the conditioned stimulus simply as $\mathbf{p}$. For our purposes we will assume that the weights associated with $\mathbf{p}^0$ are fixed, but that the weights associated with $\mathbf{p}$ are adjusted according to the relevant learning rule.

Figure 13.2 shows a network for recognizing bananas. The network has both an unconditioned stimulus (banana shape) and a conditioned stimulus (banana smell). We don't mean to imply here that smell is more conditionable than sight. In our examples in this chapter the choices of conditioned and unconditioned stimuli are arbitrary and are used simply to demonstrate the performance of the learning rules. We will use this network to demonstrate the operation of the Hebb rule in the following section.

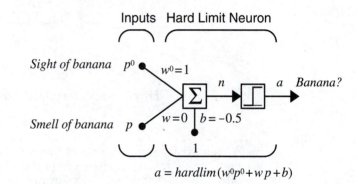

$$a = hardlim(w^0 p^0 + w p + b)$$

Figure 13.2 Banana Associator

The definitions of the unconditioned and conditioned inputs for this network are

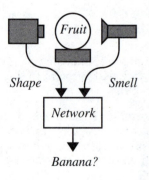

$$p^0 = \begin{cases} 1, & \text{shape detected} \\ 0, & \text{shape not detected} \end{cases} \qquad p = \begin{cases} 1, & \text{smell detected} \\ 0, & \text{smell not detected} \end{cases} . \tag{13.3}$$

At this time we would like the network to associate the shape of a banana, but the not the smell, with a response indicating the fruit is a banana. The problem is solved by assigning a value greater than $-b$ to w^0 and assigning a value less than $-b$ to w. The following values satisfy these requirements:

$$w^0 = 1, \ w = 0. \tag{13.4}$$

The banana associator's input/output function now simplifies to

$$a = hardlim(p^0 - 0.5) .\qquad(13.5)$$

Thus, the network will only respond if a banana is sighted ($p^0 = 1$), whether a banana is smelled ($p = 1$) or not ($p = 0$).

We will use this network in later sections to illustrate the performance of several associative learning rules.

Unsupervised Hebb Rule

For simple problems it is not difficult to design a network with a fixed set of associations. On the other hand, a more useful network would be able to learn associations.

When should an association be learned? It is generally accepted that both animals and humans tend to associate things that occur simultaneously. To paraphrase Hebb: if a banana smell stimulus occurs simultaneously with a banana concept response (activated by some other stimulus such as the sight of a banana shape), the network should strengthen the connection between them so that later it can activate its banana concept in response to the banana smell alone.

The unsupervised Hebb rule does just that by increasing the weight w_{ij} between a neuron's input p_j and output a_i in proportion to their product:

$$w_{ij}(q) = w_{ij}(q-1) + \alpha a_i(q) p_j(q) .\qquad(13.6)$$

(See also Eq. (7.5).) The learning rate α dictates how many times a stimulus and response must occur together before an association is made. In the network in Figure 13.2, an association will be made when $w > -b = 0.5$, since then $p = 1$ will produce the response $a = 1$, regardless of the value of p^0.

Local Learning   Note that Eq. (13.6) uses only signals available within the layer containing the weights being updated. Rules that satisfy this condition are called *local learning* rules. This is in contrast to the backpropagation rule, for example, in which the sensitivity must be propagated back from the final layer. The rules introduced in this chapter will all be local learning rules.

The unsupervised Hebb rule can also be written in vector form:

$$\mathbf{W}(q) = \mathbf{W}(q-1) + \alpha\mathbf{a}(q)\mathbf{p}^T(q) .\qquad(13.7)$$

Training Sequence   As with all unsupervised rules, learning is performed in response to a series of inputs presented in time (the *training sequence*):

$$\mathbf{p}(1), \mathbf{p}(2), \dots, \mathbf{p}(Q) .\qquad(13.8)$$

(Note that we are using the notation $\mathbf{p}(q)$, instead of $\mathbf{p}_q$, in order to emphasize the time-sequence nature of the inputs.) At each iteration, the output $\mathbf{a}$ is calculated in response to the input $\mathbf{p}$, and then the weights $\mathbf{W}$ are updated with the Hebb rule.

Let's apply the unsupervised Hebb rule to the banana associator. The associator will start with the weight values determined in our previous example, so that it will initially respond to the sight, but not the smell, of a banana.

$$w^0 = 1, w(0) = 0 \qquad (13.9)$$

The associator will be repeatedly exposed to a banana. However, while the network's smell sensor will work reliably, the shape sensor will operate only intermittently (on even time steps). Thus the training sequence will consist of repetitions of the following two sets of inputs:

$$\{p^0(1) = 0, p(1) = 1\}, \{p^0(2) = 1, p(2) = 1\}, \dots . \qquad (13.10)$$

The first weight w^0, representing the weight for the unconditioned stimulus p^0, will remain constant, while w will be updated at each iteration, using the unsupervised Hebb rule with a learning rate of 1:

$$w(q) = w(q-1) + a(q) p(q) . \qquad (13.11)$$

The output for the first iteration ($q = 1$) is

$$a(1) = hardlim(w^0 p^0(1) + w(0) p(1) - 0.5) \qquad (13.12)$$
$$= hardlim(1 \cdot 0 + 0 \cdot 1 - 0.5) = 0 \quad \text{(no response)} .$$

The smell alone did not generate a response. Without a response, the Hebb rule does not alter w.

$$w(1) = w(0) + a(1) p(1) = 0 + 0 \cdot 1 = 0 \qquad (13.13)$$

In the second iteration, both the banana's shape and smell are detected and the network responds accordingly:

$$a(2) = hardlim(w^0 p^0(2) + w(1) p(2) - 0.5) \qquad (13.14)$$
$$= hardlim(1 \cdot 1 + 0 \cdot 1 - 0.5) = 1 \quad \text{(banana)} .$$

Because the smell stimulus and the response have occurred simultaneously, the Hebb rule increases the weight between them.

$$w(2) = w(1) + a(2) p(2) = 0 + 1 \cdot 1 = 1 \qquad (13.15)$$

When the sight detector fails again, in the third iteration, the network responds anyway. It has made a useful association between the smell of a banana and its response.

$$a(3) = hardlim(w^0 p^0(3) + w(2)p(3) - 0.5) \qquad (13.16)$$
$$= hardlim(1 \cdot 0 + 1 \cdot 1 - 0.5) = 1 \quad \text{(banana)}$$

$$w(3) = w(2) + a(3)p(3) = 1 + 1 \cdot 1 = 2 \qquad (13.17)$$

From now on, the network is capable of responding to bananas that are detected either by sight or smell. Even if both detection systems suffer intermittent faults, the network will be correct most of the time.

To experiment with the unsupervised Hebb rule, use the Neural Network Design Demonstration Unsupervised Hebb Rule (**nnd13uh**).

We have seen that the unsupervised Hebb rule can learn useful associations. However, the Hebb rule, as defined in Eq. (13.6), has some practical shortcomings. The first problem becomes evident if we continue to present inputs and update w in the example above. The weight w will become arbitrarily large. This is at odds with the biological systems that inspired the Hebb rule. Synapses cannot grow without bound.

The second problem is that there is no mechanism for weights to decrease. If the inputs or outputs of a Hebb network experience any noise, every weight will grow (however slowly) until the network responds to any stimulus.

Hebb Rule with Decay

One way to improve the Hebb rule is by adding a weight decay term (Eq. (7.45)),

$$\mathbf{W}(q) = \mathbf{W}(q-1) + \alpha \mathbf{a}(q)\mathbf{p}^T(q) - \gamma \mathbf{W}(q-1)$$
$$= (1-\gamma)\mathbf{W}(q-1) + \alpha \mathbf{a}(q)\mathbf{p}^T(q) , \qquad (13.18)$$

Decay Rate   where γ, the *decay rate*, is a positive constant less than one. As γ approaches zero, the learning law becomes the standard rule. As γ approaches one, the learning law quickly forgets old inputs and remembers only the most recent patterns. This keeps the weight matrix from growing without bound. (The idea of filtering the weight changes was also discussed in Chapter 12, where we called it momentum.)

The maximum weight value w_{ij}^{max} is determined by γ. This value is found by setting both a_i and p_j to a value of 1 for all q (to maximize learning) in the scalar version of Eq. (13.18) and solving for the steady state weight (i.e. when both new and old weights are equal).

$$w_{ij} = (1 - \gamma) w_{ij} + \alpha a_i p_j$$
$$w_{ij} = (1 - \gamma) w_{ij} + \alpha \tag{13.19}$$
$$w_{ij} = \frac{\alpha}{\gamma}$$

Let's examine the operation of the Hebb rule with decay on our previous banana associator problem. We will use a decay rate γ of 0.1. The first iteration, where only the smell stimulus is presented, is the same:

$$a(1) = 0 \quad \text{(no response)}, \quad w(1) = 0. \tag{13.20}$$

The next iteration also produces identical results. Here both stimuli are presented, and the network responds to the shape. Coincidence of the smell stimulus and response create a new association:

$$a(2) = 1 \quad \text{(banana)}, \quad w(2) = 1. \tag{13.21}$$

The results of the third iteration are not the same. The network has learned to respond to the smell, and the weight continues to increase. However, this time the weight increases by only 0.9, instead of 1.0.

$$w(3) = w(2) + a(3) p(3) - 0.1 w(2) = 1 + 1 \cdot 1 - 0.1 \cdot 1 = 1.9 \tag{13.22}$$

The decay term limits the weight's value, so that no matter how often the association is reinforced, w will never increase beyond w_{ij}^{max}.

$$w_{ij}^{max} = \frac{\alpha}{\gamma} = \frac{1}{0.1} = 10 \tag{13.23}$$

The new rule also ensures that associations learned by the network will not be artifacts of noise. Any small random increases will soon decay away.

Figure 13.3 displays the response of the Hebb rule, with and without decay, for the banana recognition example. Without decay, the weight continues to increase by the same amount each time the neuron is activated. When decay is added, the weight exponentially approaches its maximum value ($w_{ij}^{max} = 10$).

To experiment with the Hebb rule with decay, use the Neural Network Design Demonstrations Hebb with Decay(**nnd13hd** *) and Effect of Decay Rate (* **nnd13edr** *).*

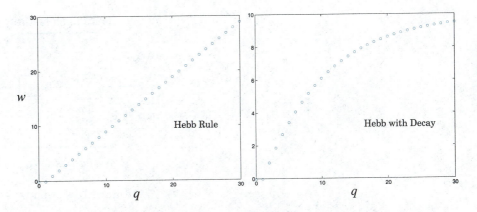

Figure 13.3 Response of the Hebb Rule, With and Without Decay

The Hebb rule with decay does solve the problem of large weights. However, it does so at a price. The environment must be counted on to occasionally present all stimuli that have associations. Without reinforcement, associations will decay away.

To illustrate this fact, consider Eq. (13.18) if $a_i = 0$:

$$w_{ij}(q) = (1 - \gamma) w_{ij}(q-1) .$$
(13.24)

If $\gamma = 0.1$, this reduces to

$$w_{ij}(q) = (0.9) w_{ij}(q-1) .$$
(13.25)

Therefore w_{ij} will be decreased by 10% at each presentation for which $a_i = 0$. Any association that was previously learned will eventually be lost. We will discuss a solution to this problem in a later section.

Simple Recognition Network

Instar So far we have considered only associations between scalar inputs and outputs. We will now examine a neuron that has a vector input. (See Figure 13.4.) This neuron, which is sometimes referred to as an *instar*, is the simplest network that is capable of pattern recognition, as we will demonstrate shortly.

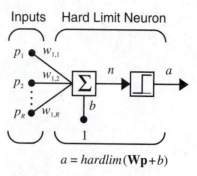

$$a = hardlim(\mathbf{Wp}+b)$$

Figure 13.4 Instar

You will notice the similarities between the instar of Figure 13.4 and the perceptron of Figure 4.2 (also the ADALINE of Figure 10.2 and the linear associator of Figure 7.1). We give these networks different names, in part for historical reasons (since they arose at different times and out of different environments), and because they perform different functions and are analyzed in different ways. For example, we will not directly consider the decision boundary of the instar, although this was an important concept for the perceptron. Instead, we will analyze the ability of the instar to recognize a pattern, as with the neurons in the first layer of the Hamming network. (See page 3-9.)

The input/output expression for the instar is

$$a = hardlim(\mathbf{Wp} + b) = hardlim({}_1\mathbf{w}^T\mathbf{p} + b) .\qquad(13.26)$$

The instar will be active whenever the inner product between the weight vector (row of the weight matrix) and the input is greater than or equal to $-b$:

$$_1\mathbf{w}^T\mathbf{p} \geq -b .\qquad(13.27)$$

From our discussion of the Hamming network on page 3-9, we know that for two vectors of constant length, the inner product will be largest when they point in the same direction. We can also show this using Eq. (5.15):

$$_1\mathbf{w}^T\mathbf{p} = \|_1\mathbf{w}\|\|\mathbf{p}\|\cos\theta \geq -b ,\qquad(13.28)$$

where θ is the angle between the two vectors. Clearly the inner product is maximized when the angle θ is 0. If $\mathbf{p}$ and $_1\mathbf{w}$ have the same length ($\|\mathbf{p}\| = \|_1\mathbf{w}\|$), then the inner product will be largest when $\mathbf{p} = {}_1\mathbf{w}$.

Based on these arguments, the instar of Figure 13.4 will be active when $\mathbf{p}$ is "close" to $_1\mathbf{w}$. By setting the bias b appropriately, we can select how close the input vector must be to the weight vector in order to activate the instar.

If we set

$$b = -\|{}_1\mathbf{w}\|\|\mathbf{p}\|,\tag{13.29}$$

then the instar will only be active when $\mathbf{p}$ points in exactly the same direction as ${}_1\mathbf{w}$ ($\theta = 0$). Thus, we will have a neuron that recognizes only the pattern ${}_1\mathbf{w}$.

If we would like the instar to respond to any pattern near ${}_1\mathbf{w}$ (θ small), then we can increase b to some value larger than $-\|{}_1\mathbf{w}\|\|\mathbf{p}\|$. The larger the value of b, the more patterns there will be that can activate the instar, thus making it the less discriminatory.

We should note that this analysis assumes that all input vectors have the same length (norm). We will revisit the question of normalization in Chapters 14–16.

We can now design a vector recognition network if we know which vector we want to recognize. However, if the network is to learn a vector without supervision, we need a new rule, since neither version of the Hebb rule produces normalized weights.

Instar Rule

One problem of the Hebb rule with decay was that it required stimuli to be repeated or associations would be lost. A better rule might allow weight decay only when the instar is active ($a \neq 0$). Weight values would still be limited, but forgetting would be minimized. Consider again the original Hebb rule:

$$w_{ij}(q) = w_{ij}(q-1) + \alpha a_i(q)\, p_j(q).\tag{13.30}$$

To get the benefits of weight decay, while limiting the forgetting problem, a decay term can be added that is proportional to $a_i(q)$:

$$w_{ij}(q) = w_{ij}(q-1) + \alpha a_i(q)\, p_j(q) - \gamma a_i(q)\, w_{ij}^{old}\tag{13.31}$$

We can simplify Eq. (13.31) by setting γ equal to α (so new weight values are learned at the same rate old values decay) and gathering terms.

$$w_{ij}(q) = w_{ij}(q-1) + \alpha a_i(q)\, (p_j(q) - w_{ij}^{old})\tag{13.32}$$

Instar Rule   This equation, called the *instar rule*, can also be rewritten in vector form:

$${}_i\mathbf{w}(q) = {}_i\mathbf{w}(q-1) + \alpha a_i(q)\, (\mathbf{p}(q) - {}_i\mathbf{w}(q-1)).\tag{13.33}$$

The performance of the instar rule can be best understood if we consider the case where the instar is active ($a_i = 1$). Eq. (13.33) can then be written

$$
\begin{aligned}
{}_i\mathbf{w}(q) &= {}_i\mathbf{w}(q-1) + \alpha\,(\mathbf{p}(q) - {}_i\mathbf{w}(q-1)) \\
&= (1-\alpha)\,{}_i\mathbf{w}(q-1) + \alpha\mathbf{p}(q) \, .
\end{aligned}
\tag{13.34}
$$

This operation is displayed graphically in Figure 13.5.

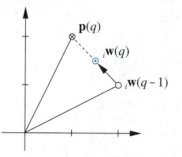

Figure 13.5 Graphical Representation of the Instar Rule

When the instar is active, the weight vector is moved toward the input vector along a line between the old weight vector and the input vector. The distance the weight vector moves depends on the value of α. When $\alpha = 0$, the new weight vector is equal to the old weight vector (no movement). When $\alpha = 1$, the new weight vector is equal to the input vector (maximum movement). If $\alpha = 0.5$, the new weight vector will be halfway between the old weight vector and the input vector.

One useful feature of the instar rule is that if the input vectors are normalized, then ${}_i\mathbf{w}$ will also be normalized once it has learned a particular vector $\mathbf{p}$. We have found a rule that not only minimizes forgetting, but results in normalized weight vectors, if the input vectors are normalized.

Let's apply the instar rule to the network in Figure 13.6. It has two inputs: one indicating whether a fruit has been visually identified as an orange (unconditioned stimulus) and another consisting of the three measurements taken of the fruit (conditioned stimulus).

The output of this network is

$$
a = hardlim\,(w^0 p^0 + \mathbf{W}\mathbf{p} + b) \, .
\tag{13.35}
$$

The elements of input $\mathbf{p}$ will be constrained to ± 1 values, as defined in Chapter 3 (Eq. (3.2)). This constraint ensures that $\mathbf{p}$ is a normalized vector with a length of $\|\mathbf{p}\| = \sqrt{3}$. The definitions of p^0 and $\mathbf{p}$ are

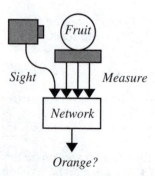

$$p^0 = \begin{cases} 1, & \text{orange detected visually} \\ 0, & \text{orange not detected} \end{cases} \qquad \mathbf{p} = \begin{bmatrix} shape \\ texture \\ weight \end{bmatrix}. \qquad (13.36)$$

The bias b is -2, a value slightly more positive than $-\|\mathbf{p}\|^2 = -3$. (See Eq. (13.29).)

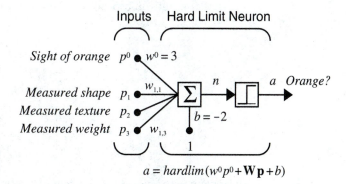

Inputs   Hard Limit Neuron

Sight of orange p^0 $w^0 = 3$

Measured shape p_1 $w_{1,1}$

Measured texture p_2 n a *Orange?*

Measured weight p_3 $w_{1,3}$ $b = -2$

$$a = hardlim(w^0 p^0 + \mathbf{W}\mathbf{p} + b)$$

Figure 13.6 Orange Recognizer

We would like the network to have a constant association between the sight of an orange and its response, so w^0 will be set greater than $-b$. But initially, the network should not respond to any combination of fruit measurements, so the measurement weights will start with values of 0.

$$w^0 = 3, \quad \mathbf{W}(0) = {}_1\mathbf{w}^T(0) = \begin{bmatrix} 0 & 0 & 0 \end{bmatrix} \qquad (13.37)$$

The measurement weights will be updated with the instar rule, using a learning rate of $\alpha = 1$.

$$ {}_1\mathbf{w}(q) = {}_1\mathbf{w}(q-1) + a(q)(\mathbf{p}(q) - {}_1\mathbf{w}(q-1)) \qquad (13.38)$$

The training sequence will consist of repeated presentations of an orange. The measurements will be given every time. However, in order to demonstrate the operation of the instar rule, we will assume that the visual system only operates correctly on even time steps, due to a fault in its construction.

$$\left\{ p^0(1) = 0, \mathbf{p}(1) = \begin{bmatrix} 1 \\ -1 \\ -1 \end{bmatrix} \right\}, \left\{ p^0(2) = 1, \mathbf{p}(2) = \begin{bmatrix} 1 \\ -1 \\ -1 \end{bmatrix} \right\}, \dots \qquad (13.39)$$

Because $\mathbf{W}$ initially contains all zeros, the instar does not respond to the measurements of an orange in the first iteration.

$$a(1) = hardlim(w^0 p^0(1) + \mathbf{W}\mathbf{p}(1) - 2)$$

$$a(1) = hardlim\left(3 \cdot 0 + \begin{bmatrix} 0 & 0 & 0 \end{bmatrix}\begin{bmatrix} 1 \\ -1 \\ -1 \end{bmatrix} - 2\right) = 0 \quad \text{(no response)} \tag{13.40}$$

Since the neuron did not respond, its weights $_1\mathbf{w}$ are not altered by the instar rule.

$$_1\mathbf{w}(1) = {}_1\mathbf{w}(0) + a(1)(\mathbf{p}(1) - {}_1\mathbf{w}(0)) \tag{13.41}$$

$$= \begin{bmatrix} 0 \\ 0 \\ 0 \end{bmatrix} + 0\left(\begin{bmatrix} 1 \\ -1 \\ -1 \end{bmatrix} - \begin{bmatrix} 0 \\ 0 \\ 0 \end{bmatrix}\right) = \begin{bmatrix} 0 \\ 0 \\ 0 \end{bmatrix}$$

However, the neuron does respond when the orange is identified visually, in addition to being measured, in the second iteration.

$$a(2) = hardlim(w^0 p^0(2) + \mathbf{W}\mathbf{p}(2) - 2) \tag{13.42}$$

$$= hardlim\left(3 \cdot 1 + \begin{bmatrix} 0 & 0 & 0 \end{bmatrix}\begin{bmatrix} 1 \\ -1 \\ -1 \end{bmatrix} - 2\right) = 1 \quad \text{(orange)}$$

The result is that the neuron learns to associate the orange's measurement vector with its response. The weight vector $_1\mathbf{w}$ becomes a copy of the orange measurement vector.

$$_1\mathbf{w}(2) = {}_1\mathbf{w}(1) + a(2)(\mathbf{p}(2) - {}_1\mathbf{w}(1)) \tag{13.43}$$

$$= \begin{bmatrix} 0 \\ 0 \\ 0 \end{bmatrix} + 1\left(\begin{bmatrix} 1 \\ -1 \\ -1 \end{bmatrix} - \begin{bmatrix} 0 \\ 0 \\ 0 \end{bmatrix}\right) = \begin{bmatrix} 1 \\ -1 \\ -1 \end{bmatrix}$$

The network can now recognize the orange by its measurements. The neuron responds in the third iteration, even though the visual detection system failed again.

$$a(3) = hardlim(w^0 p^0(3) + \mathbf{W}\mathbf{p}(3) - 2)$$

$$a(3) = hardlim\left(3 \cdot 0 + \begin{bmatrix} 1 & -1 & -1 \end{bmatrix}\begin{bmatrix} 1 \\ -1 \\ -1 \end{bmatrix} - 2\right) = 1 \quad \text{(orange)}$$

(13.44)

13

Having completely learned the measurements, the weights stop changing. (A lower learning rate would have required more iterations.)

$$_1\mathbf{w}(3) = {}_1\mathbf{w}(2) + a(3)(\mathbf{p}(3) - {}_1\mathbf{w}(2))$$

(13.45)

$$= \begin{bmatrix} 1 \\ -1 \\ -1 \end{bmatrix} + 1\left(\begin{bmatrix} 1 \\ -1 \\ -1 \end{bmatrix} - \begin{bmatrix} 1 \\ -1 \\ -1 \end{bmatrix}\right) = \begin{bmatrix} 1 \\ -1 \\ -1 \end{bmatrix}$$

The network has learned to recognize an orange by its measurements, even when its visual detection system fails.

*To experiment with the instar rule, use the Neural Network Design Demonstrations Instar (**nnd13is**) and Graphical Instar (**nnd13gis**).*

Kohonen Rule

Kohonen Rule

At this point it is appropriate to introduce another associative learning rule, which is related to the instar rule. It is the *Kohonen rule*:

$$_1\mathbf{w}(q) = {}_1\mathbf{w}(q-1) + \alpha(\mathbf{p}(q) - {}_1\mathbf{w}(q-1)), \quad \text{for } i \in X(q).$$

(13.46)

Like the instar rule, the Kohonen rule allows the weights of a neuron to learn an input vector and is therefore suitable for recognition applications. Unlike the instar rule, learning is not proportional to the neuron's output $a_i(q)$. Instead, learning occurs when the neuron's index i is a member of the set $X(q)$.

If the instar rule is applied to a layer of neurons whose transfer function only returns values of 0 or 1 (such as *hardlim*), then the Kohonen rule can be made equivalent to the instar rule by defining $X(q)$ as the set of all i such that $a_i(q) = 1$. The advantage of the Kohonen rule is that it can also be used with other definitions. It is useful for training networks such as the self-organizing feature map, which will be introduced in Chapter 14.

Simple Recall Network

Outstar We have seen that the instar network (with a vector input and a scalar output) can perform pattern recognition by associating a particular vector stimulus with a response. The *outstar* network, shown in Figure 13.7, has a scalar input and a vector output. It can perform *pattern recall* by associating a stimulus with a vector response.

The input-output expression for this network is

$$\mathbf{a} = \mathbf{satlins}\,(\mathbf{W}p)\,. \tag{13.47}$$

The symmetric saturating function **satlins** was chosen because this network will be used to recall a vector containing values of –1 or 1.

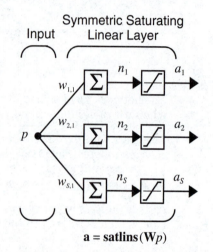

$$\mathbf{a} = \mathbf{satlins}(\mathbf{W}p)$$

Figure 13.7 Outstar Network

If we would like the network to associate a stimulus (an input of 1) with a particular output vector $\mathbf{a}^*$, we can simply set $\mathbf{W}$ (which contains only a single column vector) equal to $\mathbf{a}^*$. Then, if p is 1, the output will be $\mathbf{a}^*$:

$$\mathbf{a} = \mathbf{satlins}\,(\mathbf{W}p) = \mathbf{satlins}\,(\mathbf{a}^* \cdot 1) = \mathbf{a}^*\,. \tag{13.48}$$

(This assumes that the elements of $\mathbf{a}^*$ are less than or equal to 1 in magnitude.)

Note that we have created a recall network by setting a *column* of the weight matrix to the desired vector. Earlier we designed a recognition network by setting a *row* of the weight matrix to the desired vector.

We can now design a network that can recall a known vector $\mathbf{a}^*$, but we need a learning rule if the network is to learn a vector without supervision. We will describe such a learning rule in the next section.

Outstar Rule

To derive the instar rule, forgetting was limited by making the weight decay term of the Hebb rule proportional to the output of the network, a_i. Conversely, to obtain the outstar learning rule, we make the weight decay term proportional to the input of the network, p_j:

$$w_{ij}(q) = w_{ij}(q-1) + \alpha a_i(q) p_j(q) - \gamma p_j(q) w_{ij}(q-1) . \qquad (13.49)$$

If we set the decay rate γ equal to the learning rate α and collect terms, we get

$$w_{ij}(q) = w_{ij}(q-1) + \alpha (a_i(q) - w_{ij}(q-1)) p_j(q) . \qquad (13.50)$$

The outstar rule has properties complimentary to the instar rule. Learning occurs whenever p_j is nonzero (instead of a_i). When learning occurs, column $\mathbf{w}_j$ moves toward the output vector.

Outstar Rule   As with the instar rule, the *outstar rule* can be written in vector form:

$$\mathbf{w}_j(q) = \mathbf{w}_j(q-1) + \alpha (\mathbf{a}(q) - \mathbf{w}_j(q-1)) p_j(q) , \qquad (13.51)$$

where $\mathbf{w}_j$ is the jth column of the matrix $\mathbf{W}$.

To test the outstar rule we will train the network shown in Figure 13.8.

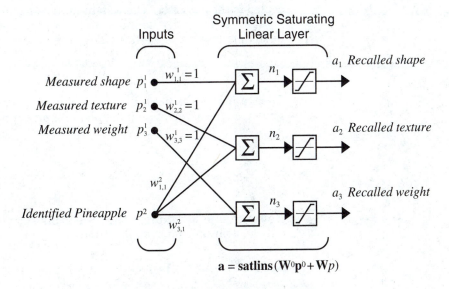

$$\mathbf{a} = \mathbf{satlins}(\mathbf{W}^0 \mathbf{p}^0 + \mathbf{W} p)$$

Figure 13.8 Pineapple Recaller

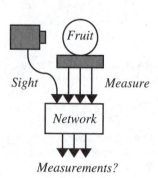

Fruit

Sight   Measure

Network

Measurements?

The outputs of the network are calculated as follows:

$$\mathbf{a} = \mathbf{satlins}\,(\mathbf{W}^0 \mathbf{p}^0 + \mathbf{W}p)\,, \tag{13.52}$$

where

$$\mathbf{W}^0 = \begin{bmatrix} 1 & 0 & 0 \\ 0 & 1 & 0 \\ 0 & 0 & 1 \end{bmatrix}. \tag{13.53}$$

The network's two inputs provide it with measurements $\mathbf{p}^0$ taken on a fruit (unconditioned stimulus), as well as a signal p indicating a pineapple has been identified visually (conditioned stimulus).

$$\mathbf{p}^0 = \begin{bmatrix} shape \\ texture \\ weight \end{bmatrix} \qquad p = \begin{cases} 1, & \text{if a pineapple can be seen} \\ 0, & \text{otherwise} \end{cases} \tag{13.54}$$

The network's output is to reflect the measurements of the fruit currently being examined, using whatever inputs are available.

The weight matrix for the unconditioned stimulus, $\mathbf{W}^0$, is set to the identity matrix, so that any set of measurements $\mathbf{p}^0$ (with ±1 values) will be copied to the output $\mathbf{a}$. The weight matrix for the conditioned stimulus, $\mathbf{W}$, is set to zero initially, so that a 1 on p will not generate a response. $\mathbf{W}$ will be updated with the outstar rule using a learning rate of 1:

$$\mathbf{w}_j\,(q) = \mathbf{w}_j\,(q-1) + (\mathbf{a}\,(q) - \mathbf{w}_j\,(q-1))\,p\,(q)\,. \tag{13.55}$$

The training sequence will consist of repeated presentations of the sight and measurements of a pineapple. The pineapple measurements are

$$\mathbf{p}^{pineapple} = \begin{bmatrix} -1 \\ -1 \\ 1 \end{bmatrix}. \tag{13.56}$$

However, due to a fault in the measuring system, measured values will only be available on even iterations.

$$\left\{ \mathbf{p}^0\,(1) = \begin{bmatrix} 0 \\ 0 \\ 0 \end{bmatrix}, p\,(1) = 1 \right\}, \left\{ \mathbf{p}^0\,(2) = \begin{bmatrix} -1 \\ -1 \\ 1 \end{bmatrix}, p\,(2) = 1 \right\}, \ldots \tag{13.57}$$

In the first iteration, the pineapple is seen, but the measurements are unavailable.

$$a(1) = \mathbf{satlins}(W^0 p^0(1) + Wp(1)), \quad (13.58)$$

$$a(1) = \mathbf{satlins}\left(\begin{bmatrix} 0 \\ 0 \\ 0 \end{bmatrix} + \begin{bmatrix} 0 \\ 0 \\ 0 \end{bmatrix} 1\right) = \begin{bmatrix} 0 \\ 0 \\ 0 \end{bmatrix} \quad \text{(no response)} \quad (13.59)$$

The network sees the pineapple but cannot output proper measurements, because it has not learned them and the measurement system is not working. The weights remain unchanged after being updated.

$$\mathbf{w}_1(1) = \mathbf{w}_1(0) + (a(1) - \mathbf{w}_1(0))p(1) = \begin{bmatrix} 0 \\ 0 \\ 0 \end{bmatrix} + \left(\begin{bmatrix} 0 \\ 0 \\ 0 \end{bmatrix} - \begin{bmatrix} 0 \\ 0 \\ 0 \end{bmatrix}\right) 1 = \begin{bmatrix} 0 \\ 0 \\ 0 \end{bmatrix} \quad (13.60)$$

In the second iteration the pineapple is seen, and the measurements are taken properly.

$$a(2) = \mathbf{satlins}\left(\begin{bmatrix} -1 \\ -1 \\ 1 \end{bmatrix} + \begin{bmatrix} 0 \\ 0 \\ 0 \end{bmatrix} 1\right) = \begin{bmatrix} -1 \\ -1 \\ 1 \end{bmatrix} \quad \text{(measurements given)} \quad (13.61)$$

The measurements are available, so the network outputs them correctly. The weights are then updated as follows:

$$\mathbf{w}_1(2) = \mathbf{w}_1(1) + (a(2) - \mathbf{w}_1(1))p(2)$$

$$= \begin{bmatrix} 0 \\ 0 \\ 0 \end{bmatrix} + \left(\begin{bmatrix} -1 \\ -1 \\ 1 \end{bmatrix} - \begin{bmatrix} 0 \\ 0 \\ 0 \end{bmatrix}\right) 1 = \begin{bmatrix} -1 \\ -1 \\ 1 \end{bmatrix}. \quad (13.62)$$

Since the sight of the pineapple and the measurements were both available, the network forms an association between them. The weight matrix is now a copy of the measurements, so they can be recalled later.

In iteration three, measurements are unavailable once again, but the output is

$$\mathbf{a}(3) = \mathbf{satlins}\left(\begin{bmatrix} 0 \\ 0 \\ 0 \end{bmatrix} + \begin{bmatrix} -1 \\ -1 \\ 1 \end{bmatrix} 1\right) = \begin{bmatrix} -1 \\ -1 \\ 1 \end{bmatrix} \quad \text{(measurements recalled)}. \quad (13.63)$$

The network is now able to recall the measurements of the pineapple when it sees it, even though the measurement system fails. From now on, the weights will no longer change values unless a pineapple is seen with different measurements.

$$\mathbf{w}_1(3) = \mathbf{w}_1(2) + (\mathbf{a}(2) - \mathbf{w}_1(2))\,p(2)$$

$$= \begin{bmatrix} -1 \\ -1 \\ 1 \end{bmatrix} + \left(\begin{bmatrix} -1 \\ -1 \\ 1 \end{bmatrix} - \begin{bmatrix} -1 \\ -1 \\ 1 \end{bmatrix}\right) 1 = \begin{bmatrix} -1 \\ -1 \\ 1 \end{bmatrix} \quad (13.64)$$

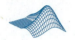

*To experiment with the outstar rule with decay, use the Neural Network Design Demonstration Outstar Rule (**nnd13os**).*

In Chapter 16 we will investigate the ART networks, which use both the instar and the outstar rules.

Summary of Results

Association

An association is a link between the inputs and outputs of a network so that when a stimulus A is presented to the network, it will output a response B.

Associative Learning Rules

Unsupervised Hebb Rule

$$\mathbf{W}(q) = \mathbf{W}(q-1) + \alpha\mathbf{a}(q)\mathbf{p}^T(q)$$

Hebb Rule with Decay

$$\mathbf{W}(q) = (1-\gamma)\mathbf{W}(q-1) + \alpha\mathbf{a}(q)\mathbf{p}^T(q)$$

Instar

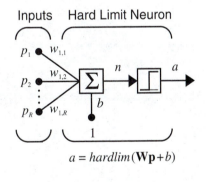

Inputs   Hard Limit Neuron

$$a = hardlim(\mathbf{W}\mathbf{p}+b)$$

$$a = hardlim({}_1\mathbf{w}^T\mathbf{p} + b)$$

The instar is activated for ${}_1\mathbf{w}^T\mathbf{p} = \|{}_1\mathbf{w}\|\|\mathbf{p}\|\cos\theta \geq -b$,

where θ is the angle between $\mathbf{p}$ and ${}_1\mathbf{w}$.

Instar Rule

$${}_i\mathbf{w}(q) = {}_i\mathbf{w}(q-1) + \alpha a_i(q)(\mathbf{p}(q) - {}_i\mathbf{w}(q-1))$$

$${}_i\mathbf{w}(q) = (1-\alpha)\mathbf{w}(q-1) + \alpha\mathbf{p}(q), \quad if\ (a_i(q) = 1)$$

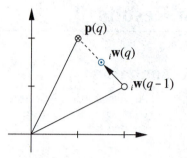

Graphical Representation of the Instar Rule ($a_i(q) = 1$)

Kohonen Rule

$$_i\mathbf{w}(q) = \mathbf{w}(q-1) + \alpha(\mathbf{p}(q) - \mathbf{w}(q-1)), \quad \text{for } i \in X(q)$$

Outstar

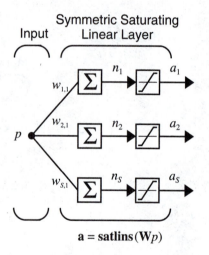

$$\mathbf{a} = \mathbf{satlins}(\mathbf{W}p)$$

Outstar Rule

$$\mathbf{w}_j(q) = \mathbf{w}_j(q-1) + \alpha(\mathbf{a}(q) - \mathbf{w}_j(q-1))p_j(q)$$

Solved Problems

P13.1 **In Eq. (13.19) the maximum weight for the Hebb rule with decay was calculated, assuming that p_j and a_i were 1 at every time step. Calculate the maximum weight resulting if p_j and a_i alternate together between values of 0 and 1.**

13

We begin with the scalar version of the Hebb rule with decay:

$$w_{ij}(q) = (1 - \gamma) w_{ij}(q - 1) + \alpha a_i(q) p_j(q) .$$

We can rewrite this expression twice using q to index the weight values as the weight is updated over two time steps.

$$w_{ij}(q + 1) = (1 - \gamma) w_{ij}(q) + \alpha a_i(q) p_j(q)$$

$$w_{ij}(q + 2) = (1 - \gamma) w_{ij}(q + 1) + \alpha a_i(q + 1) p_j(q + 1)$$

By substituting the first equation into the second, we get a single expression showing how w_{ij} is updated over two time steps.

$$w_{ij}(q + 2) = (1 - \gamma) ((1 - \gamma) w_{ij}(q) + \alpha a_i(q) p_j(q)) + \alpha a_i(q + 1) p_j(q + 1)$$

At this point we can substitute values for p_j and a_i. Because we are looking for a maximum weight, we will set $p_j(q)$ and $a_i(q)$ to 0, and $p_j(q + 1)$ and $a_i(q + 1)$ to 1. This will mean that the weight decreases in the first time step, and increases in the second, ensuring that $w_{ij}(q + 2)$ is the maximum of the two weights. If we solve for $w_{ij}(q + 2)$, we obtain

$$w_{ij}(q + 2) = (1 - \gamma)^2 w_{ij}(q) + \alpha .$$

Assuming that w_{ij} will eventually reach a steady state value, we can find it by setting both $w_{ij}(q + 2)$ and $w_{ij}(q)$ equal to w_{ij}^{max} and solving

$$w_{ij}^{max} = (1 - \gamma)^2 w_{ij}^{max} + \alpha ,$$

$$w_{ij}^{max} = \frac{\alpha}{2\gamma - \gamma^2} .$$

We can use MATLAB to make a plot of this relationship. The plot will show learning rates and decay rates at intervals of 0.025.

```
lr = 0:0.025:1;
dr = 0.025:0.025:1;
```

Here are the commands for creating a mesh plot of the maximum weight, as a function of the learning and decay rate values.

```
[LR,DR] = meshgrid(dr,lr);
MW = LR ./ (DR .* (2 - DR));
mesh(DR,LR,MW);
```

The plot shows that w_{ij}^{max} approaches infinity as the decay rate γ becomes small with respect to the learning rate α (see Figure P13.1).

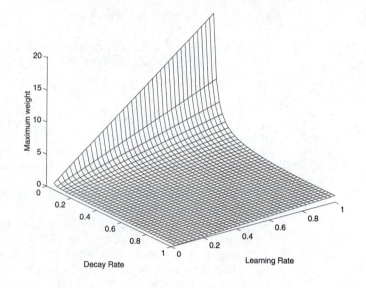

Figure P13.1 Maximum Weight w_{ij}^{max}

P13.2 **Retrain the orange recognition network on page 13-13 using the instar rule with a learning rate of 0.4. Use the same training sequence. How many time steps are required for the network to learn to recognize an orange by its measurements?**

Here is the training sequence. It is to be repeated until the network can respond to the orange measurements ($\mathbf{p} = \begin{bmatrix} 1 & -1 & -1 \end{bmatrix}^T$), even when the visual detection system fails ($p^0 = 0$).

$$\left\{ p^0(1) = 0, \mathbf{p}(1) = \begin{bmatrix} 1 \\ -1 \\ -1 \end{bmatrix} \right\}, \left\{ p^0(2) = 1, \mathbf{p}(2) = \begin{bmatrix} 1 \\ -1 \\ -1 \end{bmatrix} \right\}, \dots$$

We will use MATLAB to make the calculations. These two lines of code set the weights to their initial values.

```
w0 = 3;
W = [0 0 0];
```

We can then simulate the first time step of the network.

```
p0 = 0;
p = [1; -1; -1];
a = hardlim(w0*p0+W*p-2)
a =
        0
```

The neuron does not yet recognize the orange, so its output is 0. The weights do not change when updated with the instar rule.

```
W = W + 0.4*a*(p'-W)
W =
        0 0 0
```

The neuron begins learning the measurements in the second iteration.

```
p0 = 1;
p = [1; -1; -1];
a = hardlim(w0*p0+W*p-2)
a =
        1

W = W + 0.4*a*(p'-W)
W =
        0.4000 -0.4000 -0.4000
```

But the association is still not strong enough for a response in the third iteration.

```
p0 = 0;
p = [1; -1; -1];
a = hardlim(w0*p0+W*p-2)
a =
        0

W = W + 0.4*a*(p'-W)
W =
        0.4000 -0.4000 -0.4000
```

Here are the results of the fourth iteration:

```
a =
     1
W =
     0.6400 -0.6400 -0.6400
```

the fifth iteration:

```
a =
     0
W =
     0.6400 -0.6400 -0.6400
```

and the sixth iteration:

```
a =
     1
W =
     0.7840 -0.7840 -0.7840 .
```

By the seventh iteration the network is able to recognize the orange by its measurements alone.

```
p0 = 0;
p = [1; -1; -1];
a = hardlim(w0*p0+W*p-2)
a =
     1

W = W + 0.4*a*(p'-W)
W =
     0.8704 -0.8704 -0.8704
```

Due to the lower learning rate, the network had to experience the measurements paired with its response three times (the even numbered iterations) before it developed a strong association between them.

P13.3 **Both the recognition and recall networks used in this chapter's examples could only learn a single vector. Draw the diagram and determine the parameters of a network capable of recognizing and responding to the following two vectors:**

$$\mathbf{p}_1 = \begin{bmatrix} 5 \\ -5 \\ 5 \end{bmatrix} \qquad \mathbf{p}_2 = \begin{bmatrix} -5 \\ 5 \\ 5 \end{bmatrix} .$$

The network should only respond when an input vector is identical to one of these vectors.

We know the network must have three inputs, because it must recognize three-element vectors. We also know that it will have two outputs, one output for each response.

Such a network can be obtained by combining two instars into a single layer, as in Figure P13.2.

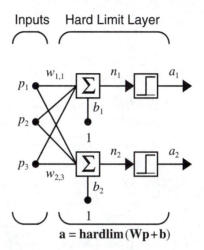

Figure P13.2 Two-Vector Recognition Network

We now set the weights $_1\mathbf{w}$ of the first neuron equal to $\mathbf{p}_1$, so that its net input will be at a maximum when an input vector points in the same direction as $\mathbf{p}_1$. Likewise, we will set $_2\mathbf{w}$ to $\mathbf{p}_2$ so that the second neuron is most sensitive to vectors in the direction of $\mathbf{p}_2$.

Combining the weight vectors gives us the weight matrix

$$\mathbf{W} = \begin{bmatrix} _1\mathbf{w}^T \\ _2\mathbf{w}^T \end{bmatrix} = \begin{bmatrix} \mathbf{p}_1^T \\ \mathbf{p}_2^T \end{bmatrix} = \begin{bmatrix} 5 & -5 & 5 \\ -5 & 5 & 5 \end{bmatrix}.$$

(Note that this is the same manner in which we determined the weight matrix for the first layer of the Hamming network. In fact, the first layer of the Hamming network is a layer of instars. More about that in the next chapter.)

The lengths of $\mathbf{p}_1$ and $\mathbf{p}_2$ are the same:

$$\|\mathbf{p}_1\| = \|\mathbf{p}_2\| = \sqrt{(5)^2 + (-5)^2 + (5)^2} = \sqrt{75}.$$

To ensure that only an exact match between an input vector and a stored vector results in a response, both biases are set as follows (Eq. (13.29)):

$$b_1 = b_2 = -\|\mathbf{p}_1\|^2 = -75.$$

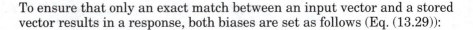

We can use MATLAB to test that the network does indeed respond to $\mathbf{p}_1$.

```
W = [5 -5 5; -5 5 5];
b = [-75; -75];
p1 = [5; -5; 5];
a = hardlim(W*p1+b)
a =

        1
        0
```

The first neuron responded, indicating that the input vector was $\mathbf{p}_1$. The second neuron did not respond, because the input was not $\mathbf{p}_2$.

We can also check that the network does not respond to a third vector $\mathbf{p}_3$ that is not equal to either of the stored vectors.

```
p3 = [-5; 5; -5];
a = hardlim(W*p3+b)
a =

        0


        0
```

Neither neuron recognizes this new vector, so they both output 0.

P13.4 **A single instar is being used for pattern recognition. Its weights and bias have the following values:**

$$\mathbf{W} = {}_1\mathbf{w}^T = \begin{bmatrix} 1 & -1 & -1 \end{bmatrix} \qquad b = -2.$$

How close must an input vector (with a magnitude of $\sqrt{3}$) be to the weight vector for the neuron to output a 1? Find a vector that occurs on the border between those vectors that are recognized and those vectors that are not.

We begin by writing the expression for the neuron's output.

$$a = hardlim\,({}_1\mathbf{w}^T\mathbf{p} + b)$$

According to the definition of *hardlim*, a will be 1 if and only if the inner product between ${}_1\mathbf{w}^T$ and $\mathbf{p}$ is greater than or equal to $-b$ (Eq. (13.28)):

$$_1\mathbf{w}^T\mathbf{p} = \|_1\mathbf{w}\|\|\mathbf{p}\|\cos\theta \geq -b\,.$$

We can find the maximum angle between $_1\mathbf{w}$ and $\mathbf{p}$ that meets this condition by substituting for the norms and solving

$$(\sqrt{3})\,(\sqrt{3})\,\cos\theta \geq 2$$

$$\theta \leq \cos^{-1}\!\left(\frac{2}{3}\right) = 48.19°\,.$$

To find a borderline vector with magnitude $\sqrt{3}$, we need a vector $\mathbf{p}$ that meets the following conditions:

$$\|\mathbf{p}_1\| = \sqrt{p_1^2 + p_2^2 + p_3^2} = \sqrt{3}\,,$$

$$_1\mathbf{w}^T\mathbf{p} = w_1 p_1 + w_2 p_2 + w_3 p_3 - b = p_1 - p_2 - p_3 - 2 = 0\,.$$

Since we have three variables and only two constraints, we can set the third variable p_1 to 0 and solve

$$\sqrt{p_1^2 + p_2^2 + p_3^2} = \sqrt{3} \quad\Rightarrow\quad p_2^2 + p_3^2 = 3\,,$$

$$p_1 - p_2 - p_3 - 2 \quad\Rightarrow\quad p_2 + p_3 = -2\,,$$

$$(p_2 + p_3)^2 = p_2^2 + p_3^2 + 2p_2 p_3 = (-2)^2 = 4\,,$$

$$3 + 2p_2 p_3 = 4 \quad\Rightarrow\quad p_2 p_3 = 0.5\,,$$

$$p_2(p_2 + p_3) = p_2^2 + p_2 p_3 = p_2^2 + 0.5 = p_2(-2) = -2p_2\,.$$

After a little work we find that there are two possible values for p_2:

$$p_2^2 + 2p_2 + 0.5 = 0\,,$$

$$p_2 = -1 \pm \sqrt{0.5}\,.$$

It turns out that if we pick p_2 to be one of these values, then p_3 will take on the other value.

$$p_2 + p_3 = -1 \pm \sqrt{0.5} + p_3 = -2$$

$$p_3 = -1 \mp \sqrt{0.5}$$

Therefore, the following vector **p** is just the right distance from **w** to be recognized.

$$\mathbf{p} = \begin{bmatrix} 0 \\ -1 + \sqrt{0.5} \\ -1 - \sqrt{0.5} \end{bmatrix}$$

We can test it by presenting it to the network.

$$a = hardlim\,(\,_1\mathbf{w}^T\mathbf{p} + b)$$

$$a = hardlim\left(\begin{bmatrix} 1 & -1 & -1 \end{bmatrix} \begin{bmatrix} 0 \\ -1 + \sqrt{0.5} \\ -1 - \sqrt{0.5} \end{bmatrix} - 2 \right)$$

$$a = hardlim\,(0) = 1$$

The vector **p** does indeed result in a net input of 0 and is therefore on the boundary of the instar's active region.

P13.5 **Consider the instar network shown in Figure P13.3. The training sequence for this network will consist of the following inputs:**

$$\left\{ p^0\,(1) = 0,\, \mathbf{p}\,(1) = \begin{bmatrix} -1 \\ 1 \end{bmatrix} \right\},\ \left\{ p^0\,(2) = 1,\, \mathbf{p}\,(2) = \begin{bmatrix} -1 \\ 1 \end{bmatrix} \right\},\ \dots.$$

These two sets of inputs are repeatedly presented to the network until the weight matrix W converges.

   i. **Perform the first four iterations of the instar rule, with learning rate $\alpha = 0.5$. Assume that the initial W matrix is set to all zeros.**

   ii. **Display the results of each iteration of the instar rule in graphical form (as in Figure 13.5).**

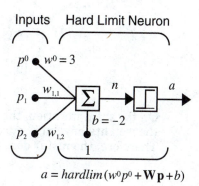

Inputs   Hard Limit Neuron

$$a = hardlim\,(w^0 p^0 + \mathbf{W} \mathbf{p} + b)$$

Figure P13.3 Instar Network for Problem P13.5

i. Because **W** initially contains all zeros, the instar does not respond to the measurements in the first iteration.

$$a\,(1) = hardlim\,(w^0 p^0\,(1) + \mathbf{W} \mathbf{p}\,(1) - 2)$$

$$a\,(1) = hardlim\left(3 \cdot 0 + \begin{bmatrix} 0 & 0 \end{bmatrix}\begin{bmatrix} -1 \\ 1 \end{bmatrix} - 2\right) = 0$$

The neuron did not respond. Therefore its weights $_1\mathbf{w}$ are not altered by the instar rule.

$$_1\mathbf{w}\,(1) \;=\; _1\mathbf{w}\,(0) + 0.5a\,(1)\,(\mathbf{p}\,(1) - {_1\mathbf{w}}\,(0))$$

$$= \begin{bmatrix} 0 \\ 0 \end{bmatrix} + 0\left(\begin{bmatrix} -1 \\ 1 \end{bmatrix} - \begin{bmatrix} 0 \\ 0 \end{bmatrix}\right) = \begin{bmatrix} 0 \\ 0 \end{bmatrix}$$

Because the unconditioned stimulus appears on the second iteration, the instar does respond.

$$a\,(2) = hardlim\,(w^0 p^0\,(2) + \mathbf{W} \mathbf{p}\,(2) - 2)$$

$$a\,(2) = hardlim\left(3 \cdot 1 + \begin{bmatrix} 0 & 0 \end{bmatrix}\begin{bmatrix} -1 \\ 1 \end{bmatrix} - 2\right) = 1$$

The neuron did respond, and its weights $_1\mathbf{w}$ are updated by the instar rule.

$$_1\mathbf{w}(2) = {}_1\mathbf{w}(1) + 0.5a(2)(\mathbf{p}(2) - {}_1\mathbf{w}(1))$$

$$= \begin{bmatrix} 0 \\ 0 \end{bmatrix} + 0.5\left(\begin{bmatrix} -1 \\ 1 \end{bmatrix} - \begin{bmatrix} 0 \\ 0 \end{bmatrix}\right) = \begin{bmatrix} -0.5 \\ 0.5 \end{bmatrix}$$

On the third iteration, the unconditioned stimulus is not presented, and the weights have not yet converged close enough to the input pattern. Therefore, the instar does not respond.

$$a(3) = hardlim(w^0 p^0(3) + \mathbf{W}\mathbf{p}(3) - 2)$$

$$a(3) = hardlim\left(3 \cdot 0 + \begin{bmatrix} -0.5 & 0.5 \end{bmatrix}\begin{bmatrix} -1 \\ 1 \end{bmatrix} - 2\right) = 0$$

Since the neuron did not respond, its weights are not updated.

$$_1\mathbf{w}(3) = {}_1\mathbf{w}(2) + 0.5a(3)(\mathbf{p}(3) - {}_1\mathbf{w}(2))$$

$$= \begin{bmatrix} -0.5 \\ 0.5 \end{bmatrix} + 0\left(\begin{bmatrix} -1 \\ 1 \end{bmatrix} - \begin{bmatrix} -0.5 \\ 0.5 \end{bmatrix}\right) = \begin{bmatrix} -0.5 \\ 0.5 \end{bmatrix}$$

Because the unconditioned stimulus again appears on the fourth iteration, the instar does respond.

$$a(4) = hardlim(w^0 p^0(4) + \mathbf{W}\mathbf{p}(4) - 2)$$

$$a(4) = hardlim\left(3 \cdot 1 + \begin{bmatrix} -0.5 & 0.5 \end{bmatrix}\begin{bmatrix} -1 \\ 1 \end{bmatrix} - 2\right) = 1$$

Since the instar was activated, its weights are updated.

$$_1\mathbf{w}(4) = {}_1\mathbf{w}(3) + 0.5a(4)(\mathbf{p}(4) - {}_1\mathbf{w}(3))$$

$$= \begin{bmatrix} -0.5 \\ 0.5 \end{bmatrix} + 0.5\left(\begin{bmatrix} -1 \\ 1 \end{bmatrix} - \begin{bmatrix} -0.5 \\ 0.5 \end{bmatrix}\right) = \begin{bmatrix} -0.75 \\ 0.75 \end{bmatrix}$$

This completes the fourth iteration. If we continue this process, $_1\mathbf{w}$ will converge to $\mathbf{p}$.

ii. Note that the weights are only updated (instar active) on iterations 2 and 4. Recall from Eq. (13.34) that when the instar is active, the learning rule can be written

$$_1\mathbf{w}(q) = {}_1\mathbf{w}(q-1) + \alpha(\mathbf{p}(q) - {}_1\mathbf{w}(q-1)) = (1-\alpha){}_1\mathbf{w}(q-1) + \alpha\mathbf{p}(q).$$

13

When the instar is active, the weight vector is moved toward the input vector along a line between the old weight vector and the input vector. Figure P13.4 displays the movement of the weight vector for this problem. The weights were updated on iterations 2 and 4. Because $\alpha = 0.5$, whenever the instar is active the weight vector moves halfway from its current position toward the input vector.

$$_1\mathbf{w}(q) = (0.5){}_1\mathbf{w}(q-1) + (0.5)\mathbf{p}(q)$$

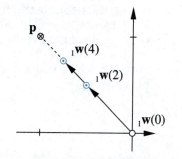

Figure P13.4 Instar Rule Example

Epilogue

In this chapter we introduced some simple networks capable of forming associations. We also developed and studied several learning rules that allowed networks to create new associations. Each rule operated by strengthening an association between any stimulus and response that occurred simultaneously.

The simple associative networks and learning rules developed in this chapter are useful in themselves, but they are also important building blocks for more powerful networks. In this chapter we introduced two networks, and associated learning rules, that will be fundamental for the development of important networks in the next three chapters: the instar and the outstar. The instar is a network that is trained to *recognize* a pattern. The outstar is a network that is trained to *recall* a pattern. We will use layers of instars in Chapters 14 and 15 to perform pattern recognition. These networks are very similar to the Hamming network of Chapter 3, whose first layer was, in fact, a layer of instars. In Chapter 16 we will introduce a more complex network, which combines both instars and outstars in order to produce stable learning.

Further Reading

[Ande72]   J. Anderson, "A simple neural network generating an interactive memory," *Mathematical Biosciences*, vol. 14, pp. 197–220, 1972.

Anderson has proposed a "linear associator" model for associative memory. The model was trained, using a generalization of the Hebb postulate, to learn an association between input and output vectors. The physiological plausibility of the network was emphasized. Kohonen published a closely related paper at the same time [Koho72], although the two researchers were working independently.

[Gros68]   S. Grossberg, "Some physiological and biochemical consequences of psychological postulates," *Proceedings of the National Academy of Sciences*, vol. 60, pp. 758–765, 1968.

This article describes early mathematical models (nonlinear differential equations) of associative learning. It synthesizes psychological, mathematical and physiological ideas.

[Gros82]   S. Grossberg, *Studies of Mind and Brain*, Boston: D. Reidel Publishing Co., 1982.

This book is a collection of Stephen Grossberg papers from the period 1968 through 1980. It covers many of the fundamental concepts which are used in later Grossberg networks, such as the Adaptive Resonance Theory networks.

[Hebb49]   D. O. Hebb, *The Organization of Behavior*, New York: Wiley, 1949.

The main premise of this seminal book was that behavior could be explained by the action of neurons. In it, Hebb proposed one of the first learning laws, which postulated a mechanism for learning at the cellular level.

[Koho72]   T. Kohonen, "Correlation matrix memories," *IEEE Transactions on Computers*, vol. 21, pp. 353–359, 1972.

Kohonen proposed a correlation matrix model for associative memory. The model was trained, using the outer product rule (also known as the Hebb rule), to learn an association between input and output vectors. The mathematical structure of the network was emphasized. Anderson published a closely related paper at the same time [Ande72], although the two researchers were working independently.

13

[Koho87]   T. Kohonen, *Self-Organization and Associative Memory*, 2nd Ed., Berlin: Springer-Verlag, 1987.

This book introduces the Kohonen rule and several networks that use it. It provides a complete analysis of linear associative models and gives many extensions and examples.

[Leib90]   D. Lieberman, *Learning, Behavior and Cognition*, Belmont, CA: Wadsworth, 1990.

Leiberman's text forms an excellent introduction to behavioral psychology. This field is of interest to anyone looking to model human (or animal) learning with neural networks.

Exercises

E13.1 The network shown in Figure E13.1 is to be trained using the Hebb rule with decay, using a learning rate α of 0.3 and a decay rate γ of 0.1.

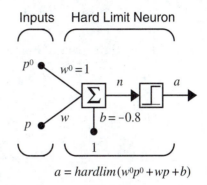

$$a = hardlim(w^0 p^0 + wp + b)$$

Figure E13.1 Associative Network

i. If w is initially set to 0, and w^0 and b remain constant (with the values shown in Figure E13.1), how many consecutive presentations of the following training set are required before the neuron will respond to the test set? Make a plot of w versus iteration number.

Training set: $\{p^0 = 1, p = 1\}$ Test set: $\{p^0 = 0, p = 1\}$

ii. Assume that w has an initial value of 1. How many consecutive presentations of the following training set are required before the neuron will no longer be able to respond to the test set? Make a plot of w versus iteration number.

Training set: $\{p^0 = 0, p = 0\}$ Test set: $\{p^0 = 0, p = 1\}$

E13.2 For Exercise E13.1 part (i), use Eq. (13.19) to determine the steady state value of w. Verify that this answer agrees with your plot from Exercise E13.1 part (i).

E13.3 Repeat Exercise E13.1, but this time use the Hebb rule without decay ($\gamma = 0$).

E13.4 The following rule looks similar to the instar rule, but it behaves quite differently:

$$\Delta w_{ij} = -\alpha a_i (p_j + w_{ij}^{old})$$

   i. Determine the conditions under which the Δw_{ij} is nonzero.

   ii. What value does the weight approach when Δw_{ij} is nonzero?

   iii. Can you think of a use for this rule?

E13.5 The instar shown in Figure E13.2 is to be used to recognize a vector.

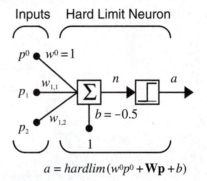

Figure E13.2 Vector Recognizer

   i. Train the network with the instar rule on the following training sequence. Apply the instar rule to the second input's weights only (which should be initialized to zeros), using a learning rate of 0.6. The other weight and the bias are to remain constant at the values in the figure. (You may wish to use MATLAB to perform the calculations.)

$$\left\{ p^0(1) = 1, \mathbf{p}(1) = \begin{bmatrix} 0.174 \\ 0.985 \end{bmatrix} \right\} \quad \left\{ p^0(2) = 0, \mathbf{p}(2) = \begin{bmatrix} -0.174 \\ 0.985 \end{bmatrix} \right\}$$

$$\left\{ p^0(3) = 1, \mathbf{p}(3) = \begin{bmatrix} 0.174 \\ 0.985 \end{bmatrix} \right\} \quad \left\{ p^0(4) = 0, \mathbf{p}(4) = \begin{bmatrix} -0.174 \\ 0.985 \end{bmatrix} \right\}$$

$$\left\{ p^0(5) = 1, \mathbf{p}(5) = \begin{bmatrix} 0.174 \\ 0.985 \end{bmatrix} \right\} \quad \left\{ p^0(6) = 0, \mathbf{p}(6) = \begin{bmatrix} -0.174 \\ 0.985 \end{bmatrix} \right\}$$

   ii. What were your final values for $\mathbf{W}$?

   iii. How do these final values compare with the vectors in the training sequence?

iv. What magnitude would you expect the weights to have after training, if the network were trained for many more iterations of the same training sequence?

13

E13.6 Consider the instar network shown in Figure E13.3. The training sequence for this network will consist of the following inputs:

$$\left\{ p^0(1) = 0, \mathbf{p}(1) = \begin{bmatrix} 1 \\ -1 \end{bmatrix} \right\}, \left\{ p^0(2) = 1, \mathbf{p}(2) = \begin{bmatrix} 1 \\ -1 \end{bmatrix} \right\}, \dots$$

These two sets of inputs are repeatedly presented to the network until the weight matrix **W** converges.

    i. Perform the first eight iterations of the instar rule, with learning rate $\alpha = 0.25$. Assume that the initial **W** matrix is set to

$$\mathbf{W} = \begin{bmatrix} 1 & 0 \end{bmatrix}.$$

    ii. Display the results of each iteration of the instar rule in graphical form (as in Figure 13.5).

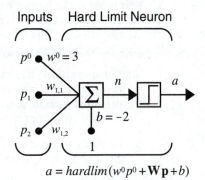

$$a = hardlim(w^0 p^0 + \mathbf{W}\mathbf{p} + b)$$

Figure E13.3 Instar Network for Exercise E13.6

E13.7 Draw a diagram of a network capable of recalling three different four-element vectors (of ±1 values) when given different stimuli (of value 1).

    i. How many inputs does your network have? How many outputs? What transfer function did you use?

    ii. Choose values for the network's weights so that it can recall each of the following vectors:

$$\mathbf{p}_1 = \begin{bmatrix} 1 \\ -1 \\ 1 \\ -1 \end{bmatrix} \qquad \mathbf{p}_2 = \begin{bmatrix} -1 \\ -1 \\ 1 \\ -1 \end{bmatrix} \qquad \mathbf{p}_3 = \begin{bmatrix} 1 \\ -1 \\ -1 \\ 1 \end{bmatrix}$$

   iii. Choose an appropriate value for the biases. Explain your choice.

   iv. Test the network with one of the vectors above. Was its response correct?

   v. Test the network with the following vector.

$$\mathbf{p}_1 = \begin{bmatrix} -1 \\ -1 \\ 1 \\ 1 \end{bmatrix}$$

Why did it respond the way it did?

E13.8 This chapter included an example of a recognition network that initially used a visual system to identify oranges. At first the network needed the visual system to tell it when an orange was present, but eventually it learned to recognize oranges from sensor measurements.

   i. Let us replace the visual system with a person. Initially, the network would depend on a person to tell it when an orange was present. Would you consider the network to be learning in a supervised or unsupervised manner?

   ii. In what ways would the input from a person resemble the targets used to train supervised networks in earlier chapters?

   iii. In what ways would it differ?

E13.9 The network shown in Figure E13.4 is installed in an elevator used by three senior executives in a plush high-security corporate building. It has buttons marked '1' through '4' for four floors above the ground floor. When an executive enters the elevator on the ground floor, it determines which person it is with a retinal scan, and then uses the network to select the floor where that person is most likely to go to. If the guess is incorrect, the person can push a different button at any time, but if the network is correct, it will save an important executive the effort of pushing a button.

13

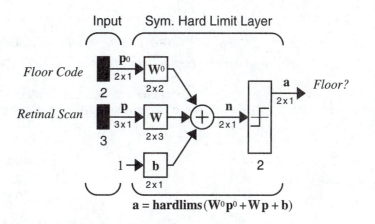

Input Sym. Hard Limit Layer

$$a = \text{hardlims}(W^0 p^0 + W p + b)$$

Figure E13.4 Elevator Network

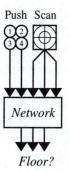

The network's input/output function is

$$a = \text{hardlims}(W^0 p^0 + W p + b).$$

The first input p^0 provides the network with a floor code, if a button has been pushed.

$$p_1^0 = \begin{bmatrix} -1 \\ -1 \end{bmatrix} \text{ (1st floor)} \quad p_2^0 = \begin{bmatrix} 1 \\ -1 \end{bmatrix} \text{ (2nd floor)}$$

$$p_3^0 = \begin{bmatrix} -1 \\ 1 \end{bmatrix} \text{ (3rd floor)} \quad p_4^0 = \begin{bmatrix} 1 \\ 1 \end{bmatrix} \text{ (4th floor)}$$

If no button is pushed, then no code is given.

$$p_0^0 = \begin{bmatrix} 0 \\ 0 \end{bmatrix} \text{ (no button pushed)}$$

The first input is weighted with an identity matrix, and the biases are set to –0.5, so that if a button is pushed the network will respond with its code.

$$W^0 = I, \ b = \begin{bmatrix} -0.5 \\ -0.5 \end{bmatrix}$$

The second input is always available. It consists of three elements that represent the three executives:

$$\mathbf{p}_1 = \begin{bmatrix} 1 \\ 0 \\ 0 \end{bmatrix} \text{ (President)}, \quad \mathbf{p}_2 = \begin{bmatrix} 0 \\ 1 \\ 0 \end{bmatrix} \text{ (Vice-President)}, \quad \mathbf{p}_3 = \begin{bmatrix} 0 \\ 0 \\ 1 \end{bmatrix} \text{ (Chairman)}.$$

The network learns to recall the executives' favorite floors by updating the second set of weights using the outstar rule (using a learning rate of 0.6). Initially those weights are set to zero:

$$\mathbf{W} = \begin{bmatrix} 0 & 0 & 0 \\ 0 & 0 & 0 \\ 0 & 0 & 0 \end{bmatrix}.$$

i. Use MATLAB to simulate the network for the following sequence of events:

> President pushes '4', Vice-President pushes '3',
> Chairman pushes '1', Vice-President pushes '3',
> Chairman pushes '2', President pushes '4'.

In other words, train the network on the following sequence:

$$\{\mathbf{p}^0 = \mathbf{p}_4^0, \mathbf{p} = \mathbf{p}_1\}, \{\mathbf{p}^0 = \mathbf{p}_3^0, \mathbf{p} = \mathbf{p}_2\}, \{\mathbf{p}^0 = \mathbf{p}_1^0, \mathbf{p} = \mathbf{p}_3\},$$

$$\{\mathbf{p}^0 = \mathbf{p}_3^0, \mathbf{p} = \mathbf{p}_2\}, \{\mathbf{p}^0 = \mathbf{p}_2^0, \mathbf{p} = \mathbf{p}_3\}, \{\mathbf{p}^0 = \mathbf{p}_4^0, \mathbf{p} = \mathbf{p}_1\}.$$

ii. What are the final weights?

iii. Now continue simulating the network on these events:

> President does not push a button,
> Vice-President does not push a button,
> Chairman does not push a button.

iv. Which floors did the network take each executive to?

v. If the executives were to push the following buttons many times, what would you expect the resulting weight matrix to look like?

> President pushes '3',
> Vice-President pushes '2',
> Chairman pushes '4'.

14 Competitive Networks

14

Objectives

The Hamming network, introduced in Chapter 3, demonstrated one technique for using a neural network for pattern recognition. It required that the prototype patterns be known beforehand and incorporated into the network as rows of a weight matrix.

In this chapter we will discuss networks that are very similar in structure and operation to the Hamming network. Unlike the Hamming network, however, they use the associative learning rules of Chapter 13 to adaptively learn to classify patterns. Three such networks are introduced in this chapter: the competitive network, the feature map and the learning vector quantization (LVQ) network.

Theory and Examples

The Hamming network is one of the simplest examples of a competitive network. The neurons in the output layer of the Hamming network compete with each other to determine a winner. The winner indicates which prototype pattern is most representative of the input pattern. The competition is implemented by lateral inhibition — a set of negative connections between the neurons in the output layer. In this chapter we will illustrate how this competition can be combined with the associative learning rules of Chapter 13 to produce powerful self-organizing (unsupervised) networks.

As early as 1959, Frank Rosenblatt created a simple "spontaneous" classifier, an unsupervised network based on the perceptron, which learned to classify input vectors into two classes with roughly equal members.

In the late 1960s and early 1970s, Stephen Grossberg introduced many competitive networks that used lateral inhibition to good effect. Some of the useful behaviors he obtained were noise suppression, contrast-enhancement and vector normalization. His networks will be examined in Chapters 15 and 16.

In 1973, Christoph von der Malsburg introduced a self-organizing learning rule that allowed a network to classify inputs in such a way that neighboring neurons responded to similar inputs. The topology of his network mimicked, in some ways, the structures previously found in the visual cortex of cats by David Hubel and Torten Wiesel. His learning rule generated a great deal of interest, but it used a nonlocal calculation to ensure that weights were normalized. This made it less biologically plausible.

Grossberg extended von der Malsburg's work by rediscovering the instar rule, examined in Chapter 13. (The instar rule had previously been introduced by Nils Nilsson in his 1965 book *Learning Machines*.) Grossberg showed that the instar rule removed the necessity of re-normalizing weights, since weight vectors that learn to recognize normalized input vectors will automatically be normalized themselves.

The work of Grossberg and von der Malsburg emphasizes the biological plausibility of their networks. Another influential researcher, Teuvo Kohonen, has also been a strong proponent of competitive networks. However, his emphasis has been on engineering applications and efficient mathematical descriptions of the networks. During the 1970s he developed a simplified version of the instar rule and also, inspired by the work of von der Malsburg and Grossberg, found an efficient way to incorporate topology into a competitive network.

In this chapter we will concentrate on the Kohonen framework for competitive networks. His models illustrate the major features of competitive networks, and yet they are mathematically more tractable than the Grossberg networks. They provide a good introduction to competitive learning.

We will begin with the simple competitive network. Next we will present the *self-organizing feature map*, which incorporates a network topology. Finally, we will discuss *learning vector quantization*, which incorporates competition within a supervised learning framework.

Hamming Network

14

Since the competitive networks discussed in this chapter are closely related to the Hamming network (shown in Figure 14.1), it is worth reviewing the key concepts of that network first.

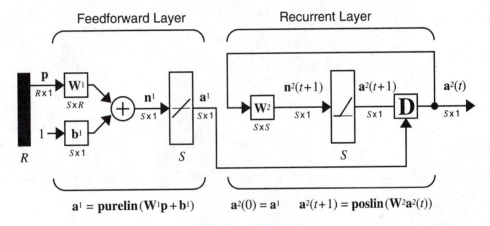

$$\mathbf{a}^1 = \mathbf{purelin}(\mathbf{W}^1\mathbf{p} + \mathbf{b}^1) \qquad \mathbf{a}^2(0) = \mathbf{a}^1 \qquad \mathbf{a}^2(t+1) = \mathbf{poslin}(\mathbf{W}^2\mathbf{a}^2(t))$$

Figure 14.1 Hamming Network

The Hamming network consists of two layers. The first layer (which is a layer of instars) performs a correlation between the input vector and the prototype vectors. The second layer performs a competition to determine which of the prototype vectors is closest to the input vector.

Layer 1

Recall from Chapter 13 (see page 13-9 and following) that a single instar is able to recognize only one pattern. In order to allow multiple patterns to be classified, we need to have multiple instars. This is accomplished in the Hamming network.

Suppose that we want the network to recognize the following prototype vectors:

$$\{\mathbf{p}_1, \mathbf{p}_2, \cdots, \mathbf{p}_Q\} \ . \tag{14.1}$$

Then the weight matrix, $\mathbf{W}^1$, and the bias vector, $\mathbf{b}^1$, for Layer 1 will be:

$$\mathbf{W}^1 = \begin{bmatrix} {}_1\mathbf{w}^T \\ {}_2\mathbf{w}^T \\ \vdots \\ {}_S\mathbf{w}^T \end{bmatrix} = \begin{bmatrix} \mathbf{p}_1^T \\ \mathbf{p}_2^T \\ \vdots \\ \mathbf{p}_Q^T \end{bmatrix}, \quad \mathbf{b}^1 = \begin{bmatrix} R \\ R \\ \vdots \\ R \end{bmatrix}, \tag{14.2}$$

where each row of $\mathbf{W}^1$ represents a prototype vector which we want to recognize, and each element of $\mathbf{b}^1$ is set equal to the number of elements in each input vector (R). (The number of neurons, S, is equal to the number of prototype vectors which are to be recognized, Q.)

Thus, the output of the first layer is

$$\mathbf{a}^1 = \mathbf{W}^1\mathbf{p} + \mathbf{b}^1 = \begin{bmatrix} \mathbf{p}_1^T\mathbf{p} + R \\ \mathbf{p}_2^T\mathbf{p} + R \\ \vdots \\ \mathbf{p}_Q^T\mathbf{p} + R \end{bmatrix}. \tag{14.3}$$

Note that the outputs of Layer 1 are equal to the inner products of the prototype vectors with the input, plus R. As we discussed in Chapter 3 (page 3-9), these inner products indicate how close each of the prototype patterns is to the input vector. (This was also discussed in our presentation of the instar on page 13-10.)

Layer 2

In the instar of Chapter 13, a *hardlim* transfer function was used to decide if the input vector was close enough to the prototype vector. In Layer 2 of the Hamming network we have multiple instars, therefore we want to decide which prototype vector is closest to the input. Instead of the *hardlim* transfer function, we will use a competitive layer to choose the closest prototype.

Layer 2 is a competitive layer. The neurons in this layer are initialized with the outputs of the feedforward layer, which indicate the correlation between the prototype patterns and the input vector. Then the neurons compete with each other to determine a winner. After the competition, only one neuron will have a nonzero output. The winning neuron indicates which category of input was presented to the network (each prototype vector represents a category).

The first-layer output $\mathbf{a}^1$ is used to initialize the second layer.

$$\mathbf{a}^2(0) = \mathbf{a}^1 \tag{14.4}$$

Then the second-layer output is updated according to the following recurrence relation:

$$\mathbf{a}^2(t+1) = \mathbf{poslin}(\mathbf{W}^2\mathbf{a}^2(t)).\tag{14.5}$$

The second-layer weights $\mathbf{W}^2$ are set so that the diagonal elements are 1, and the off-diagonal elements have a small negative value.

$$w_{ij}^2 = \begin{cases} 1, & \text{if } i = j \\ -\varepsilon, & \text{otherwise} \end{cases}, \text{ where } 0 < \varepsilon < \frac{1}{S-1}\tag{14.6}$$

Lateral Inhibition This matrix produces *lateral inhibition*, in which the output of each neuron has an inhibitory effect on all of the other neurons. To illustrate this effect, substitute weight values of 1 and $-\varepsilon$ for the appropriate elements of $\mathbf{W}^2$, and rewrite Eq. (14.5) for a single neuron.

$$a_i^2(t+1) = poslin\left(a_i^2(t) - \varepsilon \sum_{j \neq i} a_j^2(t) \right)\tag{14.7}$$

At each iteration, each neuron's output will decrease in proportion to the sum of the other neurons' outputs (with a minimum output of 0). The output of the neuron with the largest initial condition will decrease more slowly than the outputs of the other neurons. Eventually that neuron will be the only one with a positive output. At this point the network has reached steady state. The index of the second-layer neuron with a stable positive output is the index of the prototype vector that best matched the input.

Winner-Take-All This is called a *winner-take-all competition*, since only one neuron will have a nonzero output. In Chapter 15 we will discuss other types of competition.

 *You may wish to experiment with the Hamming network and the apple/orange classification problem. The Neural Network Design Demonstration Hamming Classification (**nnd3hamc**) was previously introduced in Chapter 3.*

Competitive Layer

Competition The second-layer neurons in the Hamming network are said to be in *competition* because each neuron excites itself and inhibits all the other neurons. To simplify our discussions in the remainder of this chapter, we will define a transfer function that does the job of a recurrent competitive layer:

$$\mathbf{a} = \mathbf{compet}(\mathbf{n}).\tag{14.8}$$

It works by finding the index i^* of the neuron with the largest net input, and setting its output to 1 (with ties going to the neuron with the lowest index). All other outputs are set to 0.

$$a_i = \begin{cases} 1, i = i^* \\ 0, i \neq i^* \end{cases}, \text{ where } n_{i^*} \geq n_i, \forall i, \text{ and } i^* \leq i, \forall n_i = n_{i^*} \qquad (14.9)$$

Replacing the recurrent layer of the Hamming network with a competitive transfer function on the first layer will simplify our presentations in this chapter. (We will study the competition process in more detail in Chapter 15.) A competitive layer is displayed in Figure 14.2.

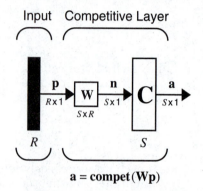

$$\mathbf{a} = \mathbf{compet}(\mathbf{Wp})$$

Figure 14.2 Competitive Layer

As with the Hamming network, the prototype vectors are stored in the rows of $\mathbf{W}$. The net input $\mathbf{n}$ calculates the distance between the input vector $\mathbf{p}$ and each prototype $_i\mathbf{w}$ (assuming vectors have normalized lengths of L). The net input n_i of each neuron i is proportional to the angle θ_i between $\mathbf{p}$ and the prototype vector $_i\mathbf{w}$:

$$\mathbf{n} = \mathbf{Wp} = \begin{bmatrix} _1\mathbf{w}^T \\ _2\mathbf{w}^T \\ \vdots \\ _S\mathbf{w}^T \end{bmatrix} \mathbf{p} = \begin{bmatrix} _1\mathbf{w}^T\mathbf{p} \\ _2\mathbf{w}^T\mathbf{p} \\ \vdots \\ _S\mathbf{w}^T\mathbf{p} \end{bmatrix} = \begin{bmatrix} L^2\cos\theta_1 \\ L^2\cos\theta_2 \\ \vdots \\ L^2\cos\theta_S \end{bmatrix}. \qquad (14.10)$$

The competitive transfer function assigns an output of 1 to the neuron whose weight vector points in the direction closest to the input vector:

$$\mathbf{a} = \mathbf{compet}(\mathbf{Wp}). \qquad (14.11)$$

To experiment with the competitive network and the apple / orange classification problem, use the Neural Network Design Demonstration Competitive Classification *(nnd14cc).*

Competitive Learning

We can now design a competitive network classifier by setting the rows of
W to the desired prototype vectors. However, we would like to have a
learning rule that could be used to train the weights in a competitive network, without knowing the prototype vectors. One such learning rule is the
instar rule from Chapter 13:

$$_i\mathbf{w}(q) = \,_i\mathbf{w}(q-1) + \alpha a_i(q)(\mathbf{p}(q) - \,_i\mathbf{w}(q-1)).$$ (14.12)

For the competitive network, **a** is only nonzero for the winning neuron
($i = i^*$). Therefore, we can get the same results using the Kohonen rule.

$$_i\mathbf{w}(q) = \,_i\mathbf{w}(q-1) + \alpha(\mathbf{p}(q) - \,_i\mathbf{w}(q-1))$$

$$= (1-\alpha)\,_i\mathbf{w}(q-1) + \alpha\mathbf{p}(q)$$ (14.13)

and

$$_i\mathbf{w}(q) = \,_i\mathbf{w}(q-1) \qquad i \neq i^*$$ (14.14)

Thus, the row of the weight matrix that is closest to the input vector (or has
the largest inner product with the input vector) moves toward the input
vector. It moves along a line between the old row of the weight matrix and
the input vector, as shown in Figure 14.3.

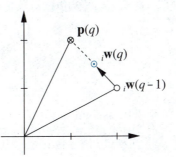

Figure 14.3 Graphical Representation of the Kohonen Rule

Let's use the six vectors in Figure 14.4 to demonstrate how a competitive
layer learns to classify vectors. Here are the six vectors:

$$\mathbf{p}_1 = \begin{bmatrix} -0.1961 \\ 0.9806 \end{bmatrix}, \mathbf{p}_2 = \begin{bmatrix} 0.1961 \\ 0.9806 \end{bmatrix}, \mathbf{p}_3 = \begin{bmatrix} 0.9806 \\ 0.1961 \end{bmatrix}$$ (14.15)

$$\mathbf{p}_4 = \begin{bmatrix} 0.9806 \\ -0.1961 \end{bmatrix}, \mathbf{p}_5 = \begin{bmatrix} -0.5812 \\ -0.8137 \end{bmatrix}, \mathbf{p}_6 = \begin{bmatrix} -0.8137 \\ -0.5812 \end{bmatrix}.$$

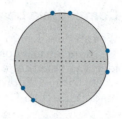

Figure 14.4 Sample Input Vectors

Our competitive network will have three neurons, and therefore it can classify vectors into three classes. Here are the "randomly" chosen normalized initial weights:

$$_1\mathbf{w} = \begin{bmatrix} 0.7071 \\ -0.7071 \end{bmatrix}, \; _2\mathbf{w} = \begin{bmatrix} 0.7071 \\ 0.7071 \end{bmatrix}, \; _3\mathbf{w} = \begin{bmatrix} -1.0000 \\ 0.0000 \end{bmatrix}, \; \mathbf{W} = \begin{bmatrix} _1\mathbf{w}^T \\ _2\mathbf{w}^T \\ _3\mathbf{w}^T \end{bmatrix}. \quad (14.16)$$

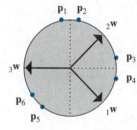

The data vectors are shown at left, with the weight vectors displayed as arrows. Let's present the vector $\mathbf{p}_2$ to the network:

$$\mathbf{a} = \mathbf{compet}\,(\mathbf{W}\mathbf{p}_2) = \mathbf{compet} \left(\begin{bmatrix} 0.7071 & -0.7071 \\ 0.7071 & 0.7071 \\ -1.0000 & 0.0000 \end{bmatrix} \begin{bmatrix} 0.1961 \\ 0.9806 \end{bmatrix} \right) \quad (14.17)$$

$$= \mathbf{compet} \left(\begin{bmatrix} -0.5547 \\ 0.8321 \\ -0.1961 \end{bmatrix} \right) = \begin{bmatrix} 0 \\ 1 \\ 0 \end{bmatrix}.$$

The second neuron's weight vector was closest to $\mathbf{p}_2$, so it won the competition ($i^* = 2$) and output a 1. We now apply the Kohonen learning rule to the winning neuron with a learning rate of $\alpha = 0.5$.

$$_2\mathbf{w}^{new} = \,_2\mathbf{w}^{old} + \alpha\,(\mathbf{p}_2 - \,_2\mathbf{w}^{old}) \quad (14.18)$$

$$= \begin{bmatrix} 0.7071 \\ 0.7071 \end{bmatrix} + 0.5 \left(\begin{bmatrix} 0.1961 \\ 0.9806 \end{bmatrix} - \begin{bmatrix} 0.7071 \\ 0.7071 \end{bmatrix} \right) = \begin{bmatrix} 0.4516 \\ 0.8438 \end{bmatrix}$$

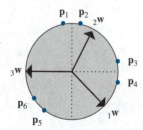

The Kohonen rule moves $_2\mathbf{w}$ closer to $\mathbf{p}_2$, as can be seen in the diagram at left. If we continue choosing input vectors at random and presenting them to the network, then at each iteration the weight vector closest to the input vector will move toward that vector. Eventually, each weight vector will point at a different cluster of input vectors. Each weight vector becomes a prototype for a different cluster.

This problem is simple enough that we can predict which weight vector will point at which cluster. The final weights will look something like those shown in Figure 14.5.

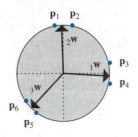

Figure 14.5 Final Weights

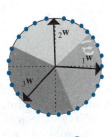

Once the network has learned to cluster the input vectors, it will classify new vectors accordingly. The diagram in the left margin uses shading to show which region each neuron will respond to. The competitive layer assigns each input vector **p** to one of these classes by producing an output of 1 for the neuron whose weight vector is closest to **p**.

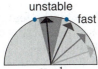

To experiment with the competitive learning use the Neural Network Design Demonstration Competitive Learning (**nnd14cl**).

Problems with Competitive Layers

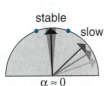

Competitive layers make efficient adaptive classifiers, but they do suffer from a few problems. The first problem is that the choice of learning rate forces a trade-off between the speed of learning and the stability of the final weight vectors. A learning rate near zero results in slow learning. However, once a weight vector reaches the center of a cluster it will tend to stay close to the center.

In contrast, a learning rate near 1.0 results in fast learning. However, once the weight vector has reached a cluster, it will continue to oscillate as different vectors in the cluster are presented.

Sometimes this trade-off between fast learning and stability can be used to advantage. Initial training can be done with a large learning rate for fast learning. Then the learning rate can be decreased as training progresses, to achieve stable prototype vectors. Unfortunately, this technique will not work if the network needs to continuously adapt to new arrangements of input vectors.

A more serious stability problem occurs when clusters are close together. In certain cases, a weight vector forming a prototype of one cluster may "invade" the territory of another weight vector, and therefore upset the current classification scheme.

The series of four diagrams in Figure 14.6 illustrate this problem. Two input vectors (shown with blue circles in diagram (a)) are presented several times. The result is that the weight vectors representing the middle and right clusters shift to the right. Eventually one of the right cluster vectors is reclassified by the center weight vector. Further presentations move the middle vector over to the right until it "loses" some of its vectors, which then become part of the class associated with the left weight vector.

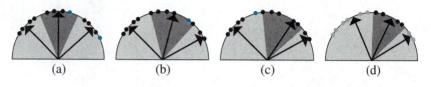

(a) (b) (c) (d)

Figure 14.6 Example of Unstable Learning

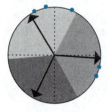

A third problem with competitive learning is that occasionally a neuron's initial weight vector is located so far from any input vectors that it never wins the competition, and therefore never learns. The result is a "dead" neuron, which does nothing useful. For example, the downward-pointing weight vector in the diagram to the left will never learn, regardless of the order in which vectors are presented. One solution to this problem consists of adding a negative bias to the net input of each neuron and then decreasing the bias each time the neuron wins. This will make it harder for a neuron to win the competition if it has won often. This mechanism is sometimes called a "conscience." (See Exercise E14.4.)

Finally, a competitive layer always has as many classes as it has neurons. This may not be acceptable for some applications, especially when the number of clusters is not known in advance. In addition, for competitive layers, each class consists of a convex region of the input space. Competitive layers cannot form classes with nonconvex regions or classes that are the union of unconnected regions.

Some of the problems discussed in this section are solved by the feature map and LVQ networks, which are introduced in later sections of this chapter, and the ART networks, which are presented in Chapter 16.

Competitive Layers in Biology

In previous chapters we have made no mention of how neurons are physically organized within a layer (the topology of the network). In biological neural networks, neurons are typically arranged in two-dimensional layers, in which they are densely interconnected through lateral feedback. The diagram to the left shows a layer of twenty-five neurons arranged in a two-dimensional grid.

Often weights vary as a function of the distance between the neurons they connect. For example, the weights for Layer 2 of the Hamming network are assigned as follows:

$$w_{ij} = \begin{cases} 1, & \text{if } i = j \\ -\varepsilon, & \text{if } i \neq j \end{cases}. \tag{14.19}$$

Eq. (14.20) assigns the same values as Eq. (14.19), but in terms of the distances d_{ij} between neurons:

neuron *j*

$$w_{ij} = \begin{cases} 1, & \text{if } d_{ij} = 0 \\ -\varepsilon, & \text{if } d_{ij} > 0 \end{cases}. \tag{14.20}$$

Either Eq. (14.19) or Eq. (14.20) will assign the weight values shown in the diagram at left. Each neuron *i* is labeled with the value of the weight w_{ij}, which comes from it to the neuron marked *j*.

On-center/off-surround

The term *on-center/off-surround* is often used to describe such a connection pattern between neurons. Each neuron reinforces itself (center), while inhibiting all other neurons (surround).

It turns out that this is a crude approximation of biological competitive layers. In biology, a neuron reinforces not only itself, but also those neurons close to it. Typically, the transition from reinforcement to inhibition occurs smoothly as the distance between neurons increases.

This transition is illustrated on the left side of Figure 14.7. This is a function that relates the distance between neurons to the weight connecting them. Those neurons that are close provide excitatory (reinforcing) connections, and the magnitude of the excitation decreases as the distance increases. Beyond a certain distance, the neurons begin to have inhibitory connections, and the inhibition increases as the distance increases. Be-

Mexican-Hat Function

cause of its shape, the function is referred to as the *Mexican-hat function*. On the right side of Figure 14.7 is a two-dimensional illustration of the Mexican-hat (on-center/off-surround) function. Each neuron *i* is marked to show the sign and relative strength of its weight w_{ij} going to neuron *j*.

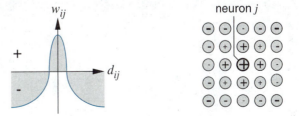

Figure 14.7 On-Center/Off-Surround Layer in Biology

Biological competitive systems, in addition to having a gradual transition between excitatory and inhibitory regions of the on-center/off-surround connection pattern, also have a weaker form of competition than the winner-take-all competition of the Hamming network. Instead of a single active neuron (winner), biological networks generally have "bubbles" of activity that are centered around the most active neuron. This is caused in part by the form of the on-center/off-surround connectivity pattern and also by nonlinear feedback connections. (See the discussion on contour enhancement in Chapter 15.)

Self-Organizing Feature Maps

In order to emulate the activity bubbles of biological systems, without having to implement the nonlinear on-center/off-surround feedback connections, Kohonen designed the following simplification. His self-organizing feature map (SOFM) network first determines the winning neuron $i*$ using the same procedure as the competitive layer. Next, the weight vectors for all neurons within a certain neighborhood of the winning neuron are updated using the Kohonen rule,

SOFM

$$_i\mathbf{w}(q) = {}_i\mathbf{w}(q-1) + \alpha(\mathbf{p}(q) - {}_i\mathbf{w}(q-1))$$
$$= (1-\alpha){}_i\mathbf{w}(q-1) + \alpha\mathbf{p}(q) \qquad i \in N_{i*}(d), \qquad (14.21)$$

Neighborhood

where the *neighborhood* $N_{i*}(d)$ contains the indices for all of the neurons that lie within a radius d of the winning neuron $i*$:

$$N_i(d) = \{j, d_{ij} \le d\}. \qquad (14.22)$$

When a vector $\mathbf{p}$ is presented, the weights of the winning neuron *and* its neighbors will move toward $\mathbf{p}$. The result is that, after many presentations, neighboring neurons will have learned vectors similar to each other.

To demonstrate the concept of a neighborhood, consider the two diagrams shown in Figure 14.8. The left diagram illustrates a two-dimensional neighborhood of radius $d = 1$ around neuron 13. The right diagram shows a neighborhood of radius $d = 2$.

The definition of these neighborhoods would be

$$N_{13}(1) = \{8, 12, 13, 14, 18\}, \qquad (14.23)$$

$$N_{13}(2) = \{3, 7, 8, 9, 11, 12, 13, 14, 15, 17, 18, 19, 23\}. \qquad (14.24)$$

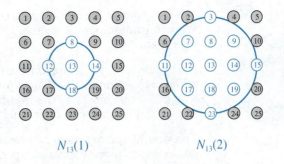

$N_{13}(1)$ $N_{13}(2)$

Figure 14.8 Neighborhoods

We should mention that the neurons in an SOFM do not have to be arranged in a two-dimensional pattern. It is possible to use a one-dimensional arrangement, or even three or more dimensions. For a one-dimensional SOFM, a neuron will only have two neighbors within a radius of 1 (or a single neighbor if the neuron is at the end of the line). It is also possible to define distance in different ways. For instance, Kohonen has suggested rectangular and hexagonal neighborhoods for efficient implementation. The performance of the network is not sensitive to the exact shape of the neighborhoods.

Now let's demonstrate the performance of an SOFM network. Figure 14.9 shows a feature map and the two-dimensional topology of its neurons.

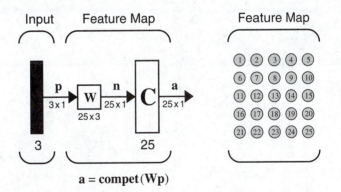

$$a = \text{compet}(Wp)$$

Figure 14.9 Self-Organizing Feature Map

The diagram in the left margin shows the initial weight vectors for the feature map. Each three-element weight vector is represented by a dot on the sphere. (The weights are normalized, therefore they will fall on the surface of a sphere.) Dots of neighboring neurons are connected by lines so you can see how the physical topology of the network is arranged in the input space.

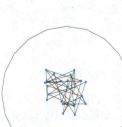

The diagram to the left shows a square region on the surface of the sphere. We will randomly pick vectors in this region and present them to the feature map.

Each time a vector is presented, the neuron with the closest weight vector will win the competition. The winning neuron and its neighbors move their weight vectors closer to the input vector (and therefore to each other). For this example we are using a neighborhood with a radius of 1.

The weight vectors have two tendencies: first, they spread out over the input space as more vectors are presented; second, they move toward the weight vectors of neighboring neurons. These two tendencies work together to rearrange the neurons in the layer so that they evenly classify the input space.

The series of diagrams in Figure 14.10 shows how the weights of the twenty-five neurons spread out over the active input space and organize themselves to match its topology.

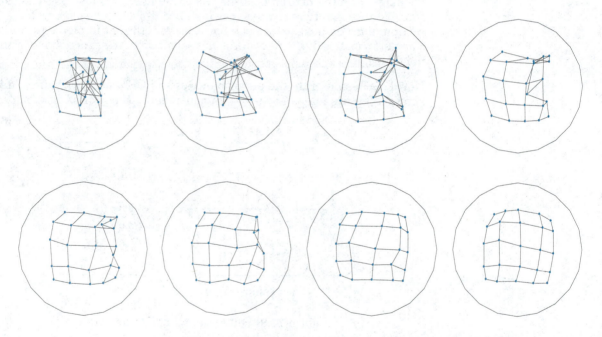

Figure 14.10 Self-Organization, 250 Iterations per Diagram

In this example, the input vectors were generated with equal probability from any point in the input space. Therefore, the neurons classify roughly equal areas of the input space.

Figure 14.11 provides more examples of input regions and the resulting feature maps after self-organization.

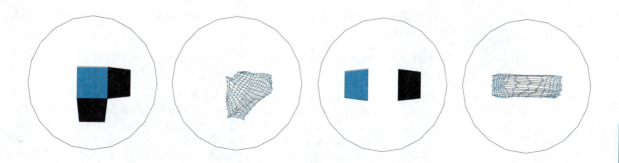

14

Figure 14.11 Other Examples of Feature Map Training

Occasionally feature maps can fail to properly fit the topology of their input space. This usually occurs when two parts of the net fit the topology of separate parts of the input space, but the net forms a twist between them. An example is given in Figure 14.12.

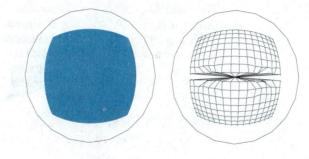

Figure 14.12 Feature Map with a Twist

It is unlikely that this twist will ever be removed, because the two ends of the net have formed stable classifications of different regions.

Improving Feature Maps

So far, we have described only the most basic algorithm for training feature maps. Now let's consider several techniques that can be used to speed up the self-organizing process and to make it more reliable.

One method to improve the performance of the feature map is to vary the size of the neighborhoods during training. Initially, the neighborhood size, d, is set large. As training progresses, d is gradually reduced, until it only includes the winning neuron. This speeds up self-organizing and makes twists in the map very unlikely.

The learning rate can also be varied over time. An initial rate of 1 allows neurons to quickly learn presented vectors. During training, the learning rate is decreased asymptotically toward 0, so that learning becomes stable.

(We discussed the use of this technique for competitive layers earlier in the chapter.)

Another alteration that speeds self-organization is to have the winning neuron use a larger learning rate than the neighboring neurons.

Finally, both competitive layers and feature maps often use an alternative expression for net input. Instead of using the inner product, they can directly compute the distance between the input vector and the prototype vectors. The advantage of using the distance is that input vectors do not need to be normalized. This alternative net input expression is introduced in the next section on LVQ networks.

*To experiment with feature maps use the Neural Network Design Demonstrations 1-D Feature Maps (*nnd14fm1*) and 2-D Feature Maps (*nnd14fm2*).*

Learning Vector Quantization

The final network we will introduce in this chapter is the learning vector quantization (LVQ) network, which is shown in Figure 14.13. The LVQ network is a hybrid network. It uses both unsupervised and supervised learning to form classifications.

In the LVQ network, each neuron in the first layer is assigned to a class, with several neurons often assigned to the same class. Each class is then assigned to one neuron in the second layer. The number of neurons in the first layer, S^1, will therefore always be at least as large as the number of neurons in the second layer, S^2, and will usually be larger.

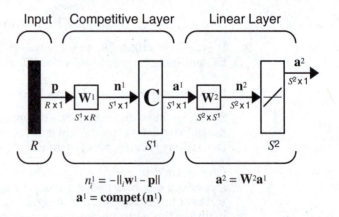

$$n_i^1 = -\|_i\mathbf{w}^1 - \mathbf{p}\|$$
$$\mathbf{a}^1 = \mathbf{compet}(\mathbf{n}^1)$$
$$\mathbf{a}^2 = \mathbf{W}^2\mathbf{a}^1$$

Figure 14.13 LVQ Network

As with the competitive network, each neuron in the first layer of the LVQ network learns a prototype vector, which allows it to classify a region of the input space. However, instead of computing the proximity of the input and weight vectors by using the inner product, we will simulate the LVQ networks by calculating the distance directly. One advantage of calculating the distance directly is that vectors need not be normalized. When the vectors are normalized, the response of the network will be the same, whether the inner product is used or the distance is directly calculated.

The net input of the first layer of the LVQ will be

$$n_i^1 = -\left\| {}_i\mathbf{w}^1 - \mathbf{p} \right\|, \tag{14.25}$$

14

or, in vector form,

$$\mathbf{n}^1 = -\begin{bmatrix} \left\| {}_1\mathbf{w}^1 - \mathbf{p} \right\| \\ \left\| {}_2\mathbf{w}^1 - \mathbf{p} \right\| \\ \vdots \\ \left\| {}_{S^1}\mathbf{w}^1 - \mathbf{p} \right\| \end{bmatrix}. \tag{14.26}$$

The output of the first layer of the LVQ is

$$\mathbf{a}^1 = \mathbf{compet}\,(\mathbf{n}^1)\,. \tag{14.27}$$

Therefore the neuron whose weight vector is closest to the input vector will output a 1, and the other neurons will output 0.

Thus far, the LVQ network behaves exactly like the competitive network (at least for normalized vectors). There is a difference in interpretation, however. In the competitive network, the neuron with the nonzero output indicates which class the input vector belongs to. For the LVQ network, the

Subclass winning neuron indicates a *subclass*, rather than a class. There may be several different neurons (subclasses) that make up each class.

The second layer of the LVQ network is used to combine subclasses into a single class. This is done with the $\mathbf{W}^2$ matrix. The columns of $\mathbf{W}^2$ represent subclasses, and the rows represent classes. $\mathbf{W}^2$ has a single 1 in each column, with the other elements set to zero. The row in which the 1 occurs indicates which class the appropriate subclass belongs to.

$$(w_{ki}^2 = 1) \Rightarrow \text{subclass } i \text{ is a part of class } k \tag{14.28}$$

The process of combining subclasses to form a class allows the LVQ network to create complex class boundaries. A standard competitive layer has the limitation that it can only create decision regions that are convex. The LVQ network overcomes this limitation.

LVQ Learning

The learning in the LVQ network combines competitive learning with supervision. As with all supervised learning algorithms, it requires a set of examples of proper network behavior:

$$\{\mathbf{p}_1, \mathbf{t}_1\}, \{\mathbf{p}_2, \mathbf{t}_2\}, \dots, \{\mathbf{p}_Q, \mathbf{t}_Q\} \ .$$

Each target vector must contain only zeros, except for a single 1. The row in which the 1 appears indicates the class to which the input vector belongs. For example, if we have a problem where we would like to classify a particular three-element vector into the second of four classes, we can express this as

$$\left\{ \mathbf{p}_1 = \begin{bmatrix} \sqrt{1/2} \\ 0 \\ \sqrt{1/2} \end{bmatrix}, \mathbf{t}_1 = \begin{bmatrix} 0 \\ 1 \\ 0 \\ 0 \end{bmatrix} \right\} . \tag{14.29}$$

Before learning can occur, each neuron in the second layer is assigned to an output neuron. This generates the matrix $\mathbf{W}^2$. Typically, equal numbers of hidden neurons are connected to each output neuron, so that each class can be made up of the same number of convex regions. All elements of $\mathbf{W}^2$ are set to zero, except for the following:

If hidden neuron i is to be assigned to class k, then set $w_{ki}^2 = 1$. \quad (14.30)

Once $\mathbf{W}^2$ is defined, it will never be altered. The hidden weights $\mathbf{W}^1$ are trained with a variation of the Kohonen rule.

The LVQ learning rule proceeds as follows. At each iteration, an input vector $\mathbf{p}$ is presented to the network, and the distance from $\mathbf{p}$ to each prototype vector is computed. The hidden neurons compete, neuron $i*$ wins the competition, and the $i*$th element of $\mathbf{a}^1$ is set to 1. Next, $\mathbf{a}^1$ is multiplied by $\mathbf{W}^2$ to get the final output $\mathbf{a}^2$, which also has only one nonzero element, $k*$, indicating that $\mathbf{p}$ is being assigned to class $k*$.

The Kohonen rule is used to improve the hidden layer of the LVQ network in two ways. First, if $\mathbf{p}$ is classified correctly, then we move the weights ${}_{i*}\mathbf{w}^1$ of the winning hidden neuron toward $\mathbf{p}$.

$${}_{i*}\mathbf{w}^1(q) = {}_{i*}\mathbf{w}^1(q-1) + \alpha(\mathbf{p}(q) - {}_{i*}\mathbf{w}^1(q-1)), \text{ if } a_{k*}^2 = t_{k*} = 1 \quad (14.31)$$

Second, if $\mathbf{p}$ was classified incorrectly, then we know that the wrong hidden neuron won the competition, and therefore we move its weights ${}_{i*}\mathbf{w}^1$ *away* from $\mathbf{p}$.

$$_{i*}\mathbf{w}^1(q) = {_{i*}\mathbf{w}^1}(q-1) - \alpha(\mathbf{p}(q) - {_{i*}\mathbf{w}^1}(q-1)), \text{ if } a_{k*}^2 = 1 \neq t_{k*} = 0 \quad (14.32)$$

The result will be that each hidden neuron moves toward vectors that fall into the class for which it forms a subclass and away from vectors that fall into other classes.

Let's take a look at an example of LVQ training. We would like to train an LVQ network to solve the following classification problem:

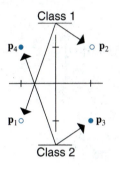

$$\text{class 1: } \left\{ \mathbf{p}_1 = \begin{bmatrix} -1 \\ -1 \end{bmatrix}, \mathbf{p}_2 = \begin{bmatrix} 1 \\ 1 \end{bmatrix} \right\}, \text{ class 2: } \left\{ \mathbf{p}_3 = \begin{bmatrix} 1 \\ -1 \end{bmatrix}, \mathbf{p}_4 = \begin{bmatrix} -1 \\ 1 \end{bmatrix} \right\}, \quad (14.33)$$

as illustrated by the figure in the left margin. We begin by assigning target vectors to each input:

$$\left\{ \mathbf{p}_1 = \begin{bmatrix} -1 \\ -1 \end{bmatrix}, \mathbf{t}_1 = \begin{bmatrix} 1 \\ 0 \end{bmatrix} \right\}, \left\{ \mathbf{p}_2 = \begin{bmatrix} 1 \\ 1 \end{bmatrix}, \mathbf{t}_2 = \begin{bmatrix} 1 \\ 0 \end{bmatrix} \right\}, \quad (14.34)$$

$$\left\{ \mathbf{p}_3 = \begin{bmatrix} 1 \\ -1 \end{bmatrix}, \mathbf{t}_3 = \begin{bmatrix} 0 \\ 1 \end{bmatrix} \right\}, \left\{ \mathbf{p}_4 = \begin{bmatrix} -1 \\ 1 \end{bmatrix}, \mathbf{t}_4 = \begin{bmatrix} 0 \\ 1 \end{bmatrix} \right\}. \quad (14.35)$$

We now must choose how many subclasses will make up each of the two classes. If we let each class be the union of two subclasses, we will end up with four neurons in the hidden layer. The output layer weight matrix will be

$$\mathbf{W}^2 = \begin{bmatrix} 1 & 1 & 0 & 0 \\ 0 & 0 & 1 & 1 \end{bmatrix}. \quad (14.36)$$

$\mathbf{W}^2$ connects hidden neurons 1 and 2 to output neuron 1. It connects hidden neurons 3 and 4 to output neuron 2. Each class will be made up of two convex regions.

The row vectors in $\mathbf{W}^1$ are initially set to random values. They can be seen in the diagram at left. The weights belonging to the two hidden neurons that define class 1 are marked with hollow circles. The weights defining class 2 are marked with solid circles. The values for these weights are

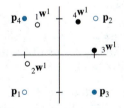

$$_1\mathbf{w}^1 = \begin{bmatrix} -0.543 \\ 0.840 \end{bmatrix}, {_2\mathbf{w}^1} = \begin{bmatrix} -0.969 \\ -0.249 \end{bmatrix}, {_3\mathbf{w}^1} = \begin{bmatrix} 0.997 \\ 0.094 \end{bmatrix}, {_4\mathbf{w}^1} = \begin{bmatrix} 0.456 \\ 0.954 \end{bmatrix}. \quad (14.37)$$

At each iteration of the training process, we present an input vector, find its response, and then adjust the weights. In this case we will begin by presenting $\mathbf{p}_3$.

$$\mathbf{a}^{1} = \mathbf{compet}\,(\mathbf{n}^{1}) = \mathbf{compet}\begin{pmatrix}\begin{bmatrix}-\|{}_{1}\mathbf{w}^{1} - \mathbf{p}_{3}\| \\ -\|{}_{2}\mathbf{w}^{1} - \mathbf{p}_{3}\| \\ -\|{}_{3}\mathbf{w}^{1} - \mathbf{p}_{3}\| \\ -\|{}_{4}\mathbf{w}^{1} - \mathbf{p}_{3}\|\end{bmatrix}\end{pmatrix} \tag{14.38}$$

$$= \mathbf{compet}\begin{pmatrix}\begin{bmatrix}-\left\|\begin{bmatrix}-0.543 & 0.840\end{bmatrix}^{T} - \begin{bmatrix}1 & -1\end{bmatrix}^{T}\right\| \\ -\left\|\begin{bmatrix}-0.969 & -0.249\end{bmatrix}^{T} - \begin{bmatrix}1 & -1\end{bmatrix}^{T}\right\| \\ -\left\|\begin{bmatrix}0.997 & 0.094\end{bmatrix}^{T} - \begin{bmatrix}1 & -1\end{bmatrix}^{T}\right\| \\ -\left\|\begin{bmatrix}0.456 & 0.954\end{bmatrix}^{T} - \begin{bmatrix}1 & -1\end{bmatrix}^{T}\right\|\end{bmatrix}\end{pmatrix} = \mathbf{compet}\begin{pmatrix}\begin{bmatrix}-2.40 \\ -2.11 \\ -1.09 \\ -2.03\end{bmatrix}\end{pmatrix} = \begin{bmatrix}0 \\ 0 \\ 1 \\ 0\end{bmatrix}$$

The third hidden neuron has the closest weight vector to $\mathbf{p}_{3}$. In order to determine which class this neuron belongs to, we multiply $\mathbf{a}^{1}$ by $\mathbf{W}^{2}$.

$$\mathbf{a}^{2} = \mathbf{W}^{2}\mathbf{a}^{1} = \begin{bmatrix}1 & 1 & 0 & 0 \\ 0 & 0 & 1 & 1\end{bmatrix}\begin{bmatrix}0 \\ 0 \\ 1 \\ 0\end{bmatrix} = \begin{bmatrix}0 \\ 1\end{bmatrix} \tag{14.39}$$

This output indicates that $\mathbf{p}_{3}$, is a member of class 2. This is correct, so $_{3}\mathbf{w}^{1}$ is updated by moving it toward $\mathbf{p}_{3}$.

$$_{3}\mathbf{w}^{1}(1) = {}_{3}\mathbf{w}^{1}(0) + \alpha\,(\mathbf{p}_{3} - {}_{3}\mathbf{w}^{1}(0)) \tag{14.40}$$

$$= \begin{bmatrix}0.997 \\ 0.094\end{bmatrix} + 0.5\begin{pmatrix}\begin{bmatrix}1 \\ -1\end{bmatrix} - \begin{bmatrix}0.997 \\ 0.094\end{bmatrix}\end{pmatrix} = \begin{bmatrix}0.998 \\ -0.453\end{bmatrix}$$

The diagram on the left side of Figure 14.14 shows the weights after $_{3}\mathbf{w}^{1}$ was updated on the first iteration. The diagram on the right side of Figure 14.14 shows the weights after the algorithm has converged.

The diagram on the right side of Figure 14.14 also indicates how the regions of the input space will be classified. The regions that will be classified as class 1 are shown in gray, and the regions that will be classified as class 2 are shown in blue.

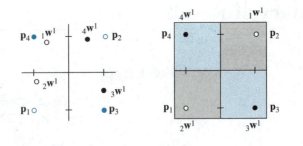

Figure 14.14 After First and Many Iterations

Improving LVQ Networks (LVQ2)

The LVQ network described above works well for many problems, but it does suffer from a couple of limitations. First, as with competitive layers, occasionally a hidden neuron in an LVQ network can have initial weight values that stop it from ever winning the competition. The result is a dead neuron that never does anything useful. This problem is solved with the use of a "conscience" mechanism, a technique discussed earlier for competitive layers, and also presented in Exercise E14.4.

Secondly, depending on how the initial weight vectors are arranged, a neuron's weight vector may have to travel through a region of a class that it doesn't represent, to get to a region that it does represent. Because the weights of such a neuron will be repulsed by vectors in the region it must cross, it may not be able to cross, and so it may never properly classify the region it is being attracted to. This is usually solved by applying the following modification to the Kohonen rule.

If the winning neuron in the hidden layer incorrectly classifies the current input, we move its weight vector away from the input vector, as before. However, we also adjust the weights of the closest neuron to the input vector that does classify it properly. The weights for this second neuron should be moved toward the input vector.

When the network correctly classifies an input vector, the weights of only one neuron are moved toward the input vector. However, if the input vector is incorrectly classified, the weights of two neurons are updated, one weight vector is moved away from the input vector, and the other one is moved toward the input vector. The resulting algorithm is called *LVQ2*.

LVQ2

*To experiment with LVQ networks use the Neural Network Design Demonstrations LVQ1 Networks (**nnd14lv1**) and LVQ2 Networks (**nnd14lv2**).*

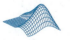

Summary of Results

Competitive Layer

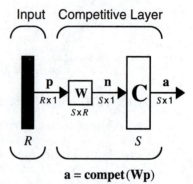

$$a = \text{compet}(\mathbf{Wp})$$

Competitive Learning with the Kohonen Rule

$${}_{i^*}\mathbf{w}(q) = {}_{i^*}\mathbf{w}(q-1) + \alpha(\mathbf{p}(q) - {}_{i^*}\mathbf{w}(q-1)) = (1-\alpha)\,{}_{i^*}\mathbf{w}(q-1) + \alpha\mathbf{p}(q)$$

$${}_{i^*}\mathbf{w}(q) = {}_{i^*}\mathbf{w}(q-1) \qquad i \neq i^*,$$

where i^* is the winning neuron.

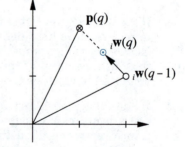

Self-Organizing Feature Map

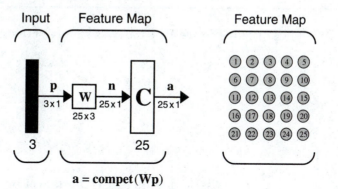

$$\mathbf{a} = \mathbf{compet}(\mathbf{Wp})$$

Self-Organizing with the Kohonen Rule

$$_i\mathbf{w}(q) = {}_i\mathbf{w}(q-1) + \alpha(\mathbf{p}(q) - {}_i\mathbf{w}(q-1))$$

$$= (1-\alpha){}_i\mathbf{w}(q-1) + \alpha\mathbf{p}(q) \qquad i \in N_{i*}(d)$$

$$N_i(d) = \{j, d_{ij} \le d\}$$

LVQ Network

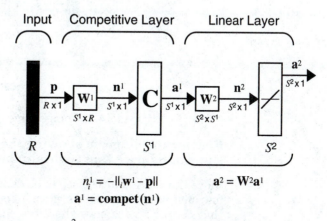

$$n_i^1 = -\|{}_i\mathbf{w}^1 - \mathbf{p}\| \qquad\qquad \mathbf{a}^2 = \mathbf{W}^2\mathbf{a}^1$$

$$\mathbf{a}^1 = \mathbf{compet}(\mathbf{n}^1)$$

$$(w_{ki}^2 = 1) \Rightarrow \text{subclass } i \text{ is a part of class } k$$

LVQ Network Learning with the Kohonen Rule

$$_{i*}\mathbf{w}^1(q) = {}_{i*}\mathbf{w}^1(q-1) + \alpha(\mathbf{p}(q) - {}_{i*}\mathbf{w}^1(q-1)), \text{ if } a_{k*}^2 = t_{k*} = 1$$

$$_{i*}\mathbf{w}^1(q) = {}_{i*}\mathbf{w}^1(q-1) - \alpha(\mathbf{p}(q) - {}_{i*}\mathbf{w}^1(q-1)), \text{ if } a_{k*}^2 = 1 \ne t_{k*} = 0$$

Solved Problems

P14.1 **Figure P14.1 shows several clusters of normalized vectors.**

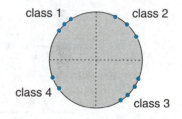

Figure P14.1 Clusters of Input Vectors for Problem P14.1

Design the weights of the competitive network shown in Figure P14.2, so that it classifies the vectors according to the classes indicated in the diagram and with the minimum number of neurons.

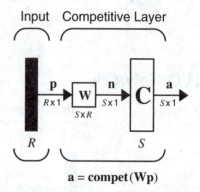

$$a = compet(Wp)$$

Figure P14.2 Competitive Network for Problem P14.1

Redraw the diagram showing the weights you chose and the decision boundaries that separate the region of each class.

Since there are four classes to be defined, the competitive layer will need four neurons. The weights of each neuron act as prototypes for the class that neuron represents. Therefore, for each neuron we will choose a prototype vector that appears to be approximately at the center of a cluster.

Classes 1, 2 and 3 each appear to be roughly centered at a multiple of $45°$. Given this, the following three vectors are normalized (as is required for the competitive layer) and point in the proper directions.

$$_1\mathbf{w} = \begin{bmatrix} -1/\sqrt{2} \\ 1/\sqrt{2} \end{bmatrix}, \; _2\mathbf{w} = \begin{bmatrix} 1/\sqrt{2} \\ 1/\sqrt{2} \end{bmatrix}, \; _3\mathbf{w} = \begin{bmatrix} 1/\sqrt{2} \\ -1/\sqrt{2} \end{bmatrix}$$

The center of the fourth cluster appears to be about twice as far from the vertical axis as it is from the horizontal axis. The resulting normalized weight vector is

$$_4\mathbf{w} = \begin{bmatrix} -2/\sqrt{5} \\ -1/\sqrt{5} \end{bmatrix}.$$

14

The weight matrix $\mathbf{W}$ for the competitive layer is simply the matrix of the transposed prototype vectors:

$$W = \begin{bmatrix} _1\mathbf{w}^T \\ _2\mathbf{w}^T \\ _3\mathbf{w}^T \\ _4\mathbf{w}^T \end{bmatrix} = \begin{bmatrix} -1/\sqrt{2} & 1/\sqrt{2} \\ 1/\sqrt{2} & 1/\sqrt{2} \\ 1/\sqrt{2} & -1/\sqrt{2} \\ -2/\sqrt{5} & -1/\sqrt{5} \end{bmatrix}.$$

We get Figure P14.3 by drawing these weight vectors with arrows and bisecting the circle between each adjacent weight vector to get the class regions.

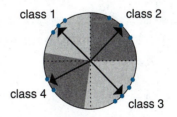

Figure P14.3 Final Classifications for Problem P14.1

P14.2 **Figure P14.4 shows three input vectors and three initial weight vectors for a three-neuron competitive layer. Here are the values of the input vectors:**

$$\mathbf{p}_1 = \begin{bmatrix} -1 \\ 0 \end{bmatrix}, \; \mathbf{p}_2 = \begin{bmatrix} 0 \\ 1 \end{bmatrix}, \; \mathbf{p}_3 = \begin{bmatrix} 1/\sqrt{2} \\ 1/\sqrt{2} \end{bmatrix}.$$

The initial values of the three weight vectors are

$$_1\mathbf{w} = \begin{bmatrix} 0 \\ -1 \end{bmatrix}, \,_2\mathbf{w} = \begin{bmatrix} -2/\sqrt{5} \\ 1/\sqrt{5} \end{bmatrix}, \,_3\mathbf{w} = \begin{bmatrix} -1/\sqrt{5} \\ 2/\sqrt{5} \end{bmatrix}.$$

Calculate the resulting weights found after training the competitive layer with the Kohonen rule and a learning rate α of 0.5, on the following series of inputs:

$$\mathbf{p}_1, \mathbf{p}_2, \mathbf{p}_3, \mathbf{p}_1, \mathbf{p}_2, \mathbf{p}_3.$$

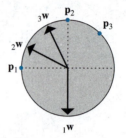

Figure P14.4 Input Vectors and Initial Weights for Problem P14.2

First we combine the weight vectors into the weight matrix $\mathbf{W}$.

$$\mathbf{W} = \begin{bmatrix} 0 & -1 \\ -2/\sqrt{5} & 1/\sqrt{5} \\ -1/\sqrt{5} & 2/\sqrt{5} \end{bmatrix}$$

Then we present the first vector $\mathbf{p}_1$.

$$\mathbf{a} = \mathbf{compet}\,(\mathbf{Wp}_1) = \mathbf{compet}\left(\begin{bmatrix} 0 & -1 \\ -2/\sqrt{5} & 1/\sqrt{5} \\ -1/\sqrt{5} & 2/\sqrt{5} \end{bmatrix}\begin{bmatrix} -1 \\ 0 \end{bmatrix}\right) = \mathbf{compet}\left(\begin{bmatrix} 0 \\ 0.894 \\ 0.447 \end{bmatrix}\right) = \begin{bmatrix} 0 \\ 1 \\ 0 \end{bmatrix}$$

The second neuron responded, since $_2\mathbf{w}$ was closest to $\mathbf{p}_1$. Therefore, we will update $_2\mathbf{w}$ with the Kohonen rule.

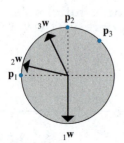

$$_2\mathbf{w}^{new} = \,_2\mathbf{w}^{old} + \alpha\,(\mathbf{p}_1 - \,_2\mathbf{w}^{old}) = \begin{bmatrix} -2/\sqrt{5} \\ 1/\sqrt{5} \end{bmatrix} + 0.5\left(\begin{bmatrix} -1 \\ 0 \end{bmatrix} - \begin{bmatrix} -2/\sqrt{5} \\ 1/\sqrt{5} \end{bmatrix}\right) = \begin{bmatrix} -0.947 \\ 0.224 \end{bmatrix}$$

The diagram at left shows that the new $_2\mathbf{w}$ moved closer to $\mathbf{p}_1$.

We will now repeat this process for $\mathbf{p}_2$.

$$\mathbf{a} = \mathbf{compet}\,(\mathbf{W}\mathbf{p}_2) = \mathbf{compet}\left(\begin{bmatrix} 0 & -1 \\ -0.947 & 0.224 \\ -1/\sqrt{5} & 2/\sqrt{5} \end{bmatrix}\begin{bmatrix} 0 \\ 1 \end{bmatrix}\right) = \mathbf{compet}\left(\begin{bmatrix} -1 \\ 0.224 \\ 0.894 \end{bmatrix}\right) = \begin{bmatrix} 0 \\ 0 \\ 1 \end{bmatrix}$$

The third neuron won, so its weights move closer to $\mathbf{p}_2$.

$$_3\mathbf{w}^{new} = {}_3\mathbf{w}^{old} + \alpha\,(\mathbf{p}_2 - {}_3\mathbf{w}^{old}) = \begin{bmatrix} -1/\sqrt{5} \\ 2/\sqrt{5} \end{bmatrix} + 0.5\left(\begin{bmatrix} 0 \\ 1 \end{bmatrix} - \begin{bmatrix} -1/\sqrt{5} \\ 2/\sqrt{5} \end{bmatrix}\right) = \begin{bmatrix} -0.224 \\ 0.947 \end{bmatrix}$$

We now present $\mathbf{p}_3$.

$$\mathbf{a} = \mathbf{compet}\,(\mathbf{W}\mathbf{p}_3) = \mathbf{compet}\left(\begin{bmatrix} 0 & -1 \\ -0.947 & 0.224 \\ -0.224 & 0.947 \end{bmatrix}\begin{bmatrix} 1/\sqrt{2} \\ 1/\sqrt{2} \end{bmatrix}\right)$$

$$= \mathbf{compet}\left(\begin{bmatrix} -0.707 \\ -0.512 \\ 0.512 \end{bmatrix}\right) = \begin{bmatrix} 0 \\ 0 \\ 1 \end{bmatrix}$$

The third neuron wins again.

$$_3\mathbf{w}^{new} = {}_3\mathbf{w}^{old} + \alpha\,(\mathbf{p}_2 - {}_3\mathbf{w}^{old}) = \begin{bmatrix} -0.224 \\ 0.947 \end{bmatrix} + 0.5\left(\begin{bmatrix} 1/\sqrt{2} \\ 1/\sqrt{2} \end{bmatrix} - \begin{bmatrix} -0.224 \\ 0.947 \end{bmatrix}\right) = \begin{bmatrix} 0.2417 \\ 0.8272 \end{bmatrix}$$

After presenting $\mathbf{p}_1$ through $\mathbf{p}_3$ again, neuron 2 will again win once and neuron 3 twice. The final weights are

$$\mathbf{W} = \begin{bmatrix} 0 & -1 \\ -0.974 & 0.118 \\ 0.414 & 0.8103 \end{bmatrix}.$$

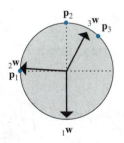

The final weights are also shown in the diagram at left.

Note that $_2\mathbf{w}$ has almost learned $\mathbf{p}_1$, and $_3\mathbf{w}$ is directly between $\mathbf{p}_2$ and $\mathbf{p}_3$. The other weight vector, $_1\mathbf{w}$, was never updated. The first neuron, which never won the competition, is a dead neuron.

P14.3 **Consider the configuration of input vectors and initial weights shown in Figure P14.5. Train a competitive network to cluster these vectors using the Kohonen rule with learning rate $\alpha = 0.5$. Find graphically the position of the weights after all of the input**

vectors (in the order shown) have been presented once.

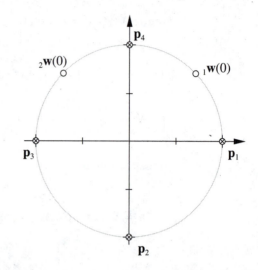

Figure P14.5 Input Vectors and Initial Weights for Problem P14.3

This problem can be solved graphically, without any computations. The results are displayed in Figure P14.6.

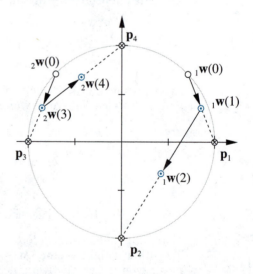

Figure P14.6 Solution for Problem P14.3

The input vector $\mathbf{p}_1$ is presented first. The weight vector ${}_1\mathbf{w}$ is closest to $\mathbf{p}_1$, therefore neuron 1 wins the competition and ${}_1\mathbf{w}$ is moved halfway to $\mathbf{p}_1$, since $\alpha = 0.5$. Next, $\mathbf{p}_2$ is presented, and again neuron 1 wins the competition and $_1\mathbf{w}$ is moved halfway to $\mathbf{p}_2$. During these first two iterations, $_2\mathbf{w}$ is not changed.

On the third iteration, $\mathbf{p}_3$ is presented. This time $_2\mathbf{w}$ wins the competition and is moved halfway to $\mathbf{p}_3$. On the fourth iteration, $\mathbf{p}_4$ is presented, and neuron 2 again wins. The weight vector $_2\mathbf{w}$ is moved halfway to $\mathbf{p}_4$.

If we continue to train the network, neuron 1 will classify the input vectors $\mathbf{p}_1$ and $\mathbf{p}_2$, and neuron 2 will classify the input vectors $\mathbf{p}_3$ and $\mathbf{p}_4$. If the input vectors were presented in a different order, would the final classification be different?

14

P14.4 **So far in this chapter we have only talked about feature maps whose neurons are arranged in two dimensions. The feature map shown in Figure P14.7 contains nine neurons arranged in one dimension.**

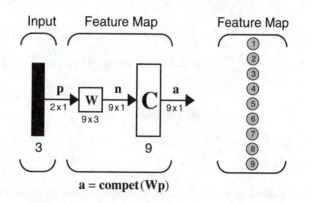

Figure P14.7 Nine-Neuron Feature Map

Given the following initial weights, draw a diagram of the weight vectors, with lines connecting weight vectors of neighboring neurons.

$$\mathbf{W} = \begin{bmatrix} 0.41 & 0.45 & 0.41 & 0 & 0 & 0 & -0.41 & -0.45 & -0.41 \\ 0.41 & 0 & -0.41 & 0.45 & 0 & -0.45 & 0.41 & 0 & -0.41 \\ 0.82 & 0.89 & 0.82 & 0.89 & 1 & 0.89 & 0.82 & 0.89 & 0.82 \end{bmatrix}^T$$

Train the feature map for one iteration, on the vector below, using a learning rate of 0.1 and a neighborhood of radius 1. Redraw the diagram for the new weight matrix.

$$\mathbf{p} = \begin{bmatrix} 0.67 \\ 0.07 \\ 0.74 \end{bmatrix}$$

The feature map diagram for the initial weights is given in Figure P14.8.

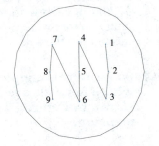

Figure P14.8 Original Feature Map

We start updating the network by presenting **p** to the network.

$$\mathbf{a} = \mathbf{compet}\,(\mathbf{Wp})$$

$$= \mathbf{compet}\left(\begin{bmatrix} 0.41 & 0.45 & 0.41 & 0 & 0 & 0 & -0.41 & -0.45 & -0.41 \\ 0.41 & 0 & -0.41 & 0.45 & 0 & -0.45 & 0.41 & 0 & -0.41 \\ 0.82 & 0.89 & 0.82 & 0.89 & 1 & 0.89 & 0.82 & 0.89 & 0.82 \end{bmatrix}^{T} \begin{bmatrix} 0.67 \\ 0.07 \\ 0.74 \end{bmatrix} \right)$$

$$= \mathbf{compet}\left(\begin{bmatrix} 0.91 & 0.96 & 0.85 & 0.70 & 0.74 & 0.63 & 0.36 & 0.36 & 0.3 \end{bmatrix}^{T} \right)$$

$$= \begin{bmatrix} 0 & 1 & 0 & 0 & 0 & 0 & 0 & 0 & 0 \end{bmatrix}^{T}$$

The second neuron won the competition. Looking at the network diagram, we see that the second neuron's neighbors, at a radius of 1, include neurons 1 and 3. We must update each of these neurons' weights with the Kohonen rule.

$$_1\mathbf{w}(1) = {}_1\mathbf{w}(0) + \alpha(\mathbf{p} - {}_1\mathbf{w}(0)) = \begin{bmatrix} 0.41 \\ 0.41 \\ 0.82 \end{bmatrix} + 0.1\left(\begin{bmatrix} 0.67 \\ 0.07 \\ 0.74 \end{bmatrix} - \begin{bmatrix} 0.41 \\ 0.41 \\ 0.82 \end{bmatrix}\right) = \begin{bmatrix} 0.43 \\ 0.37 \\ 0.81 \end{bmatrix}$$

$$_2\mathbf{w}(1) = {}_2\mathbf{w}(0) + \alpha(\mathbf{p} - {}_2\mathbf{w}(0)) = \begin{bmatrix} 0.45 \\ 0 \\ 0.89 \end{bmatrix} + 0.1\left(\begin{bmatrix} 0.67 \\ 0.07 \\ 0.74 \end{bmatrix} - \begin{bmatrix} 0.45 \\ 0 \\ 0.89 \end{bmatrix}\right) = \begin{bmatrix} 0.47 \\ 0.01 \\ 0.88 \end{bmatrix}$$

14

$$_3\mathbf{w}(1) = {}_3\mathbf{w}(0) + \alpha(\mathbf{p} - {}_3\mathbf{w}(0)) = \begin{bmatrix} 0.41 \\ -0.41 \\ 0.82 \end{bmatrix} + 0.1\left(\begin{bmatrix} 0.67 \\ 0.07 \\ 0.74 \end{bmatrix} - \begin{bmatrix} 0.41 \\ -0.41 \\ 0.82 \end{bmatrix}\right) = \begin{bmatrix} 0.43 \\ -0.36 \\ 0.81 \end{bmatrix}$$

Figure P14.9 shows the feature map after the weights were updated.

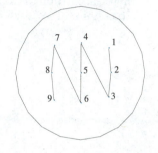

Figure P14.9 Feature Map after Update

P14.5 **Given the LVQ network shown in Figure P14.10 and the weight values shown below, draw the regions of the input space that make up each class.**

$$\mathbf{W}^1 = \begin{bmatrix} 0 & 0 \\ 1 & -1 \\ 1 & 1 \\ -1 & 1 \\ -1 & -1 \end{bmatrix}, \ \mathbf{W}^2 = \begin{bmatrix} 1 & 0 & 0 & 0 & 0 \\ 0 & 1 & 0 & 0 & 0 \\ 0 & 0 & 1 & 1 & 1 \end{bmatrix}$$

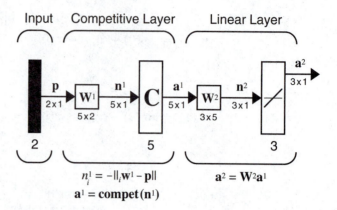

$$n_i^1 = -\|_i\mathbf{w}^1 - \mathbf{p}\|$$
$$\mathbf{a}^1 = \mathbf{compet}(\mathbf{n}^1)$$

$$\mathbf{a}^2 = \mathbf{W}^2\mathbf{a}^1$$

Figure P14.10 LVQ Network for Problem P14.5

We create the diagram shown in Figure P14.11 by marking each vector $_i\mathbf{w}$ in $\mathbf{W}^1$ according to the index k of the corresponding nonzero element in the ith column of $\mathbf{W}^2$, which indicates the class.

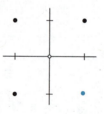

Figure P14.11 Prototype Vectors Marked by Class

The decision boundaries separating each class are found by drawing lines between each pair of prototype vectors, perpendicular to an imaginary line connecting them and equidistant from each vector.

In Figure P14.12, each convex region is colored according to the weight vector it is closest to.

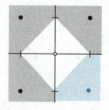

Figure P14.12 Class Regions and Decision Boundaries

P14.6 **Design an LVQ network to solve the classification problem shown in Figure P14.13. The vectors in the diagram are to be classified into one of three classes, according to their color.**

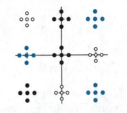

Figure P14.13 Classification Problem

When the design is complete, draw a diagram showing the region for each class.

We will begin by noting that since LVQ networks calculate the distance between vectors directly, instead of using the inner product, they can classify vectors that are not normalized, such as those above.

Next we will identify each color with a class:

- Class 1 will include all white dots.

- Class 2 will include all black dots.

- Class 3 will include all blue dots.

Now we can choose the dimensions of the LVQ network. Since there are three classes, the network must have three neurons in its output layer. There are nine subclasses (i.e., clusters). Therefore the hidden layer must have nine neurons. This gives us the network shown in Figure P14.14.

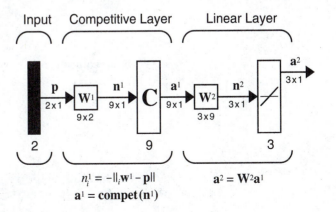

Figure P14.14 LVQ Network for Problem P14.6

We can now design the weight matrix $\mathbf{W}^1$ of the first layer by setting each row equal to a transposed prototype vector for one cluster. Picking prototype vectors at the center of each cluster gives us the following values:

$$\mathbf{W}^1 = \begin{bmatrix} -1 & 0 & 1 & -1 & 0 & 1 & -1 & 0 & 1 \\ 1 & 1 & 1 & 0 & 0 & 0 & -1 & -1 & -1 \end{bmatrix}^T .$$

Now each neuron in the first layer will respond to a different cluster.

Next we choose $\mathbf{W}^2$ so that each subclass is connected to the appropriate class. To do this we use the following rule:

If subclass i is to be assigned to class k, then set $w_{ki}^2 = 1$.

For example, the first subclass is the top-left cluster in the vector diagram. The vectors in this cluster are white, so they belong in the first class. Therefore we should set $w_{1,1}^2$ to one.

Once we have done this for all nine subclasses we end up with these values:

$$\mathbf{W}^2 = \begin{bmatrix} 1 & 0 & 0 & 0 & 0 & 1 & 0 & 1 & 0 \\ 0 & 1 & 0 & 0 & 1 & 0 & 1 & 0 & 0 \\ 0 & 0 & 1 & 1 & 0 & 0 & 0 & 0 & 1 \end{bmatrix} .$$

We can test the network by presenting a vector to it. Here we calculate the output of the first layer for $\mathbf{p} = \begin{bmatrix} 1 & 0 \end{bmatrix}^T$:

$$\mathbf{a}^1 = \mathbf{compet}\,(\mathbf{n}^1) = \mathbf{compet}\left(\begin{bmatrix} -\sqrt{5} \\ -\sqrt{2} \\ -1 \\ -2 \\ -1 \\ 0 \\ -\sqrt{5} \\ -\sqrt{2} \\ -1 \end{bmatrix} \right) = \begin{bmatrix} 0 \\ 0 \\ 0 \\ 0 \\ 0 \\ 1 \\ 0 \\ 0 \\ 0 \end{bmatrix} .$$

The network says that the vector we presented is in the sixth subclass. Let's see what the second layer says.

$$\mathbf{a}^2 = \mathbf{W}^2\mathbf{a}^1 = \begin{bmatrix} 1 & 0 & 0 & 0 & 0 & 1 & 0 & 1 & 0 \\ 0 & 1 & 0 & 0 & 1 & 0 & 1 & 0 & 0 \\ 0 & 0 & 1 & 1 & 0 & 0 & 0 & 0 & 1 \end{bmatrix} \begin{bmatrix} 0 \\ 0 \\ 0 \\ 0 \\ 0 \\ 0 \\ 1 \\ 0 \\ 0 \\ 0 \end{bmatrix} = \begin{bmatrix} 1 \\ 0 \\ 0 \end{bmatrix}$$

14

The second layer indicates that the vector is in class 1, as indeed it is. The diagram of class regions and decision boundaries is shown in Figure P14.15.

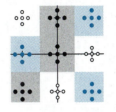

Figure P14.15 Class Regions and Decision Boundaries

P14.7 **Competitive layers and feature maps require that input vectors be normalized. But what if the available data is not normalized?**

One way to handle such data is simply to normalize it before giving it to the network. This has the disadvantage that the vector magnitude information, which may be important, is lost.

Another solution is to replace the inner product expression usually used to calculate net input,

$$\mathbf{a} = \text{compet}(\mathbf{Wp}),$$

with a direct calculation of distance,

$$n_i = -\|{}_i\mathbf{w} - \mathbf{p}\| \text{ and } \mathbf{a} = \text{compet}(\mathbf{n}),$$

as is done with the LVQ network. This works and saves the magnitude information.

However, a third solution is to append a constant of 1 to each input vector before normalizing it. Now the change in the added element will preserve the vector magnitude information.

Normalize the following vectors using this last method:

$$\mathbf{p}_1 = \begin{bmatrix} 1 \\ 1 \end{bmatrix}, \ \mathbf{p}_2 = \begin{bmatrix} 0 \\ 1 \end{bmatrix}, \ \mathbf{p}_3 = \begin{bmatrix} 0 \\ 0 \end{bmatrix}.$$

First we add an extra element with value 1 to each vector.

$$\mathbf{p}'_1 = \begin{bmatrix} 1 \\ 1 \\ 1 \end{bmatrix}, \ \mathbf{p}'_2 = \begin{bmatrix} 0 \\ 1 \\ 1 \end{bmatrix}, \ \mathbf{p}'_3 = \begin{bmatrix} 0 \\ 0 \\ 1 \end{bmatrix}$$

Then we normalize each vector.

$$\mathbf{p}''_1 = \begin{bmatrix} 1 \\ 1 \\ 1 \end{bmatrix} \Big/ \left\| \begin{bmatrix} 1 \\ 1 \\ 1 \end{bmatrix} \right\| = \begin{bmatrix} 1/\sqrt{3} \\ 1/\sqrt{3} \\ 1/\sqrt{3} \end{bmatrix}$$

$$\mathbf{p}''_2 = \begin{bmatrix} 0 \\ 1 \\ 1 \end{bmatrix} \Big/ \left\| \begin{bmatrix} 0 \\ 1 \\ 1 \end{bmatrix} \right\| = \begin{bmatrix} 0 \\ 1/\sqrt{2} \\ 1/\sqrt{2} \end{bmatrix}$$

$$\mathbf{p}''_3 = \begin{bmatrix} 0 \\ 0 \\ 1 \end{bmatrix} \Big/ \left\| \begin{bmatrix} 0 \\ 0 \\ 1 \end{bmatrix} \right\| = \begin{bmatrix} 0 \\ 0 \\ 1 \end{bmatrix}$$

Now the third element of each vector contains magnitude information, since it is equal to the inverse of the magnitude of the original vectors.

Epilogue

In this chapter we have demonstrated how the associative instar learning rule of Chapter 13 can be combined with competitive networks, similar to the Hamming network of Chapter 3, to produce powerful self-organizing networks. By combining competition with the instar rule, each of the prototype vectors that are learned by the network become representative of a particular class of input vector. Thus the competitive networks learn to divide their input space into distinct classes. Each class is represented by one of the prototype vectors (rows of the weight matrix).

Three types of networks, all developed by Tuevo Kohonen, were discussed in this chapter. The first is the standard competitive layer. Its simple operation makes it a practical network for many problems.

The self-organizing feature map is very similar to the competitive layer, but more closely models biological on-center/off-surround networks. The result is a network that not only learns to classify input vectors, but also learns the topology of the input space.

The third network, the LVQ network, uses both unsupervised and supervised learning to recognize clusters. It uses a second layer to combine multiple convex regions into classes that can have any shape. LVQ networks can even be trained to recognize classes made up of multiple unconnected regions.

Chapters 15 and 16 will build on the networks presented in this chapter. For example, Chapter 15 will carry out a more detailed examination of lateral inhibition, on-center/off-surround networks and the biology that inspired them. In Chapter 16 we discuss a modification to the standard competitive network (called adaptive resonance theory), which solves the weight stability problem that we discussed in this chapter.

14

Further Reading

[FrSk91]   J. Freeman and D. Skapura, *Neural Networks: Algorithms, Applications, and Programming Techniques*, Reading, MA: Addison-Wesley, 1991.

This text contains code fragments for network algorithms, making the details of the networks clear.

[Koho87]   T. Kohonen, *Self-Organization and Associative Memory*, 2nd Ed., Berlin: Springer-Verlag, 1987.

Kohonen introduces the Kohonen rule and several networks that use it. It provides a complete analysis of linear associative models and gives many extensions and examples.

[Hech90]   R. Hecht-Nielsen, *Neurocomputing*, Reading, MA: Addison-Wesley, 1990.

This book contains a section on the history and mathematics of competitive learning.

[RuMc86]   D. Rumelhart, J. McClelland et al., *Parallel Distributed Processing*, vol. 1, Cambridge, MA: MIT Press, 1986.

Both volumes of this set are classics in neural network literature. The first volume contains a chapter describing competitive layers and how they learn to detect features.

Exercises

E14.1 Suppose that the weight matrix for layer 2 of the Hamming network is given by

$$\mathbf{W}^2 = \begin{bmatrix} 1 & -\dfrac{3}{4} & -\dfrac{3}{4} \\[2mm] -\dfrac{3}{4} & 1 & -\dfrac{3}{4} \\[2mm] -\dfrac{3}{4} & -\dfrac{3}{4} & 1 \end{bmatrix}.$$

This matrix violates Eq. (14.6), since

$$\varepsilon = \frac{3}{4} > \frac{1}{S-1} = \frac{1}{2}.$$

Give an example of an output from Layer 1 for which Layer 2 will fail to operate correctly.

E14.2 Consider the input vectors and initial weights shown in Figure E14.1.

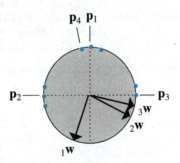

Figure E14.1 Cluster Data Vectors

i. Draw the diagram of a competitive network that could classify the data above so that each of the three clusters of vectors would have its own class.

ii. Train the network graphically (using the initial weights shown) by presenting the labeled vectors in the following order:

$$\mathbf{p}_1 , \mathbf{p}_2 , \mathbf{p}_3 , \mathbf{p}_4 .$$

Recall that the competitive transfer function chooses the neuron with the lowest index to win if more than one neuron has the same net input. The Kohonen rule is introduced graphically in Figure 14.3.

iii. Redraw the diagram in Figure E14.1, showing your final weight vectors and the decision boundaries between each region that represents a class.

E14.3 Train a competitive network using the following input patterns:

$$\mathbf{p}_1 = \begin{bmatrix} 1 \\ -1 \end{bmatrix}, \quad \mathbf{p}_2 = \begin{bmatrix} 1 \\ 1 \end{bmatrix}, \quad \mathbf{p}_3 = \begin{bmatrix} -1 \\ -1 \end{bmatrix}.$$

i. Use the Kohonen learning law with $\alpha = 0.5$, and train for one pass through the input patterns. (Present each input once, in the order given.) Display the results graphically. Assume the initial weight matrix is

$$\mathbf{W} = \begin{bmatrix} \sqrt{2} & 0 \\ 0 & \sqrt{2} \end{bmatrix}.$$

ii. After one pass through the input patterns, how are the patterns clustered? (In other words, which patterns are grouped together in the same class?) Would this change if the input patterns were presented in a different order? Explain.

iii. Repeat part (i) using $\alpha = 0.25$. How does this change affect the training?

E14.4 Earlier in this chapter the term "conscience" was used to refer to a technique for avoiding the dead neuron problem plaguing competitive layers and LVQ networks.

Neurons that are too far from input vectors to ever win the competition can be given a chance by using adaptive biases that get more negative each time a neuron wins the competition. The result is that neurons that win very often start to feel "guilty" until other neurons have a chance to win.

Figure E14.2 shows a competitive network with biases. A typical learning rule for the bias b_i of neuron i is

$$b_i^{new} = \begin{cases} 0.9 b_i^{old}, & \text{if } i = i^* \\ b_i^{old} - 0.2, & \text{if } i \neq i^* \end{cases}.$$

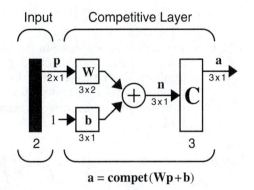

$$a = \text{compet}(Wp+b)$$

Figure E14.2 Competitive Layer with Biases

i. Examine the vectors in Figure E14.3. Is there any order in which the vectors can be presented that will cause $_1w$ to win the competition and move closer to one of the vectors? (Note: assume that adaptive biases are *not* being used.)

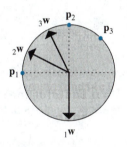

Figure E14.3 Input Vectors and Dead Neuron

ii. Given the input vectors and the initial weights and biases defined below, calculate the weights (using the Kohonen rule) and the biases (using the above bias rule). Repeat the sequence shown below until neuron 1 wins the competition.

$$\mathbf{p}_1 = \begin{bmatrix} -1 \\ 0 \end{bmatrix}, \ \mathbf{p}_2 = \begin{bmatrix} 0 \\ 1 \end{bmatrix}, \ \mathbf{p}_3 = \begin{bmatrix} 1/\sqrt{2} \\ 1/\sqrt{2} \end{bmatrix}$$

$$_1\mathbf{w} = \begin{bmatrix} 0 \\ -1 \end{bmatrix}, \ _2\mathbf{w} = \begin{bmatrix} -2/\sqrt{5} \\ -1/\sqrt{5} \end{bmatrix}, \ _3\mathbf{w} = \begin{bmatrix} -1/\sqrt{5} \\ -2/\sqrt{5} \end{bmatrix}$$

Sequence of input vectors: $\mathbf{p}_1, \mathbf{p}_2, \mathbf{p}_3, \mathbf{p}_1, \mathbf{p}_2, \mathbf{p}_3, \dots$

iii. How many presentations occur before $_1\mathbf{w}$ wins the competition?

E14.5 The net input expression for LVQ networks calculates the distance between the input and each weight vector directly, instead of using the inner product. The result is that the LVQ network does not require normalized input vectors. This technique can also be used to allow a competitive layer to classify nonnormalized vectors. Such a network is shown in Figure E14.4.

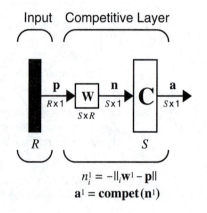

Input   Competitive Layer

$$n_i^1 = -\|_i\mathbf{w}^1 - \mathbf{p}\|$$
$$\mathbf{a}^1 = \mathbf{compet}(\mathbf{n}^1)$$

Figure E14.4 Competitive Layer with Alternate Net Input Expression

Use this technique to train a two-neuron competitive layer on the (nonnormalized) vectors below, using a learning rate, α, of 0.5.

$$\mathbf{p}_1 = \begin{bmatrix} 1 \\ 1 \end{bmatrix}, \ \mathbf{p}_2 = \begin{bmatrix} -1 \\ 2 \end{bmatrix}, \ \mathbf{p}_3 = \begin{bmatrix} -2 \\ -2 \end{bmatrix}$$

Present the vectors in the following order:

$$\mathbf{p}_1, \mathbf{p}_2, \mathbf{p}_3, \mathbf{p}_2, \mathbf{p}_3, \mathbf{p}_1.$$

Here are the initial weights of the network:

$$_1\mathbf{w} = \begin{bmatrix} 0 \\ 1 \end{bmatrix}, \ _2\mathbf{w} = \begin{bmatrix} 1 \\ 0 \end{bmatrix}.$$

E14.6 Show that the modified competitive network of Figure E14.4, which computes distance directly, will produce the same results as the standard competitive network, which uses the inner product, when the input vectors are normalized.

E14.7 We would like a classifier that divides the square region defined below into sixteen classes of roughly equal size.

$$0 \le p_1 \le 1 \,,\, 2 \le p_2 \le 3$$

  i. Use MATLAB to randomly generate 200 vectors in the region shown above.

  ii. Write a MATLAB M-file to implement a competitive layer with Kohonen learning. Calculate the net input by finding the distance between the input and weight vectors directly, as is done by the LVQ network, so the vectors do not need to be normalized. Use the M-file to train a competitive layer to classify the 200 vectors. Try different learning rates and compare performance.

  iii. Write a MATLAB M-file to implement a four-neuron by four-neuron (two-dimensional) feature map. Use the feature map to classify the same vectors. Use different learning rates and neighborhood sizes, then compare performance.

E14.8 We would like a classifier that divides the interval of the input space defined below into five classes.

$$0 \le p_1 \le 1$$

  i. Use MATLAB to randomly generate 100 values in the interval shown above with a uniform distribution.

  ii. Square each number so that the distribution is no longer uniform.

  iii. Write a MATLAB M-file to implement a competitive layer. Use the M-file to train a five-neuron competitive layer on the squared values until its weights are fairly stable.

  iv. How are the weight values of the competitive layer distributed? Is there some relationship between how the weights are distributed and how the squared input values are distributed?

E14.9 An LVQ network has the following weights:

$$\mathbf{W}^1 = \begin{bmatrix} 0 & 0 \\ 1 & 0 \\ -1 & 0 \\ 0 & 1 \\ 0 & -1 \end{bmatrix},\ \mathbf{W}^2 = \begin{bmatrix} 1 & 0 & 0 & 0 & 0 \\ 0 & 1 & 1 & 0 & 0 \\ 0 & 0 & 0 & 1 & 1 \end{bmatrix}.$$

  i. How many classes does this LVQ network have? How many subclasses?

ii. Draw a diagram showing the first-layer weight vectors and the decision boundaries that separate the input space into subclasses.

iii. Label each subclass region to indicate which class it belongs to.

E14.10 We would like an LVQ network that classifies the following vectors according to the classes indicated:

$$\text{class 1: } \left\{ \begin{bmatrix} -1 \\ 1 \\ -1 \end{bmatrix}, \begin{bmatrix} 1 \\ -1 \\ -1 \end{bmatrix} \right\}, \text{class 2: } \left\{ \begin{bmatrix} -1 \\ -1 \\ 1 \end{bmatrix}, \begin{bmatrix} 1 \\ -1 \\ 1 \end{bmatrix}, \begin{bmatrix} 1 \\ 1 \\ -1 \end{bmatrix} \right\}, \text{class 3: } \left\{ \begin{bmatrix} -1 \\ -1 \\ -1 \end{bmatrix}, \begin{bmatrix} -1 \\ 1 \\ 1 \end{bmatrix} \right\}.$$

i. How many neurons are required in each layer of the LVQ network?

ii. Define the weights for the first layer.

iii. Define the weights for the second layer.

iv. Test your network for at least one vector from each class.

E14.11 We would like an LVQ network that classifies the following vectors according to the classes indicated:

$$\text{class 1: } \left\{ \mathbf{p}_1 = \begin{bmatrix} 1 \\ 1 \end{bmatrix}, \mathbf{p}_2 = \begin{bmatrix} 0 \\ 2 \end{bmatrix} \right\}, \text{class 2: } \left\{ \mathbf{p}_3 = \begin{bmatrix} -1 \\ 1 \end{bmatrix}, \mathbf{p}_4 = \begin{bmatrix} 1 \\ 2 \end{bmatrix} \right\}$$

i. Could this classification problem be solved by a perceptron? Explain your answer.

ii. How many neurons must be in each layer of an LVQ network that can classify the above data, given that each class is made up of two convex-shaped subclasses?

iii. Define the second-layer weights for such a network.

iv. Initialize the first-layer weights of the network to all zeros and calculate the changes made to the weights by the Kohonen rule (with a learning rate α of 0.5) for the following series of vectors:

$$\mathbf{p}_4, \mathbf{p}_2, \mathbf{p}_3, \mathbf{p}_1, \mathbf{p}_2.$$

v. Draw a diagram showing the input vectors, the final weight vectors and the decision boundaries between the two classes.

15 Grossberg Network

15

Objectives

This chapter is a continuation of our discussion of associative and competitive learning algorithms in Chapters 13 and 14. The Grossberg network described in this chapter is a self-organizing continuous-time competitive network. This will be the first time we have considered continuous-time recurrent networks, and we will introduce concepts here that will be further explored in Chapters 17 and 18. This Grossberg network is also the foundation for the adaptive resonance theory (ART) networks that we will present in Chapter 16.

We will begin with a discussion of the biological motivation for the Grossberg network: the human visual system. Although we will not cover this material in any depth, the Grossberg networks are so heavily influenced by biology that it is difficult to discuss his networks without putting them in their biological context. It is also important to note that biology provided the original inspirations for the field of artificial neural networks, and we should continue to look for inspiration there, as scientists continue to develop new understanding of brain function.

Theory and Examples

During the late 1960s and the 1970s the number of researchers in the field of neural networks dropped dramatically. There were, however, a number of researchers who continued to work during this period, including Tuevo Kohonen, James Anderson, Kunihiko Fukushima and Shun-ichi Amari, among others. One of the most prolific was Stephen Grossberg.

Grossberg has been continuously active, and highly productive, in neural network research since the early 1960s. His work is characterized by the use of nonlinear mathematics to model specific functions of mind and brain, and his volume of output has been consistent with the magnitude of the task of understanding the brain. The topics of his papers have ranged from such specific areas as how competitive networks can provide contrast enhancement in vision, to such general subjects as a universal theory for human memory.

In part because of the scale of his efforts, his work has a reputation for difficulty. Each new paper is built on a foundation of 30 years of previous results, and is therefore difficult to assess on its own merits. In addition, his terminology is self-consistent, but not in standard use by other researchers. His work is also characterized by a high level of mathematical and neurophysiological sophistication. He is inspired by the interdisciplinary research into brain function by Helmholtz, Maxwell and Mach, and he brings this viewpoint to his work. His research lies at the intersection of mathematics, psychology and neurophysiology. A lack of background in these areas can make his work difficult to approach on a first reading.

This chapter will take a rudimentary look at one of the seminal networks developed by Grossberg. In order to obtain the maximum understanding of his ideas, we will begin with a brief introduction to the biological motivation for the network: the visual system. Then we will present the mathematical building block for many of Grossberg's networks: the shunting model. After understanding the function of this simple model, we will demonstrate how it can be used to build a neural network for adaptive pattern recognition. This network will then form the basis for the adaptive resonance theory networks that are discussed in Chapter 17. By building up gradually to the more complex networks, we hope to make them more easily understandable.

There is an important lesson we should take from the work described in this chapter. Although the original inspiration for the field of artificial neural networks came from biology, at times we forget to look back to biology for new ideas. It will be the blending of biology, mathematics, psychology and other disciplines that will provide the maximum growth in our understanding of neural networks.

Biological Motivation: Vision

The neural network described in this chapter was inspired by the developmental physiology of the human visual system. In this section we want to provide a brief introduction to vision, so that the function of the network will be more understandable.

In Figure 15.1 we have a schematic representation of the first stages of the visual system. Light passes through the cornea (the transparent front part of the eye) and the lens, which bends the light to focus objects on the retina (the interior layer of the external wall of the eye). It is after the light falls on the retina that the immense job of translating this information into an understandable image begins. As we will see later in this chapter, much of what we "see" is not actually present in the image projected onto the retina.

15

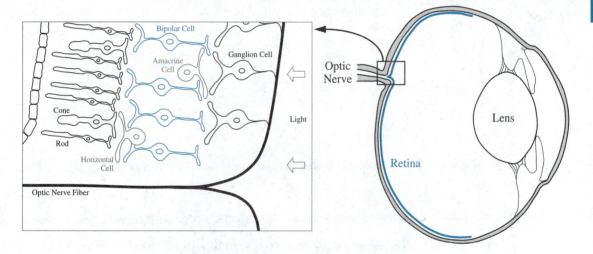

Figure 15.1 Eyeball and Retina

Retina The *retina* is actually a part of the brain. It becomes separated from the brain during fetal development, but remains connected to it through the optic nerve. The retina consists of three layers of nerve cells. The outer layer consists of the photoreceptors (rods and cones), which convert light into **Rods** electrical signals. The *rods* allow us to see in dim light, whereas the *cones* **Cones** allow us to see fine detail and color. For reasons not completely understood, light must pass through the other two layers of the retina in order to stimulate the rods and cones. As we will see later, this obstruction must be compensated for in neural processing, in order to reconstruct recognizable images.

The middle layer of the retina consists of three types of cells: bipolar cells, **Bipolar Cells** horizontal cells and amacrine cells. *Bipolar cells* receive input from the receptors and feed into the third layer of the retina, containing the ganglion

Horizontal Cells
Amacrine Cells

cells. *Horizontal cells* link the receptors and the bipolar cells, and *amacrine cells* link bipolar cells with the ganglion cells.

Ganglion Cells

The final layer of the retina contains the *ganglion cells*. The axons of the ganglion cells pass across the surface of the retina and collect in a bundle to form the optic nerve. It is interesting to note that each eye contains roughly 125 million receptors, but only 1 million ganglion cells. Clearly there is significant processing done in the retina to perform data reduction.

The axons of the ganglion cells, bundled into the optic nerve, connect to an area of the brain called the lateral geniculate nucleus, as illustrated in Figure 15.2. From this point the fibers fan out into the primary visual cortex, located at the back of the brain. The axons of the ganglion cells make synapses with lateral geniculate cells, and the axons of the lateral geniculate cells make synapses with cells in the visual cortex. The *visual cortex* is the region of the brain devoted to visual function and consists of many layers of cells.

Visual Cortex

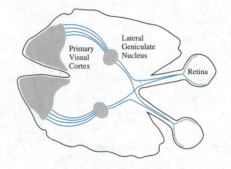

Figure 15.2 Visual Pathway

The connections along the visual pathway are far from random. The mapping from each layer to the next is highly organized. The axons from the ganglion cells in a certain part of the retina go to cells in a particular part of the lateral geniculate, which in turn go to a particular part of the visual cortex. (This topographic mapping was one of the inspirations for the self-organizing feature map described in Chapter 14.) In addition, as we can see in Figure 15.2, each hemisphere of the brain receives input from both eyes, since half of the optic nerve fibers cross and the other half stay uncrossed. It turns out that the left half of each visual field ends up in the right half of the brain, and the right half of each visual field ends up in the left half of the brain.

Illusions

We now have some idea of the general structure of the visual pathway, but how does it function? What is the purpose of the three layers of the retina? What operations are performed by the lateral geniculate? Some hints to the answers to these questions can be obtained by investigating visual illusions.

Why are there so many visual illusions? Mechanisms that overcome imperfections of the retinal uptake process imply illusions. Grossberg and others have used the vast store of known illusions to probe adaptive perceptual mechanisms [GrMi89]. If we can develop mathematical models that produce the same illusions the biological system does, then we may have a mechanism that describes how this part of the brain works. To help us understand why illusions exist, we will first consider some of the imperfections of the retinal uptake process.

Optic Disk   Figure 15.3 is the view of the retina that an ophthalmologist has when looking into the eye through the cornea. The large pale circle is the *optic disk*, where the optic nerve leaves the retina on its way to the lateral geniculate. This is also where arteries enter and veins leave the retina. The optic disk causes a blind spot in our vision, as we will discuss in a moment.

Fovea   The darker disk to the right of the optic disk is the *fovea*, which constitutes the center of our field of vision. This is a region of the retina, about half a millimeter in diameter, that contains only cones. Although cones are distributed throughout the retina, they are most densely packed in the fovea. In addition, in this area of the retina the other layers are displaced to the side, so that the cones lie at the front. The densely packed photoreceptors, and the lack of obstruction, give us our best fine-detail vision at the fovea, which allows us to precisely focus the lens.

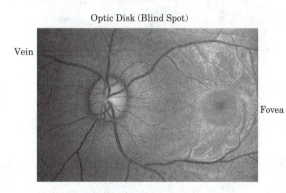

Figure 15.3 Back of the Eye (from [John01])

From Figure 15.3 we can see that there are a number of imperfections in retinal uptake. First, there are no rods and cones in the optic disk, which leaves a blind spot in our field of vision. We are not normally aware of the blind spot because of processing done in the visual pathway, but we can identify it with a simple test. Look at the blue circle on the left side of Figure 15.4, while covering your left eye. As you move your head closer to the page, then farther away, you will notice a point (about nine inches away) at which the circle on the right will disappear from your field of vision. (You are still looking at the circle on the left.) If you haven't tried this before, it can be a little disconcerting. The interesting thing is that we don't see our blind spot as a black hole. Somehow our brains fill in the missing region.

Figure 15.4 Test for the Blind Spot

Other imperfections in the retinal uptake are the arteries and veins that cross in front of the photoreceptors at the back of the retina. These obstruct the rods and cones from receiving all of the light in the visual field. In addition, because the photoreceptors are at the back of the retina, light must pass through the other two layers to reach them.

Figure 15.5 illustrates the effect of these imperfections. Here we see an edge displayed on the retina. The drawing on the right illustrates the image initially perceived by the photoreceptors. The regions covered by the blind spot and the veins are not observed by the rods and cones. (The reason we do not "see" the arteries, veins, etc., is that the vision pathway does not respond to stabilized images. The eyeballs are constantly jerking, in what are called saccadic movements, so that even fixed objects in our field of vision are moving relative to the eye. The veins are fixed relative to the eyeball, so they fade from our vision.)

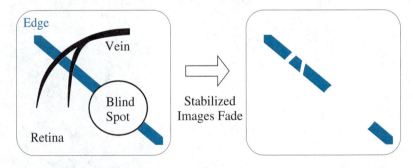

Figure 15.5 Perception of an Edge on the Retina (after [Gros90])

Because we do not see edges as displayed on the right side of Figure 15.5, the neural systems in our visual pathway must be performing some operation that compensates for the distortions and completes the image. Grossberg suggests [GrMi89] that there are two primary types of compensatory

Emergent Segmentation
Featural Filling-in

processing involved. The first, which he calls *emergent segmentation*, completes missing boundaries. The second, which he calls *featural filling-in*, fills in the color and brightness inside the resulting boundaries. These two processes are illustrated in Figure 15.6. In the top figure we see an edge as it is originally perceived by the rods and cones, with missing sections. In the lower figure we see the completed edge, after the emergent segmentation and featural filling-in.

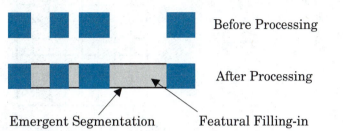

Before Processing

After Processing

Emergent Segmentation   Featural Filling-in

Figure 15.6 Compensatory Processing (after [Gros90])

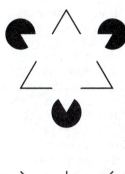

If the processing along the visual pathway is recreating missing parts of the images we see, there must be times when it makes mistakes, since it cannot know exactly those parts of a scene from which it receives no light. These mistakes are illustrated by visual illusions. Consider, for example, the two figures in the left margin. In the top figure you should be able to see a bright white triangle lying on top of several other black objects. In fact, no such triangle exists in the figure. It is purely a creation of the emergent segmentation and featural filling-in process of your visual system. The same is true of the bright white circle which appears to lie on top of the lines in the lower-left figure.

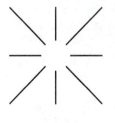

The featural filling-in process is also demonstrated in Figure 15.7. This illusion is called neon color spreading [vanT75]. In the diagram on the right you may be able to see light blue diamonds, or even wide light blue lines criss-crossing the figure. In the diagram on the left you may be able to see a light blue ring. The blue you see filling in the diamonds and the ring is not a result of the color having been smeared during the printing process, nor is it caused by the scattering of light. This effect does not appear on the retina at all. It does not exist, except in your brain. (The perception of neon color spreading can vary from individual to individual, and the strength of the perception is dependent on the colors used. If you do not notice the effect in Figure 15.7, look at the cover of any issue of the journal *Neural Networks*, Pergamon Press.)

Later in this chapter we will discuss some neural network models that can help to explain the processes that implement emergent segmentation, as well as other visual phenomena.

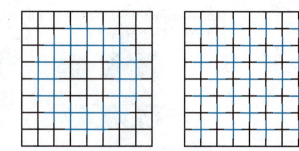

Figure 15.7 Neon Color Spreading (Featural Filling In)

Vision Normalization

In addition to emergent segmentation and featural filling-in, there are two other phenomena that give us an indication of what operations are being performed in the early vision system: *brightness constancy* and *brightness contrast*. The brightness constancy effect is evidenced by the test illustrated in Figure 15.8. In this test a subject is shown a small grey disk inside a darker grey annulus, which is illuminated by white light of a certain intensity. The subject is asked to indicate the brightness of the central disk by looking at a series of grey disks, separately illuminated, and selecting the disk with the same brightness. Next, the brightness of the light illuminating the grey disk and dark annulus is increased, and the subject is again asked to select the disk with the same brightness. This process is repeated for several different levels of illumination. It turns out that in each case the subject will choose the same disk as matching the original central disk. Even though the total light entering the subject's eye is 10 to 100 times brighter, it is only the relative brightness that registers.

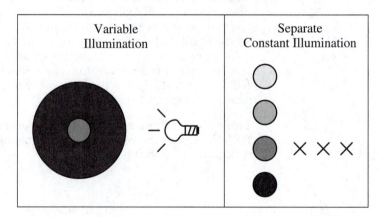

Figure 15.8 Test of Brightness Constancy (after [Gros90])

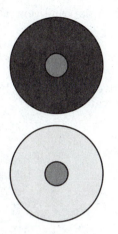

Another phenomenon of the vision system, which is closely related to brightness constancy, is brightness contrast. This effect is illustrated by the two figures in the left margin. At the centers of the two figures we have two small disks with equivalent grey scale. The small disk in the top figure is surrounded by a darker annulus, while the small disk in the lower figure is surrounded by a lighter annulus. Even though both disks have the same grey scale, the one inside the darker annulus appears brighter. This is because our vision system is sensitive to relative intensities. It would seem that the total activity across the image is held constant.

The properties of brightness constancy and brightness contrast are very important to our vision system. Since we see things in so many different lighting conditions, if we were not able to compensate for the absolute intensity of a scene, we would never learn to recognize things. Grossberg calls this process of normalization "discounting the illuminant."

In the rest of this chapter we want to present a neural network architecture that is consistent with the physical phenomena discussed in this section.

Basic Nonlinear Model

Leaky Integrator

Before we introduce the Grossberg network, we will begin by looking at some of the building blocks that make up the network. The first building block is the *"leaky"* integrator, which is shown in Figure 15.9. The basic equation for this system is

$$\varepsilon \frac{dn(t)}{dt} = -n(t) + p(t),$$ (15.1)

Time Constant

where ε is the system *time constant*.

Leaky Integrator

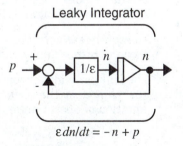

$$\varepsilon dn/dt = -n + p$$

Figure 15.9 Leaky Integrator

The response of the leaky integrator to an arbitrary input $p(t)$ is

$$n(t) = e^{-t/\varepsilon} n(0) + \frac{1}{\varepsilon} \int_0^t e^{-(t-\tau)/\varepsilon} p(t-\tau) d\tau.$$ (15.2)

For example, if the input $p(t)$ is constant and the initial condition $n(0)$ is zero, Eq. (15.2) will produce

$$n(t) = p(1 - e^{-t/\varepsilon}) . \qquad (15.3)$$

A graph of this response, for $p = 1$ and $\varepsilon = 1$, is given in Figure 15.10. The response exponentially approaches a steady state value of 1.

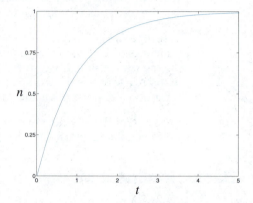

Figure 15.10 Leaky Integrator Response

There are two important properties of the leaky integrator that we want to note. First, because Eq. (15.1) is linear, if the input p is scaled, then the response $n(t)$ will be scaled by the same amount. For example, if the input is doubled, then the response will also be doubled, but will maintain the same shape. This is evident in Eq. (15.3). Second, the speed of response of the leaky integrator is determined by the time constant ε. When ε decreases, the response becomes faster; when ε increases, the response becomes slower. (See Problem P15.1.)

*To experiment with the leaky integrator, use the Neural Network Design Demonstration Leaky Integrator (**nnd15li**).*

Shunting Model

The leaky integrator forms the nucleus of one of Grossberg's fundamental neural models: the *shunting model*, which is shown in Figure 15.11. The equation of operation of this network is

$$\varepsilon\frac{dn(t)}{dt} = -n(t) + (b^+ - n(t)) p^+ - (n(t) + b^-) p^- , \qquad (15.4)$$

Excitatory

Inhibitory

where p^+ is a nonnegative value representing the *excitatory* input to the network (the input that causes the response to increase), and p^- is a nonnegative value representing the *inhibitory* input (the input that causes the response to decrease). The biases b^+ and b^- are nonnegative constants that determine the upper and lower limits on the neuron response, as we will explain next.

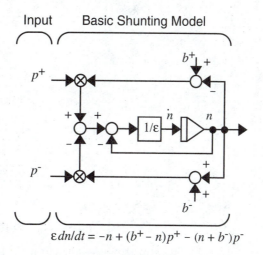

$$\varepsilon \, dn/dt = -n + (b^+ - n)p^+ - (n + b^-)p^-$$

Figure 15.11 Shunting Model

There are three terms on the right-hand side of Eq. (15.4). When the net sign of these three terms is positive, $n(t)$ will go up. When the net sign is negative, $n(t)$ will go down. To understand the performance of the network, let's investigate the three terms individually.

The first term, $-n(t)$, is a linear decay term, which is also found in the leaky integrator. It is negative whenever $n(t)$ is positive, and positive whenever $n(t)$ is negative. The second term, $(b^+ - n(t))\, p^+$, provides nonlinear gain control. This term will be positive while $n(t)$ is less than b^+, but will become zero when $n(t) = b^+$. This effectively sets an upper limit on $n(t)$ of b^+. The third term, $-(n(t) + b^-)\, p^-$, also provides nonlinear gain control. It sets a lower limit on $n(t)$ of $-b^-$.

Figure 15.12 illustrates the performance of the shunting network when $b^+ = 1$, $b^- = 0$ and $\varepsilon = 1$. In the left graph we see the network response when the excitatory input $p^+ = 1$ and the inhibitory input $p^- = 0$. For the right graph $p^+ = 5$ and $p^- = 0$. Notice that even though the excitatory input is increased by a factor of 5, the steady state network response is increased by less than a factor of 2. If we were to continue to increase the excitatory input, we would find that the steady state network response would increase, but would always be less than $b^+ = 1$.

If we apply an inhibitory input to the shunting network, the steady state network response will decrease, but will remain greater than $-b^-$. To summarize the operation of the shunting model, if $n(0)$ falls between b^+ and $-b^-$, then $n(t)$ will remain between these limits, as shown in the figure in the left margin.

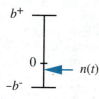

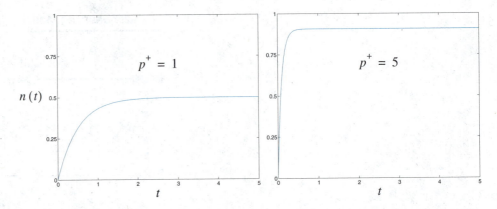

Figure 15.12 Shunting Network Response

The shunting model will form the basis for the Grossberg competitive network, which we will discuss in the next section. The nonlinear gain control will be used to normalize input patterns and to maintain relative intensities over a wide range of total intensity.

*To experiment with the shunting network, use the Neural Network Design Demonstration Shunting Network (*nnd15sn*).*

Two-Layer Competitive Network

We are now ready to present the Grossberg competitive network. This network was inspired by the operation of the mammalian visual system, which we discussed in the opening section of this chapter. (Grossberg was influenced by the work of Chistoph von der Malsburg [vond73], which was influenced in turn by the Nobel-prize-winning experimental work of David Hubel and Torsten Wiesel [HuWi62].) A block diagram of the network is shown in Figure 15.13.

There are three components to the Grossberg network: Layer 1, Layer 2 and the adaptive weights. Layer 1 is a rough model of the operation of the retina, while Layer 2 represents the visual cortex. These models do not fully explain the complexity of the human visual system, but they do illustrate a number of its characteristics. The network includes *short-term memory* (STM) and *long-term memory* (LTM) mechanisms, and performs adaptation, filtering, normalization and contrast enhancement. In the following subsections we will discuss the operation of each of the components of the network.

Short-Term Memory
Long-Term Memory

As we analyze the various elements of the Grossberg network, you will notice the similarity to the Kohonen competitive network of the previous chapter.

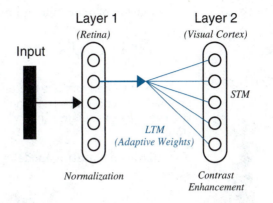

Figure 15.13 Grossberg Competitive Network

15

Layer 1

Layer 1 of the Grossberg network receives external inputs and normalizes the intensity of the input pattern. (Recall from Chapter 14 that the Kohonen network performs best when the input patterns are normalized. For the Grossberg network the normalization is accomplished by the first layer of the network.) A block diagram of this layer is given in Figure 15.14. Note that it uses the shunting model, with the excitatory and inhibitory inputs computed from the input vector **p** .

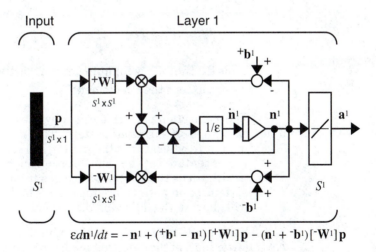

$$\varepsilon d\mathbf{n}^1/dt = -\mathbf{n}^1 + (^+\mathbf{b}^1 - \mathbf{n}^1)[^+\mathbf{W}^1]\mathbf{p} - (\mathbf{n}^1 + {}^-\mathbf{b}^1)[^-\mathbf{W}^1]\mathbf{p}$$

Figure 15.14 Layer 1 of the Grossberg Network

The equation of operation of Layer 1 is

$$\varepsilon\frac{d\mathbf{n}^1(t)}{dt} = -\mathbf{n}^1(t) + (^+\mathbf{b}^1 - \mathbf{n}^1(t))\,[^+\mathbf{W}^1]\,\mathbf{p} - (\mathbf{n}^1(t) + {}^-\mathbf{b}^1)\,[^-\mathbf{W}^1]\,\mathbf{p}. \quad (15.5)$$

As we mentioned earlier, the parameter ε determines the speed of response. It is chosen so that the neuron responses will be much faster than the changes in the adaptive weights, which we will discuss in a later section.

Eq. (15.5) is a shunting model with excitatory input $[^+\mathbf{W}^1]\,\mathbf{p}$, where

$$^+\mathbf{W}^1 = \begin{bmatrix} 1 & 0 & \cdots & 0 \\ 0 & 1 & \cdots & 0 \\ \vdots & \vdots & & \vdots \\ 0 & 0 & \cdots & 1 \end{bmatrix}. \quad (15.6)$$

Therefore the excitatory input to neuron i is the ith element of the input vector.

The inhibitory input to Layer 1 is $[^-\mathbf{W}^1]\,\mathbf{p}$, where

$$^-\mathbf{W}^1 = \begin{bmatrix} 0 & 1 & \cdots & 1 \\ 1 & 0 & \cdots & 1 \\ \vdots & \vdots & & \vdots \\ 1 & 1 & \cdots & 0 \end{bmatrix}. \quad (15.7)$$

Thus the inhibitory input to neuron i is the sum of all elements of the input vector, except the ith element.

On-Center/Off-Surround

The connection pattern defined by the matrices $^+\mathbf{W}^1$ and $^-\mathbf{W}^1$ is called an *on-center/off-surround* pattern. This is because the excitatory input for neuron i (which turns the neuron on) comes from the element of the input vector centered at the same location (element i), while the inhibitory input (which turns the neuron off) comes from surrounding locations. This type of connection pattern produces a normalization of the input pattern, as we will show in the following discussion.

For simplicity, we will set the inhibitory bias $^-\mathbf{b}^1$ to zero, which sets the lower limit of the shunting model to zero, and we will set all elements of the excitatory bias $^+\mathbf{b}^1$ to the same value, i.e.,

$$^+b_i^1 = {}^+b^1,\ i = 1, 2, \dots, S^1, \quad (15.8)$$

so that the upper limit for all neurons will be the same.

To investigate the normalization effect of Layer 1, consider the response of neuron i:

$$\varepsilon \frac{dn_i^1(t)}{dt} = -n_i^1(t) + ({}^+b^1 - n_i^1(t))\, p_i - n_i^1(t) \sum_{j \ne i} p_j \,. \tag{15.9}$$

In the steady state $(dn_i^1(t)/dt = 0)$ we have

$$0 = -n_i^1 + ({}^+b^1 - n_i^1)\, p_i - n_i^1 \sum_{j \ne i} p_j \,. \tag{15.10}$$

If we solve for the steady state neuron output n_i^1 we find

$$n_i^1 = \frac{{}^+b^1 \, p_i}{1 + \sum\limits_{j=1}^{S^1} p_j} \,. \tag{15.11}$$

We now define the relative intensity of input i to be

$$\bar{p}_i = \frac{p_i}{P} \text{ where } P = \sum_{j=1}^{S^1} p_j \,. \tag{15.12}$$

Then the steady state neuron activity can be written

$$n_i^1 = \left(\frac{{}^+b^1 P}{1 + P} \right) \bar{p}_i \,. \tag{15.13}$$

Therefore n_i^1 will be proportional to the relative intensity $\bar{p}_i$, regardless of the magnitude of the total input P. In addition, the total neuron activity is bounded:

$$\sum_{j=1}^{S^1} n_j^1 = \sum_{j=1}^{S^1} \left(\frac{{}^+b^1 P}{1 + P} \right) \bar{p}_j = \left(\frac{{}^+b^1 P}{1 + P} \right) \le {}^+b^1 \,. \tag{15.14}$$

The input vector is normalized so that the total activity is less than ${}^+b^1$, while the relative intensities of the individual elements of the input vector are maintained. Therefore, the outputs of Layer 1, n_i^1, code the relative input intensities, $\bar{p}_i$, rather than the instantaneous fluctuations in the total input activity, P. This result is produced by the on-center/off-surround connection pattern of the inputs and the nonlinear gain control of the shunting model.

Note that Layer 1 of the Grossberg network explains the brightness constancy and brightness contrast characteristics of the human visual system,

15

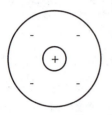

which we discussed on page 15-8. The network is sensitive to the relative intensities of an image, rather than absolute intensities. In addition, experimental evidence has shown that the on-center/off-surround connection pattern is a characteristic feature of the receptive fields of retinal ganglion cells [Hube88]. (The receptive field is an area of the retina in which the photoreceptors feed into a given cell. The figure in the left margin illustrates the on-center/off-surround receptive field of a typical retinal ganglion cell. A "+" indicates an excitatory region, and a "-" indicates an inhibitory region. It is a two-dimensional pattern, as opposed to the one-dimensional connections of Eq. (15.6) and Eq. (15.7).)

To illustrate the performance of Layer 1, consider the case of two neurons, with $^+b^1 = 1$, $\varepsilon = 0.1$:

$$(0.1) \frac{dn_1^1(t)}{dt} = -n_1^1(t) + (1 - n_1^1(t)) p_1 - n_1^1(t) p_2 , \tag{15.15}$$

$$(0.1) \frac{dn_2^1(t)}{dt} = -n_2^1(t) + (1 - n_2^1(t)) p_2 - n_2^1(t) p_1 . \tag{15.16}$$

The response of this network, for two different input vectors, is shown in Figure 15.15. For both input vectors, the second element is four times as large as the first element, although the total intensity of the second input vector is five times as large as that of the first input vector (50 vs. 10). From Figure 15.15 we can see that the response of the network maintains the relative intensities of the inputs, while limiting the total response. The total response $(n_1^1(t) + n_2^1(t))$ will always be less than 1.

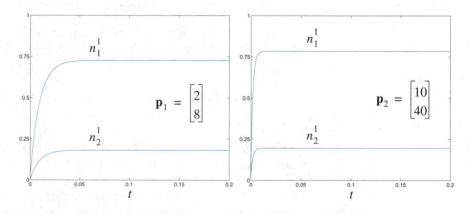

Figure 15.15 Layer 1 Response

To experiment with Layer 1 of the Grossberg network, use the Neural Network Design Demonstration Grossberg Layer 1 *(**nnd15gl1**).*

Layer 2

Layer 2 of the Grossberg network, which is a layer of continuous-time instars, performs several functions. First, like Layer 1, it normalizes total activity in the layer. Second, it contrast enhances its pattern, so that the neuron that receives the largest input will dominate the response. (This is closely related to the winner-take-all competition in the Hamming network and the Kohonen network.) Finally, it operates as a *short-term memory* (STM) by storing the contrast-enhanced pattern.

Short-Term Memory

Figure 15.16 is a diagram of Layer 2. As with Layer 1, the shunting model forms the basis for Layer 2. The main difference between Layer 2 and Layer 1 is that Layer 2 uses feedback connections. The feedback enables the network to store a pattern, even after the input has been removed. The feedback also performs the competition that causes the contrast enhancement of the pattern. We will demonstrate these properties in the following discussion.

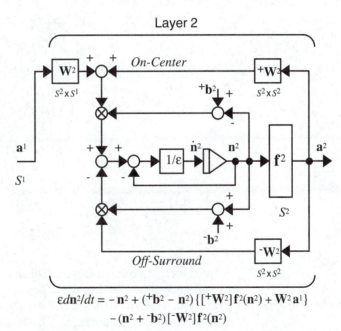

$$\epsilon d\mathbf{n}^2/dt = -\mathbf{n}^2 + (^+\mathbf{b}^2 - \mathbf{n}^2)\{[^+\mathbf{W}^2]\mathbf{f}^2(\mathbf{n}^2) + \mathbf{W}^2\mathbf{a}^1\}$$
$$- (\mathbf{n}^2 + {}^-\mathbf{b}^2)[^-\mathbf{W}^2]\mathbf{f}^2(\mathbf{n}^2)$$

Figure 15.16 Layer 2 of the Grossberg Network

The equation of operation of Layer 2 is

$$\epsilon\frac{d\mathbf{n}^2(t)}{dt} = -\mathbf{n}^2(t) + (^+\mathbf{b}^2 - \mathbf{n}^2(t))\{[^+\mathbf{W}^2]\mathbf{f}^2(\mathbf{n}^2(t)) + \mathbf{W}^2\mathbf{a}^1\} \qquad (15.17)$$
$$- (\mathbf{n}^2(t) + {}^-\mathbf{b}^2)[^-\mathbf{W}^2]\mathbf{f}^2(\mathbf{n}^2(t))$$

This is a shunting model with excitatory input $\{\, [\,^{+}\mathbf{W}^2]\,\mathbf{f}^2(\mathbf{n}^2(t)) + \mathbf{W}^2\mathbf{a}^1\,\}$, where $^{+}\mathbf{W}^2 = \,^{+}\mathbf{W}^1$ provides on-center feedback connections, and $\mathbf{W}^2$ consists of adaptive weights, analogous to the weights in the Kohonen network. The rows of $\mathbf{W}^2$, after training, will represent the prototype patterns. The inhibitory input to the shunting model is $[\,^{-}\mathbf{W}^2]\,\mathbf{f}^2(\mathbf{n}^2(t))$, where $^{-}\mathbf{W}^2 = \,^{-}\mathbf{W}^1$ provides off-surround feedback connections.

To illustrate the performance of Layer 2, consider a two-neuron layer with

$$\varepsilon = 0.1 \,,\; ^{+}\mathbf{b}^2 = \begin{bmatrix} 1 \\ 1 \end{bmatrix},\; ^{-}\mathbf{b}^2 = \begin{bmatrix} 0 \\ 0 \end{bmatrix},\; \mathbf{W}^2 = \begin{bmatrix} (_1\mathbf{w}^2)^T \\ (_2\mathbf{w}^2)^T \end{bmatrix} = \begin{bmatrix} 0.9 & 0.45 \\ 0.45 & 0.9 \end{bmatrix},\quad (15.18)$$

and

$$f^2(n) = \frac{10\,(n)^2}{1 + (n)^2}. \tag{15.19}$$

The equations of operation of the layer will be

$$(0.1)\,\frac{dn_1^2(t)}{dt} = -n_1^2(t) + (1 - n_1^2(t))\,\{f^2(n_1^2(t)) + (_1\mathbf{w}^2)^T\mathbf{a}^1\} \tag{15.20}$$

$$- n_1^2(t)\,f^2(n_2^2(t))$$

$$(0.1)\,\frac{dn_2^2(t)}{dt} = -n_2^2(t) + (1 - n_2^2(t))\,\{f^2(n_2^2(t)) + (_2\mathbf{w}^2)^T\mathbf{a}^1\} \tag{15.21}$$

$$- n_2^2(t)\,f^2(n_1^2(t))\,.$$

Note the relationship between these equations and the Hamming and Kohonen networks. The inputs to Layer 2 are the inner products between the prototype patterns (rows of the weight matrix $\mathbf{W}^2$) and the output of Layer 1 (normalized input pattern). The largest inner product will correspond to the prototype pattern closest to the input pattern. Layer 2 then performs a competition between the neurons, which tends to *contrast enhance* the output pattern — maintaining large outputs while attenuating small outputs. This contrast enhancement is generally milder than the winner-take-all competition of the Hamming and Kohonen networks. In the Hamming and Kohonen networks, the competition drives all but one of the neuron outputs to zero. The exception is the one with the largest input. In the Grossberg network, the competition maintains large values and attenuates

Contrast Enhance

small values, but does not necessarily drive all small values to zero. The amount of contrast enhancement is determined by the transfer function f^2, as we will see in the next section.

Figure 15.17 illustrates the response of Layer 2 when the input vector $\mathbf{a}^1 = \begin{bmatrix} 0.2 & 0.8 \end{bmatrix}^T$ (the steady state result obtained from our Layer 1 example) is applied for 0.25 seconds and then removed.

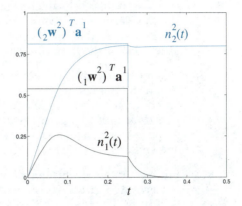

Figure 15.17 Layer 2 Response

There are two important characteristics of this response. First, even before the input is removed, some contrast enhancement is performed. The inputs to Layer 2 are

$$\left({}_1\mathbf{w}^2 \right)^T \mathbf{a}^1 = \begin{bmatrix} 0.9 & 0.45 \end{bmatrix} \begin{bmatrix} 0.2 \\ 0.8 \end{bmatrix} = 0.54 , \tag{15.22}$$

$$\left({}_2\mathbf{w}^2 \right)^T \mathbf{a}^1 = \begin{bmatrix} 0.45 & 0.9 \end{bmatrix} \begin{bmatrix} 0.2 \\ 0.8 \end{bmatrix} = 0.81 . \tag{15.23}$$

Therefore the second neuron has 1.5 times as much input as the first neuron. However, after 0.25 seconds the output of the second neuron is 6.34 times the output of the first neuron. The contrast between high and low has been increased dramatically.

The second characteristic of the response is that after the input has been set to zero, the network further enhances the contrast and stores the pattern. In Figure 15.17 we can see that after the input is removed (at 0.25 seconds) the output of the first neuron decays to zero, while the output of the second neuron reaches a steady state value of 0.79. This output is maintained, even after the input is removed. (Grossberg calls this behavior *reverberation* [Gross76].) It is the nonlinear feedback that enables the network to store the pattern, and the on-center/off-surround connection pattern (determined by $^+\mathbf{W}^2$ and $^-\mathbf{W}^2$) that causes the contrast enhancement.

As an aside, note that we have used the on-center/off-surround structure in both layers of the Grossberg network. There are other connection patterns that could be used for different applications. Recall, for instance, the emergent segmentation problem discussed earlier in this chapter. A structure that has been proposed to implement this mechanism is the *oriented receptive field* [GrMi89], which is shown in the left margin. For this structure, the "on" (excitatory) connections come from one side of the field (indicated by the blue region), and the "off" (inhibitory) connections come from the other side of the field (indicated by the white region).

Oriented Receptive Field

The operation of the oriented receptive field is illustrated in Figure 15.18. When the field is aligned with an edge, the corresponding neuron is activated (large response). When the field is not aligned with an edge, then the neuron is inactive (small response). This explains why we might perceive an edge where none exists, as can be seen in the right-most receptive field shown in Figure 15.18.

For a complete discussion of oriented receptive fields and how they can be incorporated into a neural network architecture for preattentive vision, see [GrMi89]. This paper also discusses a mechanism for featural filling-in.

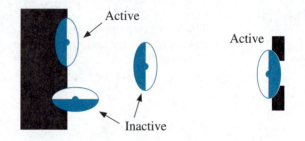

Figure 15.18 Operation of Oriented Receptive Field

Choice of Transfer Function

The behavior of Layer 2 of the Grossberg network depends very much on the transfer function $f^2(n)$. For example, suppose that an input has been applied for some length of time, so that the output has stabilized to the pattern shown in the left margin. (Each point represents the output of an individual neuron.) If the input is then removed, Figure 15.19 demonstrates how the choice of $f^2(n)$ will affect the steady state response of the network. (See [Gross82].)

$n^2_i(0)$

i

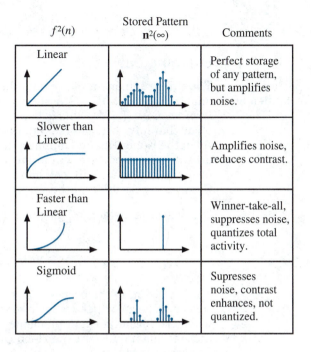

$f^2(n)$	Stored Pattern $\mathbf{n}^2(\infty)$	Comments
Linear		Perfect storage of any pattern, but amplifies noise.
Slower than Linear		Amplifies noise, reduces contrast.
Faster than Linear		Winner-take-all, suppresses noise, quantizes total activity.
Sigmoid		Supresses noise, contrast enhances, not quantized.

Figure 15.19 Effect of Transfer Function $f^2(n)$ (after [Gross82])

If the transfer function is *linear*, the pattern is perfectly stored. Unfortunately, the noise in the pattern will be amplified and stored as easily as the significant inputs. (See Problem P15.6.) If the transfer function is *slower-than-linear* (e.g., $f^2(n) = 1 - e^{-n}$), the steady state response is independent of the initial conditions; all neurons that begin with nonzero values will come to the same level in the steady state. All contrast is eliminated, and noise is amplified.

Faster-than-linear transfer functions (e.g., $f^2(n) = (n)^2$) produce a winner-take-all competition. Only those neurons with the largest initial values are stored; all others are driven to zero. This minimizes the effect of noise, but quantizes the response into an all-or-nothing signal (as in the Hamming and Kohonen networks).

A *sigmoid* function is faster-than-linear for small signals, approximately linear for intermediate signals and slower-than-linear for large signals. When a sigmoid transfer function is used in Layer 2, the pattern is contrast enhanced; larger values are amplified, and smaller values are attenuated. All initial neuron outputs that are less than a certain level (called the *quenching threshold* by Grossberg [Gros76]) decay to zero. This merges the noise suppression of the faster-than-linear transfer functions with the perfect storage produced by linear transfer functions.

To experiment with Layer 2 of the Grossberg network, use the Neural Network Design Demonstration Grossberg Layer 2 (`nnd15gl2`).

Learning Law

Long-Term Memory

The third component of the Grossberg network is the learning law for the adaptive weights $\mathbf{W}^2$. Grossberg calls these adaptive weights the *long-term memory* (LTM). This is because the rows of $\mathbf{W}^2$ will represent patterns that have been stored and that the network will be able to recognize. As in the Kohonen and Hamming networks, the stored pattern that is closest to an input pattern will produce the largest output in Layer 2. In the next subsection we will look more closely at the relationship between the Grossberg network and the Kohonen network.

One learning law for $\mathbf{W}^2$ is given by

$$\frac{dw_{i,j}^2(t)}{dt} = \alpha \{ -w_{i,j}^2(t) + n_i^2(t)n_j^1(t) \} . \tag{15.24}$$

The first term in the bracket on the right-hand side of Eq. (15.24) is a passive decay term, which we have seen in the Layer 1 and Layer 2 equations, while the second term implements a Hebbian-type learning. Together, these terms implement the Hebb rule with decay, which was discussed in Chapter 13.

Recall from Chapter 13 that it is often useful to turn off learning (and forgetting) when $n_i^2(t)$ is not active. This can be accomplished by the following learning law:

$$\frac{dw_{i,j}^2(t)}{dt} = \alpha n_i^2(t) \{ -w_{i,j}^2(t) + n_j^1(t) \} , \tag{15.25}$$

or, in vector form,

$$\frac{d [_i\mathbf{w}^2(t)]}{dt} = \alpha n_i^2(t) \{ -[_i\mathbf{w}^2(t)] + \mathbf{n}^1(t) \} , \tag{15.26}$$

where $_i\mathbf{w}^2(t)$ is a vector composed of the elements of the ith row of $\mathbf{W}^2$ (see Eq. (4.4)).

The terms on the right-hand side of Eq. (15.25) are multiplied (gated) by $n_i^2(t)$, which allows learning (and forgetting) to occur only when $n_i^2(t)$ is not zero. This is the continuous-time implementation of the instar learning rule, which we introduced in Chapter 13 (Eq. (13.32)). In the following subsection we will demonstrate the equivalence of Eq. (15.25) and Eq. (13.32).

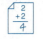

To illustrate the performance of the Grossberg learning law, consider a network with two neurons in each layer. The weight update equations would be

$$\frac{dw^2_{1,1}(t)}{dt} = n^2_1(t)\,\{-w^2_{1,1}(t) + n^1_1(t)\}\,, \tag{15.27}$$

$$\frac{dw^2_{1,2}(t)}{dt} = n^2_1(t)\,\{-w^2_{1,2}(t) + n^1_2(t)\}\,, \tag{15.28}$$

$$\frac{dw^2_{2,1}(t)}{dt} = n^2_2(t)\,\{-w^2_{2,1}(t) + n^1_1(t)\}\,, \tag{15.29}$$

$$\frac{dw^2_{2,2}(t)}{dt} = n^2_2(t)\,\{-w^2_{2,2}(t) + n^1_2(t)\}\,, \tag{15.30}$$

where the learning rate coefficient α has been set to 1. To simplify our example, we will assume that two different input patterns are alternately presented to the network for periods of 0.2 seconds at a time. We will also assume that Layer 1 and Layer 2 converge very quickly, in comparison with the convergence of the weights, so that the neuron outputs are effectively constant over the 0.2 seconds. The Layer 1 and Layer 2 outputs for the two different input patterns will be

$$\text{for pattern 1: } \mathbf{n}^1 = \begin{bmatrix} 0.9 \\ 0.45 \end{bmatrix},\ \mathbf{n}^2 = \begin{bmatrix} 1 \\ 0 \end{bmatrix}, \tag{15.31}$$

$$\text{for pattern 2: } \mathbf{n}^1 = \begin{bmatrix} 0.45 \\ 0.9 \end{bmatrix},\ \mathbf{n}^2 = \begin{bmatrix} 0 \\ 1 \end{bmatrix}. \tag{15.32}$$

Pattern 1 is coded by the first neuron in Layer 2, and pattern 2 is coded by the second neuron in Layer 2.

Figure 15.20 illustrates the response of the adaptive weights, beginning with all weights set to zero. Note that the first row of the weight matrix ($w^2_{1,1}(t)$ and $w^2_{1,2}(t)$) is only adjusted during those periods when $n^2_1(t)$ is nonzero, and that it converges to the corresponding $\mathbf{n}^1$ pattern ($n^1_1(t) = 0.9$ and $n^1_2(t) = 0.45$). (The elements in the first row of the weight matrix are indicated by the blue lines in Figure 15.20.) Also, the second row of the weight matrix ($w^2_{2,1}(t)$ and $w^2_{2,2}(t)$) is only adjusted during those periods when $n^2_2(t)$ is nonzero, and it converges to the corresponding $\mathbf{n}^1$ pattern ($n^1_1(t) = 0.45$

and $n_2^1(t) = 0.9$). (The elements in the second row of the weight matrix are indicated by the black lines in Figure 15.20.)

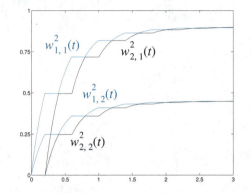

Figure 15.20 Response of the Adaptive Weights

*To experiment with the adaptive weights, use the Neural Network Design Demonstration Adaptive Weights (**nnd15aw**).*

Relation to Kohonen Law

In the previous section we indicated that the Grossberg learning law was a continuous-time version of the instar learning law, which we discussed in Chapter 13. Now we want to demonstrate this fact. We will also show that the Grossberg network is, in its simplest form, a continuous-time version of the Kohonen competitive network of Chapter 14.

To begin, let's repeat the Grossberg learning law of Eq. (15.25):

$$\frac{d[_i\mathbf{w}^2(t)]}{dt} = \alpha n_i^2(t)\{-[_i\mathbf{w}^2(t)] + \mathbf{n}^1(t)\} \ . \tag{15.33}$$

If we approximate the derivative by

$$\frac{d[_i\mathbf{w}^2(t)]}{dt} \approx \frac{_i\mathbf{w}^2(t+\Delta t) - _i\mathbf{w}^2(t)}{\Delta t}, \tag{15.34}$$

then we can rewrite Eq. (15.33) as

$$_i\mathbf{w}^2(t+\Delta t) = _i\mathbf{w}^2(t) + \alpha(\Delta t)n_i^2(t)\{-_i\mathbf{w}^2(t) + \mathbf{n}^1(t)\} \ . \tag{15.35}$$

(Compare this equation with the instar rule that was presented in Chapter 13 in Eq. (13.33).) If we rearrange terms, this can be reduced to

$$_i\mathbf{w}^2(t+\Delta t) \;=\; \{1 - \alpha(\Delta t)\, n_i^2(t)\} \,_i\mathbf{w}^2(t) + \alpha(\Delta t)\, n_i^2(t)\,\{\mathbf{n}^1(t)\}\,. \qquad (15.36)$$

To simplify the analysis further, assume that a faster-than-linear transfer function is used in Layer 2, so that only one neuron in that layer will have a nonzero output; call it neuron i^*. Then only row i^* of the weight matrix will be updated:

$$_{i^*}\mathbf{w}^2(t+\Delta t) \;=\; \{1 - \alpha'\}\,_{i^*}\mathbf{w}^2(t) + \{\alpha\}\,'\mathbf{n}^1(t), \qquad (15.37)$$

where $\alpha' = \alpha(\Delta t)\, n_{i^*}^2(t)$.

This is almost identical to the Kohonen rule for the competitive network that we introduced in Chapter 14 in Eq. (14.13). The weight vector for the winning neuron (with nonzero output) will be moved toward $\mathbf{n}^1$, which is a normalized version of the current input pattern.

There are three major differences between the Grossberg network that we have presented in this chapter and the basic Kohonen competitive network. First, the Grossberg network is a continuous-time network (satisfies a set of nonlinear differential equations). Second, Layer 1 of the Grossberg network automatically normalizes the input vectors. Third, Layer 2 of the Grossberg network can perform a "soft" competition, rather than the winner-take-all competition of the Kohonen network. This soft competition allows more than one neuron in Layer 2 to learn. This causes the Grossberg network to operate as a feature map.

15

Summary of Results

Basic Nonlinear Model

Leaky Integrator

$$\varepsilon \frac{dn(t)}{dt} = -n(t) + p(t)$$

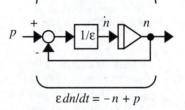

Leaky Integrator

$$\varepsilon\, dn/dt = -n + p$$

Shunting Model

$$\varepsilon \frac{dn(t)}{dt} = -n(t) + (b^+ - n(t))\, p^+ - (n(t) + b^-)\, p^-$$

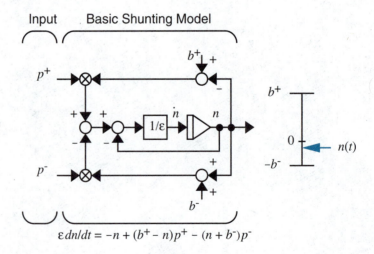

$$\varepsilon\, dn/dt = -n + (b^+ - n)p^+ - (n + b^-)p^-$$

Two-Layer Competitive Network

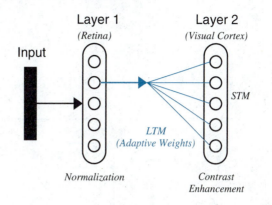

Input

Layer 1
(Retina)

Layer 2
(Visual Cortex)

STM

LTM
(Adaptive Weights)

Normalization

Contrast Enhancement

Layer 1

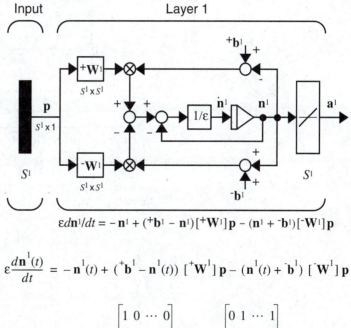

$$\varepsilon d\mathbf{n}^1/dt = -\mathbf{n}^1 + ({}^+\mathbf{b}^1 - \mathbf{n}^1)[{}^+\mathbf{W}^1]\mathbf{p} - (\mathbf{n}^1 + {}^-\mathbf{b}^1)[{}^-\mathbf{W}^1]\mathbf{p}$$

$$\varepsilon\frac{d\mathbf{n}^1(t)}{dt} = -\mathbf{n}^1(t) + ({}^+\mathbf{b}^1 - \mathbf{n}^1(t))[{}^+\mathbf{W}^1]\mathbf{p} - (\mathbf{n}^1(t) + {}^-\mathbf{b}^1)[{}^-\mathbf{W}^1]\mathbf{p}$$

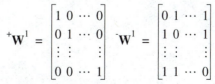

$${}^+\mathbf{W}^1 = \begin{bmatrix} 1 & 0 & \cdots & 0 \\ 0 & 1 & \cdots & 0 \\ \vdots & \vdots & & \vdots \\ 0 & 0 & \cdots & 1 \end{bmatrix} \quad {}^-\mathbf{W}^1 = \begin{bmatrix} 0 & 1 & \cdots & 1 \\ 1 & 0 & \cdots & 1 \\ \vdots & \vdots & & \vdots \\ 1 & 1 & \cdots & 0 \end{bmatrix}$$

On-Center   *Off-Surround*

Steady State Neuron Activity

$$n_i^1 = \left(\frac{{}^+b^1 P}{1 + P}\right)\bar{p}_i, \text{ where } \bar{p}_i = \frac{p_i}{P} \text{ and } P = \sum_{j=1}^{S^1} p_j$$

Layer 2

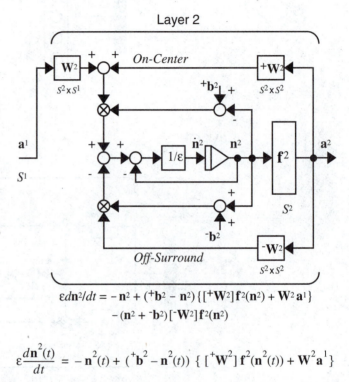

Layer 2

$$\epsilon d\mathbf{n}^2/dt = -\mathbf{n}^2 + ({}^+\mathbf{b}^2 - \mathbf{n}^2)\{[{}^+\mathbf{W}^2]\mathbf{f}^2(\mathbf{n}^2) + \mathbf{W}^2\mathbf{a}^1\}$$
$$- (\mathbf{n}^2 + {}^-\mathbf{b}^2)[{}^-\mathbf{W}^2]\mathbf{f}^2(\mathbf{n}^2)$$

$$\epsilon\frac{d\mathbf{n}^2(t)}{dt} = -\mathbf{n}^2(t) + ({}^+\mathbf{b}^2 - \mathbf{n}^2(t))\{[{}^+\mathbf{W}^2]\mathbf{f}^2(\mathbf{n}^2(t)) + \mathbf{W}^2\mathbf{a}^1\}$$

$$- (\mathbf{n}^2(t) + {}^-\mathbf{b}^2)[{}^-\mathbf{W}^2]\mathbf{f}^2(\mathbf{n}^2(t))$$

Choice of Transfer Function

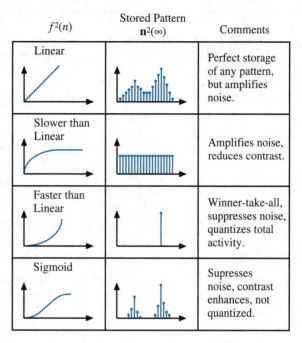

$f^2(n)$	Stored Pattern $\mathbf{n}^2(\infty)$	Comments
Linear		Perfect storage of any pattern, but amplifies noise.
Slower than Linear		Amplifies noise, reduces contrast.
Faster than Linear		Winner-take-all, suppresses noise, quantizes total activity.
Sigmoid		Supresses noise, contrast enhances, not quantized.

Learning Law

$$\frac{d\,[_i\mathbf{w}^2(t)]}{dt} = \alpha n_i^2(t)\,\{-\,[_i\mathbf{w}^2(t)] + \mathbf{n}^1(t)\}$$

(Continuous-Time Instar Learning)

15

Solved Problems

P15.1 **Demonstrate the effect of the coefficient ε on the performance of the leaky integrator, which is shown in Figure P15.1, with the input $p = 1$.**

Leaky Integrator

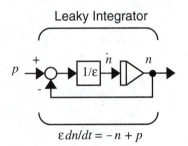

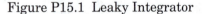

$$\varepsilon \, dn/dt = -n + p$$

Figure P15.1 Leaky Integrator

The equation of operation for the leaky integrator is

$$\varepsilon \frac{dn(t)}{dt} = -n(t) + p(t).$$

The solution to this differential equation, for an arbitrary input $p(t)$, is

$$n(t) = e^{-t/\varepsilon} n(0) + \frac{1}{\varepsilon} \int_0^t e^{-(t-\tau)/\varepsilon} p(t-\tau) d\tau.$$

If $p(t) = 1$, the solution will be

$$n(t) = e^{-t/\varepsilon} n(0) + \frac{1}{\varepsilon} \int_0^t e^{-(t-\tau)/\varepsilon} d\tau.$$

We want to show how this response changes as a function of ε. The response will be

$$n(t) = e^{-t/\varepsilon} n(0) + (1 - e^{-t/\varepsilon}) = e^{-t/\varepsilon}(n(0) - 1) + 1.$$

This response begins at $n(0)$, and then grows exponentially (or decays exponentially, depending on whether or not $n(0)$ is greater than or less than 1), approaching the steady state response of $n(\infty) = 1$. As ε is decreased, the response becomes faster (since $e^{-t/\varepsilon}$ decays more quickly), while the steady state value remains constant. Figure P15.2 illustrates the responses for $\varepsilon = 1, 0.5, 0.25, 0.125$, with $n(0) = 0$. Notice that the steady state value remains 1 for each case. Only the speed of response changes.

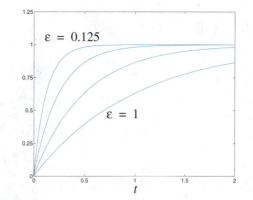

Figure P15.2 Effect of ε on Leaky Integrator Response

15

P15.2 Again using the leaky integrator of Figure P15.1, set $\varepsilon = 1$.

    i. Find a difference equation approximation to the leaky integrator differential equation by approximating the derivative using

$$\frac{dn(t)}{dt} \approx \frac{n(t + \Delta t) - n(t)}{\Delta t}.$$

    ii. Using $\Delta t = 0.1$, compare the response of this difference equation with the response of the differential equation for $p(t) = 1$ and $n(0) = 0$. Compare the two over the range $0 < t < 1$.

    iii. Using the difference equation model for the leaky integrator, show that the response is a weighted average of previous inputs.

i. If we make the approximation to the derivative, we find

$$\frac{n(t + \Delta t) - n(t)}{\Delta t} = -n(t) + p(t)$$

or

$$n(t + \Delta t) = n(t) + \Delta t \{-n(t) + p(t)\} = (1 - \Delta t)\, n(t) + (\Delta t)\, p(t).$$

ii. If we let $\Delta t = 0.1$ we obtain the difference equation

$$n(t + 0.1) = 0.9 n(t) + 0.1 p(t).$$

If we let $p(t) = 1$ and $n(0) = 0$, then we can solve for $n(t)$:

$$n(0.1) = 0.9n(0) + 0.1p(0) = 0.1$$

$$n(0.2) = 0.9n(0.1) + 0.1p(0.1) = 0.9(0.1) + 0.1(1) = 0.19,$$

$$n(0.3) = 0.9n(0.2) + 0.1p(0.2) = 0.9(0.19) + 0.1(1) = 0.271,$$

$$n(0.4) = 0.9n(0.3) + 0.1p(0.3) = 0.9(0.271) + 0.1(1) = 0.3439,$$

$$n(0.5) = 0.9n(0.4) + 0.1p(0.4) = 0.9(0.3439) + 0.1(1) = 0.4095,$$

$$n(0.6) = 0.4686, \ n(0.7) = 0.5217, \ n(0.8) = 0.5695,$$

$$n(0.9) = 0.6126, \ n(1.0) = 0.6513.$$

From Problem P15.1, the solution to the differential equation is

$$n(t) = e^{-t/\varepsilon}n(0) + (1 - e^{-t/\varepsilon}) = (1 - e^{-t}).$$

Figure P15.3 illustrates the relationship between the difference equation solution and the differential equation solution. The black line represents the differential equation solution, and the blue circles represent the difference equation solution. The two solutions are very close, and can be made arbitrarily close by decreasing the interval Δt.

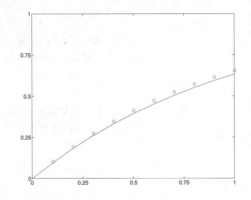

Figure P15.3 Comparison of Difference and Differential Equations

iii. Consider again the difference equation model of the leaky integrator, which we developed in part (ii):

$$n(t + 0.1) = 0.9n(t) + 0.1p(t).$$

If we start from a zero initial condition we find

$$n(0.1) = 0.9n(0) + 0.1p(0) = 0.1p(0),$$

$$n(0.2) = 0.9n(0.1) + 0.1p(0.1) = 0.9\{0.1p(0)\} + 0.1p(0.1) = 0.09p(0) + 0.1p(0.1)$$

$$n(0.3) = 0.9n(0.2) + 0.1p(0.2) = 0.081p(0) + 0.09p(0.1) + 0.1p(0.2)$$

$$\vdots$$

$$n(k0.1) = 0.1\{(0.9)^{k-1}p(0) + (0.9)^{k-2}p(0.1) + \cdots + p((k-1)0.1)\}.$$

Therefore the response of the leaky integrator is a weighted average of previous inputs, $p(0), p(0.1), \ldots, p((k-1)0.1)$. Note that the recent inputs contribute more to the response than the early inputs.

P15.3 **Find the response of the shunting network shown in Figure P15.4 for $\varepsilon = 1$, $b^+ = 1$, $b^- = 1$, $p^+ = 0$, $p^- = 10$ and $n(0) = 0.5$.**

15

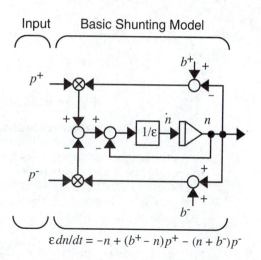

Input   Basic Shunting Model

$$\varepsilon\, dn/dt = -n + (b^+ - n)p^+ - (n + b^-)p^-$$

Figure P15.4 Shunting Network

The equation of operation of the shunting network is

$$\varepsilon\frac{dn(t)}{dt} = -n(t) + (b^+ - n(t))p^+ - (n(t) + b^-)p^-.$$

For the given parameter values this becomes

$$\frac{dn(t)}{dt} = -n(t) - (n(t) + 1)10 = -11n(t) - 10.$$

The solution to this equation is

$$n(t) = e^{-11t}n(0) + \int_0^t e^{-11(t-\tau)}(-10)\,d\tau,$$

or

$$n(t) = e^{-11t}0.5 + \left(-\frac{10}{11}\right)(1 - e^{-11t}).$$

The response is plotted in Figure P15.5.

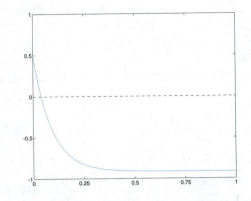

Figure P15.5 Shunting Network Response

There are two things to note about this response. First, as with all shunting networks, the response will never drop below $-{}^-b$, which in this case is -1. As the inhibitory input p^- is increased, the steady state response will decrease, but it can never be less than $-{}^-b$. The second characteristic of the response is that the speed of the response will increase as the input is increased. For instance, if the input were changed from $p^- = 10$ to $p^- = 100$, the response would be

$$n(t) = e^{-101t}0.5 + \left(-\frac{100}{101}\right)(1 - e^{-101t}).$$

Since e^{-101t} decays more rapidly than e^{-11t}, the response will be faster.

P15.4 **Find the response of Layer 1 of the Grossberg network for the case of two neurons, with ${}^+b^1 = 1$, ${}^-b^1 = 0$, $\varepsilon = 1$ and input vector $\mathbf{p} = \begin{bmatrix} c & 2c \end{bmatrix}^T$. Assume that the initial conditions are set to zero. Demonstrate the effect of c on the response.**

The Layer 1 differential equations for this case are

$$\frac{dn_1^1(t)}{dt} = -n_1^1(t) + (1 - n_1^1(t))(c) - n_1^1(t)(2c) = -(1 + 3c)\,n_1^1(t) + c,$$

$$\frac{dn_2^1(t)}{dt} = -n_2^1(t) + (1 - n_2^1(t))(2c) - n_2^1(t)(c) = -(1 + 3c)n_2^1(t) + 2c.$$

The solutions to these equations would be

$$n_1^1(t) = e^{-(1+3c)t}n_1^1(0) + \int_0^t e^{-(1+3c)(t-\tau)}(c)\,d\tau,$$

$$n_2^1(t) = e^{-(1+3c)t}n_2^1(0) + \int_0^t e^{-(1+3c)(t-\tau)}(2c)\,d\tau.$$

If the initial conditions are set to zero, these equations reduce to

$$n_1^1(t) = \left(\frac{c}{1+3c}\right)(1 - e^{-(1+3c)t}),$$

$$n_2^1(t) = \left(\frac{2c}{1+3c}\right)(1 - e^{-(1+3c)t}).$$

Note that the outputs of Layer 1 retain the same relative intensities as the inputs; the output of neuron 2 is always twice the output of neuron 1. This behavior is consistent with Eq. (15.13). In addition, the total output intensity ($n_1^1(t) + n_2^1(t)$) is never larger than $^+b^1 = 1$, as predicted in Eq. (15.14).

As c is increased, it has two effects on the response. First, the steady state values increase slightly. Second, the response becomes faster, since $e^{-(1+3c)t}$ decays more rapidly as c increases.

P15.5 **Consider Layer 2 of the Grossberg network. Assume that the input to Layer 2 is applied for some length of time and then removed (set to zero).**

   i. **Find a differential equation that describes the variation in the total output of Layer 2,**

   $$N^2(t) = \sum_{k=1}^{S^2} n_k^2(t),$$

   after the input to Layer 2 has been removed.

   ii. **Find a differential equation that describes the variation in the relative outputs of Layer 2,**

   $$\bar{n}_i^2(t) = \frac{n_i^2(t)}{N^2(t)},$$

   after the input to Layer 2 has been removed.

i. The operation of Layer 2 is described by Eq. (15.17):

$$\varepsilon\frac{d\mathbf{n}^2(t)}{dt} = -\mathbf{n}^2(t) + (^+\mathbf{b}^2 - \mathbf{n}^2(t))\ \{\ [^+\mathbf{W}^2]\ \mathbf{f}^2(\mathbf{n}^2(t)) + \mathbf{W}^2\mathbf{a}^1\}$$

$$-\ (\mathbf{n}^2(t) + {^-\mathbf{b}}^2)\ [^-\mathbf{W}^2]\ \mathbf{f}^2(\mathbf{n}^2(t))\ .$$

If the input is removed, then $\mathbf{W}^2\mathbf{a}^1$ is zero. For simplicity, we will set the inhibitory bias $^-\mathbf{b}^2$ to zero, and we will set all elements of the excitatory bias $^+\mathbf{b}^2$ to $^+b^2$. The response of neuron i is then given by

$$\varepsilon\frac{dn_i^2(t)}{dt} = -n_i^2(t) + (^+b^2 - n_i^2(t))\ \{f^2(n_i^2(t))\} - n_i^2(t)\ \{\sum_{k \neq i} f^2(n_k^2(t))\}\ .$$

This can be rearranged to produce

$$\varepsilon\frac{dn_i^2(t)}{dt} = -n_i^2(t) + {^+b}^2\ \{f^2(n_i^2(t))\} - n_i^2(t)\left\{\sum_{k=1}^{S^2} f^2(n_k^2(t))\right\}\ .$$

If we then make the definition

$$F^2(t) = \sum_{k=1}^{S^2} f^2(n_k^2(t))\ ,$$

we can simplify the equation to

$$\varepsilon\frac{dn_i^2(t)}{dt} = -\ (1 + F^2(t))\ n_i^2(t) + {^+b}^2\ \{f^2(n_i^2(t))\}\ .$$

To get the total activity, sum this equation over i to produce

$$\varepsilon\frac{dN^2(t)}{dt} = -\ (1 + F^2(t))\ N^2(t) + {^+b}^2\ \{F^2(t)\}\ .$$

This equation describes the variation in the total activity in Layer 2 over time.

ii. The derivative of the relative activity is

$$\frac{d}{dt}[\bar{n}_i^2(t)] = \frac{d}{dt}\left[\frac{n_i^2(t)}{N^2(t)}\right] = \frac{1}{N^2(t)}\frac{d}{dt}[n_i^2(t)] - \left[\frac{n_i^2(t)}{(N^2(t))^2}\right]\frac{d}{dt}[N^2(t)]\ .$$

If we then substitute our previous equations for these derivatives, we find

$$\varepsilon\frac{d}{dt}[\bar{n}_i^2(t)] = \frac{1}{N^2(t)}\left[\{-(1+F^2(t))\,n_i^2(t) + {}^+b^2\{f^2(n_i^2(t))\}\}\right.$$
$$\left. - \frac{n_i^2(t)}{N^2(t)}\{-(1+F^2(t))\,N^2(t) + {}^+b^2\{F^2(t)\}\}\right].$$

Two terms on the right-hand side will cancel to produce

$$\varepsilon\frac{d}{dt}[\bar{n}_i^2(t)] = \frac{1}{N^2(t)}\left[\{{}^+b^2\{f^2(n_i^2(t))\}\} - \frac{n_i^2(t)}{N^2(t)}\{{}^+b^2\{F^2(t)\}\}\right],$$

or

$$\varepsilon\frac{d}{dt}[\bar{n}_i^2(t)] = \frac{{}^+b^2 F^2(t)}{N^2(t)}\left[\frac{f^2(n_i^2(t))}{F^2(t)} - \frac{n_i^2(t)}{N^2(t)}\right].$$

We can put this in a more useful form if we expand the terms in the brackets:

$$\left[\frac{f^2(n_i^2(t))}{F^2(t)} - \frac{n_i^2(t)}{N^2(t)}\right] = \frac{1}{F^2(t)N^2(t)}[f^2(n_i^2(t))N^2(t) - n_i^2(t)F^2(t)]$$

$$= \frac{1}{F^2(t)N^2(t)}\left[g^2(n_i^2(t))n_i^2(t)\sum_{k=1}^{s^2} n_k^2(t) - n_i^2(t)\sum_{k=1}^{s^2} g^2(n_k^2(t))n_k^2(t)\right]$$

$$= \frac{n_i^2(t)}{F^2(t)N^2(t)}\left[\sum_{k=1}^{s^2} n_k^2(t)[g^2(n_i^2(t)) - g^2(n_k^2(t))]\right],$$

where

$$g^2(n_i^2(t)) = \frac{f^2(n_i^2(t))}{n_i^2(t)}.$$

Combining this expression with our previous equation, we obtain

$$\varepsilon\frac{d}{dt}[\bar{n}_i^2(t)] = {}^+b^2\bar{n}_i^2(t)\left[\sum_{k=1}^{s^2} \bar{n}_k^2(t)[g^2(n_i^2(t)) - g^2(n_k^2(t))]\right].$$

This form of the differential equation describing the evolution of the relative outputs is very useful in demonstrating the characteristics of Layer 2, as we will see in the next solved problem.

15

P15.6 Suppose that the transfer function in Layer 2 of the Grossberg network is linear.

  i. Show that the relative outputs of Layer 2 will not change after the input has been removed.

  ii. Under what conditions will the total output of Layer 2 decay to zero after the input has been removed?

i. From Problem P15.5 we know that the relative outputs of Layer 2, after the input has been removed, evolve according to

$$\varepsilon \frac{d}{dt}[\bar{n}_i^2(t)] = {}^+b^2\bar{n}_i^2(t)\left[\sum_{k=1}^{S^2} \bar{n}_k^2(t)\,[g^2(n_i^2(t)) - g^2(n_k^2(t))]\right].$$

If the transfer function for Layer 2, $f^2(n)$, is linear, then

$$f^2(n) = c\,n.$$

Therefore

$$g^2(n) = \frac{f^2(n)}{n} = \frac{c\,n}{n} = c.$$

If we substitute this expression into our differential equation, we find

$$\varepsilon \frac{d}{dt}[\bar{n}_i^2(t)] = {}^+b^2\bar{n}_i^2(t)\left[\sum_{k=1}^{S^2} \bar{n}_k^2(t)\,[c - c]\right] = 0.$$

Therefore the relative outputs do not change.

ii. From Problem P15.5, the total output of Layer 2, after the input has been removed, evolves according to

$$\varepsilon\frac{dN^2(t)}{dt} = -(1 + F^2(t))\,N^2(t) + {}^+b^2\,\{F^2(t)\}.$$

If $f^2(n)$ is linear, then

$$F^2(t) = \sum_{k=1}^{S^2} f^2(n_k^2(t)) = \sum_{k=1}^{S^2} c\,n_k^2(t) = c\sum_{k=1}^{S^2} n_k^2(t) = c\,N^2(t).$$

Therefore the differential equation can be written

$$\varepsilon\frac{dN^2(t)}{dt} = -(1 + c\,N^2(t))\,N^2(t) + {}^+b^2\,\{c\,N^2(t)\} = -\{1 - {}^+b^2c + c\,N^2(t)\}\,N^2(t).$$

To find the equilibrium solutions of this equation, we set the derivative to zero:

$$0 = -\{1 - {}^{+}b^2 c + c\, N^2(t)\}\, N^2(t).$$

Therefore there are two equilibrium solutions:

$$N^2(t) = 0 \text{ or } N^2(t) = \frac{{}^{+}b^2 c - 1}{c}.$$

We want to know the conditions under which the total output will converge to each of these possible solutions. Consider two cases:

1. $1 \ge {}^{+}b^2 c$

   For this case, the derivative of the total output,

   $$\varepsilon \frac{d N^2(t)}{dt} = -\{1 - {}^{+}b^2 c + c\, N^2(t)\}\, N^2(t),$$

   will always be negative for positive $N^2(t)$. (Recall that the outputs of Layer 2 are never negative.) Therefore, the total output will decay to zero.

   $$\lim_{t \to \infty} N^2(t) = 0$$

2. $1 < {}^{+}b^2 c$

   (a) If $N^2(0) > ({}^{+}b^2 c - 1)/c$, then the derivative of the total output will be negative until $N^2(t) = ({}^{+}b^2 c - 1)/c$, when the derivative will be zero. Therefore,

   $$\lim_{t \to \infty} N^2(t) = \frac{({}^{+}b^2 c - 1)}{c}.$$

   (b) If $N^2(0) < ({}^{+}b^2 c - 1)/c$, then the derivative of the total output will be positive until $N^2(t) = ({}^{+}b^2 c - 1)/c$, when the derivative will be zero. Therefore,

   $$\lim_{t \to \infty} N^2(t) = \frac{({}^{+}b^2 c - 1)}{c}.$$

Therefore, if the transfer function of Layer 2 is linear, the total output will decay to zero if $1 \ge {}^{+}b^2 c$. If $1 < {}^{+}b^2 c$, then the total output will converge to $({}^{+}b^2 c - 1)/c$. In any case, the relative outputs will remain constant.

15

As an example of these results, consider the following Layer 2 equations:

$$\frac{dn_1^2(t)}{dt} = -n_1^2(t) + (1.5 - n_1^2(t)) \, \{n_1^2(t)\} - n_1^2(t) \, \{n_2^2(t)\} \, ,$$

$$\frac{dn_2^2(t)}{dt} = -n_2^2(t) + (1.5 - n_2^2(t)) \, \{n_2^2(t)\} - n_2^2(t) \, \{n_1^2(t)\} \, .$$

For this case, $\varepsilon = 1$, ${}^+b^2 = 1.5$ and $c = 1$, therefore $1 < {}^+b^2 c$. The total output will converge to

$$\lim_{t \to \infty} N^2(t) = \frac{({}^+b^2 c - 1)}{c} = \frac{(1.5 - 1)}{1} = 0.5 \, .$$

In Figure P15.6 we can see the response of Layer 2 for two different sets of initial conditions:

$$\mathbf{n}^2(0) = \begin{bmatrix} 0.75 \\ 0.5 \end{bmatrix} \text{ and } \mathbf{n}^2(0) = \begin{bmatrix} 0.15 \\ 0.1 \end{bmatrix} .$$

As expected, the total output converges to 0.5 for both initial conditions. In addition, since the relative values of the initial conditions are the same for the two cases, the outputs converge to the same values in both cases.

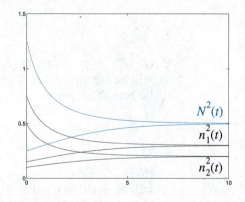

Figure P15.6 Response of Layer 2 for Linear $f^2(n)$

P15.7 **Show that the continuous-time Hebb rule with decay, given by Eq. (15.24), is equivalent to the discrete-time version given by Eq. (13.18).**

The continuous-time Hebb rule with decay is

$$\frac{dw_{i,j}^2(t)}{dt} = \alpha\{-w_{i,j}^2(t) + n_i^2(t)n_j^1(t)\}\ .$$

If we approximate the derivative by

$$\frac{dw_{i,j}^2(t)}{dt} \approx \frac{w_{i,j}^2(t+\Delta t) - w_{i,j}^2(t)}{\Delta t}\ ,$$

the Hebb rule becomes

$$w_{i,j}^2(t+\Delta t) = w_{i,j}^2(t) + \alpha\Delta t\{-w_{i,j}^2(t) + n_i^2(t)n_j^1(t)\}\ .$$

This can be rearranged to obtain

$$w_{i,j}^2(t+\Delta t) = [1 - \alpha\Delta t]\,w_{i,j}^2(t) + \alpha\Delta t\{n_i^2(t)n_j^1(t)\}\ .$$

In vector form this would be

$$\mathbf{W}^2(t+\Delta t) = [1 - \alpha\Delta t]\,\mathbf{W}^2(t) + \alpha\Delta t\{\mathbf{n}^2(t)\,(\mathbf{n}^1(t))^T\}\ .$$

If we compare this with Eq. (13.18),

$$\mathbf{W}(q) = (1 - \gamma)\,\mathbf{W}(q-1) + \alpha\mathbf{a}(q)\,\mathbf{p}^T(q)\ ,$$

we can see that they have the identical form.

15

Epilogue

The Grossberg network presented in this chapter was inspired by the visual system of higher vertebrates. To motivate the network, we presented a brief description of the primary visual pathway. We also discussed some visual illusions, which help us to understand the mechanisms underlying the visual system.

The Grossberg network is a two-layer, continuous-time competitive network, which is very similar in structure and operation to the Kohonen competitive network presented in Chapter 14. The first layer of the Grossberg network normalizes the input pattern. It demonstrates how the visual system can use on-center/off-surround connection patterns and a shunting model to implement an automatic gain control, which normalizes total activity.

The second layer of the Grossberg network performs a competition, which contrast enhances the output pattern and stores it in short-term memory. It uses nonlinear feedback and the on-center/off-surround connection pattern to produce the competition and the storage. The choice of the transfer function and the feedback connection pattern determines the degree of competition (e.g., winner-take-all, mild contrast enhancement, or no change in the pattern).

The adaptive weights in the Grossberg network use an instar learning rule, which stores prototype patterns in long-term memory. When a winner-take-all competition is performed in the second layer, this learning rule is equivalent to the Kohonen learning rule used in Chapter 14.

As with the Kohonen network, one key problem of the Grossberg network is the stability of learning; as more inputs are applied to the network, the weight matrix may never converge. This problem was discussed extensively in Chapter 14. In Chapter 16 we will present a class of networks that is designed to overcome this difficulty: the Adaptive Resonance Theory (ART) networks. The ART networks are direct descendents of the Grossberg network presented in this chapter.

Another problem with the Grossberg network, which we have not discussed in this chapter, is the stability of the differential equations that implement the network. In Layer 2, for example, we have a set of differential equations with nonlinear feedback. Can we make some general statement about the stability of such systems? Chapter 17 will present a comprehensive discussion of this problem.

Further Reading

[GrMi89]   S. Grossberg, E. Mingolla and D. Todorovic, "A neural network architecture for preattentive vision," *IEEE Transactions on Biomedical Engineering*, vol. 36, no. 1, pp. 65–84, 1989.

The objective of this paper is to develop a neural network for general purpose preattentive vision. The network consists of two main subsystems: a boundary contour system and a feature contour system.

[Gros76]   S. Grossberg, "Adaptive pattern classification and universal recoding: I. Parallel development and coding of neural feature detectors," *Biological Cybernetics*, vol. 23, pp. 121–134, 1976.

Grossberg describes a continuous-time competitive network, inspired by the developmental physiology of the visual cortex. The structure of this network forms the foundation for other important networks.

[Gros82]   S. Grossberg, *Studies of Mind and Brain*, Boston: D. Reidel Publishing Co., 1982.

This book is a collection of Stephen Grossberg papers from the period 1968 through 1980. It covers many of the fundamental concepts that are used in later Grossberg networks, such as the adaptive resonance theory networks.

[Hube88]   D.H. Hubel, *Eye, Brain, and Vision*, New York: Scientific American Library, 1988.

David Hubel has been at the center of research in this area for 30 years, and his book provides an excellent introduction to the human visual system. He explains the current view of the visual system in a way that is easily accessible to anyone with some scientific training.

[vanT75]   H. F. J. M. van Tuijl, "A new visual illusion: Neonlike color spreading and complementary color induction between subjective contours," *Acta Psychologica*, vol. 39, pp. 441–445, 1975.

This paper describes the original discovery of the illusion in which crosses of certain colors, when placed inside Ehrenstein figures, appear to spread into solid shapes.

15

[vond73]   C. von der Malsburg, "Self-organization of orientation sensitive cells in the striate cortex," *Kybernetic*, vol. 14, pp. 85–100, 1973.

Malsberg's is one of the first papers to present a self-organizing feature map neural network. The network is a model for the visual cortex of higher vertebrates. This paper influenced the work of Kohonen and Grossberg on feature maps.

Exercises

E15.1 Consider the leaky integrator shown in Figure E15.1.

    i. Find the response $n(t)$ if $\varepsilon = 1$, $n(0) = 1$ and $p(t) = 0.5$.

    ii. Find the response $n(t)$ if $\varepsilon = 1$, $n(0) = 1$ and $p(t) = 2$.

    iii. Find the response $n(t)$ if $\varepsilon = 4$, $n(0) = 1$ and $p(t) = 2$.

    iv. Check your answers to the previous parts by writing a MATLAB M-file to simulate the leaky integrator. Use the **ode45** routine. Plot the response for each case.

Leaky Integrator

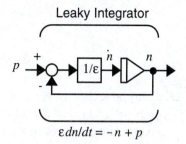

$$\varepsilon \, dn/dt = -n + p$$

Figure E15.1 Leaky Integrator

E15.2 Consider the shunting network shown in Figure E15.2.

    i. Find the response of the shunting network if $\varepsilon = 2$, $b^+ = 3$, $b^- = 1$, $p^+ = 0$, $p^- = 5$ and $n(0) = 1$.

    ii. Find the response of the shunting network if $\varepsilon = 2$, $b^+ = 3$, $b^- = 1$, $p^+ = 0$, $p^- = 50$ and $n(0) = 1$.

    iii. Find the response of the shunting network if $\varepsilon = 2$, $b^+ = 3$, $b^- = 1$, $p^+ = 50$, $p^- = 0$ and $n(0) = 1$.

    iv. Check your answers to the previous parts by writing a MATLAB M-file to simulate the shunting network. Use the **ode45** routine. Plot the response for each case.

    v. Explain the differences in operation of the leaky integrator and the shunting network.

15

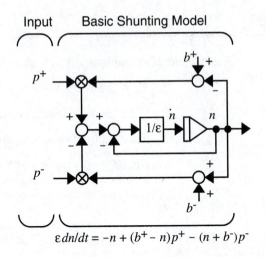

Input   Basic Shunting Model

$$\varepsilon\, dn/dt = -n + (b^+ - n)p^+ - (n + b^-)p^-$$

Figure E15.2 Shunting Network

E15.3 Suppose that Layer 1 of the Grossberg network has two neurons, with $^+b^1 = 0.5$, $\varepsilon = 0.5$ and input vector $\mathbf{p} = \begin{bmatrix} 2 & 1 \end{bmatrix}^T$. Assume that the initial conditions are set to zero.

    i. Find the steady state response of Layer 1, using Eq. (15.13).

    ii. Find the solution to the differential equation for Layer 1. Verify that the steady state response agrees with your answer to part (i).

    iii. Check your answer by writing a MATLAB M-file to simulate Layer 1 of the Grossberg network. Use the **ode45** routine. Plot the response.

E15.4 Repeat Exercise E15.3 for input vector $\mathbf{p} = \begin{bmatrix} 20 & 10 \end{bmatrix}^T$.

E15.5 Find the differential equation that describes the variation in the total output of Layer 1,

$$N^1(t) = \sum_{i=1}^{s^1} n_i^1(t).$$

(Use the technique presented in Problem P15.5.)

E15.6 Assume that Layer 2 of the Grossberg network has two neurons, with $f^2(n) = 2n$, $\varepsilon = 1$, ${}^+b^2 = 1$ and ${}^-b^2 = 0$. The inputs have been applied for some length of time, then removed.

  i. What will be the steady state total output, $\lim_{t \to \infty} N^2(t)$?

  ii. Repeat part (i) if ${}^+b^2 = 0.25$.

```
» 2 + 2
ans =
   4
```

  iii. Check your answers to the previous parts by writing a MATLAB M-file to simulate Layer 2 of the Grossberg network. Use the **ode45** routine. Plot the responses for the following initial conditions:

$$\mathbf{n}^2(0) = \begin{bmatrix} 2 \\ 1 \end{bmatrix} \text{ and } \mathbf{n}^2(0) = \begin{bmatrix} 0.2 \\ 0.1 \end{bmatrix}.$$

15

E15.7 Suppose that the transfer function for Layer 2 of the Grossberg network is $f^2(n) = c \times (n)^2$, and $\varepsilon = 1$, ${}^+b^2 = 1$.

  i. Using the results of Problem P15.5, show that, after the inputs have been removed, all of the relative outputs of Layer 2 will decay to zero, except the one with the largest initial condition (winner-take-all competition).

  ii. For what values of c will the total output $N^2(t)$ have a nonzero stable point (steady state value)?

  iii. If the condition of part (ii) is satisfied, what will be the steady state value of $N^2(t)$? Will this depend on the initial condition $N^2(0)$?

```
» 2 + 2
ans =
   4
```

  iv. Check your answers to the previous parts by writing a MATLAB M-file and simulating the total response of Layer 2 for $c = 4$ and $N^2(0) = 3$.

E15.8 Simulate the response of the adaptive weights for the Grossberg network. Assume that the coefficient ε is 1. Assume that two different input patterns are alternately presented to the network for periods of 0.2 seconds at a time. Also, assume that Layer 1 and Layer 2 converge very quickly, in comparison with the convergence of the weights, so that the neuron outputs are effectively constant over the 0.2 seconds. The Layer 2 and Layer 1 outputs for the two different input patterns will be:

```
» 2 + 2
ans =
   4
```

$$\text{for pattern 1: } \mathbf{n}^1 = \begin{bmatrix} 0.8 \\ 0.2 \end{bmatrix}, \mathbf{n}^2 = \begin{bmatrix} 1 \\ 0 \end{bmatrix},$$

$$\text{for pattern 2: } \mathbf{n}^1 = \begin{bmatrix} 0.5 \\ 0.5 \end{bmatrix}, \mathbf{n}^2 = \begin{bmatrix} 0 \\ 1 \end{bmatrix}.$$

E15.9 Repeat Exercise E15.8, but use the Hebb rule with decay, Eq. (15.24), instead of the instar learning of Eq. (15.25). Explain the differences between the two responses.

16 Adaptive Resonance Theory

16

Objectives

In Chapters 14 and 15 we learned that one key problem of competitive networks is the stability of learning. There is no guarantee that, as more inputs are applied to the network, the weight matrix will eventually converge. In this chapter we will present a modified type of competitive learning, called adaptive resonance theory (ART), which is designed to overcome the problem of learning stability.

Theory and Examples

A key problem of the Grossberg network presented in Chapter 15, and the competitive networks of Chapter 14, is that they do not always form stable clusters (or categories). Grossberg did show [Gros76] that if the number of input patterns is not too large, or if the input patterns do not form too many clusters relative to the number of neurons in Layer 2, then the learning eventually stabilizes. However, he also showed that the standard competitive networks do not have stable learning in response to arbitrary input patterns. The learning instability occurs because of the network's adaptability (or plasticity), which causes prior learning to be eroded by more recent learning.

Stability/Plasticity Grossberg refers to this problem as the "*stability / plasticity dilemma*." How can a system be receptive to significant new patterns and yet remain stable in response to irrelevant patterns? We know that biological systems are very good at this. For example, you can easily recognize your mother's face, even if you have not seen her for a long time and have met many new people in the mean time.

Grossberg and Gail Carpenter developed a theory, called adaptive resonance theory (ART), to address the stability/plasticity dilemma (see [CaGr87a], [CaGr87b], [CaGr90], [CaGrRe91] and [CaGrMa92]). The ART networks are based on the Grossberg network of Chapter 15. The key innovation of ART is the use of "expectations." As each input pattern is presented to the network, it is compared with the prototype vector that it most closely matches (the expectation). If the match between the prototype and the input vector is not adequate, a new prototype is selected. In this way, previously learned memories (prototypes) are not eroded by new learning.

It is beyond the scope of this text to discuss all of the variations of adaptive resonance theory. Instead, we will present one of the ART networks in detail — ART1 (see [CaGr87a]). This particular network is designed for binary input vectors only. However, from this one architecture, the key features of adaptive resonance theory can be understood.

Overview of Adaptive Resonance

The basic ART architecture is shown in Figure 16.1. It is a modification of the Grossberg network of Chapter 15 (compare with Figure 15.13), which is designed to stabilize the learning process. The innovations of the ART architecture consist of three parts: Layer 2 (L2) to Layer 1 (L1) expectations, the orienting subsystem and gain control. In this section we will describe the general operation of the ART system; then, in later sections, we will discuss each subsystem in detail.

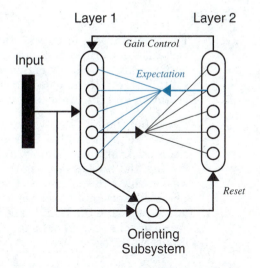

Figure 16.1 Basic ART Architecture

Recall from Chapter 15 that the L1-L2 connections of the Grossberg network are instars, which perform a clustering (or categorization) operation. When an input pattern is presented to the network, it is multiplied (after normalization) by the L1-L2 weight matrix. Then, a competition is performed at Layer 2 to determine which row of the weight matrix is closest to the input vector. That row is then moved toward the input vector. After learning is complete, each row of the L1-L2 weight matrix is a prototype pattern, which represents a cluster (or category) of input vectors.

In the ART networks, learning also occurs in a set of feedback connections from Layer 2 to Layer 1. These connections are outstars (see Chapter 13), which perform pattern recall. When a node in Layer 2 is activated, this reproduces a prototype pattern (the expectation) at Layer 1. Layer 1 then performs a comparison between the expectation and the input pattern.

When the expectation and the input pattern are not closely matched, the orienting subsystem causes a reset in Layer 2. This reset disables the current winning neuron, and the current expectation is removed. A new competition is then performed in Layer 2, while the previous winning neuron is disabled. The new winning neuron in Layer 2 projects a new expectation to Layer 1, through the L2-L1 connections. This process continues until the L2-L1 expectation provides a close enough match to the input pattern.

In the following sections we will investigate each of the subsystems of the ART system, as they apply to one particular ART network — ART1 ([CaGr87a]). We will first describe the differential equations that describe the subsystem operations. Then we will derive the steady state responses of each subsystem. Finally, we will summarize the overall operation of the ART1 system.

16

Layer 1

The main purpose of Layer 1 is to compare the input pattern with the expectation pattern from Layer 2. (*Both patterns are binary in ART1.*) If the patterns are not closely matched, the orienting subsystem will cause a reset in Layer 2. If the patterns are close enough, Layer 1 combines the expectation and the input to form a new prototype pattern.

Layer 1 of the ART1 network, which is displayed in Figure 16.2, is very similar to Layer 1 of the Grossberg network (see Figure 15.14). The differences occur at the excitatory and inhibitory inputs to the shunting model. For the ART1 network, no normalization is performed at Layer 1; therefore we don't have the on-center/off-surround connections from the input vector. The excitatory input to Layer 1 of ART1 consists of a combination of the input pattern and the L1-L2 expectation. The inhibitory input consists of the gain control signal from Layer 2. In the following we will explain how these inputs work together.

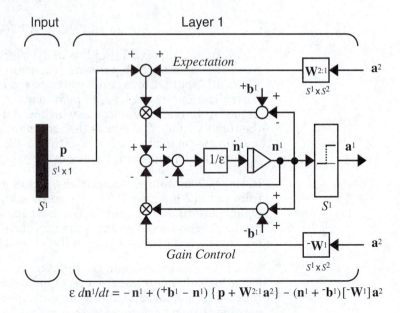

$$\varepsilon \, d\mathbf{n}^1/dt = -\mathbf{n}^1 + ({}^+\mathbf{b}^1 - \mathbf{n}^1)\{\mathbf{p} + \mathbf{W}^{2:1}\mathbf{a}^2\} - (\mathbf{n}^1 + {}^-\mathbf{b}^1)[{}^-\mathbf{W}^1]\mathbf{a}^2$$

Figure 16.2 Layer 1 of the ART1 Network

The equation of operation of Layer 1 is

$$\varepsilon \frac{d\mathbf{n}^1(t)}{dt} = -\mathbf{n}^1(t) + ({}^+\mathbf{b}^1 - \mathbf{n}^1(t))\{\mathbf{p} + \mathbf{W}^{2:1}\mathbf{a}^2(t)\} \qquad (16.1)$$

$$- (\mathbf{n}^1(t) + {}^-\mathbf{b}^1)[{}^-\mathbf{W}^1]\mathbf{a}^2(t)$$

and the output of Layer 1 is computed

$$\mathbf{a}^1 = \mathbf{hardlim}^+(\mathbf{n}^1),\tag{16.2}$$

where

$$hardlim^+(n) = \begin{cases} 1, & n > 0 \\ 0, & n \le 0 \end{cases}.\tag{16.3}$$

Eq. (16.1) is a shunting model with excitatory input $\mathbf{p} + \mathbf{W}^{2:1}\mathbf{a}^2(t)$, which is the sum of the input vector and the L2-L1 expectation. For example, assume that the jth neuron in Layer 2 has won the competition, so that its output is 1, and the other neurons have zero output. For this case we have

$$\mathbf{W}^{2:1}\mathbf{a}^2 = \begin{bmatrix} \mathbf{w}_1^{2:1} & \mathbf{w}_2^{2:1} & \cdots & \mathbf{w}_j^{2:1} & \cdots & \mathbf{w}_{S^2}^{2:1} \end{bmatrix} \begin{bmatrix} 0 \\ 0 \\ \vdots \\ 1 \\ \vdots \end{bmatrix} = \mathbf{w}_j^{2:1},\tag{16.4}$$

16

where $\mathbf{w}_j^{2:1}$ is the jth column of the matrix $\mathbf{W}^{2:1}$. (The $\mathbf{W}^{2:1}$ matrix is trained using an outstar rule, as we will show in a later section.) Now we can see that

$$\mathbf{p} + \mathbf{W}^{2:1}\mathbf{a}^2 = \mathbf{p} + \mathbf{w}_j^{2:1}.\tag{16.5}$$

Therefore the excitatory input to Layer 1 is the sum of the input pattern and the L2-L1 expectation. Each column of the L2-L1 matrix represents a different expectation (prototype pattern). Layer 1 combines the input pattern with the expectation using an AND operation, as we will see later.

The inhibitory input to Layer 1 is the gain control term $[\,\mathbf{^-W}^1]\,\mathbf{a}^2(t)$, where

$$\mathbf{^-W}^1 = \begin{bmatrix} 1 & 1 & \cdots & 1 \\ 1 & 1 & \cdots & 1 \\ \vdots & \vdots & & \vdots \\ 1 & 1 & \cdots & 1 \end{bmatrix}.\tag{16.6}$$

Therefore, the inhibitory input to each neuron in Layer 1 is the sum of all of the outputs of Layer 2. Since we will be using a winner-take-all competition in Layer 2, whenever Layer 2 is active there will be one, and only one, nonzero element of $\mathbf{a}^2$ after the competition. Therefore the gain control input to Layer 1 will be one when Layer 2 is active, and zero when Layer 2 is inactive (all neurons having zero output). The purpose of this gain control will become apparent as we analyze the steady state behavior of Layer 1.

Steady State Analysis

The response of neuron i in Layer 1 is described by

$$\varepsilon \frac{dn_i^1}{dt} = -n_i^1 + ({}^+b^1 - n_i^1)\left\{ p_i + \sum_{j=1}^{S^2} w_{i,j}^{2:1} a_j^2 \right\} - (n_i^1 + {}^-b^1) \sum_{j=1}^{S^2} a_j^2, \qquad (16.7)$$

where $\varepsilon \ll 1$ so that the short-term memory traces (the neuron outputs) change much faster than the long-term memory traces (the weight matrices).

We want to investigate the steady state response of this system for two different cases. In the first case Layer 2 is inactive, therefore $a_j^2 = 0$ for all j. In the second case Layer 2 is active, and therefore one neuron has an output of 1, and all other neurons output 0.

Consider first the case where Layer 2 is inactive. Since each $a_j^2 = 0$, Eq. (16.7) simplifies to

$$\varepsilon \frac{dn_i^1}{dt} = -n_i^1 + ({}^+b^1 - n_i^1)\{p_i\}. \qquad (16.8)$$

In the steady state $(dn_i^1(t)/dt = 0)$ we have

$$0 = -n_i^1 + ({}^+b^1 - n_i^1) p_i = -(1 + p_i) n_i^1 + {}^+b^1 p_i. \qquad (16.9)$$

If we solve for the steady state neuron output n_i^1 we find

$$n_i^1 = \frac{{}^+b^1 p_i}{1 + p_i}. \qquad (16.10)$$

Therefore, if $p_i = 0$ then $n_i^1 = 0$, and if $p_i = 1$ then $n_i^1 = {}^+b^1/2 > 0$. Since we chose the transfer function for Layer 1 to be the *hardlim*$^+$ function, then we have

$$\mathbf{a}^1 = \mathbf{p}. \qquad (16.11)$$

Therefore, when Layer 2 is inactive, the output of Layer 1 is the same as the input pattern.

Now let's consider the second case, where Layer 2 is active. Assume that neuron j is the winning neuron in Layer 2. Then $a_j^2 = 1$ and $a_k^2 = 0$ for $k \neq j$. For this case Eq. (16.7) simplifies to

$$\varepsilon \frac{dn_i^1}{dt} = -n_i^1 + (^+b^1 - n_i^1)\{p_i + w_{i,j}^{2:1}\} - (n_i^1 + ^-b^1). \qquad (16.12)$$

In the steady state $(dn_i^1(t)/dt = 0)$ we have

$$0 = -n_i^1 + (^+b^1 - n_i^1)\{p_i + w_{i,j}^{2:1}\} - (n_i^1 + ^-b^1) \qquad (16.13)$$

$$= -(1 + p_i + w_{i,j}^{2:1} + 1)n_i^1 + (^+b^1 (p_i + w_{i,j}^{2:1}) - ^-b^1).$$

If we solve for the steady state neuron output n_i^1 we find

$$n_i^1 = \frac{^+b^1 (p_i + w_{i,j}^{2:1}) - ^-b^1}{2 + p_i + w_{i,j}^{2:1}}. \qquad (16.14)$$

Recall that Layer 1 should combine the input vector with the expectation from Layer 2 (represented by $\mathbf{w}_j^{2:1}$). Since we are dealing with binary patterns (both the input and the expectation), we will use a logical AND operation to combine the two vectors. In other words, we want n_i^1 to be less than zero when either p_i or $w_{i,j}^{2:1}$ is equal to zero, and we want n_i^1 to be greater than zero when both p_i and $w_{i,j}^{2:1}$ are equal to one.

If we apply these conditions to Eq. (16.14), we obtain the following equations:

$$^+b^1 (2) - ^-b^1 > 0, \qquad (16.15)$$

$$^+b^1 - ^-b^1 < 0, \qquad (16.16)$$

which we can combine to produce

$$^+b^1 (2) > ^-b^1 > ^+b^1. \qquad (16.17)$$

For example, we can use $^+b^1 = 1$ and $^-b^1 = 1.5$ to satisfy these conditions.

Therefore, if Eq. (16.17) is satisfied, and neuron j of Layer 2 is active, then the output of Layer 1 will be

$$\mathbf{a}^1 = \mathbf{p} \cap \mathbf{w}_j^{2:1}, \qquad (16.18)$$

where $\cap$ represents the logical AND operation.

Notice that we needed the gain control in order to implement the AND operation. Consider the numerator of Eq. (16.14):

16

$$^{+}b^{1}\,(p_{i}+w_{i,j}^{2:1})-\,^{-}b^{1}\,. \tag{16.19}$$

The term $^{-}b^{1}$ is multiplied by the gain control term, which in this case is 1. If this term did not exist, then Eq. (16.19) would be greater than zero (and therefore n_{i}^{1} would be greater than zero) whenever either p_{i} or $w_{i,j}^{2:1}$ was greater than zero. This would represent an OR operation, rather than an AND operation. As we will see when we discuss the orienting subsystem, it is critical that Layer 1 perform an AND operation.

When Layer 2 is inactive, the gain control term is zero. This is necessary because in that case we want Layer 1 to respond to the input pattern alone, since no expectation will be activated by Layer 2.

To summarize the steady state operation of Layer 1:

If Layer 2 is not active (i.e., each $a_{j}^{2}=0$),

$$\mathbf{a}^{1}=\mathbf{p}\,. \tag{16.20}$$

If Layer 2 is active (i.e., one $a_{j}^{2}=1$),

$$\mathbf{a}^{1}=\mathbf{p}\cap\mathbf{w}_{j}^{2:1}\,. \tag{16.21}$$

To demonstrate the operation of Layer 1, assume the following network parameters:

$$\varepsilon=0.1,\ ^{+}b^{1}=1\ \text{and}\ ^{-}b^{1}=1.5\,. \tag{16.22}$$

Assume also that we have two neurons in Layer 2, two elements in the input vector and the following weight matrix and input:

$$\mathbf{W}^{2:1}=\begin{bmatrix}1&1\\0&1\end{bmatrix}\ \text{and}\ \mathbf{p}=\begin{bmatrix}0\\1\end{bmatrix}. \tag{16.23}$$

If we take the case where Layer 2 is active, and neuron 2 of Layer 2 wins the competition, the equations of operation of Layer 1 are

$$(0.1)\frac{dn_{1}^{1}}{dt}=-n_{1}^{1}+(1-n_{1}^{1})\,\{p_{1}+w_{1,2}^{2:1}\}-(n_{1}^{1}+1.5) \tag{16.24}$$

$$=-n_{1}^{1}+(1-n_{1}^{1})\,\{0+1\}-(n_{1}^{1}+1.5)\ =\ -3n_{1}^{1}-0.5$$

$$(0.1)\frac{dn_2^1}{dt} = -n_2^1 + (1-n_2^1)\{p_2 + w_{2,2}^{2:1}\} - (n_2^1 + 1.5) \tag{16.25}$$

$$= -n_2^1 + (1-n_2^1)\{1+1\} - (n_2^1 + 1.5) = -4n_2^1 + 0.5.$$

These can be simplified to obtain

$$\frac{dn_1^1}{dt} = -30n_1^1 - 5, \tag{16.26}$$

$$\frac{dn_2^1}{dt} = -40n_2^1 + 5. \tag{16.27}$$

In this simple case we can find closed-form solutions for these equations. If we assume that both neurons start with zero initial conditions, the solutions are

$$n_1^1(t) = -\frac{1}{6}[1 - e^{-30t}], \tag{16.28}$$

$$n_2^1(t) = \frac{1}{8}[1 - e^{-40t}]. \tag{16.29}$$

These are displayed in Figure 16.3.

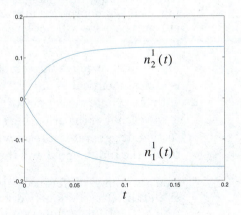

Figure 16.3 Response of Layer 1

Note that $n_1^1(t)$ converges to a negative value, and $n_2^1(t)$ converges to a positive value. Therefore, $a_1^1(t)$ converges to 0, and $a_2^1(t)$ converges to 1 (recall that the transfer function for Layer 1 is *hardlim*$^+$). This agrees with our steady state analysis (see Eq. (16.21)), since

$$\mathbf{p} \cap \mathbf{w}_2^{2:1} = \begin{bmatrix} 0 \\ 1 \end{bmatrix} \cap \begin{bmatrix} 1 \\ 1 \end{bmatrix} = \begin{bmatrix} 0 \\ 1 \end{bmatrix} = \mathbf{a}^1 . \tag{16.30}$$

To experiment with Layer 1 of the ART1 network, use the Neural Network Design Demonstration ART1 Layer 1 (`nnd16al1`*).*

Layer 2

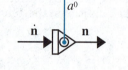

Layer 2 of the ART1 network is almost identical to Layer 2 of the Grossberg network of Chapter 15. Its main purpose is to contrast enhance its output pattern. For our implementation of the ART1 network, the contrast enhancement will be a winner-take-all competition, so only the neuron that receives the largest input will have a nonzero output.

There is one major difference between the second layers of the Grossberg and the ART1 networks. Layer 2 of the ART1 network uses an integrator that can be reset. In this type of integrator, whose symbol is shown in the left margin, any positive outputs are reset to zero whenever the a^0 signal becomes positive. The outputs that are reset remain inhibited for a long period of time, so that they cannot be driven above zero. (By a "long" period of time we mean until an adequate match has occurred and the weights have been updated.)

In the original ART1 paper, Carpenter and Grossberg suggested that the reset mechanism could be implemented using a gated dipole field [CaGr87]. They later suggested a more sophisticated biological model, using chemical neurotransmitters, in their ART3 architecture [CaGr90]. For our purposes we will not be concerned with the specific biological implementation.

Figure 16.4 displays the complete Layer 2 of the ART1 network. Again, it is almost identical to Layer 2 of the Grossberg network (see Figure 15.16), with the primary exception of the resetable integrator. The reset signal, a^0, is the output of the orienting subsystem, which we will discuss in the next section. It generates a reset whenever there is a mismatch at Layer 1 between the input signal and the L2-L1 expectation.

One other small difference between Layer 2 of the ART1 network and Layer 2 of the Grossberg network is that two transfer functions are used in ART1. The transfer function $\mathbf{f}^2(\mathbf{n}^2)$ is used for the on-center/off-surround feedback connections, while the output of Layer 2 is computed as $\mathbf{a}^2 = \mathbf{hardlim}^+(\mathbf{n}^2)$. The reason for the second transfer function is that we want the output of Layer 2 to be a binary signal.

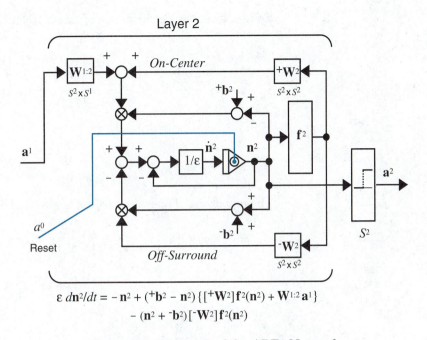

$$\varepsilon\, d\mathbf{n}^2/dt = -\mathbf{n}^2 + (^+\mathbf{b}^2 - \mathbf{n}^2)\{[^+\mathbf{W}^2]\mathbf{f}^2(\mathbf{n}^2) + \mathbf{W}^{1:2}\mathbf{a}^1\}$$
$$- (\mathbf{n}^2 + {}^-\mathbf{b}^2)[^-\mathbf{W}^2]\mathbf{f}^2(\mathbf{n}^2)$$

Figure 16.4 Layer 2 of the ART1 Network

The equation of operation of Layer 2 is

$$\varepsilon\frac{d\mathbf{n}^2(t)}{dt} = -\mathbf{n}^2(t) + (^+\mathbf{b}^2 - \mathbf{n}^2(t))\, \{\, [^+\mathbf{W}^2]\, \mathbf{f}^2(\mathbf{n}^2(t)) + \mathbf{W}^{1:2}\mathbf{a}^1 \} \qquad (16.31)$$

$$- (\mathbf{n}^2(t) + {}^-\mathbf{b}^2)\, [^-\mathbf{W}^2]\, \mathbf{f}^2(\mathbf{n}^2(t))\, .$$

This is a shunting model with excitatory input $\{\, [^+\mathbf{W}^2]\, \mathbf{f}^2(\mathbf{n}^2(t)) + \mathbf{W}^{1:2}\mathbf{a}^1 \}$, where $^+\mathbf{W}^2$ provides on-center feedback connections (identical to Layers 1 and 2 of the Grossberg network of Chapter 15, Eq. (15.6)), and $\mathbf{W}^{1:2}$ consists of adaptive weights, analogous to the weights in the Kohonen network. They are trained according to an instar rule, as we will see in a later section. The rows of $\mathbf{W}^{1:2}$, after training, will represent the prototype patterns.

The inhibitory input to the shunting model is $[^-\mathbf{W}^2]\, \mathbf{f}^2(\mathbf{n}^2(t))$, where $^-\mathbf{W}^2$ provides off-surround feedback connections (identical to Layers 1 and 2 of the Grossberg network — Eq. (15.7)).

To illustrate the performance of Layer 2, consider a two-neuron layer with

$$\varepsilon = 0.1, \ {}^{+}\mathbf{b}^2 = \begin{bmatrix} 1 \\ 1 \end{bmatrix}, \ {}^{-}\mathbf{b}^2 = \begin{bmatrix} 1 \\ 1 \end{bmatrix}, \ \mathbf{W}^{1:2} = \begin{bmatrix} ({}_{1}\mathbf{w}^{1:2})^T \\ ({}_{2}\mathbf{w}^{1:2})^T \end{bmatrix} = \begin{bmatrix} 0.5 & 0.5 \\ 1 & 0 \end{bmatrix}, \quad (16.32)$$

and

$$f^2(n) = \begin{cases} 10 \, (n)^2, & n \geq 0 \\ 0, & n < 0 \end{cases}. \quad (16.33)$$

The equations of operation of the layer will be

$$(0.1) \frac{dn_1^2(t)}{dt} = -n_1^2(t) + (1 - n_1^2(t)) \, \{ f^2(n_1^2(t)) + ({}_{1}\mathbf{w}^{1:2})^T \mathbf{a}^1 \} \quad (16.34)$$

$$- (n_1^2(t) + 1) \, f^2(n_2^2(t))$$

$$(0.1) \frac{dn_2^2(t)}{dt} = -n_2^2(t) + (1 - n_2^2(t)) \, \{ f^2(n_2^2(t)) + ({}_{2}\mathbf{w}^{1:2})^T \mathbf{a}^1 \} \quad (16.35)$$

$$- (n_2^2(t) + 1) \, f^2(n_1^2(t)) .$$

This is identical in form to the Grossberg Layer 2 example in Chapter 15 (see Eq. (15.20) and Eq. (15.21)), except that ${}^{-}b^2 = 1$. This will allow $n_1^2(t)$ and $n_2^2(t)$ to range between –1 and +1.

The inputs to Layer 2 are the inner products of the prototype patterns (rows of the weight matrix $\mathbf{W}^{1:2}$) with the output of Layer 1. (The rows of this weight matrix are normalized, as will be explained in a later section.) The largest inner product will correspond to the prototype pattern that is closest to the output of Layer 1. Layer 2 then performs a competition between the neurons. The transfer function $f^2(n)$ is chosen to be a faster-than-linear transfer function (see Chapter 15, page 15-20, for a discussion of the effect of $f^2(n)$). This choice will force the neuron with largest input to have a positive n, and the other neuron to have a negative n (with appropriate choice of network parameters). After the competition, one neuron output will be 1, and the other neuron output will be zero, since we are using the $hardlim^+$ transfer function to compute the layer output.

Figure 16.5 illustrates the response of Layer 2 when the input vector is $\mathbf{a}^1 = \begin{bmatrix} 1 & 0 \end{bmatrix}^T$. The second row of $\mathbf{W}^{1:2}$ has a larger inner product with $\mathbf{a}^1$

than the second row, therefore neuron 2 wins the competition. At steady state, $n_2^2(t)$ has a positive value, and $n_1^2(t)$ has a negative value. The steady state Layer 2 output will then be

$$\mathbf{a}^2 = \begin{bmatrix} 0 \\ 1 \end{bmatrix}. \tag{16.36}$$

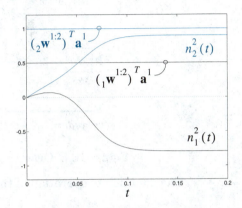

Figure 16.5 Response of Layer 2

We can summarize the steady state operation of Layer 2 as follows:

$$a_i^2 = \begin{cases} 1, & \text{if } ((_i\mathbf{w}^{1:2})^T\mathbf{a}^1 = max\,[\,(_j\mathbf{w}^{1:2})^T\mathbf{a}^1]) \\ 0, & \text{otherwise} \end{cases} \tag{16.37}$$

To experiment with Layer 2 of the ART1 network, use the Neural Network Design Demonstration ART1 Layer 2 (**nnd16al2**)*.*

Orienting Subsystem

One of the key elements of the ART architecture is the Orienting Subsystem. Its purpose is to determine if there is a sufficient match between the L2-L1 expectation and the input pattern. When there is not enough of a match, the Orienting Subsystem should send a reset signal to Layer 2. The reset signal will cause a long-lasting inhibition of the previous winning neuron, and thus allow another neuron to win the competition.

Figure 16.6 displays the Orienting Subsystem.

16

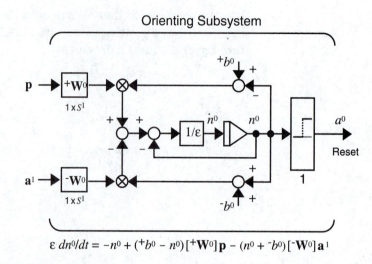

$$\varepsilon \, dn^0/dt = -n^0 + (^+b^0 - n^0)\,[^+\mathbf{W}^0]\,\mathbf{p} - (n^0 + {}^-b^0)\,[^-\mathbf{W}^0]\,\mathbf{a}^1$$

Figure 16.6 Orienting Subsystem of the ART1 Network

The equation of operation of the Orienting Subsystem is

$$\varepsilon\frac{dn^0(t)}{dt} = -n^0(t) + (^+b^0 - n^0(t))\,\{^+\mathbf{W}^0\mathbf{p}\} - (n^0(t) + {}^-b^0)\,\{^-\mathbf{W}^0\mathbf{a}^1\}\ . \quad (16.38)$$

This is a shunting model, with excitatory input $^+\mathbf{W}^0\mathbf{p}$, where

$$^+\mathbf{W}^0 = \begin{bmatrix} \alpha & \alpha & \dots & \alpha \end{bmatrix}\ . \quad (16.39)$$

Therefore, the excitatory input can be written

$$^+\mathbf{W}^0\mathbf{p} = \begin{bmatrix} \alpha & \alpha & \dots & \alpha \end{bmatrix}\mathbf{p} = \alpha \sum_{j=1}^{S^1} p_j = \alpha\|\mathbf{p}\|^2\ , \quad (16.40)$$

where the last equality holds because $\mathbf{p}$ is a binary vector.

The inhibitory input to the Orienting Subsystem is $^-\mathbf{W}^0\mathbf{a}^1$, where

$$^-\mathbf{W}^0 = \begin{bmatrix} \beta & \beta & \dots & \beta \end{bmatrix}\ . \quad (16.41)$$

Therefore, the inhibitory input can be written

$$^-\mathbf{W}^0\mathbf{a}^1 = \begin{bmatrix} \beta & \beta & \dots & \beta \end{bmatrix}\mathbf{a}^1 = \beta \sum_{j=1}^{S^1} a_j^1(t) = \beta\|\mathbf{a}^1\|^2\ . \quad (16.42)$$

Whenever the excitatory input is larger than the inhibitory input, the Orienting Subsystem will be driven on. Consider the following steady state operation:

$$0 = -n^0 + ({}^+b^0 - n^0) \{\alpha \|\mathbf{p}\|^2\} - (n^0 + {}^-b^0) \{\beta \|\mathbf{a}^1\|^2\} \qquad (16.43)$$

$$= -(1 + \alpha \|\mathbf{p}\|^2 + \beta \|\mathbf{a}^1\|^2) n^0 + {}^+b^0 (\alpha \|\mathbf{p}\|^2) - {}^-b^0 (\beta \|\mathbf{a}^1\|^2) .$$

If we solve for n^0, we find

$$n^0 = \frac{{}^+b^0 (\alpha \|\mathbf{p}\|^2) - {}^-b^0 (\beta \|\mathbf{a}^1\|^2)}{(1 + \alpha \|\mathbf{p}\|^2 + \beta \|\mathbf{a}^1\|^2)} . \qquad (16.44)$$

Let ${}^+b^0 = {}^-b^0 = 1$, then $n^0 > 0$ if $\alpha \|\mathbf{p}\|^2 - \beta \|\mathbf{a}^1\|^2 > 0$, or in other words:

$$n^0 > 0 \text{ if } \frac{\|\mathbf{a}^1\|^2}{\|\mathbf{p}\|^2} < \frac{\alpha}{\beta} = \rho . \qquad (16.45)$$

Vigilance

This is the condition that will cause a reset of Layer 2, since $a^0 = hardlim^+(n^0)$. The term ρ is called the *vigilance* parameter, and must fall in the range $0 < \rho < 1$. If the vigilance is close to 1, a reset will occur unless $\mathbf{a}^1$ is close to $\mathbf{p}$. If the vigilance is close to 0, $\mathbf{a}^1$ need not be close to $\mathbf{p}$ to prevent a reset. The vigilance parameter determines the coarseness of the categorization (or clustering) created by the prototype vectors.

Recall from Eq. (16.21) that $\mathbf{a}^1 = \mathbf{p} \cap \mathbf{w}_j^{2:1}$ whenever Layer 2 is active. Therefore, $\|\mathbf{p}\|^2$ will always be greater than or equal to $\|\mathbf{a}^1\|^2$. They will be equal when the expectation $\mathbf{w}_j^{2:1}$ has a 1 wherever the input $\mathbf{p}$ has a 1. Therefore, the orienting subsystem will cause a reset when there is enough of a mismatch between $\mathbf{p}$ and $\mathbf{w}_j^{2:1}$. The amount of mismatch required for a reset is determined by the vigilance parameter ρ.

To demonstrate the operation of the Orienting Subsystem, suppose that $\varepsilon = 0.1$, $\alpha = 3$, $\beta = 4$ ($\rho = 0.75$),

$$\mathbf{p} = \begin{bmatrix} 1 \\ 1 \end{bmatrix} \text{ and } \mathbf{a}^1 = \begin{bmatrix} 1 \\ 0 \end{bmatrix} . \qquad (16.46)$$

The equation of operation becomes

$$(0.1) \frac{dn^0(t)}{dt} = -n^0(t) + (1 - n^0(t)) \{3 (p_1 + p_2)\}$$

$$- (n^0(t) + 1) \{4 (a_1^1 + a_2^1)\}$$ (16.47)

or

$$\frac{dn^0(t)}{dt} = -110 n^0(t) + 20 .$$ (16.48)

The response is plotted in Figure 16.7. In this case a reset signal will be sent to Layer 2, since $n^0(t)$ is positive. In this example, because the vigilance parameter is set to $\rho = 0.75$, and **p** has only two elements, we will have a reset whenever **p** and $\mathbf{a}^1$ are not identical. (If the vigilance parameter were set to $\rho = 0.25$, we would not have had a reset for the **p** and $\mathbf{a}^1$ of Eq. (16.46), since $\|\mathbf{a}^1\|^2 / \|\mathbf{p}\|^2 = 1/2$.)

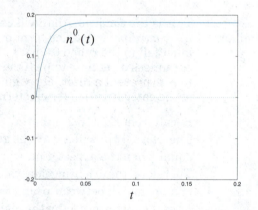

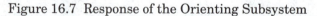

Figure 16.7 Response of the Orienting Subsystem

The steady state operation of the Orienting Subsystem can be summarized as follows:

$$a^0 = \begin{cases} 1 , & \text{if } [\|\mathbf{a}^1\|^2 / \|\mathbf{p}\|^2 < \rho] \\ 0 , & \text{otherwise} \end{cases} .$$ (16.49)

To experiment with the Orienting Subsystem, use the Neural Network Design Demonstration Orienting Subsystem *(***nnd16os***).*

Learning Law: L1-L2

The ART1 network has two separate learning laws: one for the L1-L2 connections, and another for the L2-L1 connections. The L1-L2 connections use a type of instar learning to learn to *recognize* a set of prototype patterns. The L2-L1 connections use outstar learning in order to *reproduce* (or recall) a set of prototype patterns. In this section we will describe the L1-L2 instar learning law, and in the following section we will present the L2-L1 outstar learning law.

We should note that the L1-L2 connections and the L2-L1 connections are updated at the same time. Whenever the input pattern and the expectation have an adequate match, as determined by the Orienting Subsystem, both $\mathbf{W}^{1:2}$ and $\mathbf{W}^{2:1}$ are adapted. This process of matching, and subsequent adaptation, is referred to as *resonance*, hence the name adaptive resonance theory.

Resonance

Subset/Superset Dilemma

The learning in the L1-L2 connections of the ART1 network is very close to the learning in the Grossberg network of Chapter 15, with one major difference. In the Grossberg network, the input patterns are normalized in Layer 1, and therefore all of the prototype patterns will have the same length. In the ART1 network no normalization takes place in Layer 1. Therefore a problem can occur when one prototype pattern is a subset of another. For example, suppose that the L1-L2 connection matrix is

$$\mathbf{W}^{1:2} = \begin{bmatrix} 1 & 1 & 0 \\ 1 & 1 & 1 \end{bmatrix}, \tag{16.50}$$

so that the prototype patterns are

$${}_1\mathbf{w}^{1:2} = \begin{bmatrix} 1 \\ 1 \\ 0 \end{bmatrix} \text{ and } {}_2\mathbf{w}^{1:2} = \begin{bmatrix} 1 \\ 1 \\ 1 \end{bmatrix}. \tag{16.51}$$

We say that ${}_1\mathbf{w}^{1:2}$ is a subset of ${}_2\mathbf{w}^{1:2}$, since ${}_2\mathbf{w}^{1:2}$ has a 1 wherever ${}_1\mathbf{w}^{1:2}$ has a 1.

If the output of Layer 1 is

$$\mathbf{a}^1 = \begin{bmatrix} 1 \\ 1 \\ 0 \end{bmatrix}, \tag{16.52}$$

16

then the input to Layer 2 will be

$$\mathbf{W}^{1:2}\mathbf{a}^1 = \begin{bmatrix} 1 & 1 & 0 \\ 1 & 1 & 1 \end{bmatrix} \begin{bmatrix} 1 \\ 1 \\ 0 \end{bmatrix} = \begin{bmatrix} 2 \\ 2 \end{bmatrix}. \tag{16.53}$$

Both prototype vectors have the same inner product with $\mathbf{a}^1$, even though the first prototype is identical to $\mathbf{a}^1$ and the second prototype is not. This is called the subset/superset dilemma.

One solution to the subset/superset dilemma is to normalize the prototype patterns. That is, when a prototype pattern has a large number of nonzero entries, the magnitude of each entry should be reduced. For example, using our preceding problem, we could modify the L1-L2 matrix as follows:

$$\mathbf{W}^{1:2} = \begin{bmatrix} \dfrac{1}{2} & \dfrac{1}{2} & 0 \\[6pt] \dfrac{1}{3} & \dfrac{1}{3} & \dfrac{1}{3} \end{bmatrix}. \tag{16.54}$$

The input to Layer 2 will then be

$$\mathbf{W}^{1:2}\mathbf{a}^1 = \begin{bmatrix} \dfrac{1}{2} & \dfrac{1}{2} & 0 \\[6pt] \dfrac{1}{3} & \dfrac{1}{3} & \dfrac{1}{3} \end{bmatrix} \begin{bmatrix} 1 \\ 1 \\ 0 \end{bmatrix} = \begin{bmatrix} 1 \\[4pt] \dfrac{2}{3} \end{bmatrix}. \tag{16.55}$$

Now we have the desired result: the first prototype has the largest inner product with $\mathbf{a}^1$. The first neuron in Layer 2 will be activated.

In the Grossberg network of Chapter 15 we obtained normalized prototype patterns by normalizing the input patterns in Layer 1. In the ART1 network we will normalize the prototype patterns by using an on-center/off-surround competition in the L1-L2 learning law.

Learning Law

The learning law for $\mathbf{W}^{1:2}$ is

$$\frac{d[_i\mathbf{w}^{1:2}(t)]}{dt} = a_i^2(t) \left[\{^+\mathbf{b} - _i\mathbf{w}^{1:2}(t)\} \zeta [^+\mathbf{W}] \mathbf{a}^1(t) \right. \tag{16.56}$$

$$\left. - \{_i\mathbf{w}^{1:2}(t) + ^-\mathbf{b}\} [^-\mathbf{W}] \mathbf{a}^1(t) \right],$$

where

$$
{}^+\mathbf{b} = \begin{bmatrix} 1 \\ 1 \\ \vdots \\ 1 \end{bmatrix}, \quad {}^-\mathbf{b} = \begin{bmatrix} 0 \\ 0 \\ \vdots \\ 0 \end{bmatrix}, \quad {}^+\mathbf{W} = \begin{bmatrix} 1 & 0 & \cdots & 0 \\ 0 & 1 & \cdots & 0 \\ \vdots & \vdots & & \vdots \\ 0 & 0 & \cdots & 1 \end{bmatrix} \text{ and } {}^-\mathbf{W} = \begin{bmatrix} 0 & 1 & \cdots & 1 \\ 1 & 0 & \cdots & 1 \\ \vdots & \vdots & & \vdots \\ 1 & 1 & \cdots & 0 \end{bmatrix}. \quad (16.57)
$$

This is a modified form of instar learning. When neuron i of Layer 2 is active, the ith row of $\mathbf{W}^{1:2}$, ${}_i\mathbf{w}^{1:2}$, is moved in the direction of $\mathbf{a}^1$. The difference between Eq. (16.56) and the standard instar learning is that the elements of ${}_i\mathbf{w}^{1:2}$ compete, and therefore ${}_i\mathbf{w}^{1:2}$ is normalized. In the bracket on the right side of Eq. (16.56) we can see that it has the form of a shunting model, with on-center/off-surround input connections from $\mathbf{a}^1$. The excitatory bias is ${}^+\mathbf{b} = \mathbf{1}$ (a vector of 1's), and the inhibitory bias is ${}^-\mathbf{b} = \mathbf{0}$, which ensures that the elements of ${}_i\mathbf{w}^{1:2}$ remain between 0 and 1. (Recall our discussion of the shunting model in Chapter 15.)

To verify that Eq. (16.56) causes normalization of the prototype patterns, let's investigate the steady state operation. For this analysis we will assume that the outputs of Layer 1 and Layer 2 remain constant until the weights reach steady state. This is called *fast learning*.

Fast Learning

The equation for element $w_{i,j}^{1:2}$ is

$$
\frac{dw_{i,j}^{1:2}(t)}{dt} = a_i^2(t) \left[(1 - w_{i,j}^{1:2}(t)) \zeta a_j^1(t) - w_{i,j}^{1:2}(t) \sum_{k \neq j} a_k^1(t) \right]. \quad (16.58)
$$

If we assume that neuron i is active in Layer 2 ($a_i^2(t) = 1$) and set the derivative to zero in Eq. (16.58), we see that

$$
0 = \left[(1 - w_{i,j}^{1:2}) \zeta a_j^1 - w_{i,j}^{1:2} \sum_{k \neq j} a_k^1 \right]. \quad (16.59)
$$

To find the steady state value of $w_{i,j}^{1:2}$, we will consider two cases. First, assume that $a_j^1 = 1$. Then we have

$$
0 = (1 - w_{i,j}^{1:2}) \zeta - w_{i,j}^{1:2} (\|\mathbf{a}^1\|^2 - 1) = -(\zeta + \|\mathbf{a}^1\|^2 - 1) w_{i,j}^{1:2} + \zeta, \quad (16.60)
$$

or

$$
w_{i,j}^{1:2} = \frac{\zeta}{\zeta + \|\mathbf{a}^1\|^2 - 1}. \quad (16.61)
$$

(Note that $\sum_{k=1}^{s^1} a_k^1 = \|\mathbf{a}^1\|^2$, since $\mathbf{a}^1$ is a binary vector.)

On the other hand, if $a_j^1 = 0$, then Eq. (16.59) reduces to

$$0 = -w_{i,j}^{1:2} \|\mathbf{a}^1\|^2 , \tag{16.62}$$

or

$$w_{i,j}^{1:2} = 0 . \tag{16.63}$$

To summarize Eq. (16.61) and Eq. (16.63):

$$_i\mathbf{w}^{1:2} = \frac{\zeta \mathbf{a}^1}{\zeta + \|\mathbf{a}^1\|^2 - 1} , \tag{16.64}$$

where $\zeta > 1$ to ensure that the denominator will never equal zero.

Therefore the prototype patterns will be normalized, and this will solve the subset/superset dilemma. (By "normalized" here we do not mean that all prototype vectors will have unit length in Euclidean distance, but simply that the rows of $\mathbf{W}^{1:2}$ that have more nonzero entries will have elements with smaller magnitudes. In this case, vectors with more nonzero entries may actually have a smaller length than vectors with fewer nonzero entries.)

Learning Law: L2-L1

The L2-L1 connections, $\mathbf{W}^{2:1}$, in the ART1 architecture are trained using an outstar learning rule. The purpose of the L2-L1 connections is to recall an appropriate prototype pattern (the expectation), so that it can be compared and combined, in Layer 1, with the input pattern. When the expectation and the input pattern do not match, a reset is sent to Layer 2, so that a new prototype pattern can be chosen (as we have discussed in previous sections).

The learning law for $\mathbf{W}^{2:1}$ is a typical outstar equation:

$$\frac{d[\mathbf{w}_j^{2:1}(t)]}{dt} = a_j^2(t) [-\mathbf{w}_j^{2:1}(t) + \mathbf{a}^1(t)] . \tag{16.65}$$

Therefore, if neuron j in Layer 2 is active (has won the competition), then column j of $\mathbf{W}^{2:1}$ is moved toward the $\mathbf{a}^1$ pattern. To illustrate this, let's investigate the steady state operation of Eq. (16.65).

For this analysis we will assume the fast learning scenario, where the outputs of Layer 1 and Layer 2 remain constant until the weights reach steady state. Assume that neuron j in Layer 2 is active, so that $a_j^2 = 1$. Setting the derivative in Eq. (16.65) to zero, we find

$$0 = -\mathbf{w}_j^{2:1} + \mathbf{a}^1, \text{ or } \mathbf{w}_j^{2:1} = \mathbf{a}^1. \tag{16.66}$$

Therefore column j of $\mathbf{W}^{2:1}$ converges to the output of Layer 1, $\mathbf{a}^1$. Recall from Eq. (16.20) and Eq. (16.21) that $\mathbf{a}^1$ is a combination of the input pattern and the appropriate prototype pattern. Therefore the prototype pattern is modified to incorporate the current input pattern (if there is a close enough match).

Keep in mind that $\mathbf{W}^{1:2}$ and $\mathbf{W}^{2:1}$ are updated at the same time. When neuron j of Layer 2 is active and there is a sufficient match between the expectation and the input pattern (which indicates a resonance condition), then row j of $\mathbf{W}^{1:2}$ and column j of $\mathbf{W}^{2:1}$ are adapted. In fast learning, column j of $\mathbf{W}^{2:1}$ is set to $\mathbf{a}^1$, while row j of $\mathbf{W}^{1:2}$ is set to a normalized version of $\mathbf{a}^1$.

ART1 Algorithm Summary

Now that we have investigated each of the subsystems of the ART1 architecture, we can gain some insight into its overall operation if we summarize the key steady state equations and organize them into an algorithm.

Initialization

The ART1 algorithm begins with an initialization of the weight matrices $\mathbf{W}^{1:2}$ and $\mathbf{W}^{2:1}$. The initial $\mathbf{W}^{2:1}$ matrix is set to all 1's. Thus, the first time a new neuron in Layer 2 wins a competition, resonance will occur, since $\mathbf{a}^1 = \mathbf{p} \cap \mathbf{w}_j^{2:1} = \mathbf{p}$ and therefore $\|\mathbf{a}^1\|^2 / \|\mathbf{p}\|^2 = 1 > \rho$. This means that any untrained column in $\mathbf{W}^{2:1}$ is effectively a blank slate and will cause a match with any input pattern.

Since the rows of the $\mathbf{W}^{1:2}$ matrix should be normalized versions of the columns of $\mathbf{W}^{2:1}$, every element of the initial $\mathbf{W}^{1:2}$ matrix is set to $\zeta / (\zeta + S^1 - 1)$.

Algorithm

After initialization, the ART1 algorithm proceeds as follows:

1. First, we present an input pattern to the network. Since Layer 2 is not active on initialization (i.e., each $a_j^2 = 0$), the output of Layer 1 is (Eq. (16.20))

$$\mathbf{a}^1 = \mathbf{p}. \tag{16.67}$$

16

2. Next, we compute the input to Layer 2,

$$\mathbf{W}^{1:2}\mathbf{a}^1 ,$$ (16.68)

and activate the neuron in Layer 2 with the largest input (Eq. (16.37)):

$$a_i^2 = \begin{cases} 1, & \text{if } (({}_i\mathbf{w}^{1:2})^T \mathbf{a}^1 = max\,[\, ({}_k\mathbf{w}^{1:2})^T \mathbf{a}^1]\,) \\ 0, & \text{otherwise} \end{cases} .$$ (16.69)

In case of a tie, the neuron with the smallest index is declared the winner.

3. We then compute the L2-L1 expectation (where we assume neuron j of Layer 2 is activated):

$$\mathbf{W}^{2:1}\mathbf{a}^2 = \mathbf{w}_j^{2:1} .$$ (16.70)

4. Now that Layer 2 is active, we adjust the Layer 1 output to include the L2-L1 expectation (Eq. (16.21)):

$$\mathbf{a}^1 = \mathbf{p} \cap \mathbf{w}_j^{2:1} .$$ (16.71)

5. Next, the Orienting Subsystem determines the degree of match between the expectation and the input pattern (Eq. (16.49)):

$$a^0 = \begin{cases} 1, & \text{if } [\,\|\mathbf{a}^1\|^2 / \|\mathbf{p}\|^2 < \rho\,] \\ 0, & \text{otherwise} \end{cases} .$$ (16.72)

6. If $a^0 = 1$, then we set $a_j^2 = 0$, inhibit it until an adequate match occurs (resonance), and return to step 1. If $a^0 = 0$, we continue with step 7.

7. Resonance has occurred. Therefore we update row j of $\mathbf{W}^{1:2}$ (Eq. (16.61)):

$$_j\mathbf{w}^{1:2} = \frac{\zeta\mathbf{a}^1}{\zeta + \|\mathbf{a}^1\|^2 - 1} .$$ (16.73)

8. We now update column j of $\mathbf{W}^{2:1}$ (Eq. (16.66)):

$$\mathbf{w}_j^{2:1} = \mathbf{a}^1 .$$ (16.74)

9. We remove the input pattern, restore all inhibited neurons in Layer 2, and return to step 1 with a new input pattern.

The input patterns continue to be applied to the network until the weights stabilize (do not change). Carpenter and Grossberg have shown [CaGr87a] that the ART1 algorithm will always form stable clusters for any set of input patterns.

See Problems P16.5, P16.6 and P16.7 for detailed examples of the ART1 algorithm.

 *To experiment with the ART1 algorithm, use the Neural Network Design Demonstration ART1 (*nnd16a1*).*

Other ART Architectures

The ART1 network is just one example of adaptive resonance theory. Carpenter and Grossberg, and others in their research group, have developed many variations on this theme.

One disadvantage of the ART1 network is that it can only be used for binary input patterns. Carpenter and Grossberg developed a variation of ART1, called ART2, to handle either analog or binary patterns [CaGr87b]. The basic structure of ART2 is very similar to ART1, with the exception of Layer 1. In ART2 several sublayers take the place of Layer 1. These sublayers are needed because analog vectors, unlike binary vectors, can be arbitrarily close together. The sublayers perform a combination of normalization and noise suppression, in addition to the comparison of the input vector and the expectation that is needed by the orienting subsystem.

Carpenter and Grossberg later developed the ART3 network [CaGr90], which introduced a more sophisticated biological model for the reset mechanism required for ART. Up to the present time, this network has not been widely applied.

In 1991 Carpenter, Grossberg and Reynolds introduced the ARTMAP network [CaGrRe91]. In contrast with all of the previous ART networks, it is a supervised network. The ARTMAP architecture consists of two ART modules that are connected by an "inter-ART" associative memory. One ART module receives the input vector, while the other ART module receives the desired output vector. The network learns to predict the correct output vector whenever the input vector is presented.

More recently, Carpenter, Grossberg, Markuzon, Reynolds and Rosen have modified the ARTMAP architecture to incorporate fuzzy logic. The result is referred to as Fuzzy ARTMAP [CaGrMa92]. It seems to improve performance, especially with noisy input patterns.

All of these ART architectures incorporate the key modules discussed in this chapter, including:

- L1-L2 instars for pattern recognition.

- L2-L1 outstars for pattern recall.

- Layer 2 for contrast enhancement (competition).

- Layer 1 for comparison of input and expectation.

- Orienting Subsystem for resetting when a pattern mismatch occurs.

Summary of Results

Basic ART Architecture

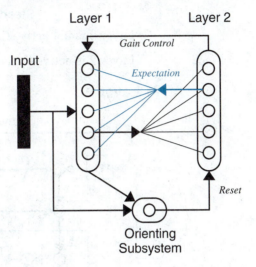

ART1 Network (Binary Patterns)

ART1 Layer 1

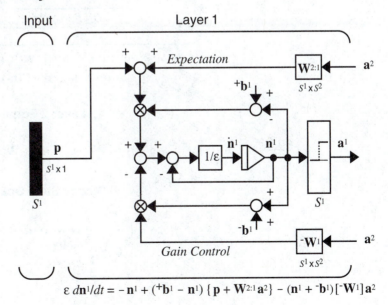

$$\varepsilon \, d\mathbf{n}^1/dt = -\mathbf{n}^1 + ({}^+\mathbf{b}^1 - \mathbf{n}^1)\{\mathbf{p} + \mathbf{W}^{2:1}\mathbf{a}^2\} - (\mathbf{n}^1 + {}^-\mathbf{b}^1)[{}^-\mathbf{W}^1]\mathbf{a}^2$$

Layer 1 Equation

$$\varepsilon \frac{d\mathbf{n}^1(t)}{dt} = -\mathbf{n}^1(t) + (^+\mathbf{b}^1 - \mathbf{n}^1(t)) \{ \mathbf{p} + \mathbf{W}^{2:1} \mathbf{a}^2(t) \} - (\mathbf{n}^1(t) + ^-\mathbf{b}^1) [^-\mathbf{W}^1] \mathbf{a}^2(t)$$

Steady State Operation

If Layer 2 is not active (i.e., each $a_j^2 = 0$), $\mathbf{a}^1 = \mathbf{p}$.

If Layer 2 is active (i.e., one $a_j^2 = 1$), $\mathbf{a}^1 = \mathbf{p} \cap \mathbf{w}_j^{2:1}$.

ART1 Layer 2

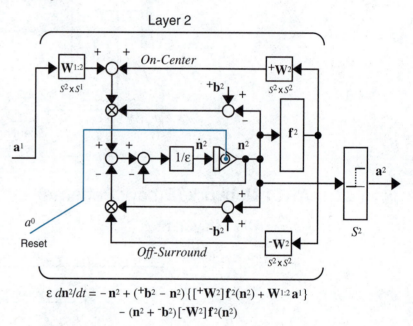

Layer 2

$$\varepsilon \, d\mathbf{n}^2/dt = -\mathbf{n}^2 + (^+\mathbf{b}^2 - \mathbf{n}^2) \{ [^+\mathbf{W}^2] \mathbf{f}^2(\mathbf{n}^2) + \mathbf{W}^{1:2} \mathbf{a}^1 \}$$
$$- (\mathbf{n}^2 + ^-\mathbf{b}^2) [^-\mathbf{W}^2] \mathbf{f}^2(\mathbf{n}^2)$$

Layer 2 Equation

$$\varepsilon \frac{d\mathbf{n}^2(t)}{dt} = -\mathbf{n}^2(t) + (^+\mathbf{b}^2 - \mathbf{n}^2(t)) \{ [^+\mathbf{W}^2] \mathbf{f}^2(\mathbf{n}^2(t)) + \mathbf{W}^{1:2} \mathbf{a}^1 \} - (\mathbf{n}^2(t) + ^-\mathbf{b}^2) [^-\mathbf{W}^2] \mathbf{f}^2(\mathbf{n}^2(t))$$

Steady State Operation

$$a_i^2 = \begin{cases} 1, & \text{if } ((_i\mathbf{w}^{1:2})^T \mathbf{a}^1 = max [(_j\mathbf{w}^{1:2})^T \mathbf{a}^1]) \\ 0, & \text{otherwise} \end{cases}$$

Orienting Subsystem

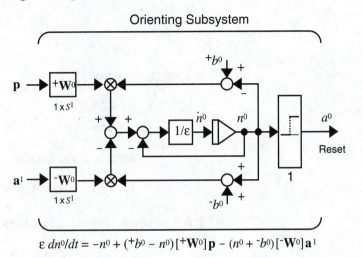

Orienting Subsystem

$$\varepsilon\, dn^0/dt = -n^0 + (^+b^0 - n^0)\,[^+\mathbf{W}^0]\,\mathbf{p} - (n^0 + {}^-b^0)\,[^-\mathbf{W}^0]\,\mathbf{a}^1$$

Orienting Subsystem Equation

$$\varepsilon\frac{dn^0(t)}{dt} = -n^0(t) + (^+b^0 - n^0(t))\,\{^+\mathbf{W}^0\mathbf{p}\} - (n^0(t) + {}^-b^0)\,\{^-\mathbf{W}^0\mathbf{a}^1\}$$

where $^+\mathbf{W}^0 = \begin{bmatrix} \alpha & \alpha & \cdots & \alpha \end{bmatrix}$, $^-\mathbf{W}^0 = \begin{bmatrix} \beta & \beta & \cdots & \beta \end{bmatrix}$, $^+b^0 = {}^-b^0 = 1$

Steady State Operation

$$a^0 = \begin{cases} 1, & \text{if } [\,\lVert \mathbf{a}^1 \rVert^2 / \lVert \mathbf{p} \rVert^2 < \rho\,] \\ 0, & \text{otherwise} \end{cases}$$

L1-L2 Learning Law

$$\frac{d\,[\,_i\mathbf{w}^{1:2}(t)\,]}{dt} = a_i^2(t)\left[\,\{^+\mathbf{b} - {}_i\mathbf{w}^{1:2}(t)\}\,\zeta\,[^+\mathbf{W}]\,\mathbf{a}^1(t) - \{_i\mathbf{w}^{1:2}(t) + {}^-\mathbf{b}\}\,[^-\mathbf{W}]\,\mathbf{a}^1(t)\,\right]$$

$$^+\mathbf{b} = \begin{bmatrix} 1 \\ 1 \\ \vdots \\ 1 \end{bmatrix} \quad ^-\mathbf{b} = \begin{bmatrix} 0 \\ 0 \\ \vdots \\ 0 \end{bmatrix} \quad ^+\mathbf{W} = \begin{bmatrix} 1 & 0 & \cdots & 0 \\ 0 & 1 & \cdots & 0 \\ \vdots & \vdots & & \vdots \\ 0 & 0 & \cdots & 1 \end{bmatrix} \quad ^-\mathbf{W} = \begin{bmatrix} 0 & 1 & \cdots & 1 \\ 1 & 0 & \cdots & 1 \\ \vdots & \vdots & & \vdots \\ 1 & 1 & \cdots & 0 \end{bmatrix}$$

16

Steady State Operation (Fast Learning)

$$_i\mathbf{w}^{1:2} = \frac{\zeta \mathbf{a}^1}{\zeta + \|\mathbf{a}^1\|^2 - 1} \quad \text{(Neuron } i \text{ in Layer 2 Active)}$$

L2-L1 Learning Law

$$\frac{d\,[\,\mathbf{w}_j^{2:1}(t)\,]}{dt} = a_j^2(t)\,[\,-\mathbf{w}_j^{2:1}(t) + \mathbf{a}^1(t)\,]$$

Steady State Operation (Fast Learning)

$$\mathbf{w}_j^{2:1} = \mathbf{a}^1 \quad \text{(Neuron } j \text{ in Layer 2 Active)}$$

ART1 Algorithm (Fast Learning) Summary

Initialization

The initial $\mathbf{W}^{2:1}$ matrix is set to all 1's.

Every element of the initial $\mathbf{W}^{1:2}$ matrix is set to $\zeta/(\zeta + S^1 - 1)$.

Algorithm

1. First, we present an input pattern to the network. Since Layer 2 is not active on initialization (i.e., each $a_j^2 = 0$), the output of Layer 1 is

$$\mathbf{a}^1 = \mathbf{p}.$$

2. Next, we compute the input to Layer 2,

$$\mathbf{W}^{1:2}\mathbf{a}^1,$$

and activate the neuron in Layer 2 with the largest input:

$$a_i^2 = \begin{cases} 1, & \text{if } ((_i\mathbf{w}^{1:2})^T\mathbf{a}^1 = max\,[\,(_k\mathbf{w}^{1:2})^T\mathbf{a}^1\,]) \\ 0, & \text{otherwise} \end{cases}.$$

In case of a tie, the neuron with the smallest index is declared the winner.

3. We then compute the L2-L1 expectation (where we assume neuron j of Layer 2 is activated):

$$\mathbf{W}^{2:1}\mathbf{a}^2 = \mathbf{w}_j^{2:1}.$$

4. Now that Layer 2 is active, we adjust the Layer 1 output to include the L2-L1 expectation:

$$\mathbf{a}^1 = \mathbf{p} \cap \mathbf{w}_j^{2:1}.$$

5. Next, the Orienting Subsystem determines the degree of match between the expectation and the input pattern:

$$a^0 = \begin{cases} 1, & \text{if } [\|\mathbf{a}^1\|^2 / \|\mathbf{p}\|^2 < \rho] \\ 0, & \text{otherwise} \end{cases}.$$

6. If $a^0 = 1$, then we set $a_j^2 = 0$, inhibit it until an adequate match occurs (resonance), and return to step 1. If $a^0 = 0$, we continue with step 7.

7. Resonance has occurred, therefore we update row j of $\mathbf{W}^{1:2}$:

$$_j\mathbf{w}^{1:2} = \frac{\zeta \mathbf{a}^1}{\zeta + \|\mathbf{a}^1\|^2 - 1}.$$

8. We now update column j of $\mathbf{W}^{2:1}$:

$$\mathbf{w}_j^{2:1} = \mathbf{a}^1.$$

9. We remove the input pattern, restore all inhibited neurons in Layer 2, and return to step 1 with a new input pattern.

16

Solved Problems

P16.1 **Consider Layer 1 of the ART1 network with the following parameters:**

$$\varepsilon = 0.01 \quad {}^{+}b^{1} = 2 \quad {}^{-}b^{1} = 3 \,.$$

Assume two neurons in Layer 2, two elements in the input vector and the following weight matrix and input:

$$\mathbf{W}^{2:1} = \begin{bmatrix} 0 & 1 \\ 1 & 1 \end{bmatrix} \quad \mathbf{p} = \begin{bmatrix} 1 \\ 1 \end{bmatrix} \,.$$

Also, assume that neuron 1 of Layer 2 is active.

   i. **Find and plot the response $\mathbf{n}^{1}$.**

   ii. **Check to see that the answer to part (i) satisfies the steady state response predicted by Eq. (16.21).**

i.   Since Layer 2 is active, and neuron 1 of Layer 2 wins the competition, the equations of operation of Layer 1 are

$$(0.01)\frac{dn_{1}^{1}}{dt} = -n_{1}^{1} + (2 - n_{1}^{1})\{p_{1} + w_{1,1}^{2:1}\} - (n_{1}^{1} + 3)$$

$$= -n_{1}^{1} + (2 - n_{1}^{1})\{1 + 0\} - (n_{1}^{1} + 3) = -3n_{1}^{1} - 1$$

$$(0.01)\frac{dn_{2}^{1}}{dt} = -n_{2}^{1} + (2 - n_{2}^{1})\{p_{2} + w_{2,1}^{2:1}\} - (n_{2}^{1} + 3)$$

$$= -n_{2}^{1} + (2 - n_{2}^{1})\{1 + 1\} - (n_{2}^{1} + 3) = -4n_{2}^{1} + 1 \,.$$

These can be simplified to obtain

$$\frac{dn_{1}^{1}}{dt} = -300n_{1}^{1} - 100 \,,$$

$$\frac{dn_{2}^{1}}{dt} = -400n_{2}^{1} + 100 \,.$$

If we assume that both neurons start with zero initial condition, the solutions are

$$n_1^1(t) = -\frac{1}{3}[1 - e^{-300t}],$$

$$n_2^1(t) = \frac{1}{4}[1 - e^{-400t}].$$

These are displayed in Figure P16.1.

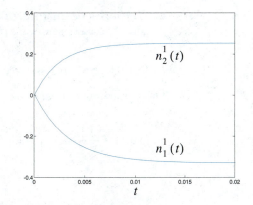

Figure P16.1 Response of Layer 1

ii. Note that $n_1^1(t)$ converges to a negative value, and $n_2^1(t)$ converges to a positive value. Therefore, $a_1^1(t)$ converges to 0, and $a_2^1(t)$ converges to 1 (recall that the transfer function for Layer 1 is $hardlim^+$). This agrees with our steady state analysis (see Eq. (16.21)), since

$$\mathbf{p} \cap \mathbf{w}_1^{2:1} = \begin{bmatrix} 1 \\ 1 \end{bmatrix} \cap \begin{bmatrix} 0 \\ 1 \end{bmatrix} = \begin{bmatrix} 0 \\ 1 \end{bmatrix} = \mathbf{a}^1. \tag{16.75}$$

P16.2 **Consider Layer 2 of the ART1 network with the following parameters:**

$$\varepsilon = 0.1 \quad {}^+\mathbf{b}^2 = \begin{bmatrix} 2 \\ 2 \end{bmatrix} \quad {}^-\mathbf{b}^2 = \begin{bmatrix} 2 \\ 2 \end{bmatrix} \quad \mathbf{W}^{1:2} = \begin{bmatrix} ({}_1\mathbf{w}^{1:2})^T \\ ({}_2\mathbf{w}^{1:2})^T \end{bmatrix} = \begin{bmatrix} 0.5 & 0.5 \\ 1 & 0 \end{bmatrix}$$

and

$$f^2(n) = \begin{cases} 10\,(n)^2 & n \geq 0 \\ 0 & n < 0 \end{cases}.$$

16

Assume that the output of Layer 1 is

$$\mathbf{a}^1 = \begin{bmatrix} 1 \\ 0 \end{bmatrix}.$$

This is equivalent to the Layer 2 example in the text (page 16-12), with the exception of the bias values.

    i. **Write the equations of operation of Layer 2 and simulate and plot the response. Explain the effect of increasing the bias values.**

    ii. **Verify that the steady state operation of Layer 2 is correct.**

i.   The equations of operation of the layer will be

$$(0.1)\frac{dn_1^2(t)}{dt} = -n_1^2(t) + (2 - n_1^2(t))\,\{f^2(n_1^2(t)) + (\,_1\mathbf{w}^{1:2})^T\mathbf{a}^1\}$$

$$- (n_1^2(t) + 2)\,f^2(n_2^2(t))\,,$$

$$(0.1)\frac{dn_2^2(t)}{dt} = -n_2^2(t) + (2 - n_2^2(t))\,\{f^2(n_2^2(t)) + (\,_2\mathbf{w}^{1:2})^T\mathbf{a}^1\}$$

$$- (n_2^2(t) + 2)\,f^2(n_1^2(t))\,.$$

Figure P16.2 illustrates the response of Layer 2 when the input vector is $\mathbf{a}^1 = \begin{bmatrix} 1 & 0 \end{bmatrix}^T$. The second row of $\mathbf{W}^{1:2}$ has a larger inner product with $\mathbf{a}^1$ than the first row, therefore neuron 2 wins the competition.

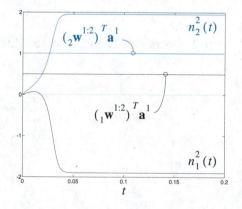

Figure P16.2 Response of Layer 2

If we compare Figure P16.2 with Figure 16.5, we can see that the bias value has three effects. First, the speed of response is increased; the neuron outputs move more quickly to their steady state values. Second, the range of the response is increased from $[-1, 1]$ to $[-2, 2]$. (Recall from Chapter 15 that for the shunting model the upper limit will be the excitatory bias ^+b. The lower limit will be the inhibitory bias ^-b.) Third, the neuron responses move closer to the upper and lower limits.

ii. At steady state, $n_1^2(t)$ has a positive value, and $n_2^2(t)$ has a negative value. The steady state Layer 2 output will then be

$$\mathbf{a}^2 = \begin{bmatrix} 1 \\ 0 \end{bmatrix}.$$

This agrees with the desired steady state response characteristics of Layer 2:

$$a_i^2 = \begin{cases} 1, & \text{if } ((_i\mathbf{w}^{1:2})^T \mathbf{a}^1 = max[(_j\mathbf{w}^{1:2})^T \mathbf{a}^1]) \\ 0, & \text{otherwise} \end{cases}.$$

16

P16.3 **Consider the Orienting Subsystem of the ART1 network with the following parameters:**

$$\varepsilon = 0.1 \quad \alpha = 0.5 \quad \beta = 2 \quad (\rho = 0.25) \quad ^+b^0 = {^-b^0} = 0.5.$$

The inputs to the Orienting Subsystem are

$$\mathbf{p} = \begin{bmatrix} 1 \\ 1 \\ 1 \\ 1 \end{bmatrix} \quad \mathbf{a}^1 = \begin{bmatrix} 1 \\ 0 \\ 0 \\ 1 \end{bmatrix}.$$

i. **Find and plot the response of the Orienting Subsystem $n^0(t)$.**

ii. **Verify that the steady state conditions are satisfied.**

The equation of operation of the Orienting Subsystem is

$$(0.1)\frac{dn^0(t)}{dt} = -n^0(t) + (0.5 - n^0(t)) \{0.5(p_1 + p_2 + p_3)\}$$

$$- (n^0(t) + 0.5) \{2(a_1^1 + a_2^1 + a_3^1)\}$$

or

$$\frac{dn^0(t)}{dt} = -65n^0(t) - 12.5 .$$

The response is then

$$n^0(t) = -0.1923 \, [1 - e^{-65t}]$$

This response is plotted in Figure P16.3. In this case, since $n^0(t)$ is negative, $a^0 = hardlim^+(n^0) = 0$, and therefore a reset signal will not be sent to Layer 2.

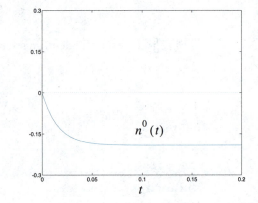

Figure P16.3 Response of the Orienting Subsystem

ii. The steady state operation of the Orienting Subsystem can be summarized as follows:

$$a^0 = \begin{cases} 1, & \text{if } [\|\mathbf{a}^1\|^2 / \|\mathbf{p}\|^2 < \rho] \\ 0, & \text{otherwise} \end{cases} .$$

For this problem

$$\|\mathbf{a}^1\|^2 / \|\mathbf{p}\|^2 = \left\|\begin{bmatrix} 1 \\ 0 \\ 1 \end{bmatrix}\right\|^2 / \left\|\begin{bmatrix} 1 \\ 1 \\ 1 \end{bmatrix}\right\|^2 = \frac{2}{3} > \rho = 0.25 .$$

Therefore $a^0 = 0$, which agrees with the results of part (i).

P16.4 Show that the learning equation for the L2-L1 connections is equivalent to the outstar equation described in Chapter 13.

The L2-L1 learning law (Eq. (16.65)) is

$$\frac{d\left[\mathbf{w}_j^{2:1}(t)\right]}{dt} = a_j^2(t)\left[-\mathbf{w}_j^{2:1}(t) + \mathbf{a}^1(t)\right].$$

If we approximate the derivative by

$$\frac{d\left[\mathbf{w}_j^{2:1}(t)\right]}{dt} \approx \frac{\mathbf{w}_j^{2:1}(t+\Delta t) - \mathbf{w}_j^{2:1}(t)}{\Delta t},$$

then we can rewrite Eq. (16.65) as

$$\mathbf{w}_j^{2:1}(t+\Delta t) = \mathbf{w}_j^{2:1}(t) + (\Delta t)\, a_j^2(t)\left\{-\mathbf{w}_j^{2:1}(t) + \mathbf{a}^1(t)\right\}.$$

This is equivalent to the outstar rule of Chapter 13 (Eq. (13.51)). Here the input to the L2-L1 connections is $a_j^2(t)$, and the output of the L2-L1 connections is $\mathbf{a}^1$.

16

P16.5 Train an ART1 network using the following input vectors:

$$\mathbf{p}_1 = \begin{bmatrix} 0 \\ 1 \\ 0 \end{bmatrix},\ \mathbf{p}_2 = \begin{bmatrix} 1 \\ 0 \\ 0 \end{bmatrix},\ \mathbf{p}_3 = \begin{bmatrix} 1 \\ 1 \\ 0 \end{bmatrix}.$$

Use the parameters $\zeta = 2$, and $\rho = 0.4$, and choose $S^2 = 3$ (3 categories).

Our initial weights will be

$$\mathbf{W}^{2:1} = \begin{bmatrix} 1 & 1 & 1 \\ 1 & 1 & 1 \\ 1 & 1 & 1 \end{bmatrix},\ \mathbf{W}^{2:1} = \begin{bmatrix} 0.5 & 0.5 & 0.5 \\ 0.5 & 0.5 & 0.5 \\ 0.5 & 0.5 & 0.5 \end{bmatrix}.$$

We now begin the algorithm.

1. Compute the Layer 1 response:

$$\mathbf{a}^1 = \mathbf{p}_1 = \begin{bmatrix} 0 \\ 1 \\ 0 \end{bmatrix}.$$

2. Next, compute the input to Layer 2:

$$\mathbf{W}^{1:2}\mathbf{a}^1 = \begin{bmatrix} 0.5 & 0.5 & 0.5 \\ 0.5 & 0.5 & 0.5 \\ 0.5 & 0.5 & 0.5 \end{bmatrix} \begin{bmatrix} 0 \\ 1 \\ 0 \end{bmatrix} = \begin{bmatrix} 0.5 \\ 0.5 \\ 0.5 \end{bmatrix}.$$

Since all neurons have the same input, pick the first neuron as the winner. (In case of a tie, pick the neuron with the smallest index.)

$$\mathbf{a}^2 = \begin{bmatrix} 1 \\ 0 \\ 0 \end{bmatrix}$$

3. Now compute the L2-L1 expectation:

$$\mathbf{W}^{2:1}\mathbf{a}^2 = \begin{bmatrix} 1 & 1 & 1 \\ 1 & 1 & 1 \\ 1 & 1 & 1 \end{bmatrix} \begin{bmatrix} 1 \\ 0 \\ 0 \end{bmatrix} = \begin{bmatrix} 1 \\ 1 \\ 1 \end{bmatrix} = \mathbf{w}_1^{2:1}.$$

4. Adjust the Layer 1 output to include the L2-L1 expectation:

$$\mathbf{a}^1 = \mathbf{p}_1 \cap \mathbf{w}_1^{2:1} = \begin{bmatrix} 0 \\ 1 \\ 0 \end{bmatrix} \cap \begin{bmatrix} 1 \\ 1 \\ 1 \end{bmatrix} = \begin{bmatrix} 0 \\ 1 \\ 0 \end{bmatrix}.$$

5. Next, the Orienting Subsystem determines the degree of match between the expectation and the input pattern:

$$\|\mathbf{a}^1\|^2 / \|\mathbf{p}_1\|^2 = \frac{1}{1} > \rho = 0.4, \text{ therefore } a^0 = 0 \text{ (no reset).}$$

6. Since $a^0 = 0$, continue with step 7.

7. Resonance has occurred, therefore update row 1 of $\mathbf{W}^{1:2}$:

$$_1\mathbf{w}^{1:2} = \frac{2\mathbf{a}^1}{2 + \|\mathbf{a}^1\|^2 - 1} = \mathbf{a}^1 = \begin{bmatrix} 0 \\ 1 \\ 0 \end{bmatrix}, \ \mathbf{W}^{1:2} = \begin{bmatrix} 0 & 1 & 0 \\ 0.5 & 0.5 & 0.5 \\ 0.5 & 0.5 & 0.5 \end{bmatrix}.$$

8. Update column 1 of $\mathbf{W}^{2:1}$:

$$\mathbf{w}_1^{2:1} = \mathbf{a}^1 = \begin{bmatrix} 0 \\ 1 \\ 0 \end{bmatrix}, \ \mathbf{W}^{2:1} = \begin{bmatrix} 0 & 1 & 1 \\ 1 & 1 & 1 \\ 0 & 1 & 1 \end{bmatrix}.$$

9. Remove $\mathbf{p}_1$, and return to step 1 with input pattern $\mathbf{p}_2$.

1. Compute the new Layer 1 response (Layer 2 inactive):

$$\mathbf{a}^1 = \mathbf{p}_2 = \begin{bmatrix} 1 \\ 0 \\ 0 \end{bmatrix}.$$

2. Next, compute the input to Layer 2:

$$\mathbf{W}^{1:2}\mathbf{a}^1 = \begin{bmatrix} 0 & 1 & 0 \\ 0.5 & 0.5 & 0.5 \\ 0.5 & 0.5 & 0.5 \end{bmatrix} \begin{bmatrix} 1 \\ 0 \\ 0 \end{bmatrix} = \begin{bmatrix} 0 \\ 0.5 \\ 0.5 \end{bmatrix}.$$

Since neurons 2 and 3 have the same input, pick the second neuron as the winner:

$$\mathbf{a}^2 = \begin{bmatrix} 0 \\ 1 \\ 0 \end{bmatrix}. \tag{16.76}$$

3. Now compute the L2-L1 expectation:

$$\mathbf{W}^{2:1}\mathbf{a}^2 = \begin{bmatrix} 0 & 1 & 1 \\ 1 & 1 & 1 \\ 0 & 1 & 1 \end{bmatrix} \begin{bmatrix} 0 \\ 1 \\ 0 \end{bmatrix} = \mathbf{w}_2^{2:1} = \begin{bmatrix} 1 \\ 1 \\ 1 \end{bmatrix}.$$

4. Adjust the Layer 1 output to include the L2-L1 expectation:

$$\mathbf{a}^1 = \mathbf{p}_2 \cap \mathbf{w}_2^{2:1} = \begin{bmatrix} 1 \\ 0 \\ 0 \end{bmatrix} \cap \begin{bmatrix} 1 \\ 1 \\ 1 \end{bmatrix} = \begin{bmatrix} 1 \\ 0 \\ 0 \end{bmatrix}.$$

5. Next, the Orienting Subsystem determines the degree of match between the expectation and the input pattern:

$$\|\mathbf{a}^1\|^2 / \|\mathbf{p}_2\|^2 = \frac{1}{1} > \rho = 0.4, \text{ therefore } a^0 = 0 \text{ (no reset).}$$

16

6. Since $a^0 = 0$, continue with step 7.

7. Resonance has occurred, therefore update row 2 of $\mathbf{W}^{1:2}$:

$$_2\mathbf{w}^{1:2} = \frac{2\mathbf{a}^1}{2 + \left\|\mathbf{a}^1\right\|^2 - 1} = \mathbf{a}^1 = \begin{bmatrix} 1 \\ 0 \\ 0 \end{bmatrix}, \mathbf{W}^{1:2} = \begin{bmatrix} 0 & 1 & 0 \\ 1 & 0 & 0 \\ 0.5 & 0.5 & 0.5 \end{bmatrix}.$$

8. Update column 2 of $\mathbf{W}^{2:1}$:

$$\mathbf{w}_2^{2:1} = \mathbf{a}^1 = \begin{bmatrix} 1 \\ 0 \\ 0 \end{bmatrix}, \mathbf{W}^{2:1} = \begin{bmatrix} 0 & 1 & 1 \\ 1 & 0 & 1 \\ 0 & 0 & 1 \end{bmatrix}.$$

9. Remove $\mathbf{p}_2$, and return to step 1 with input pattern $\mathbf{p}_3$.

1. Compute the Layer 1 response with the new input vector:

$$\mathbf{a}^1 = \mathbf{p}_3 = \begin{bmatrix} 1 \\ 1 \\ 0 \end{bmatrix}.$$

2. Next, compute the input to Layer 2:

$$\mathbf{W}^{1:2}\mathbf{a}^1 = \begin{bmatrix} 0 & 1 & 0 \\ 1 & 0 & 0 \\ 0.5 & 0.5 & 0.5 \end{bmatrix}\begin{bmatrix} 1 \\ 1 \\ 0 \end{bmatrix} = \begin{bmatrix} 1 \\ 1 \\ 1 \end{bmatrix}.$$

Since all neurons have the same input, pick the first neuron as the winner:

$$\mathbf{a}^2 = \begin{bmatrix} 1 \\ 0 \\ 0 \end{bmatrix}.$$

3. Now compute the L2-L1 expectation:

$$\mathbf{W}^{2:1}\mathbf{a}^2 = \begin{bmatrix} 0 & 1 & 1 \\ 1 & 0 & 1 \\ 0 & 0 & 1 \end{bmatrix}\begin{bmatrix} 1 \\ 0 \\ 0 \end{bmatrix} = \mathbf{w}_1^{2:1} = \begin{bmatrix} 0 \\ 1 \\ 0 \end{bmatrix}.$$

4. Adjust the Layer 1 output to include the L2-L1 expectation:

$$\mathbf{a}^1 = \mathbf{p}_3 \cap \mathbf{w}_1^{2:1} = \begin{bmatrix} 1 \\ 1 \\ 0 \end{bmatrix} \cap \begin{bmatrix} 0 \\ 1 \\ 0 \end{bmatrix} = \begin{bmatrix} 0 \\ 1 \\ 0 \end{bmatrix}.$$

5. Next, the Orienting Subsystem determines the degree of match between the expectation and the input pattern:

$$\|\mathbf{a}^1\|^2 / \|\mathbf{p}_3\|^2 = \frac{1}{2} > \rho = 0.4 \text{, therefore } a^0 = 0 \text{ (no reset).}$$

6. Since $a^0 = 0$, continue with step 7.

7. Resonance has occurred, therefore update row 1 of $\mathbf{W}^{1:2}$:

$$_1\mathbf{w}^{1:2} = \frac{2\mathbf{a}^1}{2 + \|\mathbf{a}^1\|^2 - 1} = \mathbf{a}^1 = \begin{bmatrix} 0 \\ 1 \\ 0 \end{bmatrix}, \ \mathbf{W}^{1:2} = \begin{bmatrix} 0 & 1 & 0 \\ 1 & 0 & 0 \\ 0.5 & 0.5 & 0.5 \end{bmatrix}.$$

8. Update column 1 of $\mathbf{W}^{2:1}$:

$$\mathbf{w}_2^{2:1} = \mathbf{a}^1 = \begin{bmatrix} 0 \\ 1 \\ 0 \end{bmatrix}, \ \mathbf{W}^{2:1} = \begin{bmatrix} 0 & 1 & 1 \\ 1 & 0 & 1 \\ 0 & 0 & 1 \end{bmatrix}.$$

This completes the training, since if you apply any of the three patterns again they will not change the weights. These patterns have been successfully clustered. This type of result (stable learning) is guaranteed for the ART1 algorithm, since it has been proven to always produce stable clusters.

P16.6 **Repeat Problem P16.5, but change the vigilance parameter to** $\rho = 0.6$**.**

The training will proceed exactly as in Problem P16.5, until pattern $\mathbf{p}_3$ is presented, so let's pick up the algorithm at that point.

1. Compute the Layer 1 response:

$$\mathbf{a}^1 = \mathbf{p}_3 = \begin{bmatrix} 1 \\ 1 \\ 0 \end{bmatrix}.$$

2. Next, compute the input to Layer 2:

16

$$\mathbf{W}^{1:2}\mathbf{a}^1 = \begin{bmatrix} 0 & 1 & 0 \\ 1 & 0 & 0 \\ 0.5 & 0.5 & 0.5 \end{bmatrix} \begin{bmatrix} 1 \\ 1 \\ 0 \end{bmatrix} = \begin{bmatrix} 1 \\ 1 \\ 1 \end{bmatrix} .$$

Since all neurons have the same input, pick the first neuron as the winner:

$$\mathbf{a}^2 = \begin{bmatrix} 1 \\ 0 \\ 0 \end{bmatrix} .$$

3. Now compute the L2-L1 expectation:

$$\mathbf{W}^{2:1}\mathbf{a}^2 = \begin{bmatrix} 0 & 1 & 1 \\ 1 & 0 & 1 \\ 0 & 0 & 1 \end{bmatrix} \begin{bmatrix} 1 \\ 0 \\ 0 \end{bmatrix} = \mathbf{w}_1^{2:1} = \begin{bmatrix} 0 \\ 1 \\ 0 \end{bmatrix} .$$

4. Adjust the Layer 1 output to include the L2-L1 expectation:

$$\mathbf{a}^1 = \mathbf{p}_3 \cap \mathbf{w}_1^{2:1} = \begin{bmatrix} 1 \\ 1 \\ 0 \end{bmatrix} \cap \begin{bmatrix} 0 \\ 1 \\ 0 \end{bmatrix} = \begin{bmatrix} 0 \\ 1 \\ 0 \end{bmatrix} .$$

5. Next, the Orienting Subsystem determines the degree of match between the expectation and the input pattern:

$$\|\mathbf{a}^1\|^2 / \|\mathbf{p}_3\|^2 = \frac{1}{2} < \rho = 0.6 \text{, therefore } a^0 = 1 \text{ (reset).}$$

6. Since $a^0 = 1$, set $a_1^2 = 0$, inhibit it until an adequate match occurs (resonance), and return to step 1.

1. Recompute the Layer 1 response (Layer 2 inactive):

$$\mathbf{a}^1 = \mathbf{p}_3 = \begin{bmatrix} 1 \\ 1 \\ 0 \end{bmatrix} .$$

2. Next, compute the input to Layer 2:

$$\mathbf{W}^{1:2}\mathbf{a}^{1} = \begin{bmatrix} 0 & 1 & 0 \\ 1 & 0 & 0 \\ 0.5 & 0.5 & 0.5 \end{bmatrix} \begin{bmatrix} 1 \\ 1 \\ 0 \end{bmatrix} = \begin{bmatrix} 1 \\ 1 \\ 1 \end{bmatrix} .$$

Since neuron 1 is inhibited, neuron 2 is the winner:

$$\mathbf{a}^{2} = \begin{bmatrix} 0 \\ 1 \\ 0 \end{bmatrix} .$$

3. Now compute the L2-L1 expectation:

$$\mathbf{W}^{2:1}\mathbf{a}^{2} = \begin{bmatrix} 0 & 1 & 1 \\ 1 & 0 & 1 \\ 0 & 0 & 1 \end{bmatrix} \begin{bmatrix} 0 \\ 1 \\ 0 \end{bmatrix} = \mathbf{w}_{2}^{2:1} = \begin{bmatrix} 1 \\ 0 \\ 0 \end{bmatrix} .$$

4. Adjust the Layer 1 output to include the L2-L1 expectation:

$$\mathbf{a}^{1} = \mathbf{p}_{3} \cap \mathbf{w}_{2}^{2:1} = \begin{bmatrix} 1 \\ 1 \\ 0 \end{bmatrix} \cap \begin{bmatrix} 1 \\ 0 \\ 0 \end{bmatrix} = \begin{bmatrix} 1 \\ 0 \\ 0 \end{bmatrix} .$$

5. Next, the Orienting Subsystem determines the degree of match between the expectation and the input pattern:

$$\|\mathbf{a}^{1}\|^{2}/\|\mathbf{p}_{3}\|^{2} = \frac{1}{2} < \rho = 0.6 , \text{ therefore } a^{0} = 1 \text{ (reset).}$$

6. Since $a^{0} = 1$, set $a_{2}^{2} = 0$, inhibit it until an adequate match occurs (resonance), and return to step 1.

1. Recompute the Layer 1 response:

$$\mathbf{a}^{1} = \mathbf{p}_{3} = \begin{bmatrix} 1 \\ 1 \\ 0 \end{bmatrix} .$$

2. Next, compute the input to Layer 2:

$$\mathbf{W}^{1:2}\mathbf{a}^{1} = \begin{bmatrix} 0 & 1 & 0 \\ 1 & 0 & 0 \\ 0.5 & 0.5 & 0.5 \end{bmatrix} \begin{bmatrix} 1 \\ 1 \\ 0 \end{bmatrix} = \begin{bmatrix} 1 \\ 1 \\ 1 \end{bmatrix} .$$

16

Since neurons 1 and 2 are inhibited, neuron 3 is the winner:

$$\mathbf{a}^2 = \begin{bmatrix} 0 \\ 0 \\ 1 \end{bmatrix}.$$

3. Now compute the L2-L1 expectation:

$$\mathbf{W}^{2:1}\mathbf{a}^2 = \begin{bmatrix} 0 & 1 & 1 \\ 1 & 0 & 1 \\ 0 & 0 & 1 \end{bmatrix} \begin{bmatrix} 0 \\ 0 \\ 1 \end{bmatrix} = \mathbf{w}_3^{2:1} = \begin{bmatrix} 1 \\ 1 \\ 1 \end{bmatrix}.$$

4. Adjust the Layer 1 output to include the L2-L1 expectation:

$$\mathbf{a}^1 = \mathbf{p}_3 \cap \mathbf{w}_3^{2:1} = \begin{bmatrix} 1 \\ 1 \\ 0 \end{bmatrix} \cap \begin{bmatrix} 1 \\ 1 \\ 1 \end{bmatrix} = \begin{bmatrix} 1 \\ 1 \\ 0 \end{bmatrix}.$$

5. Next, the Orienting Subsystem determines the degree of match between the expectation and the input pattern:

$$\|\mathbf{a}^1\|^2 / \|\mathbf{p}_3\|^2 = \frac{2}{2} > \rho = 0.6 \text{, therefore } a^0 = 0 \text{ (no reset)}.$$

6. Since $a^0 = 0$, continue with step 7.

7. Resonance has occurred, therefore update row 3 of $\mathbf{W}^{1:2}$:

$$_1\mathbf{w}^{1:2} = \frac{2\mathbf{a}^1}{2 + \|\mathbf{a}^1\|^2 - 1} = \frac{2}{3}\mathbf{a}^1 = \begin{bmatrix} \frac{2}{3} \\ \frac{2}{3} \\ 0 \end{bmatrix}, \quad \mathbf{W}^{1:2} = \begin{bmatrix} 0 & 1 & 0 \\ 1 & 0 & 0 \\ \frac{2}{3} & \frac{2}{3} & 0 \end{bmatrix}.$$

8. Update column 3 of $\mathbf{W}^{2:1}$:

$$\mathbf{w}_3^{2:1} = \mathbf{a}^1 = \begin{bmatrix} 1 \\ 1 \\ 0 \end{bmatrix}, \quad \mathbf{W}^{2:1} = \begin{bmatrix} 0 & 1 & 1 \\ 1 & 0 & 1 \\ 0 & 0 & 0 \end{bmatrix}.$$

This completes the training, since if you apply any of the three patterns again they will not change the weights. (Verify this for yourself by applying each input pattern to the network.) These patterns have been successfully clustered.

Note that in Problem P16.5, where the vigilance was $\rho = 0.4$, the patterns were clustered into two categories. In this problem, with vigilance $\rho = 0.6$, the patterns were clustered into three categories. The closer the vigilance is to 1, the more categories will be used. This is because an input pattern must be closer to a prototype in order to be incorporated into that proto-type. When the vigilance is close to zero, many different input patterns can be incorporated into one prototype. The vigilance parameter adjusts the coarseness of the categorization.

P16.7 **Train an ART1 network using the following input vectors (see [CaGr87a]):**

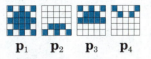

$$\mathbf{p}_1 \qquad \mathbf{p}_2 \qquad \mathbf{p}_3 \qquad \mathbf{p}_4$$

Present the vectors in the order $\mathbf{p}_1 - \mathbf{p}_2 - \mathbf{p}_3 - \mathbf{p}_1 - \mathbf{p}_4$ (i.e., $\mathbf{p}_1$ is presented twice in each epoch). Use the parameters $\zeta = 2$ and $\rho = 0.6$, and choose $S^2 = 3$ (3 categories). Train the network until the weights have converged.

We begin by initializing the weight matrices. The initial $\mathbf{W}^{2:1}$ matrix is an $S^1 \times S^2 = 25 \times 3$ matrix of 1's. The initial $\mathbf{W}^{1:2}$ matrix is normalized, therefore it is an $S^2 \times S^1 = 3 \times 25$ matrix, with each element equal to

$$\frac{\zeta}{(\zeta + S^1 - 1)} = \frac{2}{(2 + 25 - 1)} = 0.0769 .$$

To create the input vectors we will scan each pattern row-by-row, where each blue square will be represented by a 1 and each white square will be represented by a 0. Since the input patterns are 5×5 grids, this will create 25-dimensional input vectors.

We now begin the training. Since it is not practical to display all of the calculations when the vectors are so large, we have summarized the results of the algorithm in Figure P16.4. Each row represents one iteration of the ART1 algorithm (presentation of one input vector). The left-most pattern in each row is the input vector. The remainder of the patterns represent the three columns of the $\mathbf{W}^{2:1}$ matrix. At each iteration, a star indicates the resonance point — the column of $\mathbf{W}^{2:1}$ that matched with the input pattern. Whenever a reset occurred, it is represented by a check mark. When more than one reset occurred in a given iteration, the number beside the check mark indicates the order in which the reset occurred.

16

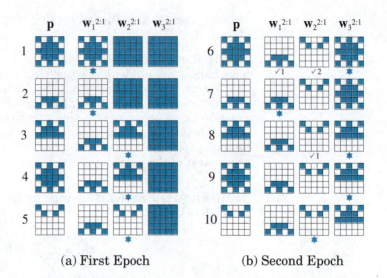

(a) First Epoch   (b) Second Epoch

Figure P16.4 ART1 Iterations for Problem

A total of 10 iterations of the algorithm were performed (two epochs of the sequence $p_1-p_2-p_3-p_1-p_4$). The weights are now stable. (You may want to check this by presenting each input pattern.)

There are several interesting points to notice in this example. First, notice that at iteration 4 both p_1 and p_3 are coded by $w_2^{2:1}$. However, on iteration 5, when p_4 is presented, $w_2^{2:1}$ is modified to include p_4. This new $w_2^{2:1}$ no longer provides an adequate match with p_1 and p_3, as we can see at iterations 6 and 8. This requires them to take over neuron 3, which was unused during the first epoch.

The results of the algorithm could be modified by changing the vigilance parameter. How small would you have to make the vigilance, so that only two neurons in Layer 2 would be required to code all 4 input vectors? How large would the vigilance have to be before a fourth Layer 2 neuron was needed?

Epilogue

Competitive learning, and many other types of neural network training algorithms, suffer from a problem called the stability/plasticity dilemma. If a learning algorithm is sensitive to new inputs (plastic), then it runs the risk of forgetting prior learning (unstable). The ART networks were designed to achieve learning stability while maintaining sensitivity to novel inputs.

In this chapter, the ART1 network was used to illustrate the key concepts of adaptive resonance theory. The ART1 network is based on the Grossberg competitive network of Chapter 15, with a few modifications. The key innovation of ART is the use of "expectations." As each input pattern is presented to the network, it is compared with the prototype vector that it most closely matches (the expectation). If the match between the prototype and the input vector is not adequate, a new prototype is selected. In this way, previously learned memories (prototypes) are not eroded by new learning.

One important point to keep in mind when analyzing ART networks, is that they were designed to be biologically plausible mechanisms for learning. They have as much to do with understanding how the brain works as they do with inspiring practical pattern recognition systems. For this reason, the learning mechanisms are required to use only local information at each neuron. This is not true of all of the learning rules discussed in this text.

Although the ART networks solve the problem of learning instability, in which the network weights never stabilize, there is another stability problem that we have not yet discussed. This is the stability of the differential equations that implement the short-term memory equations of the network. In Layer 2, for example, we have a set of differential equations with nonlinear feedback. Can we make some general statement about the stability of such systems? Chapter 17 will present a comprehensive discussion of this problem.

16

Further Reading

[CaGr87a]   G. A. Carpenter and S. Grossberg, "A massively parallel architecture for a self-organizing neural pattern recognition machine," *Computer Vision, Graphics, and Image Processing*, vol. 37, pp. 54–115, 1987.

In this original presentation of the ART1 architecture, Carpenter and Grossberg demonstrate that the architecture self-organizes and self-stabilizes in response to an arbitrary number of binary input patterns. The key feature of ART is a top-down matching mechanism.

[CaGr87b]   G. A. Carpenter and S. Grossberg, "ART2: Self-organization of stable category recognition codes for analog input patterns," *Applied Optics*, vol. 26, no. 23, pp. 4919–4930, 1987.

This article describes an extension of the ART1 architecture that is designed to handle analog input patterns.

[CaGr90]   G. A. Carpenter and S. Grossberg, "ART3: Hierarchical search using chemical transmitters in self-organizing pattern recognition architectures," *Neural Networks*, vol. 3, no. 23, pp. 129–152, 1990.

This article demonstrates how the Orienting Subsystem of the ART networks could be implemented in biological neurons through the use of chemical transmitters.

[CaGrMa92]   G. A. Carpenter, S. Grossberg, N. Markuzon, J. Reynolds and D. Rosen, "Fuzzy ARTMAP: An adaptive resonance architecture for incremental learning of analog maps," *Proceedings of the International Joint Conference on Neural Networks*, Baltimore, MD, vol. 3, no. 5, pp. 309–314, 1992.

The authors present a modification of the ARTMAP architecture to include fuzzy logic that enables better performance in a noisy environment.

[CaGrRe91]   G. A. Carpenter, S. Grossberg and J. Reynolds, "ARTMAP: Supervised real-time learning and classification of nonstationary data by a self-organizing neural network," *Neural Networks*, vol. 4, no. 5, pp. 169–181, 1991.

This article presents an adaptive resonance theory network for supervised learning. The network consists of two interconnected ART modules. One module receives the input vector, and the other module receives the desired output vector.

[Gros76]   S. Grossberg, "Adaptive pattern classification and universal recoding: I. Parallel development and coding of neural feature detectors," *Biological Cybernetics*, vol. 23, pp. 121–134, 1976.

Grossberg describes a continuous-time competitive network, inspired by the developmental physiology of the visual cortex. The structure of this network forms the foundation for other important networks.

[Gros82]   S. Grossberg, *Studies of Mind and Brain*, Boston: D. Reidel Publishing Co., 1982.

This book is a collection of Stephen Grossberg papers from the period 1968 through 1980. It covers many of the fundamental concepts used in later Grossberg networks, such as the adaptive resonance theory networks.

16

Exercises

E16.1 Consider Layer 1 of the ART1 network with $\varepsilon = 0.02$. Assume two neurons in Layer 2, two elements in the input vector and the following weight matrix and input:

$$\mathbf{W}^{2:1} = \begin{bmatrix} 0 & 1 \\ 1 & 1 \end{bmatrix} \quad \mathbf{p} = \begin{bmatrix} 0 \\ 1 \end{bmatrix}.$$

Also assume that neuron 2 of Layer 2 is active.

   i. Find and plot the response $\mathbf{n}^1$ if ${}^+b^1 = 2$ and ${}^-b^1 = 3$.

   ii. Find and plot the response $\mathbf{n}^1$ if ${}^+b^1 = 4$ and ${}^-b^1 = 5$.

   iii. Find and plot the response $\mathbf{n}^1$ if ${}^+b^1 = 4$ and ${}^-b^1 = 4$.

   iv. Check to see that the answers to parts (i)–(iii) satisfy the steady state response predicted by Eq. (16.21). Explain any inconsistencies.

   v. Check your answers to parts (i)–(iii) by writing a MATLAB M-file to simulate Layer 1 of the ART1 network. Use the **ode45** routine. Plot the response for each case.

E16.2 Consider Layer 2 of the ART1 network with the following parameters:

$$\varepsilon = 0.1 \quad \mathbf{W}^{1:2} = \begin{bmatrix} \left({}_1\mathbf{w}^{1:2} \right)^T \\ \left({}_2\mathbf{w}^{1:2} \right)^T \end{bmatrix} = \begin{bmatrix} 0.5 & 0.5 \\ 1 & 0 \end{bmatrix}$$

and

$$f^2(n) = \begin{cases} 10\,(n)^2, & n \geq 0 \\ 0, & n < 0 \end{cases}.$$

Assume that the output of Layer 1 is

$$\mathbf{a}^1 = \begin{bmatrix} 1 \\ 1 \end{bmatrix}.$$

   i. Write the equations of operation of Layer 2, and simulate and plot the response if the following bias vectors are used:

$$^+\mathbf{b}^2 = \begin{bmatrix} 2 \\ 2 \end{bmatrix} \quad ^-\mathbf{b}^2 = \begin{bmatrix} 2 \\ 2 \end{bmatrix}.$$

ii. Repeat part (i) for the following bias vectors:

$$^+\mathbf{b}^2 = \begin{bmatrix} 3 \\ 3 \end{bmatrix} \quad ^-\mathbf{b}^2 = \begin{bmatrix} 3 \\ 3 \end{bmatrix}.$$

iii. Repeat part (i) for the following bias vectors:

$$^+\mathbf{b}^2 = \begin{bmatrix} 3 \\ 3 \end{bmatrix} \quad ^-\mathbf{b}^2 = \begin{bmatrix} 0 \\ 0 \end{bmatrix}.$$

iv. Do the results of all of the previous parts satisfy the desired steady state response described in Eq. (16.37)? If not, explain why.

E16.3 Consider the Orienting Subsystem of the ART1 network with the following parameters:

$$\varepsilon = 0.1 \quad ^+b^0 = \, ^-b^0 = 2 \,.$$

The inputs to the Orienting Subsystem are

$$\mathbf{p} = \begin{bmatrix} 1 \\ 1 \\ 1 \end{bmatrix} \quad \mathbf{a}^1 = \begin{bmatrix} 0 \\ 0 \\ 1 \end{bmatrix}.$$

i. Find and plot the response of the Orienting Subsystem $n^0(t)$, for $\alpha = 0.5 \quad \beta = 4 \quad (\rho = 0.125)$.

ii. Find and plot the response of the Orienting Subsystem $n^0(t)$, for $\alpha = 0.5 \quad \beta = 2 \quad (\rho = 0.25)$.

iii. Verify that the steady state conditions are satisfied in parts (i) and (ii).

iv. Check your answers to parts (i) and (ii) by writing a MATLAB M-file to simulate the Orienting Subsystem.

16

E16.4 To derive the steady state conditions for the L1-L2 and L2-L1 learning rules, we have made the assumption that the input pattern and the neuron outputs remain constant until the weight matrices converge. This is called "fast learning." Show that this fast learning assumption is equivalent to setting the learning rate α to 1 in the instar and outstar learning rules presented in Chapter 13 and the Kohonen competitive learning rule in Chapter 14.

E16.5 Train an ART1 network using the following input vectors:

$$\mathbf{p}_1 = \begin{bmatrix} 0 \\ 1 \\ 0 \\ 1 \end{bmatrix}, \ \mathbf{p}_2 = \begin{bmatrix} 1 \\ 0 \\ 0 \\ 1 \end{bmatrix}, \ \mathbf{p}_3 = \begin{bmatrix} 1 \\ 1 \\ 0 \\ 0 \end{bmatrix}, \ \mathbf{p}_3 = \begin{bmatrix} 1 \\ 1 \\ 1 \\ 1 \end{bmatrix}.$$

Use the parameter $\zeta = 2$, and choose $S^2 = 3$ (3 categories).

   i. Train the network to convergence using $\rho = 0.3$.

  ii. Repeat part (i) using $\rho = 0.6$.

 iii. Repeat part (ii) using $\rho = 0.9$.

E16.6 The ART1 algorithm can be modified to add a new neuron in Layer 2 whenever there is no adequate match between the existing prototypes and the input pattern. This involves creating a new row of the $\mathbf{W}^{1:2}$ matrix and a new column of the $\mathbf{W}^{2:1}$ matrix. Describe how this would be done.

E16.7 Write a Matlab M-file to implement the ART1 algorithm (with the modification described in Exercise E16.6). Use this M-file to train an ART1 network using the following input vectors (see Problem P16.7):

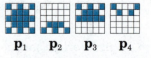

$\mathbf{p}_1$ $\mathbf{p}_2$ $\mathbf{p}_3$ $\mathbf{p}_4$

Present the vectors in the order $\mathbf{p}_1 - \mathbf{p}_2 - \mathbf{p}_3 - \mathbf{p}_1 - \mathbf{p}_4$ (i.e., $\mathbf{p}_1$ is presented twice in each epoch). Use the parameters $\zeta = 2$ and $\rho = 0.9$, and choose $S^2 = 3$ (3 categories). Train the network until the weights have converged. Compare your results with Problem P16.7.

E16.8 Recall the digit recognition problem described in Chapter 7 (page 7-10). Train an ART1 network using the digits $0-9$, as displayed below:

$\mathbf{p}_1 \quad \mathbf{p}_2 \quad \mathbf{p}_3 \quad \mathbf{p}_4 \quad \mathbf{p}_5 \quad \mathbf{p}_6 \quad \mathbf{p}_7 \quad \mathbf{p}_8 \quad \mathbf{p}_9 \quad \mathbf{p}_{10}$

Use the parameter $\zeta = 2$, and choose $S^2 = 5$ (5 categories). Use the Matlab M-file from Exercise E16.7.

 i. Train the network to convergence using $\rho = 0.3$.

 ii. Train the network to convergence using $\rho = 0.6$.

 iii. Train the network to convergence using $\rho = 0.9$.

 iv. Discuss the results of parts (i)–(iii). Explain the effect of the vigilance parameter.

16

17 Stability

17

Objectives

The problem of "convergence" in a recurrent network was first raised in our discussion of the Hopfield network, in Chapter 3. It was noted there that the output of a recurrent network could converge to a stable point, oscillate, or perhaps even diverge. The "stability" of the steepest descent process and of the LMS algorithm were discussed in Chapters 9 and 10, respectively. The stability of Grossberg's continuous-time recurrent networks was discussed in Chapter 15.

In this chapter we will define stability more carefully. Our objective is to determine whether a particular set of nonlinear equations has points (or trajectories) to which its output might converge. To help us study this topic we will introduce Lyapunov's Stability Theorem and apply it to a simple, but instructive, problem. Then, we will present a generalization of the Lyapunov Theory: LaSalle's Invariance Theorem. This will set the stage for Chapter 18, where LaSalle's theorem is used to prove the stability of Hopfield networks.

Theory and Examples

Recurrent Networks

We first discussed recurrent neural networks, which have feedback connections from their outputs to their inputs, when we introduced the Hamming and Hopfield networks in Chapter 3. The Grossberg networks of Chapters 15 and 16 also contain recurrent connections. Recurrent networks are potentially more powerful than feedforward networks, since they are able to recognize and recall temporal, as well as spatial, patterns. However, the behavior of these recurrent networks is much more complex than that of feedforward networks.

For feedforward networks, the output is constant (for a fixed input) and is a function only of the network input. For recurrent networks, however, the output of the network is a function of time. For a given input and a given initial network output, the response of the network may converge to a stable output. However, it may also oscillate, explode to infinity, or follow a chaotic pattern. In the remainder of this chapter we want to investigate general nonlinear recurrent networks, in order to determine their long-term behavior.

We will consider recurrent networks that can be described by nonlinear differential equations of the form:

$$\frac{d}{dt}\mathbf{a}(t) = \mathbf{g}(\mathbf{a}(t), \mathbf{p}(t), t). \tag{17.1}$$

Here $\mathbf{p}(t)$ is the input to the network, and $\mathbf{a}(t)$ is the output of the network. (See Figure 17.1.)

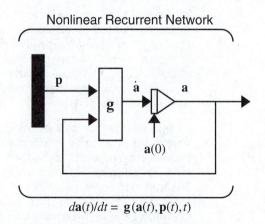

Figure 17.1 Nonlinear, Continuous-Time, Recurrent Network

We want to know how these systems perform in the steady state. We will be most interested in those cases where the network converges to a constant output — a stable equilibrium point. A nonlinear system can have many stable points. For some neural networks these stable points represent stored prototype patterns. When possible, we would like to know where the stable points are, and which initial conditions $a(0)$ converge to a given stable point (i.e., what is the basin of attraction for a given stable point?).

Stability Concepts

To begin our discussion, let's introduce some basic stability concepts with a simple, intuitive example. Consider the motion of a ball bearing, with dissipative friction, in a gravity field. In the adjacent figure, we have a ball bearing at the bottom of a trough (point $a*$). If we move the bearing to a different position, it will oscillate back and forth in the trough, but, because of friction, it will eventually settle back to the bottom of the trough. We will call this position an *asymptotically stable* point, which we will define more precisely in the next section.

Consider now the second figure in the left margin. Here we have a ball bearing positioned at the center of a flat surface. If we place the bearing in a different position, it will not move. The position at the center of the surface is not asymptotically stable, since the bearing does not move back to the center if it is moved away. However, it is stable in a certain sense, because at least the ball does not roll farther away from the center point. We call this kind of point *stable in the sense of Lyapunov*, which we will define in the next section.

Now consider the third figure in the left margin. The ball bearing is positioned at the top of a hill. This is an equilibrium point, since the ball will remain at the top of the hill, if we position it carefully. However, if the bearing is given the slightest disturbance, it will roll down the hill. This is an *unstable* equilibrium point.

In the next chapter we will try to design Hopfield neural networks, in which the stored prototype patterns will be asymptotically stable equilibrium points. We would also like the basins of attraction for these stable points to be as large as possible.

For example, consider Figure 17.2. We would like to design neural networks with large basins of attraction such as those of Case A. One can certainly imagine that if a ball that rolls with high friction is placed (with zero velocity) in any one of the basins of Case A, it will remain in that basin and will eventually find its way to the bottom (stable point). However, Case B is more complicated. If, for instance, one places a ball with friction at point P, it is not clear which stable point will eventually capture the ball. The ball may not come to rest at the stable point closest to P. It is also difficult to tell how large the basin of attraction is for a specific stable point.

17

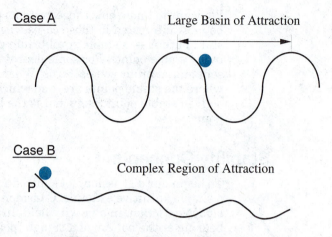

Figure 17.2 Basins of Attraction

Now that we have presented some intuitive notions of stability, we will pursue them with mathematical rigor in the remainder of this chapter.

Definitions

Equilibrium Point

We will begin with specific mathematical definitions of the different types of stability discussed in the previous section. In these definitions we will be talking about the stability of an *equilibrium point*; a point **a*** where the derivative in Eq. (17.1) is zero. For simplicity, we will talk specifically about the point **a*** = **0**, which is referred to as the origin. This restriction does not affect the generality of our discussion.

Stability

Definition 1: *Stability* (in the sense of Lyapunov)

The origin is a stable equilibrium point if for any given value $\varepsilon > 0$ there exists a number $\delta(\varepsilon) > 0$ such that if $\|\mathbf{a}(0)\| < \delta$, then the resulting motion $\mathbf{a}(t)$ satisfies $\|\mathbf{a}(t)\| < \varepsilon$ for $t > 0$.

This definition says that the system output is not going to move too far away from a given stable point, so long as it is initially close to the stable point. Let's say that you want the system output to remain within a distance ε of the origin. If the origin is stable, then you can always find a distance δ (which may be a function of ε), such that if the system output is within δ of the origin at time $t = 0$, then it will always remain within ε of the origin. The position of the ball (with zero velocity) in the figure to the left is stable in the sense of Lyapunov, so long as the ball bearing has friction. If the ball bearing did not have friction, then any initial velocity would produce a trajectory $\mathbf{a}(t)$ in which the position would go to infinity. (The vector $\mathbf{a}(t)$ in this case would consist of the position and the velocity of the ball.)

Next, let's consider the stronger concept of asymptotic stability.

Asymptotic Stability   Definition 2: *Asymptotic Stability*

The origin is an asymptotically stable equilibrium point if there exists a number $\delta > 0$ such that whenever $\|\mathbf{a}(0)\| < \delta$ the resulting motion satisfies $\|\mathbf{a}(t)\| \to 0$ as $t \to \infty$.

This is a stronger definition of stability. It says that as long as the output of the system is initially within some distance δ of the stable point, the output will eventually converge to the stable point. The position of the ball (with zero velocity) in the diagram in the left margin is asymptotically stable, so long as the ball bearing has friction. If there is no friction, the position is only stable in the sense of Lyapunov.

We would like to build neural networks that have many specified asymptotically stable points, each of which represents a prototype pattern. This is the design objective we will use for building Hopfield networks in Chapter 18.

In addition to the stability definitions, there is another concept we will use in analyzing stability. It is the concept of a *definite* function. The next two definitions will clarify this concept.

Positive Definite   Definition 3: *Positive Definite*

A scalar function $V(\mathbf{a})$ is positive definite if $V(\mathbf{0}) = 0$ and $V(\mathbf{a}) > 0$ for $\mathbf{a} \neq \mathbf{0}$.

Positive Semidefinite   Definition 4: *Positive Semidefinite*

A scalar function $V(\mathbf{a})$ is positive semidefinite if $V(\mathbf{a}) \geq 0$ for all $\mathbf{a}$.

(These definitions can be modified appropriately to define the concepts *negative definite* and *negative semidefinite*.) Now that we have defined stability, let's consider a method for testing stability.

Lyapunov Stability Theorem

One of the most important approaches for investigating the stability of nonlinear systems is the theory introduced by Alexandr Mikhailovich Lyapunov, a Russian mathematician. Although his major work was first published in 1892, it received little attention outside Russia until much later. In this section we will discuss one of Lyapunov's most powerful techniques for stability analysis — the so-called *direct method*.

17

Consider the autonomous (unforced, no explicit time dependence) system:

$$\frac{d\mathbf{a}}{dt} = \mathbf{g}(\mathbf{a}) . \tag{17.2}$$

The Lyapunov stability theorem can then be stated as follows.

Theorem 1: *Lyapunov Stability Theorem*

If a positive definite function $V(\mathbf{a})$ can be found such that $dV(\mathbf{a})/dt$ is negative semidefinite, then the origin ($\mathbf{a} = \mathbf{0}$) is stable for the system of Eq. (17.2). If a positive definite function $V(\mathbf{a})$ can be found such that $dV(\mathbf{a})/dt$ is negative definite, then the origin ($\mathbf{a} = \mathbf{0}$) is asymptotically stable. In each case, V is called a Lyapunov function of the system.

You can think of $V(\mathbf{a})$ as a generalized energy function. The concept of the theorem is that if the energy of a system is continually decreasing ($dV(\mathbf{a})/dt$ negative definite), then it will eventually settle at some minimum energy state. Lyapunov's insight was to generalize the concept of energy, so that the theorem could be applied to systems where the energy is difficult to express or has no meaning.

We should note that the theorem only states that if a suitable Lyapunov function $V(\mathbf{a})$ can be found, the system is stable. It gives us no information about the stability of the system in those situations where we are unable to find such a function.

Pendulum Example

We can gain some insight into Lyapunov's stability theorem by applying it to a simple mechanical system. This system is very simple, and its operation is easy to visualize, and yet it illustrates important concepts that we will apply to neural network design in the next chapter. The example system we will use is the pendulum shown in Figure 17.3.

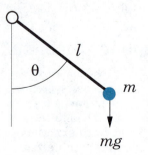

Figure 17.3 Pendulum

Using Newton's second law ($F = ma$), we can write the equation of operation of the pendulum as

$$ml\,\frac{d^2}{dt^2}(\theta) = -c\frac{d\theta}{dt} - mg\sin(\theta)\,, \tag{17.3}$$

or

$$ml\,\frac{d^2\theta}{dt^2} + c\frac{d\theta}{dt} + mg\sin(\theta) = 0\,, \tag{17.4}$$

where θ is the angle of the pendulum, m is the mass of the pendulum, l is the length of the pendulum, c is the damping coefficient, and g is the gravitational constant.

The first term on the right side of Eq. (17.3) is the damping force, which is proportional to the velocity of the pendulum. It is this term that represents the energy dissipation in the system. The second term on the right side of Eq. (17.3) is the gravitational force, which is proportional to the sine of the angle of the pendulum. It is equal to zero when the pendulum is straight down and has its maximum value when the pendulum is horizontal.

If the damping coefficient is not zero, the pendulum will eventually come to rest hanging down in the vertical position. This solution might be viewed as $\theta = 0$, but more generally it is $\theta = 2\pi n$, where $n = 0, \pm 1, \pm 2, \pm 3, \ldots$. That is, given the appropriate initial conditions, the pendulum might simply settle to $\theta = 0$ or it might rotate once to give a solution of $\theta = 2\pi$, etc. There are many possible equilibrium solutions. (The positions $\theta = \pi n$, for odd values of n, are also equilibrium points, but they are not stable.)

To analyze the stability of this system, we will write the pendulum equation in state variable form, where it will appear as a pair of first-order differential equations. Let's choose the following state variables:

$$a_1 = \theta \text{ and } a_2 = \frac{d\theta}{dt}\,. \tag{17.5}$$

We can write equations for the pendulum in terms of these state variables as follows:

$$\frac{da_1}{dt} = a_2\,, \tag{17.6}$$

$$\frac{da_2}{dt} = -\frac{g}{l}\sin(a_1) - \frac{c}{ml}a_2\,. \tag{17.7}$$

17

Now we want to investigate the stability of the origin ($\mathbf{a} = \mathbf{0}$) for this pendulum system. (The origin corresponds to a pendulum angle of zero and a pendulum velocity of zero.) We first want to check that the origin is an equilibrium point. We do this by substituting $\mathbf{a} = \mathbf{0}$ into the state equations.

$$\frac{da_1}{dt} = a_2 = 0, \tag{17.8}$$

$$\frac{da_2}{dt} = -\frac{g}{l}\sin(a_1) - \frac{c}{ml}a_2 = -\frac{g}{l}\sin(0) - \frac{c}{ml}(0) = 0 \tag{17.9}$$

Since the derivatives are zero, the origin is an equilibrium point.

Next we need to find a Lyapunov function for the pendulum. For this example we will use the energy of the system as the Lyapunov function V. To obtain the total energy of the pendulum, we add the kinetic and potential energies.

$$V(\mathbf{a}) = \frac{1}{2}ml^2(a_2)^2 + mgl(1 - \cos(a_1)) \tag{17.10}$$

In order to test the stability of the system, we need to evaluate the derivative of V with respect to time.

$$\frac{d}{dt}V(\mathbf{a}) = [\nabla V(\mathbf{a})]^T g(\mathbf{a}) = \frac{\partial V}{\partial a_1}\left(\frac{da_1}{dt}\right) + \frac{\partial V}{\partial a_2}\left(\frac{da_2}{dt}\right) \tag{17.11}$$

The partial derivatives of $V(\mathbf{a})$ can be obtained from Eq. (17.10), and the derivatives of the two state variables are given by Eq. (17.6) and Eq. (17.7). Thus we have

$$\frac{d}{dt}V(\mathbf{a}) = (mgl\sin(a_1))a_2 + (ml^2a_2)\left(-\frac{g}{l}\sin(a_1) - \frac{c}{ml}a_2\right). \tag{17.12}$$

The $(mgl\sin(a_1))a_2$ terms cancel, which leaves only

$$\frac{d}{dt}V(\mathbf{a}) = -cl(a_2)^2 \le 0. \tag{17.13}$$

In order to prove that the origin ($\mathbf{a} = \mathbf{0}$) is asymptotically stable, we must show that this derivative is negative definite. The derivative is zero at the origin, but it also is zero for any value of a_1, as long as $a_2 = 0$. Thus, $dV(\mathbf{a})/dt$ is negative semidefinite, rather than negative definite. From Lyapunov's theorem, then, we know that the origin is a stable point. However, we *cannot* say, from the theorem and this Lyapunov function, that the origin is asymptotically stable.

In this case we know that as long as the pendulum has friction, it will eventually settle in a vertical position, and, therefore, that the origin is asymptotically stable. However, Lyapunov's theorem, using our Lyapunov function, can only tell us that the origin is stable. To prove that the origin is asymptotically stable, we will need a refinement of Lyapunov's theorem, LaSalle's Invariance Theorem. We will discuss LaSalle's theorem in the next section.

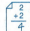

First, let's investigate the pendulum further, by taking a specific numerical example. Let $g = 9.8$, $m = 1$, $l = 9.8$, $c = 1.96$. Now we can rewrite the state equations for the pendulum as

$$\frac{da_1}{dt} = a_2, \tag{17.14}$$

$$\frac{da_2}{dt} = -\sin(a_1) - 0.2a_2. \tag{17.15}$$

Expressions for V and its derivative follow:

$$V = (9.8)^2 \left[\frac{1}{2}(a_2)^2 + (1 - \cos(a_1)) \right], \tag{17.16}$$

$$\frac{dV}{dt} = -(19.208)(a_2)^2. \tag{17.17}$$

Note that dV/dt is zero for any value of a_1 as long as $a_2 = 0$.

Figure 17.4 displays the 3-D and contour plots of the energy surface, V, as the angle varies between -10 and $+10$ radians and the angular velocity varies between -2 and 2 radians per second. Note that in this range there are three possible minimum points of the energy surface, at 0 and $\pm 2\pi$.

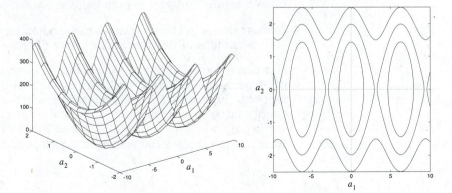

Figure 17.4 Pendulum Energy Surface

(We will find in Chapter 18 that the minimum points of the Lyapunov function can correspond to prototype patterns in an autoassociative neural network. The pendulum system, like recurrent neural networks, has many minimum points.)

Of course, the energy plots shown in Figure 17.4 do not tell us in what way, or by what route, the pendulum finds a particular energy minimum. To show this, we have plotted the energy contours, and one particular path for the pendulum, in Figure 17.5. The response trajectory, shown by the blue line, starts from an initial position, $a_1(0)$, of 1.3 radians (74°) and an initial velocity, $a_2(0)$, of 1.3 radians per second. The trajectory converges to the equilibrium point $\mathbf{a} = \mathbf{0}$.

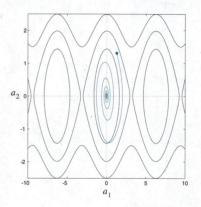

Figure 17.5 Pendulum Response on State Variable Plane

A time response plot of the two state variables is shown in Figure 17.6. Notice that, because the initial velocity is positive, the pendulum continues to move up initially. (Check to see if this agrees with Figure 17.5.) It reaches a maximum angle of about 2 radians before falling back down. The oscillations continue to decay as both state variables converge to zero.

In this case, both state variables converge to zero. However, this is not the only possible equilibrium point, as we will show later.

It is also interesting to plot the pendulum energy, V, as in Figure 17.7. Recall from Eq. (17.17) that the energy should never increase; this is consistent with Figure 17.7. Eq. (17.17) also predicts that the derivative of the energy curve should only be zero when the velocity, a_2, is zero. This is also verified if we compare Figure 17.7 with Figure 17.6. At those times where the a_2 graph crosses the zero axis, the slope of the energy curve is zero.

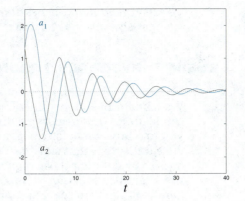

Figure 17.6 State Variables a_1 (blue) and a_2 vs. Time

Notice that, although there are points where the derivative of the energy curve is zero, the derivative does not remain zero until the energy is also zero. This observation will lead to LaSalle's Invariance Theorem, which we will discuss in the next section. The key idea of that theorem is to identify those points where the derivative of the Lyapunov function is zero, and then to determine if the system will be trapped at those points. (Those places where a trajectory can be trapped are called invariant sets.) If the only point that can trap the trajectory, and that has zero derivative, is the origin, then the origin is asymptotically stable.

17

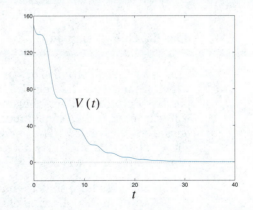

Figure 17.7 Pendulum Lyapunov Function (Energy) vs. Time

The particular pendulum behavior shown in the graphs in this section depends on the initial conditions of the two state variables. The choice of a different set of initial conditions may give results entirely different from those shown in these plots. We will expand on this in the next section.

*To experiment with the pendulum, use the Neural Network Design Demonstration Dynamic System (**nnd17ds**).*

LaSalle's Invariance Theorem

The pendulum example demonstrated a problem with Lyapunov's theorem. We found a Lyapunov function whose derivative was only negative semidefinite (not negative definite), and yet we know that the origin is asymptotically stable for the pendulum system. In this section we will introduce a theorem that clarifies this uncertainty in Lyapunov's theorem. It does so by defining those regions of the state space where the derivative of the Lyapunov function is zero, and then identifying those parts of that region that can trap the trajectory.

Before we discuss LaSalle's Invariance Theorem, we first need to introduce the following definitions.

Definitions

Lyapunov Function

Definition 5: *Lyapunov Function*

Let V be a continuously differentiable function from $\Re^n$ to $\Re$. If G is any subset of $\Re^n$, we say that V is a Lyapunov function on G for the system $d\mathbf{a}/dt = \mathbf{g}(\mathbf{a})$ if

$$\frac{dV(\mathbf{a})}{dt} = (\nabla V(\mathbf{a}))^T \mathbf{g}(\mathbf{a}) \tag{17.18}$$

does not change sign on G.

This is a generalization of our previous definition of the Lyapunov function, which we used in Theorem 1. Here we do not require that the function be positive definite. In fact, there is no direct requirement on the function itself (except that it be continuously differentiable). The only requirement is on the derivative of V. The derivative cannot change sign anywhere on the set G. Note that the derivative will not change sign if it is negative semidefinite or if it is positive semidefinite.

We should note here that we have not yet explained how to choose the set G. We will use the following definitions and theorems to help us select the best G for a given system.

Set Z

Definition 6: *Set Z*

$$Z = \{\mathbf{a}: dV(\mathbf{a})/dt = 0, \ \mathbf{a} \text{ in the closure of } G\}. \tag{17.19}$$

Here "the closure of G" includes the interior and the boundary of G. This is a key set. It contains all of those points where the derivative of the Lyapunov function is zero. Later we will want to determine where in this set the system trajectory can be trapped.

Invariant Set   Definition 7: *Invariant Set*

A set of points in $\Re^n$ is *invariant* with respect to $d\mathbf{a}/dt = \mathbf{g}(\mathbf{a})$ if every solution of $d\mathbf{a}/dt = \mathbf{g}(\mathbf{a})$ starting in that set remains in the set for all time.

If the system gets into an invariant set, then it can't get out.

Set L Definition 8: *Set L*

L is defined as the largest invariant set in Z.

This set includes all possible points at which the solution might converge. The Lyapunov function does not change in L (because its derivative is zero), and the trajectory will be trapped in L (because it is an invariant set). Now, if this set has only one stable point, then that point is asymptotically stable. This is, in essence, what LaSalle's theorem will say.

Theorem

LaSalle's Invariance Theorem extends the Lyapunov Stability Theorem. We will use it to design Hopfield networks in the next chapter. The theorem proceeds as follows [Lasa67].

Theorem 2: *LaSalle's Invariance Theorem*

If V is a Lyapunov function on G for $d\mathbf{a}/dt = \mathbf{g}(\mathbf{a})$, then each solution $\mathbf{a}(t)$ that remains in G for all $t > 0$ approaches $L^\circ = L \cup \{\infty\}$ as $t \to \infty$. (G is a basin of attraction for L, which has all of the stable points.) If all trajectories are bounded, then $\mathbf{a}(t) \to L$ as $t \to \infty$.

If a trajectory stays in G, then it will either converge to L, or it will go to infinity. If all trajectories are bounded, then all trajectories will converge to L.

There is a corollary to LaSalle's theorem that we will use extensively. It involves choosing the set G in a special way.

17

Corollary 1: *LaSalle's Corollary*

Let G be a component (one connected subset) of

$$\Omega_\eta \;=\; \{\mathbf{a} : V(\mathbf{a}) < \eta\}\,. \qquad (17.20)$$

Assume that G is bounded, $dV(\mathbf{a})/dt \le 0$ on the set G, and let the set $L^\circ = closure\,(L \cap G)$ be a subset of G. Then L° is an attractor, and G is in its region of attraction.

LaSalle's theorem, and its corollary, are very powerful. Not only can they tell us which points are stable (L°), but they can also provide us with a partial region of attraction (G). (Note that L° is constructed differently in the corollary than in the theorem.)

To clarify LaSalle's Invariance Theorem, let's return to the pendulum example we discussed earlier.

Example

Let's apply Corollary 1 to the pendulum example. The first step in using the corollary will be to choose the set Ω_η. This set will then be used to select the set G (a component of Ω_η).

For this example we will use the value $\eta = 100$, therefore Ω_{100} will be the set of points where the energy is less than or equal to 100.

$$\Omega_{100} \;=\; \{\mathbf{a} : V(\mathbf{a}) \le 100\} \qquad (17.21)$$

This set is displayed in blue in Figure 17.8.

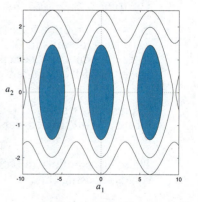

Figure 17.8 Illustration of the Set Ω_{100}

The next step in our analysis is to choose a component (connected subset) of Ω_{100} for the set G. Since we have been investigating the stability of the origin, let's choose the component of Ω_{100} that contains $\mathbf{a} = \mathbf{0}$. The resulting set is shown in Figure 17.9.

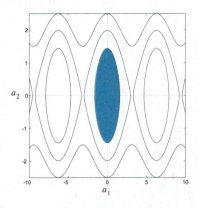

Figure 17.9 Illustration of the Set G

Now that we have chosen G, we need to check that the derivative of the Lyapunov function is less than or equal to zero on G. From Eq. (17.17) we know that $dV(\mathbf{a})/dt$ is negative semidefinite. Therefore it will certainly be less than or equal to zero on G.

We are now ready to determine the attractor set L°. We begin with the set L, which is the largest invariant set in Z.

$$Z = \{\mathbf{a}: dV(\mathbf{a})/dt = 0, \ \mathbf{a} \text{ in the closure of } G\}$$

$$= \{\mathbf{a}: a_2 = 0, \ \mathbf{a} \text{ in the closure of } G\} \ . \tag{17.22}$$

This can also be written as

$$Z = \{\mathbf{a}: a_2 = 0, -1.6 \le a_1 \le 1.6\} \ . \tag{17.23}$$

We know from Eq. (17.17) that the derivative of $V(\mathbf{a})$ is only zero when the velocity is zero, which corresponds to the a_2 axis. Therefore Z consists of the segment of the a_2 axis that falls within G. The set Z is displayed in Figure 17.10.

The set L is the largest invariant set in Z. To find L we need to answer the question: If we start the pendulum from an initial position between -1.6 and 1.6 radians, with zero initial velocity, will the velocity of the pendulum remain zero? Clearly the only such initial condition would be 0 radians (straight down). If we start the pendulum from any other position in Z, the pendulum will start to fall, so the velocity will not remain zero and the trajectory will move out of Z. Therefore, the set L consists only of the origin:

$$L = \{\mathbf{a}: \mathbf{a} = \mathbf{0}\} \ . \tag{17.24}$$

17

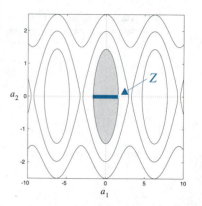

Figure 17.10 Illustration of the Set Z

The set $L°$ is the closure of the intersection of L and G, which in this case is simply L:

$$L° = closure\,(L \cap G) = L = \{\mathbf{a}: \mathbf{a} = 0\}\,.\tag{17.25}$$

Therefore, based on LaSalle's corollary, $L°$ is an attractor (asymptotically stable point) and G is in its region of attraction. This means that any trajectory that starts in G will decay to the origin.

Now suppose that we had taken a bigger region for Ω_η, such as

$$\Omega_{300} = \{\mathbf{a}: V(\mathbf{a}) \leq 300\}\,.\tag{17.26}$$

This set is shown in gray in Figure 17.11.

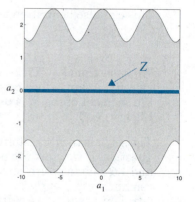

Figure 17.11 Illustration of $G = \Omega_{300}$ (Gray) and Z

We let $G = \Omega_{300}$, since Ω_{300} has only one component. The set Z is given by

$$Z = \{\mathbf{a}: a_2 = 0\}, \tag{17.27}$$

which is shown by the blue bar on the horizontal axis of Figure 17.11. Thus, it follows that

$$L^\circ = L = \{\mathbf{a}: a_1 = \pm n\pi, a_2 = 0\}. \tag{17.28}$$

This is because there are now several different positions within the set Z where we can place the pendulum, without causing the velocity to become nonzero. The pendulum can be pointing directly up or directly down. This corresponds to the positions $\pm n\pi$ for any integer n. If we place the pendulum in any of these positions, with zero velocity, then the pendulum will remain stationary. We can show this by setting the derivatives equal to zero in Eq. (17.14) and Eq. (17.15).

$$\frac{da_1}{dt} = a_2 = 0, \tag{17.29}$$

$$\left(\frac{da_2}{dt} = -\sin(a_1) - 0.2a_2 = -\sin(a_1) = 0 \right) \Rightarrow (a_1 = \pm n\pi) \tag{17.30}$$

For this choice of $G = \Omega_{300}$ we can say very little about where the trajectory will converge. We tried to increase the size of our known region of attraction for the origin, but this G is a region of attraction for all of the equilibrium points. We made G too large. The set L° is illustrated by the blue dots in Figure 17.12.

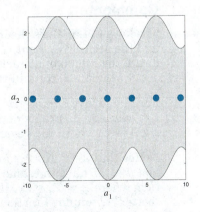

Figure 17.12 The Set L°

We cannot tell which of the equilibrium points (blue dots) will attract the trajectory. All we can say is that if we start somewhere in Ω_{300}, one of the equilibrium points will attract the system solution, but we cannot say for sure which one it will be. Consider, for instance, the trajectory shown in

Figure 17.13. This shows the pendulum response for an initial position of 2 radians and an initial velocity of 1.5 radians per second. This time the pendulum had enough velocity to go over the top, and it converged to the equilibrium point at 2π radians.

Now that we have discussed LaSalle's Invariance Theorem, you might want to experiment some more with the pendulum, in order to investigate the regions of attraction for the various stable points. To experiment with the pendulum, use the Neural Network Design Demonstration Dynamic System *(*nnd17ds*).*

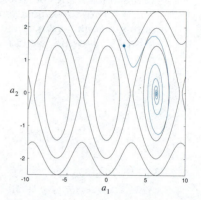

Figure 17.13 Pendulum Trajectory for Different Starting Conditions

Comments

The keys to LaSalle's theorem are the choices of the Lyapunov function V and the set G. We want G to be as large as possible, because that will indicate the region of attraction. However, we want to choose V so that the set Z, which will contain the attractor set, is as small as possible.

For instance, we could try $V = 0$. This is a Lyapunov function for the entire space $\Re^n$, since its derivative is zero (and therefore doesn't change sign) everywhere. However, it gives us no information since $Z = \Re^n$.

Notice that if V_1 and V_2 are both Lyapunov functions on G, and dV_1/dt and dV_2/dt have the same sign, then $V = V_1 + V_2$ is also a Lyapunov function, where $Z = Z_1 \cap Z_2$. If Z is smaller than both Z_1 and Z_2, then Z is a "better" Lyapunov function than either V_1 or V_2. V is always at least as good as either V_1 or V_2, since Z can never be larger than the smaller of Z_1 and Z_2. Therefore, if you have found two different Lyapunov functions and their derivatives have the same sign, then add them together and you may have a better function. The best Lyapunov function for a given system is the one that has the smallest attractor set and the largest region of attraction.

Summary of Results

Stability Concepts

Definitions

Definition 1: *Stability* (in the sense of Lyapunov)

The origin is a stable equilibrium point if for any given value $\varepsilon > 0$ there exists a number $\delta(\varepsilon) > 0$ such that if $\|\mathbf{a}(0)\| < \delta$, then the resulting motion $\mathbf{a}(t)$ satisfies $\|\mathbf{a}(t)\| < \varepsilon$ for $t > 0$.

Definition 2: *Asymptotic Stability*

The origin is an asymptotically stable equilibrium point if there exists a number $\delta > 0$ such that whenever $\|\mathbf{a}(0)\| < \delta$ the resulting motion satisfies $\|\mathbf{a}(0)\| \to 0$ as $t \to \infty$.

Definition 3: *Positive Definite*

A scalar function $V(\mathbf{a})$ is positive definite if $V(\mathbf{0}) = 0$ and $V(\mathbf{a}) > 0$ for $\mathbf{a} \neq \mathbf{0}$.

Definition 4: *Positive Semidefinite*

A scalar function $V(\mathbf{a})$ is positive semidefinite if $V(\mathbf{a}) \geq 0$ for all $\mathbf{a}$.

Lyapunov Stability Theorem

Consider the autonomous (unforced, no explicit time dependence) system

$$\frac{d\mathbf{a}}{dt} = \mathbf{g}(\mathbf{a}).$$

The Lyapunov stability theorem can then be stated as follows.

Theorem 1: *Lyapunov Stability Theorem*

If a positive definite function $V(\mathbf{a})$ can be found such that $dV(\mathbf{a})/dt$ is negative semidefinite, then the origin $(\mathbf{a} = \mathbf{0})$ is stable for this system. If a positive definite function $V(\mathbf{a})$ can be found such that $dV(\mathbf{a})/dt$ is negative definite, then the origin $(\mathbf{a} = \mathbf{0})$ is asymptotically stable. In each case, V is called a Lyapunov function of the system.

17

LaSalle's Invariance Theorem

Definitions

Definition 5: *Lyapunov Function*

Let V be a continuously differentiable function from $\Re^n$ to $\Re$. If G is any subset of $\Re^n$, we say that V is a Lyapunov function on G for the system $d\mathbf{a}/dt = \mathbf{g}(\mathbf{a})$ if

$$\frac{dV(\mathbf{a})}{dt} = (\nabla V(\mathbf{a}))^T \mathbf{g}(\mathbf{a})$$

does not change sign on G.

Definition 6: *Set Z*

$$Z = \{\mathbf{a}: dV(\mathbf{a})/dt = 0, \ \mathbf{a} \text{ in the closure of } G\}. \qquad (17.31)$$

Definition 7: *Invariant Set*

A set of points G in $\Re^n$ is *invariant* with respect to $d\mathbf{a}/dt = \mathbf{g}(\mathbf{a})$ if every solution of $d\mathbf{a}/dt = \mathbf{g}(\mathbf{a})$ starting in G remains in G for all time.

Definition 8: *Set L*

L is defined as the largest invariant set in Z.

Theorem

Theorem 2: *LaSalle's Invariance Theorem*

If V is a Lyapunov function on G for $d\mathbf{a}/dt = \mathbf{g}(\mathbf{a})$, then each solution $\mathbf{a}(t)$ that remains in G for all $t > 0$ approaches $L^\circ = L \cup \{\infty\}$ as $t \to \infty$. (G is a basin of attraction for L, which has all of the stable points.) If all trajectories are bounded, then $\mathbf{a}(t) \to L$ as $t \to \infty$.

Corollary 1: *LaSalle's Corollary*

Let G be a component (one connected subset) of

$$\Omega_\eta = \{\mathbf{a}: V(\mathbf{a}) < \eta\}. \qquad (17.32)$$

Assume that G is bounded, $dV(\mathbf{a})/dt \leq 0$ on the set G, and let the set $L^\circ = closure\,(L \cap G)$ be a subset of G. Then L° is an attractor, and G is in its region of attraction.

Solved Problems

P17.1 **Test the stability of the origin for the following system.**

$$da_1/dt = -a_1 + (a_2)^2$$

$$da_2/dt = -a_2(a_1 + 1)$$

The basic job here is to find a Lyapunov $V(\mathbf{a})$ that is positive definite and has a derivative that is negative semidefinite or, better yet, negative definite. (The latter is a stronger condition.)

Let us try $V(\mathbf{a}) = (a_1)^2 + (a_2)^2$. The derivative of $V(\mathbf{a})$ is

$$\frac{dV(\mathbf{a})}{dt} = (\nabla V)^T\left(\frac{d\mathbf{a}}{dt}\right) = \frac{\partial V}{\partial a_1}\left(\frac{da_1}{dt}\right) + \frac{\partial V}{\partial a_2}\left(\frac{da_2}{dt}\right),$$

or

$$\frac{dV(\mathbf{a})}{dt} = 2a_1(-a_1 + (a_2)^2) + 2a_2(-a_2(a_1+1)) = -2(a_1)^2 - 2(a_2)^2.$$

The derivative $dV(\mathbf{a})/dt$ is negative definite. Therefore, the origin is asymptotically stable.

17

P17.2 **Test the stability of the origin for the following system.**

$$da_1/dt = -(a_1)^5$$

$$da_2/dt = -5(a_2)^7$$

Let us try $V(\mathbf{a}) = (a_1)^2 + (a_2)^2$. Then we have

$$\frac{dV(\mathbf{a})}{dt} = 2a_1(-(a_1)^5) + 2a_2(-5(a_2)^7) = -2(a_1)^6 - 10(a_2)^8.$$

Here again, $dV(\mathbf{a})/dt$ is negative definite, and therefore the origin is asymptotically stable.

P17.3 **Consider the mechanical system shown in Figure P17.1. This is a spring-mass-damper system, with a nonlinear spring. We will define $a_1 = x$ and $a_2 = dx/dt$. Then the equations of motion are**

$$da_1/dt = a_2,$$

$$da_2/dt = -(a_1)^3 - a_2 \quad \text{(nonlinear spring)}.$$

Consider the candidate Lyapunov function

$$V(\mathbf{a}) = \frac{1}{4}(a_1)^4 + \frac{1}{2}(a_2)^2.$$

Use the corollary to LaSalle's invariance theorem to provide as much information as possible about the equilibrium points and basins of attraction.

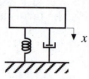

Figure P17.1 Mechanical System

First calculate the derivative of $V(\mathbf{a})$ as

$$\frac{dV(\mathbf{a})}{dt} = \frac{\partial V}{\partial a_1}\left(\frac{da_1}{dt}\right) + \frac{\partial V}{\partial a_2}\left(\frac{da_2}{dt}\right) = (a_1)^3 a_2 + a_2\left(-(a_1)^3 - a_2\right) = -(a_2)^2.$$

Thus, dV/dt does not change sign on $\Re^2$.

Now let us define

$$G = \Omega_\eta = \{\mathbf{a}: V(\mathbf{a}) \le \eta\}$$

and consider the case for $\eta = 1$. A contour plot of $V(\mathbf{a})$ is shown in Figure P17.2. The set Ω_1 is indicated in blue on the plot.

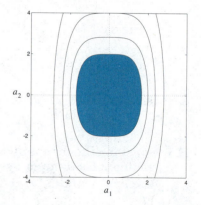

Figure P17.2 Contour Plot of $V(\mathbf{a})$ and Ω_1

Now we need to determine the set Z.

$Z = \{\mathbf{a}: dV/dt = 0, \mathbf{a}$ in the closure of $G\} = \{\mathbf{a}: a_2 = 0, \mathbf{a}$ in the closure of $G\}$

or

$$Z = \{\mathbf{a}: a_2 = 0, \ -\sqrt{2} \leq a_1 \leq \sqrt{2}\}$$

Next we find the set L. Since $\mathbf{a} = 0$ is the only invariant set,

$$L = \{\mathbf{a}: \ a_1 = 0, \ a_2 = 0\} \ .$$

Therefore, the origin,

$$\mathbf{a} = \begin{bmatrix} 0 \\ 0 \end{bmatrix},$$

is an attractor and Ω_1 is in its region of attraction.

Further, we can increase η to show that the entire $\Re^2$ is the basin of attraction for the origin.

Figure P17.3 shows the response of the spring-mass-damper from an initial position of 2 and an initial velocity of 2. Note that the trajectory is parallel to the contour lines when the trajectory crosses the a_2 axis. This agrees with our earlier result, which showed that the derivative of the Lyapunov function was zero whenever $a_2 = 0$. Fortunately, the a_2 axis is not an invariant set (except for the origin); therefore the trajectory is only attracted to the origin.

17

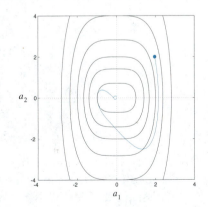

Figure P17.3 Spring-Mass-Damper Response

P17.4 **Consider the following nonlinear system:**

$$da_1/dt = a_1((a_1)^2 + (a_2)^2 - 4) - a_2$$

$$da_2/dt = a_1 + a_2((a_1)^2 + (a_2)^2 - 4) .$$

This system has two invariant sets, the origin

$$\{\mathbf{a}: \mathbf{a} = \mathbf{0} \},$$

and the circle

$$\{\mathbf{a}: (a_1)^2 + (a_2)^2 = 4 \} .$$

Assuming the candidate Lyapunov function

$$V(\mathbf{a}) = (a_1)^2 + (a_2)^2,$$

use LaSalle's Invariance Theorem to find out as much as you can about the region of attraction for the origin.

Our job, then, is to determine whether or not the given invariant sets represent a stable point or a stable trajectory. Let's first take a look at dV/dt. We recall that

$$\frac{dV(\mathbf{a})}{dt} = \frac{\partial V}{\partial a_1}\left(\frac{da_1}{dt}\right) + \frac{\partial V}{\partial a_2}\left(\frac{da_2}{dt}\right),$$

and substitute for the various terms to give

$$\frac{dV(\mathbf{a})}{dt} = 2a_1[a_1((a_1)^2 + (a_2)^2 - 4) - a_2] + 2a_2[a_1 + a_2((a_1)^2 + (a_2)^2 - 4)] .$$

This can be simplified to

$$\frac{dV(\mathbf{a})}{dt} = 2((a_1)^2 + (a_2)^2)((a_1)^2 + (a_2)^2 - 4) .$$

Thus, dV/dt is zero at $\mathbf{a} = \mathbf{0}$ and on the circle $(a_1)^2 + (a_2)^2 = 4$.

We now pick G, a region of attraction. Is there a change of sign of dV/dt over all $\Re^2$? Yes, there is. As we go from outside the circle of radius 2 to its interior, the sign of dV/dt changes from positive to negative. So dV/dt is negative semidefinite inside the circle $(a_1)^2 + (a_2)^2 = 4$. Let's pick a G inside this circle, so that the circle will not be included. The following set will do.

$$G = \Omega_1 = \{\mathbf{a}: V(\mathbf{a}) \le 1\}$$

Now we consider Ω_1. There are just two places that $dV/dt = 0$, and the only point inside Ω_1 is $\mathbf{a} = \mathbf{0}$. Therefore,

$$Z = \{\mathbf{a}: \ a_1 = 0, a_2 = 0\}$$

and

$$L^\circ = L = Z.$$

The origin is the attractor, and Ω_1 is in its region of attraction. We can use the same arguments to show that the region of attraction for the origin includes all points inside the circle $(a_1)^2 + (a_2)^2 = 4$.

Figure P17.4 displays two trajectories for this system, one that begins inside the circle $(a_1)^2 + (a_2)^2 = 4$, and one that begins outside the circle. Although the circle is an invariant set, it is not an attractor. The only attractor for this system is the origin.

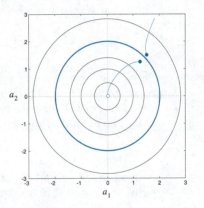

Figure P17.4 Sample Trajectories for Problem P17.4

P17.5 Consider the following nonlinear system.

$$da(t)/(dt) = -(a(t) - 1)(a(t) - 2)$$

   i. **Find any equilibrium points for this system.**

  ii. **Use the following candidate Lyapunov function to obtain whatever information you can about the regions of attraction for the equilibrium points found in part (i). (Hint: Use the corollary to LaSalle's Invariance Theorem.)**

$$V(\mathbf{a}) = (a-2)^2$$

i. To find the equilibrium points, we set $da(t)/dt = 0$.

$$0 = -(a-1)(a-2) \quad \Rightarrow \quad a = 1, a = 2 \quad \text{are equilibrium points}$$

ii. To use LaSalle's corollary, we need to find dV/dt.

$$\frac{dV}{dt} = \frac{\partial V}{\partial a}\left(\frac{da}{dt}\right) = 2(a-2)\,[-(a-1)(a-2)] = -2(a-1)(a-2)^2$$

Now we let

$$G = \Omega_\eta = \{a: V(a) < \eta\}\,.$$

For example, try $\eta = 0.5$. This gives

$$G = \Omega_{0.5} = \{a: (a-2)^2 < 0.5\}\,.$$

Note that a solution of $(a-2)^2 < 0.5$ yields

$$\pm(a-2) < \sqrt{0.5} \quad \text{or} \quad 1.3 < a < 2.7\,.$$

Thus, dV/dt is negative definite on G.

Next we need to find the set Z, which contains those points within G where dV/dt is zero. There are two points where dV/dt is zero, $a = 1$ and $a = 2$. Only one of these falls within G. Therefore

$$Z = \{a: \ a = 2\}\,.$$

Now we need to find L, the largest invariant set in Z. There is only one point in Z, and it is an equilibrium point. Thus

$$L° = L = Z\,.$$

This means that G is in the region of attraction for 2.

We can use the same arguments with values of η up to 1.0. So we can say that the region for attraction for $a = 2$ must include at least

$$\{a: \ 1 < a < 3\}\,.$$

What if we consider those regions where $\eta \geq 1$? Then Z includes both 1 and 2, and dV/dt will change sign on G. Therefore we cannot say anything about the region of attraction for $a = 1$, using this Lyapunov function and the corollary to LaSalle's Invariance Theorem.

Figure P17.5 displays some typical responses for this system. Here we can see that the equilibrium point $a = 1$ is actually unstable. Any initial condition above $a = 1$ converges to $a = 2$. Anything less than $a = 1$ goes to minus infinity.

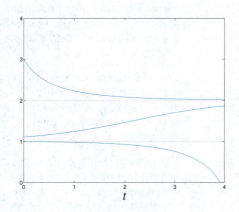

Figure P17.5 Stable and Unstable Responses for Problem P17.5

Epilogue

In this chapter we have presented the concept of stability, as applied to dynamic systems. For nonlinear dynamic systems, like recurrent neural networks, we do not talk about the stability of the system. Rather, we discuss the stability of certain system trajectories and, in particular, equilibrium points.

There were two main stability theorems discussed in this chapter. The first is the Lyapunov Stability Theorem, which introduces the concept of generalized energy — the Lyapunov function. The concept behind this theorem is that if a system's "energy" is always decreasing, then it will eventually stabilize at a point of minimum "energy."

The second theorem presented was LaSalle's Invariance Theorem, which is an enhancement of the Lyapunov Stability Theorem. There are two key improvements made by LaSalle. The first is a clarification of the cases in which the Lyapunov function does not decrease throughout the state space, but stays constant in some regions. LaSalle's theorem introduced the concept of an invariant set to identify those regions that can trap the system trajectory. The second improvement made by LaSalle's theorem is that, in addition to indicating the stability of equilibrium points, it also gave information about the regions of attraction of each stable point.

The ideas presented in this chapter are important tools for the analysis of recurrent neural networks, like the Grossberg networks of Chapters 15 and 16. (See [CoGr83] for an application of LaSalle's Invariance Theorem to recurrent neural networks.) In Chapter 18 we will use LaSalle's theorem to explain the operation of the Hopfield network.

Further Reading

[Brog91]   W. L. Brogan, *Modern Control Theory,* 3rd Ed., Englewood Cliffs, NJ: Prentice-Hall, 1991.

This is a well-written book on the subject of linear systems. The first half of the book is devoted to linear algebra. It also has good sections on the solution of linear differential equations and the stability of linear and nonlinear systems. It has many worked problems.

[CoGr83]   M. A. Cohen and S. Grossberg, "Absolute stability of global pattern formation and parallel memory storage by competitive neural networks," *IEEE Transactions on Systems, Man and Cybernetics*, vol. 13, no. 5, pp. 815–826, 1983.

Cohen and Grossberg apply LaSalle's Invariance Theorem to the analysis of the stability of competitive neural networks. The network description is very general, and the authors show how their analysis can be applied to many different types of recurrent neural networks.

[Lasa67]   J. P. LaSalle, "An invariance principle in the theory of stability," in *Differential Equations and Dynamic Systems*, J. K. Hale and J. P. LaSalle, eds., New York: Academic Press, pp. 277–286, 1967.

This article provides a unified presentation of Lyapunov's stability theory, including several extensions. It introduces LaSalle's Invariance Theorem and various corollaries.

[SlLi91]   J.-J. E. Slotine and W. Li, *Applied Nonlinear Control*, Englewood Cliffs, NJ: Prentice-Hall, 1991.

This text is an introduction to nonlinear control systems. A significant portion of the book is devoted to the analysis of nonlinear dynamic systems. A number of stability theorems are presented and demonstrated.

17

Exercises

E17.1 Use Lyapunov's Stability Theorem to test the stability of the origin for the following systems.

   i.
$$da_1/dt = -(a_1)^3 + a_2$$
$$da_2/dt = -a_1 - a_2$$

   ii.
$$da_1/dt = -a_1 + (a_2)^2$$
$$da_2/dt = -a_2(a_1 + 1)$$

E17.2 Consider the following nonlinear system:

$$da_1/dt = a_2 - 2a_1((a_1)^2 + (a_2)^2),$$

$$da_2/dt = -a_1 - 2a_2((a_1)^2 + (a_2)^2).$$

   i. Use Lyapunov's Stability Theorem and the candidate Lyapunov function shown below to investigate the stability of the origin.

$$V(\mathbf{a}) = \alpha(a_1)^2 + \beta(a_2)^2$$

   ii. Check your stability result from part (i) by writing a MATLAB M-file to simulate the response of this system for several different initial conditions. Use the **ode45** routine. Plot the responses.

E17.3 For the nonlinear system $da/dt = \sin(a)$,

   i. Find any invariant sets.

   ii. Find a Lyapunov function and identify attractors and basins of attraction.

E17.4 Consider the following nonlinear system:

$$da_1/dt = a_2,$$

$$da_2/dt = -a_1 - (a_2)^3.$$

i. Find any equilibrium points.

ii. Find as much information about the stability of the equilibrium points as possible, using the corollary to LaSalle's theorem and the candidate Lyapunov function

$$V(\mathbf{a}) = (a_1)^2 + (a_2)^2.$$

iii. Check your results from parts (i) and (ii) by writing a MATLAB M-file to simulate the response of this system for several different initial conditions. Use the **ode45** routine. Plot the responses.

E17.5 Consider the following nonlinear system

$$da/dt = (1-a)(1+a) = 1 - a^2.$$

i. Find any equilibrium points.

ii. Find a suitable Lyapunov function. (Hint: Start with a form for dV/dt and work backward to find V.)

iii. Sketch the Lyapunov function.

iv. Use the corollary to LaSalle's theorem and the Lyapunov function of part (ii) to find as much information as possible about regions of attraction. Use graphs wherever possible.

(Hint: The graph shown in Figure E17.1 may be helpful.)

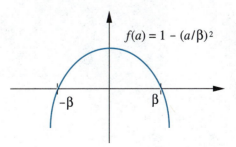

Figure E17.1 Helpful Function for Exercise E17.5

E17.6 Consider the system

$$da_1/dt = a_2 - a_1 ((a_1)^4 + 2(a_2)^2 - 10),$$

$$da_2/dt = -(a_1)^3 - 3(a_2)^5 ((a_1)^4 + 2(a_2)^2 - 10).$$

i. Find any invariant sets. (You may want to simulate this system using MATLAB in order to help identify the invariant sets.)

ii. Using the candidate Lyapunov function shown below and the corollary to LaSalle's theorem, investigate the stability of the invariant sets you found in part (i).

$$V(\mathbf{a}) = ((a_1)^4 + 2(a_2)^2 - 10)^2$$

18 Hopfield Network

18

Objectives

This chapter will discuss the Hopfield recurrent neural network — a network that was highly influential in bringing about the resurgence of neural network research in the early 1980s. We will begin with a description of the network, and then we will show how Lyapunov stability theory can be used to analyze the network operation. Finally, we will demonstrate how the network can be designed to behave as an associative memory.

This chapter brings together many topics discussed in previous chapters: the discrete-time Hopfield network (Chapter 3), eigenvalues and eigenvectors (Chapter 6); associative memory and the Hebb rule (Chapter 7); Hessian matrices, conditions for optimality, quadratic functions and surface and contour plots (Chapter 8); steepest descent and phase plane trajectories (Chapter 9); continuous-time recurrent networks (Chapter 15); and Lyapunov's Stability Theorem and LaSalle's Invariance Theorem (Chapter 17). This chapter is, in some ways, a culmination of all our previous efforts.

Theory and Examples

Much of the resurgence of interest in neural networks during the early 1980s can be attributed to the work of John Hopfield. As a well-known Cal. Tech. physicist, Hopfield's visibility and scientific credentials lent renewed credibility to the neural network field, which had been tarnished by the hype of the mid-1960s. Early in his career he studied the interaction between light and solids. Later he focused on the mechanism of electron transfer between biological molecules. One can imagine that his academic study in physics and mathematics, combined with his later experiences in biology, prepared him uniquely for the conception and presentation of his neural network contribution.

Hopfield wrote two highly influential papers in 1982 [Hopf82] and 1984 [Hopf84]. Many of the ideas in these papers were based on the previous work of other researchers, such as the neuron model of McCulloch and Pitts [McPi43], the additive model of Grossberg [Gros67], the linear associator of Anderson [Ande72] and Kohonen [Koho72] and the Brain-State-in-a-Box network of Anderson, Silverstein, Ritz and Jones [AnSi77]. However, Hopfield's papers are very readable, and they bring together a number of important ideas and present them with a clear mathematical analysis (including the application of Lyapunov stability theory).

There are several other reasons why Hopfield's papers have had such an impact. First, he identified a close analogy between his neural network and the Ising model of magnetic materials, which is used in statistical physics. This brought a significant amount of existing theory to bear on the analysis of neural networks, and it encouraged many physicists, as well as other scientists and engineers, to turn their attention to neural network research.

Hopfield also had close contacts with VLSI chip designers, because of his long association with AT&T Bell Laboratories. As early as 1987, Bell Labs had successfully developed neural network chips based on the Hopfield network. One of the main promises of neural networks is their suitability for parallel implementation in VLSI and optical devices. The fact that Hopfield addressed the implementation issues of his networks distinguished him from most previous neural network researchers.

Hopfield emphasized practicality, both in the implementation of his networks and in the types of problems they solved. Some of the applications that he described in his early papers include content-addressable memory (which we will discuss later in this chapter), analog-to-digital conversion [TaHo86], and optimization [HoTa85] (as in the traveling salesman problem).

In the next section we will present the Hopfield model. We will use the continuous-time model from the 1984 paper [Hopf84]. Then we will apply Lyapunov stability theory and LaSalle's Invariance Theorem to the analysis of the Hopfield model. In the final section we will demonstrate how the Hebb rule can be used to design Hopfield networks as content-addressable memories.

Hopfield Model

Hopfield Model

In keeping with his practical viewpoint, Hopfield presented his model as an electrical circuit. The basic *Hopfield model* (see [Hopf84]) is shown in Figure 18.1.

Amplifier

Inverting
Output

Resistor

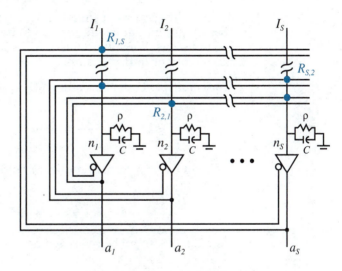

Figure 18.1 Hopfield Model

18

Each neuron is represented by an operational amplifier and its associated resistor/capacitor network. There are two sets of inputs to the neurons. The first set, represented by the currents $I_1, I_2, \ldots$, are constant external inputs. The other set consists of feedback connections from other op-amps. For instance, the second output, a_2, is fed to resistor $R_{S,2}$, which is connected, in turn, to the input of amplifier S. Resistors are, of course, only positive, but a negative input to a neuron can be obtained by selecting the inverted output of a particular amplifier. (In Figure 18.1, the inverting output of the first amplifier is connected to the input of the second amplifier through resistor $R_{2,1}$.)

The equation of operation for the Hopfield model, derived using Kirchhoff's current law, is

$$C\frac{dn_i(t)}{dt} = \sum_{j=1}^{S} T_{i,j}a_j(t) - \frac{n_i(t)}{R_i} + I_i,$$ (18.1)

where n_i is the input voltage to the ith amplifier, a_i is the output voltage of the ith amplifier, C is the amplifier input capacitance and I_i is a fixed input current to the ith amplifier. Also,

$$|T_{i,j}| = \frac{1}{R_{i,j}}, \ \frac{1}{R_i} = \frac{1}{\rho} + \sum_{j=1}^{S} \frac{1}{R_{i,j}}, \ n_i = f^{-1}(a_i) \ (\text{or } a_i = f(n_i)), \quad (18.2)$$

where $f(n)$ is the amplifier characteristic. Here and in what follows we will assume that the circuit is symmetric, so that $T_{i,j} = T_{j,i}$.

The amplifier transfer function, $a_i = f(n_i)$, is ordinarily a sigmoid function. Both this sigmoid function and its inverse are assumed to be increasing functions. We will provide a specific example of a suitable transfer function later in this chapter.

If we multiply both sides of Eq. (18.1) by R_i, we obtain

$$R_i C \frac{dn_i(t)}{dt} = \sum_{j=1}^{S} R_i T_{i,j} a_j(t) - n_i(t) + R_i I_i. \quad (18.3)$$

This can be transformed into our standard neural network notation if we define

$$\varepsilon = R_i C, \ w_{i,j} = R_i T_{i,j} \text{ and } b_i = R_i I_i. \quad (18.4)$$

Now Eq. (18.3) can be rewritten as

$$\varepsilon \frac{dn_i(t)}{dt} = -n_i(t) + \sum_{j=1}^{S} w_{i,j} a_j(t) + b_i. \quad (18.5)$$

In vector form we have

$$\varepsilon \frac{d\mathbf{n}(t)}{dt} = -\mathbf{n}(t) + \mathbf{W}\mathbf{a}(t) + \mathbf{b}. \quad (18.6)$$

and

$$\mathbf{a}(t) = \mathbf{f}(\mathbf{n}(t)). \quad (18.7)$$

The resulting Hopfield network is displayed in Figure 18.2.

Thus, Hopfield's original network of S operational amplifier circuits can be represented conveniently in our standard network notation. Note that the input vector $\mathbf{p}$ determines the initial network output. This form of the Hopfield network is used for associative memory networks, as will be discussed at the end of this chapter.

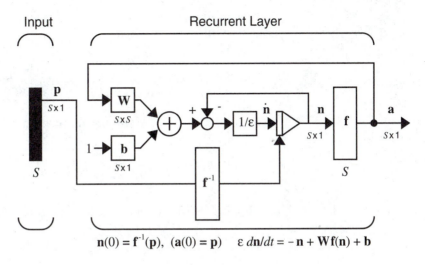

$$n(0) = f^{-1}(p), \quad (a(0) = p) \quad \varepsilon \, dn/dt = -n + Wf(n) + b$$

Figure 18.2 Hopfield Network

Lyapunov Function

The application of Lyapunov stability theory to the analysis of recurrent networks was one of the key contributions of Hopfield. (Cohen and Grossberg also used Lyapunov theory for the analysis of competitive networks at about the same time [CoGr83].) In this section we will demonstrate how LaSalle's Invariance Theorem, which was presented in Chapter 17, can be used with the Hopfield network. The first step in using LaSalle's theorem is to choose a Lyapunov function. Hopfield suggested the following function:

$$V(\mathbf{a}) \;=\; -\frac{1}{2}\mathbf{a}^T \mathbf{W} \mathbf{a} + \sum_{i=1}^{S} \left\{ \int_0^{a_i} f^{-1}(u)\, du \right\} - \mathbf{b}^T \mathbf{a}. \tag{18.8}$$

Hopfield's choice of this particular Lyapunov candidate is one of his key contributions. Notice that the first and third terms make up a quadratic function. In a later section of this chapter we will use our previous results on quadratic functions to help develop some insight into this Lyapunov function.

To use LaSalle's theorem, we will need to evaluate the derivative of $V(\mathbf{a})$. For clarity, we will consider each of the three terms of $V(\mathbf{a})$ separately. Using Eq. (8.37), the derivative of the first term is

$$\frac{d}{dt}\left\{-\frac{1}{2}\mathbf{a}^T \mathbf{W} \mathbf{a}\right\} \;=\; -\frac{1}{2}\nabla[\mathbf{a}^T \mathbf{W} \mathbf{a}]^T \frac{d\mathbf{a}}{dt} \;=\; -[\mathbf{W}\mathbf{a}]^T \frac{d\mathbf{a}}{dt} \;=\; -\mathbf{a}^T \mathbf{W} \frac{d\mathbf{a}}{dt}. \tag{18.9}$$

18

The second term in $V(\mathbf{a})$ consists of a sum of integrals. If we consider one of these integrals, we find

$$\frac{d}{dt}\left\{\int_{0}^{a_i} f^{-1}(u)\,du\right\} = \frac{d}{da_i}\left\{\int_{0}^{a_i} f^{-1}(u)\,du\right\}\frac{da_i}{dt} = f^{-1}(a_i)\frac{da_i}{dt} = n_i\frac{da_i}{dt}. \quad (18.10)$$

The total derivative of the second term in $V(\mathbf{a})$ is then

$$\frac{d}{dt}\left[\sum_{i=1}^{S}\left\{\int_{0}^{a_i} f^{-1}(u)\,du\right\}\right] = \mathbf{n}^T\frac{d\mathbf{a}}{dt}. \quad (18.11)$$

Using Eq. (8.36), we can find the derivative of the third term in $V(\mathbf{a})$.

$$\frac{d}{dt}\{-\mathbf{b}^T\mathbf{a}\} = -\nabla[\mathbf{b}^T\mathbf{a}]^T\frac{d\mathbf{a}}{dt} = -\mathbf{b}^T\frac{d\mathbf{a}}{dt} \quad (18.12)$$

Therefore, the total derivative of $V(\mathbf{a})$ is

$$\frac{d}{dt}V(\mathbf{a}) = -\mathbf{a}^T\mathbf{W}\frac{d\mathbf{a}}{dt} + \mathbf{n}^T\frac{d\mathbf{a}}{dt} - \mathbf{b}^T\frac{d\mathbf{a}}{dt} = [-\mathbf{a}^T\mathbf{W} + \mathbf{n}^T - \mathbf{b}^T]\frac{d\mathbf{a}}{dt}. \quad (18.13)$$

From Eq. (18.6) we know that

$$[-\mathbf{a}^T\mathbf{W} + \mathbf{n}^T - \mathbf{b}^T] = -\varepsilon\left[\frac{d\mathbf{n}(t)}{dt}\right]^T. \quad (18.14)$$

This allows us to rewrite Eq. (18.13) as

$$\frac{d}{dt}V(\mathbf{a}) = -\varepsilon\left[\frac{d\mathbf{n}(t)}{dt}\right]^T\frac{d\mathbf{a}}{dt} = -\varepsilon\sum_{i=1}^{S}\left(\frac{dn_i}{dt}\right)\left(\frac{da_i}{dt}\right). \quad (18.15)$$

Since $n_i = f^{-1}(a_i)$, we can expand the derivative of n_i as follows:

$$\frac{dn_i}{dt} = \frac{d}{dt}[f^{-1}(a_i)] = \frac{d}{da_i}[f^{-1}(a_i)]\frac{da_i}{dt}. \quad (18.16)$$

Now Eq. (18.15) can be rewritten

$$\frac{d}{dt}V(\mathbf{a}) = -\varepsilon\sum_{i=1}^{S}\left(\frac{dn_i}{dt}\right)\left(\frac{da_i}{dt}\right) = -\varepsilon\sum_{i=1}^{S}\left(\frac{d}{da_i}[f^{-1}(a_i)]\right)\left(\frac{da_i}{dt}\right)^2. \quad (18.17)$$

If we assume that $f^{-1}(a_i)$ is an increasing function, as it would be for an operational amplifier, then

$$\frac{d}{da_i}[f^{-1}(a_i)] > 0. \tag{18.18}$$

From Eq. (18.17), this implies that

$$\frac{d}{dt}V(\mathbf{a}) \le 0. \tag{18.19}$$

Thus, if $f^{-1}(a_i)$ is an increasing function, $dV(\mathbf{a})/dt$ is a negative semidefinite function. Therefore, $V(\mathbf{a})$ is a valid Lyapunov function.

Invariant Sets

Now we want to apply LaSalle's Invariance Theorem to determine equilibrium points for the Hopfield network. The first step is to find the set Z (Eq. (17.19)).

$$Z = \{\mathbf{a}: dV(\mathbf{a})/dt = 0, \ \mathbf{a} \text{ in the closure of } G\} \tag{18.20}$$

This set includes all points at which the derivative of the Lyapunov function is zero. For now, let's assume that G is all of $\Re^S$.

We can see from Eq. (18.17) that such derivatives will be zero if the derivatives of all of the neuron outputs are zero.

$$\frac{d\mathbf{a}}{dt} = \mathbf{0} \tag{18.21}$$

However, when the derivatives of the outputs are zero, the circuit is at equilibrium. Thus, those points where the system "energy" is not changing are also points where the circuit is at equilibrium.

This means that the set L, the largest invariant set in Z, is exactly equal to Z.

$$L = Z \tag{18.22}$$

Thus, all points in Z are potential attractors.

Some of these features will be illustrated in the following example.

Example

Consider the following example from Hopfield's original paper [Hopf84]. We will examine a system having an amplifier characteristic

$$a = f(n) = \frac{2}{\pi}\tan^{-1}\left(\frac{\gamma\pi n}{2}\right). \tag{18.23}$$

We can also write this expression as

$$n = \frac{2}{\gamma\pi}\tan\left(\frac{\pi}{2}a\right).$$ (18.24)

Assume two amplifiers, with the output of each connected to the input of the other through a unit resistor, so that

$$R_{1,2} = R_{2,1} = 1 \text{ and } T_{1,2} = T_{2,1} = 1.$$ (18.25)

Thus we have a weight matrix

$$\mathbf{W} = \begin{bmatrix} 0 & 1 \\ 1 & 0 \end{bmatrix}.$$ (18.26)

If the amplifier input capacitance is also set to 1, we have

$$\varepsilon = R_i C = 1.$$ (18.27)

Let us also take $\gamma = 1.4$ and $I_1 = I_2 = 0$. Therefore

$$\mathbf{b} = \begin{bmatrix} 0 \\ 0 \end{bmatrix}.$$ (18.28)

Recall from Eq. (18.8) that the Lyapunov function is

$$V(\mathbf{a}) = -\frac{1}{2}\mathbf{a}^T\mathbf{W}\mathbf{a} + \sum_{i=1}^{S}\left\{\int_0^{a_i} f^{-1}(u)\,du\right\} - \mathbf{b}^T\mathbf{a}.$$ (18.29)

The first term of the Lyapunov function, for this example, is

$$-\frac{1}{2}\mathbf{a}^T\mathbf{W}\mathbf{a} = -\frac{1}{2}\begin{bmatrix} a_1 & a_2 \end{bmatrix}\begin{bmatrix} 0 & 1 \\ 1 & 0 \end{bmatrix}\begin{bmatrix} a_1 \\ a_2 \end{bmatrix} = -a_1 a_2.$$ (18.30)

The third term is zero, because the biases are zero. The ith part of the second term is

$$\int_0^{a_i} f^{-1}(u)\,du = \frac{2}{\gamma\pi}\int_0^{a_i}\tan\left(\frac{\pi}{2}u\right)du = \frac{2}{\gamma\pi}\left[-\log\left[\cos\left(\frac{\pi}{2}u\right)\right]\frac{2}{\pi}\right]_0^{a_i}.$$ (18.31)

This expression can be simplified to

$$\int_0^{a_i} f^{-1}(u)\,du = -\frac{4}{\gamma\pi^2}\log\left[\cos\left(\frac{\pi}{2}a_i\right)\right].$$ (18.32)

Finally, substituting all three terms into Eq. (18.29), we have our Lyapunov function:

$$V(\mathbf{a}) = -a_1 a_2 - \frac{4}{1.4\pi^2}\left[\log\left\{\cos\left(\frac{\pi}{2}a_1\right)\right\} + \log\left\{\cos\left(\frac{\pi}{2}a_2\right)\right\}\right]. \quad (18.33)$$

Now let's write out the network equation (Eq. (18.6)). With $\varepsilon = 1$ and $\mathbf{b} = \mathbf{0}$, it is

$$\frac{d\mathbf{n}}{dt} = -\mathbf{n} + \mathbf{W}\mathbf{f}(\mathbf{n}) = -\mathbf{n} + \mathbf{W}\mathbf{a}. \quad (18.34)$$

If we substitute the weight matrix of Eq. (18.26), this expression can be written as the following pair of equations:

$$dn_1/dt = a_2 - n_1, \quad (18.35)$$

$$dn_2/dt = a_1 - n_2. \quad (18.36)$$

The neuron outputs are

$$a_1 = \frac{2}{\pi}\tan^{-1}\left(\frac{1.4\pi}{2}n_1\right), \quad (18.37)$$

$$a_2 = \frac{2}{\pi}\tan^{-1}\left(\frac{1.4\pi}{2}n_2\right). \quad (18.38)$$

Now that we have found expressions for the system Lyapunov function and the network equation of operation, let's investigate the network behavior. The Lyapunov function contour and a sample trajectory are shown in Figure 18.3.

18

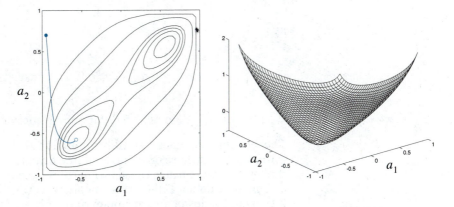

Figure 18.3 Hopfield Example Lyapunov Function and Trajectory

The contour lines in this figure represent constant values of the Lyapunov function. The system has two attractors, one in the lower left and one in the upper right of Figure 18.3. Starting from the upper left, the system converges, as shown by the blue line, to the stable point at the lower left.

Figure 18.4 displays the time response of the two neuron outputs.

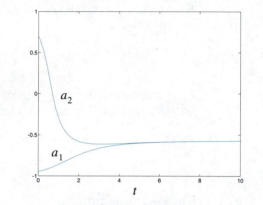

Figure 18.4 Hopfield Example Time Response

Figure 18.5 displays the time response of the Lyapunov function. As expected, it decreases continuously as the equilibrium point is approached.

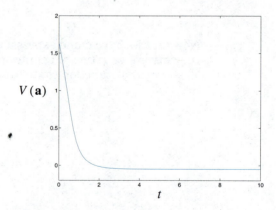

Figure 18.5 Lyapunov Function Response

The system also has an equilibrium point at the origin. If the network is initialized anywhere on a diagonal line drawn from the upper-left corner to the lower-right corner, the solution converges to the origin. Any initial conditions that do not fall on this line, however, will converge to one of the solutions in the lower-left or upper-right corner. The solution at the origin is a saddle point of the Lyapunov function, not a local minimum. We will discuss this problem in a later section. Figure 18.6 displays a trajectory that converges to the saddle point.

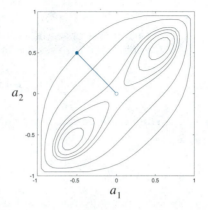

Figure 18.6 Hopfield Convergence to a Saddle Point

To experiment with the Hopfield network, use the Neural Network Design Demonstration Hopfield Network (nnd18hn).

This example has provided some insight into the Hopfield attractors. In the next section we will analyze them more carefully.

Hopfield Attractors

In the example network in the previous section we found that the Hopfield network attractors were stationary points of the Lyapunov function. Now we want to show that this is true in the general case. Recall from Eq. (18.21) that the potential attractors of the Hopfield network satisfy

$$\frac{d\mathbf{a}}{dt} = \mathbf{0}.$$ (18.39)

How are these points related to the minima of the Lyapunov function $V(\mathbf{a})$? In Chapter 8 (Eq. (8.27)) we showed that the minima of a function must be stationary points (i.e., gradient equal to zero). The stationary points of $V(\mathbf{a})$ will satisfy

$$\nabla V = \left[\frac{\partial V}{\partial a_1} \frac{\partial V}{\partial a_2} \cdots \frac{\partial V}{\partial a_S} \right]^T = \mathbf{0},$$ (18.40)

where

$$V(\mathbf{a}) = -\frac{1}{2}\mathbf{a}^T\mathbf{W}\mathbf{a} + \sum_{i=1}^{S}\left\{\int_0^{a_i} f^{-1}(u)\,du\right\} - \mathbf{b}^T\mathbf{a}. \qquad (18.41)$$

If we follow steps similar to those we used to derive Eq. (18.13), we can find the following expression for the gradient:

$$\nabla V(\mathbf{a}) = [-\mathbf{W}\mathbf{a} + \mathbf{n} - \mathbf{b}] = -\varepsilon\left[\frac{d\mathbf{n}(t)}{dt}\right]. \qquad (18.42)$$

The *i*th element of the gradient is therefore

$$\frac{\partial}{\partial a_i}V(\mathbf{a}) = -\varepsilon\frac{dn_i}{dt} = -\varepsilon\frac{d}{dt}([f^{-1}(a_i)]) = -\varepsilon\frac{d}{da_i}[f^{-1}(a_i)]\frac{da_i}{dt}. \qquad (18.43)$$

Notice, incidentally, that if $f^{-1}(a)$ is linear, Eq. (18.43) implies that

$$\frac{d\mathbf{a}}{dt} = -\alpha\nabla V(\mathbf{a}). \qquad (18.44)$$

Therefore, the response of the Hopfield network is steepest descent. Thus, if you are in a region where $f^{-1}(\mathbf{a})$ is approximately linear, the network solution approximates steepest descent.

We have assumed that the transfer function and its inverse are monotonic increasing functions. Therefore,

$$\frac{d}{da_i}[f^{-1}(a_i)] > 0. \qquad (18.45)$$

From Eq. (18.43), this implies that those points for which

$$\frac{d\mathbf{a}(t)}{dt} = \mathbf{0}, \qquad (18.46)$$

will also be points where

$$\nabla V(\mathbf{a}) = \mathbf{0}. \qquad (18.47)$$

Therefore, the attractors, which are members of the set L and satisfy Eq. (18.39), will also be stationary points of the Lyapunov function $V(\mathbf{a})$.

Effect of Gain

The Hopfield Lyapunov function can be simplified if we consider those cases where the amplifier gain γ is large. Recall that the nonlinear amplifier characteristic for our previous example was

$$a = f(n) = \frac{2}{\pi} \tan^{-1}\left(\frac{\gamma \pi n}{2}\right). \tag{18.48}$$

This function is displayed in Figure 18.7 for four different gain values.

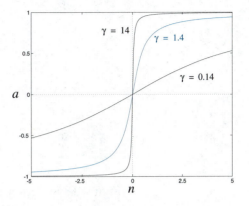

Figure 18.7 Inverse Tangent Amplifier Characteristic

The gain γ determines the steepness of the curve at $n = 0$. As γ increases, the slope of the curve at the origin increases. As γ goes to infinity, $f(n)$ approaches a signum (step) function.

Now recall from Eq. (18.8) that the general Lyapunov function is

$$V(\mathbf{a}) = -\frac{1}{2}\mathbf{a}^T\mathbf{W}\mathbf{a} + \sum_{i=1}^{S}\left\{\int_0^{a_i} f^{-1}(u)\,du\right\} - \mathbf{b}^T\mathbf{a}. \tag{18.49}$$

For our previous example,

$$f^{-1}(u) = \frac{2}{\gamma\pi}\tan\left(\frac{\pi u}{2}\right). \tag{18.50}$$

Therefore, the second term in the Lyapunov function takes the form

$$\int_0^{a_i} f^{-1}(u)\,du = \frac{2}{\gamma\pi}\left[\frac{2}{\pi}\log\left(\cos\left(\frac{\pi a_i}{2}\right)\right)\right] = -\frac{4}{\gamma\pi^2}\log\left[\cos\left(\frac{\pi a_i}{2}\right)\right]. \tag{18.51}$$

A graph of this function is shown in Figure 18.8 for three different values of the gain. Note that as γ increases the function flattens and is close to 0 most of the time. Thus, as the gain γ goes to infinity, the integral in the second term of the Lyapunov function will be close to zero in the range $-1 < a_i < 1$. This allows us to eliminate that term, and the *high-gain Lyapunov function* then reduces to

High-Gain Lyapunov Function

18

$$V(\mathbf{a}) = -\frac{1}{2}\mathbf{a}^T\mathbf{W}\mathbf{a} - \mathbf{b}^T\mathbf{a}. \tag{18.52}$$

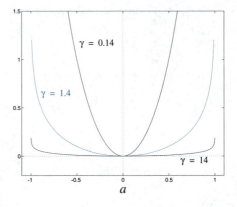

Figure 18.8 Second Term in the Lyapunov Function

By comparing Eq. (18.52) with Eq. (8.35), we can see that the high-gain Lyapunov function is, in fact, a quadratic function:

$$V(\mathbf{a}) = -\frac{1}{2}\mathbf{a}^T\mathbf{W}\mathbf{a} - \mathbf{b}^T\mathbf{a} = \frac{1}{2}\mathbf{a}^T\mathbf{A}\mathbf{a} + \mathbf{d}^T\mathbf{a} + c, \tag{18.53}$$

where

$$\nabla^2 V(\mathbf{a}) = \mathbf{A} = -\mathbf{W}, \mathbf{d} = -\mathbf{b} \text{ and } c = 0. \tag{18.54}$$

This is an important development, for now we can apply our results from Chapter 8 on quadratic functions to the understanding of the operation of Hopfield networks.

Recall that the shape of the surface of a quadratic function is determined by the eigenvalues and eigenvectors of its Hessian matrix. The Hessian matrix for our example Lyapunov function is

$$\nabla^2 V(\mathbf{a}) = -\mathbf{W} = \begin{bmatrix} 0 & -1 \\ -1 & 0 \end{bmatrix}. \tag{18.55}$$

The eigenvalues of this Hessian matrix are computed as follows:

$$\left| \nabla^2 V(\mathbf{a}) - \lambda I \right| = \begin{vmatrix} -\lambda & -1 \\ -1 & -\lambda \end{vmatrix} = \lambda^2 - 1 = (\lambda + 1)(\lambda - 1). \tag{18.56}$$

Thus, the eigenvalues are $\lambda_1 = -1$ and $\lambda_2 = 1$. It follows that the eigenvectors are

$$\mathbf{z}_1 = \begin{bmatrix} 1 \\ 1 \end{bmatrix} \text{ and } \mathbf{z}_2 = \begin{bmatrix} 1 \\ -1 \end{bmatrix}. \tag{18.57}$$

What does the surface of the high-gain Lyapunov function look like? We know, since the Hessian matrix has one positive and one negative eigenvalue, that we have a saddle point condition. The surface will have a negative curvature along the first eigenvector and a positive curvature along the second eigenvector. The surface is shown in Figure 18.9.

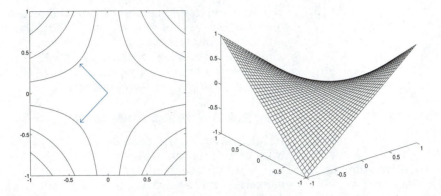

Figure 18.9 Example High Gain Lyapunov Function

The function does not have a minimum. However, the network is constrained to the hypercube $\{\mathbf{a}: -1 < a_i < 1\}$ by the amplifier transfer function. Therefore, there will be constrained minima at the two corners of the hypercube

$$\mathbf{a} = \begin{bmatrix} 1 \\ 1 \end{bmatrix} \text{ and } \mathbf{a} = \begin{bmatrix} -1 \\ -1 \end{bmatrix}. \tag{18.58}$$

When the gain is very small, there is a single minimum at the origin (see Exercise E18.1). As the gain is increased, two minima move out from the origin toward the two corners given by Eq. (18.58). Figure 18.3 displays an intermediate case, where the gain is $\gamma = 1.4$. The minima in that figure occur at

$$\mathbf{a} = \begin{bmatrix} 0.57 \\ 0.57 \end{bmatrix} \text{ and } \mathbf{a} = \begin{bmatrix} -0.57 \\ -0.57 \end{bmatrix}. \tag{18.59}$$

In the general case, where there are more than two neurons in the network, the high-gain minima will fall in certain corners of the hypercube $\{\mathbf{a}: -1 < a_i < 1\}$. We will discuss the general case in more detail in later sections, after we describe the Hopfield design process.

18

Hopfield Design

The Hopfield network does not have a learning law associated with it. It is not trained, nor does it learn on its own. Instead, a design procedure based on the Lyapunov function is used to determine the weight matrix.

Consider again the high-gain Lyapunov function

$$V(\mathbf{a}) = -\frac{1}{2}\mathbf{a}^T\mathbf{W}\mathbf{a} - \mathbf{b}^T\mathbf{a}. \tag{18.60}$$

The Hopfield design technique is to choose the weight matrix $\mathbf{W}$ and the bias vector $\mathbf{b}$ so that V takes on the form of a function that you want to minimize. Convert whatever problem you want to solve into a quadratic minimization problem. Since the Hopfield network will minimize V, it will also solve the original problem. The trick, of course, is in the conversion, which is generally not straightforward.

Content-Addressable Memory

In this section we will describe how a Hopfield network can be designed to work as an associative memory. The type of associative memory we will design is called a *content-addressable memory*, because it retrieves stored memories on the basis of part of the contents. This is in contrast to standard computer memories, where items are retrieved based on their addresses. For example, if we have a content-addressable data base that contains names, addresses and phone numbers of employees, we can retrieve a complete data entry simply by providing the employee name (or perhaps a partial name). The content-addressable memory is effectively the same as the autoassociative memory described in Chapter 7 (see page 7-10), except that in this chapter we will use the recurrent Hopfield network instead of the linear associator.

Suppose that we want to store a set of prototype patterns in a Hopfield network. When an input pattern is presented to the network, the network should produce the stored pattern that most closely resembles the input pattern. The initial network output is assigned to the input pattern. The network output should then converge to the prototype pattern closest to the input pattern. For this to happen, the prototype patterns must be minima of the Lyapunov function.

Let's assume that the prototype patterns are

$$\{\mathbf{p}_1, \mathbf{p}_2, \cdots, \mathbf{p}_Q\}. \tag{18.61}$$

Each of these vectors consists of S elements, having the values 1 or -1. Assume further that $Q \ll S$, so that the state space is large, and that the prototype patterns are well distributed in this space, and so will not be close to each other.

Content-Addressable Memory

In order for a Hopfield network to be able to recall the prototype patterns, the patterns must be minima of the Lyapunov function. Since the high-gain Lyapunov function is quadratic, we need the prototype patterns to be (constrained) minima of an appropriate quadratic function. We propose the following quadratic performance index:

$$J(\mathbf{a}) = -\frac{1}{2} \sum_{q=1}^{Q} \left([\mathbf{p}_q]^T \mathbf{a}\right)^2. \tag{18.62}$$

If the elements of the vectors $\mathbf{a}$ are restricted to be ± 1, this function is minimized at the prototype patterns, as we will now show.

Assume that the prototype patterns are orthogonal. If we evaluate the performance index at one of the prototype patterns, we find

$$J(\mathbf{p}_j) = -\frac{1}{2} \sum_{q=1}^{Q} \left([\mathbf{p}_q]^T \mathbf{p}_j\right)^2 = -\frac{1}{2}\left([\mathbf{p}_j]^T \mathbf{p}_j\right)^2 = -\frac{S}{2}. \tag{18.63}$$

The second equality follows from the orthogonality of the prototype patterns. The last equality follows because all elements of $\mathbf{p}_j$ are ± 1.

Next, evaluate the performance index at a random input pattern $\mathbf{a}$, which is presumably not close to any prototype pattern. Each element in the sum in Eq. (18.62) is an inner product between a prototype pattern and the input. The inner product will increase as the input moves closer to a prototype pattern. However, if the input is not close to any prototype pattern, then all terms of the sum in Eq. (18.62) will be small. Therefore, $J(\mathbf{a})$ will be largest (least negative) when $\mathbf{a}$ is not close to any prototype pattern, and will be smallest (most negative) when $\mathbf{a}$ is equal to any one of the prototype patterns.

We have now found a quadratic function that accurately indicates the performance of the content-addressable memory. The next step is to choose the weight matrix $\mathbf{W}$ and bias $\mathbf{b}$ so that the Hopfield Lyapunov function V will be equivalent to the quadratic performance index J.

If we use the supervised Hebb rule to compute the weight matrix (with target patterns being the same as input patterns) as

$$\mathbf{W} = \sum_{q=1}^{Q} \mathbf{p}_q (\mathbf{p}_q)^T, \tag{18.64}$$

and set the bias to zero

$$\mathbf{b} = \mathbf{0}, \tag{18.65}$$

then the Lyapunov function is

18

$$V(\mathbf{a}) = -\frac{1}{2}\mathbf{a}^T\mathbf{W}\mathbf{a} = -\frac{1}{2}\mathbf{a}^T\left[\sum_{q=1}^{Q}\mathbf{p}_q(\mathbf{p}_q)^T\right]\mathbf{a} = -\frac{1}{2}\sum_{q=1}^{Q}\mathbf{a}^T\mathbf{p}_q(\mathbf{p}_q)^T\mathbf{a}.\quad (18.66)$$

This can be rewritten

$$V(\mathbf{a}) = -\frac{1}{2}\sum_{q=1}^{Q}[(\mathbf{p}_q)^T\mathbf{a}]^2 = J(\mathbf{a}).\quad\quad (18.67)$$

Therefore, the Lyapunov function is indeed equal to the quadratic performance index for the content-addressable memory problem. The Hopfield network output will tend to converge to the stored prototype patterns (among other possible equilibrium points, as we will discuss later).

As noted in Chapter 7, the supervised Hebb rule does not work well if there is significant correlation between the prototype patterns. In that case the pseudoinverse technique has been suggested. Another design technique, which is beyond the scope of this text, is given in [LiMi89].

In the best situation, where the prototype patterns are orthogonal, every prototype pattern will be an equilibrium point of the network. However, there will be many other equilibrium points as well. The network may well converge to a pattern that is not one of the prototype patterns. A general rule is that, when using the Hebb rule, the number of stored patterns can be no more than 15% of the number of neurons.The reference [LiMi89] discusses more complex design procedures, which minimize the number of spurious equilibrium points.

In the next section we will analyze the location of the equilibrium points more closely.

Hebb Rule

Let's take a closer look at the operation of the Hopfield network when the Hebb rule is used to compute the weight matrix and the prototype patterns are orthogonal. (The following analysis follows the discussion in the Chapter 7, Problem P7.5.) The supervised Hebb rule is given by

$$\mathbf{W} = \sum_{q=1}^{Q}\mathbf{p}_q(\mathbf{p}_q)^T.\quad\quad (18.68)$$

If we apply the prototype vector $\mathbf{p}_j$ to the network, then

$$\mathbf{W}\mathbf{p}_j = \sum_{q=1}^{Q}\mathbf{p}_q(\mathbf{p}_q)^T\mathbf{p}_j = \mathbf{p}_j(\mathbf{p}_j)^T\mathbf{p}_j = S\mathbf{p}_j,\quad\quad (18.69)$$

where the second equality holds because the prototype patterns are orthogonal, and the third equality holds because each element of $\mathbf{p}_j$ is either 1 or -1. Eq. (18.69) is of the form

$$\mathbf{W}\mathbf{p}_j = \lambda\mathbf{p}_j. \tag{18.70}$$

Therefore, each prototype vector is an eigenvector of the weight matrix and they have a common eigenvalue of $\lambda = S$. The eigenspace X for the eigenvalue $\lambda = S$ is therefore

$$X = \text{span}\{\mathbf{p}_1, \mathbf{p}_2, \dots, \mathbf{p}_Q\}. \tag{18.71}$$

This space contains all vectors that can be written as linear combinations of the prototype vectors. That is, any vector $\mathbf{a}$ that is a linear combination of the prototype vectors is an eigenvector.

$$\begin{aligned}
\mathbf{W}\mathbf{a} &= \mathbf{W}\{\alpha_1\mathbf{p}_1 + \alpha_2\mathbf{p}_2 + \cdots + \alpha_Q\mathbf{p}_Q\} \\
&= \{\alpha_1\mathbf{W}\mathbf{p}_1 + \alpha_2\mathbf{W}\mathbf{p}_2 + \cdots + \alpha_Q\mathbf{W}\mathbf{p}_Q\} \\
&= \{\alpha_1 S\mathbf{p}_1 + \alpha_2 S\mathbf{p}_2 + \cdots + \alpha_Q S\mathbf{p}_Q\} \\
&= S\{\alpha_1\mathbf{p}_1 + \alpha_2\mathbf{p}_2 + \cdots + \alpha_Q\mathbf{p}_Q\} = S\mathbf{a}
\end{aligned} \tag{18.72}$$

The eigenspace for the eigenvalue $\lambda = S$ is Q-dimensional (assuming that the prototype vectors are independent).

The entire space R^S can be divided into two disjoint sets [Brog85],

$$R^S = X \cup X^\perp, \tag{18.73}$$

where $X^\perp$ is the orthogonal complement of X. (This is true for any set X, not just the one we are considering here.) Every vector in $X^\perp$ is orthogonal to every vector in X. This means that for any vector $\mathbf{a} \in X^\perp$,

$$(\mathbf{p}_q)^T\mathbf{a} = 0, \quad q = 1, 2, \dots, Q. \tag{18.74}$$

Therefore, if $\mathbf{a} \in X^\perp$,

$$\mathbf{W}\mathbf{a} = \sum_{q=1}^{Q}\mathbf{p}_q(\mathbf{p}_q)^T\mathbf{a} = \sum_{q=1}^{Q}(\mathbf{p}_q \cdot 0) = \mathbf{0} = 0 \cdot \mathbf{a}. \tag{18.75}$$

So $X^\perp$ defines an eigenspace for the repeated eigenvalue $\lambda = 0$.

18

To summarize, the weight matrix has two eigenvalues, S and 0. The eigenspace for the eigenvalue S is the space spanned by the prototype vectors. The eigenspace for the eigenvalue 0 is the orthogonal complement of the space spanned by the prototype vectors.

Since (from Eq. (18.54)) the Hessian matrix for the high-gain Lyapunov function V is

$$\nabla^2 V = -\mathbf{W}, \tag{18.76}$$

the eigenvalues for $\nabla^2 V$ will be $-S$ and 0.

The high-gain Lyapunov function is a quadratic function. Therefore, the eigenvalues of the Hessian matrix determine its shape. Because the first eigenvalue is negative, V will have negative curvature in X. Because the second eigenvalue is zero, V will have zero curvature in $X^\perp$.

What do these results say about the response of the Hopfield network? Because V has negative curvature in X, the trajectories of the Hopfield network will tend to fall into the corners of the hypercube $\{\mathbf{a}: -1 < a_i < 1\}$ that are contained in X.

Note that if we compute the weight matrix using the Hebb rule, there will be at least two minima of the Lyapunov function for each prototype vector. If $\mathbf{p}_q$ is a prototype vector, then $-\mathbf{p}_q$ will also be in the space spanned by the prototype vectors, X. Therefore, the negative of each prototype vector will be one of the corners of the hypercube $\{\mathbf{a}: -1 < a_i < 1\}$ that are contained in X. There will also be a number of other minima of the Lyapunov function that do not correspond to prototype patterns.

Spurious Patterns

The minima of V are in the corners of the hypercube $\{\mathbf{a}: -1 < a_i < 1\}$ that are contained in X. These corners will include the prototype patterns, but they will also include some linear combinations of the prototype patterns. Those minima that are not prototype patterns are often referred to as *spurious patterns*. The objective of Hopfield network design is to minimize the number of spurious patterns and to make the basins of attraction for each of the prototype patterns as large as possible. A design method that is guaranteed to minimize the number of spurious patterns is described in [LiMi89].

To illustrate these principles, consider again the second-order example we have been discussing, where the connection matrix is

$$\mathbf{W} = \begin{bmatrix} 0 & 1 \\ 1 & 0 \end{bmatrix}. \tag{18.77}$$

Suppose that this had been designed using the Hebb rule with one prototype pattern (obviously not an interesting practical case):

$$\mathbf{p}_1 = \begin{bmatrix} 1 \\ 1 \end{bmatrix}. \tag{18.78}$$

Then

$$\mathbf{W} = \mathbf{p}_1(\mathbf{p}_1)^T = \begin{bmatrix} 1 \\ 1 \end{bmatrix}\begin{bmatrix} 1 & 1 \end{bmatrix} = \begin{bmatrix} 1 & 1 \\ 1 & 1 \end{bmatrix}. \tag{18.79}$$

Notice that

$$\mathbf{W}' = \mathbf{W} - \mathbf{I} = \begin{bmatrix} 0 & 1 \\ 1 & 0 \end{bmatrix} \tag{18.80}$$

corresponds to our original connection matrix. More about this in the next section.

The high-gain Lyapunov function is

$$V(\mathbf{a}) = -\frac{1}{2}\mathbf{a}^T\mathbf{W}\mathbf{a} = -\frac{1}{2}\mathbf{a}^T\begin{bmatrix} 1 & 1 \\ 1 & 1 \end{bmatrix}\mathbf{a}. \tag{18.81}$$

The Hessian matrix for $V(\mathbf{a})$ is

$$\nabla^2 V(\mathbf{a}) = -\mathbf{W} = \begin{bmatrix} -1 & -1 \\ -1 & -1 \end{bmatrix}. \tag{18.82}$$

Its eigenvalues are

$$\lambda_1 = -S = -2 \text{, and } \lambda_2 = 0, \tag{18.83}$$

and the corresponding eigenvectors are

$$\mathbf{z}_1 = \begin{bmatrix} 1 \\ 1 \end{bmatrix} \text{ and } \mathbf{z}_2 = \begin{bmatrix} 1 \\ -1 \end{bmatrix}. \tag{18.84}$$

The first eigenvector, corresponding to the eigenvalue $-S$, represents the space spanned by the prototype vector:

$$X = \{\mathbf{a}: a_1 = a_2\}. \tag{18.85}$$

The second eigenvector, corresponding to the eigenvalue 0, represents the orthogonal complement of the first eigenvector:

18

$$X^{\perp} = \{ \mathbf{a} : a_1 = -a_2 \} .$$ (18.86)

The Lyapunov function is displayed in Figure 18.10.

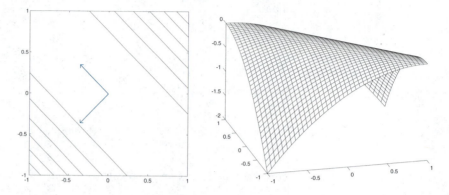

Figure 18.10 Example Lyapunov Function

This surface has a straight ridge from the upper-left to the lower-right corner. This represents the zero curvature region of $X^{\perp}$. Initial conditions to the left or to the right of the ridge will converge to the points

$$\mathbf{a} = \begin{bmatrix} 1 \\ 1 \end{bmatrix} \text{ or } \mathbf{a} = \begin{bmatrix} -1 \\ -1 \end{bmatrix} ,$$ (18.87)

respectively. Initial conditions exactly on this ridge will stabilize where they start. This situation is the same as that for our original example (see Figure 18.9), except that in that case, initial points on the sloping ridge converged to the origin, instead of remaining where they started (see Figure 18.6). Initial points to the right or to the left of the ridge, in both systems, converge to the prototype design points. Thus, the convergence of our original system, and the convergence of the system with zero diagonal elements, are identical in every important aspect. We will investigate this further in the next section.

Lyapunov Surface

In many discussions of the Hopfield network the diagonal elements of the weight matrix are set to zero. In this section we will analyze the effect of this operation on the Lyapunov surface. (See also Chapter 7, Exercise E7.5.)

For the content-addressable memory network, all of the diagonal elements of the weight matrix will be equal to Q (the number of prototype patterns), since the elements of each $\mathbf{p}_q$ are ± 1 . Therefore, we can zero the diagonal by subtracting Q times the identity matrix:

$$\mathbf{W'} = \mathbf{W} - Q\mathbf{I}. \qquad (18.88)$$

Let's investigate how this change affects the form of the Lyapunov function. If we multiply this new weight matrix times one of the prototype vectors we find

$$\mathbf{W'p}_q = [\mathbf{W} - Q\mathbf{I}]\mathbf{p}_q = S\mathbf{p}_q - Q\mathbf{p}_q = (S-Q)\mathbf{p}_q. \qquad (18.89)$$

Therefore, $(S-Q)$ is an eigenvalue of $\mathbf{W'}$, and the corresponding eigenspace is X, the space spanned by the prototype vectors.

If we multiply the new weight matrix times a vector from the orthogonal complement space, $\mathbf{a} \in X^{\perp}$, we find

$$\mathbf{W'a} = [\mathbf{W} - Q\mathbf{I}]\mathbf{a} = \mathbf{0} - Q\mathbf{a} = -Q\mathbf{a}. \qquad (18.90)$$

Therefore, $-Q$ is an eigenvalue of $\mathbf{W'}$, and the corresponding eigenspace is $X^{\perp}$.

To summarize, the eigenvectors of $\mathbf{W'}$ are the same as the eigenvectors of $\mathbf{W}$, but the eigenvalues are now $(S-Q)$ and $-Q$, instead of S and 0. Therefore, the eigenvalues of the Hessian matrix of the modified Lyapunov function, $\nabla^2 V'(\mathbf{a}) = -\mathbf{W'}$, are $-(S-Q)$ and $-Q$.

This implies that the energy surface will have negative curvature in X and positive curvature in $X^{\perp}$, in contrast with the original Lyapunov function, which had negative curvature in X and zero curvature in $X^{\perp}$.

A comparison of Figure 18.9 and Figure 18.10 demonstrates the effect on the Lyapunov function of setting the diagonal elements of the weight matrix to zero. In terms of system performance, the change has little effect. If the initial condition of the Hopfield network falls anywhere off of the line $a_1 = -a_2$, then, in either case, the output of the network will converge to one of the corners of the hypercube $\{\mathbf{a}: -1 < a_i < 1\}$, which consists of the two points $\mathbf{a} = \begin{bmatrix} 1 & 1 \end{bmatrix}^T$ and $\mathbf{a} = \begin{bmatrix} -1 & -1 \end{bmatrix}^T$.

If the initial condition falls exactly on the line $a_1 = -a_2$, and the weight matrix $\mathbf{W}$ is used, then the network output will remain constant. If the initial condition falls exactly on the line $a_1 = -a_2$, and the weight matrix $\mathbf{W'}$ is used, then the network output will converge to the saddle point at the origin (as in Figure 18.6). Neither of these results is desirable, since the network output does not converge to a minimum of the Lyapunov function. Of course, the only case in which the network converges to a saddle point is when the initial condition falls exactly on the line $a_1 = -a_2$, which would be highly unlikely in practice.

18

Summary of Results

Hopfield Model

$$\varepsilon \frac{d\mathbf{n}(t)}{dt} = -\mathbf{n}(t) + \mathbf{W}\mathbf{a}(t) + \mathbf{b}$$

$$\mathbf{a}(t) = \mathbf{f}(\mathbf{n}(t))$$

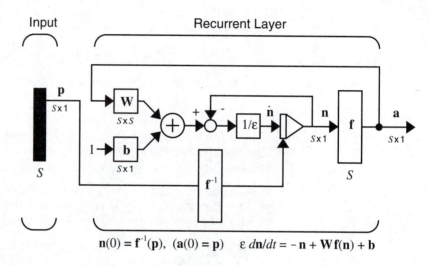

$$\mathbf{n}(0) = \mathbf{f}^{-1}(\mathbf{p}), \quad (\mathbf{a}(0) = \mathbf{p}) \qquad \varepsilon \, d\mathbf{n}/dt = -\mathbf{n} + \mathbf{W}\mathbf{f}(\mathbf{n}) + \mathbf{b}$$

Lyapunov Function

$$V(\mathbf{a}) = -\frac{1}{2}\mathbf{a}^T\mathbf{W}\mathbf{a} + \sum_{i=1}^{S}\left\{\int_0^{a_i} f^{-1}(u)\,du\right\} - \mathbf{b}^T\mathbf{a}$$

$$\frac{d}{dt}V(\mathbf{a}) = -\varepsilon \sum_{i=1}^{S}\left(\frac{d}{da_i}[f^{-1}(a_i)]\right)\left(\frac{da_i}{dt}\right)^2$$

$$\text{If } \frac{d}{da_i}[f^{-1}(a_i)] > 0, \text{ then } \frac{d}{dt}V(\mathbf{a}) \le 0.$$

Invariant Sets

The Invariant Set Consists of the Equilibrium Points.

$$L = Z = \{\mathbf{a}:d\mathbf{a}/dt = \mathbf{0}, \ \mathbf{a} \text{ in the closure of } G\}$$

Hopfield Attractors

The Equilibrium Points Are Stationary Points.

$$\text{If } \frac{d\mathbf{a}(t)}{dt} = \mathbf{0}, \text{ then } \nabla V(\mathbf{a}) = \mathbf{0}.$$

$$\nabla V(\mathbf{a}) = [-\mathbf{W}\mathbf{a} + \mathbf{n} - \mathbf{b}] = -\varepsilon\left[\frac{d\mathbf{n}(t)}{dt}\right]$$

High-Gain Lyapunov Function

$$V(\mathbf{a}) = -\frac{1}{2}\mathbf{a}^T\mathbf{W}\mathbf{a} - \mathbf{b}^T\mathbf{a}$$

$$\nabla^2 V(\mathbf{a}) = -\mathbf{W}$$

Content-Addressable Memory

$$\mathbf{W} = \sum_{q=1}^{Q} \mathbf{p}_q (\mathbf{p}_q)^T \text{ and } \mathbf{b} = \mathbf{0}$$

Energy Surface (Orthogonal Prototype Patterns)

Eigenvalues/Eigenvectors of $\nabla^2 V(\mathbf{a}) = -\mathbf{W}$ Are

$$\lambda_1 = -S, \text{ with eigenspace } X = \text{span}\{\mathbf{p}_1, \mathbf{p}_2, \dots, \mathbf{p}_Q\}.$$

$$\lambda_2 = 0, \text{ with eigenspace } X^{\perp}.$$

$X^{\perp}$ is defined such that for any vector $\mathbf{a} \in X^{\perp}$, $(\mathbf{p}_q)^T\mathbf{a} = 0$, $q = 1, 2, \dots, Q$

Trajectories (Orthogonal Prototype Patterns)

Because the first eigenvalue is negative, $V(\mathbf{a})$ will have negative curvature in X. Because the second eigenvalue is zero, $V(\mathbf{a})$ will have zero curvature in $X^{\perp}$. Because $V(\mathbf{a})$ has negative curvature in X, the trajectories of the Hopfield network will tend to fall into the corners of the hypercube $\{\mathbf{a}: -1 < a_i < 1\}$ that are contained in X.

18

Solved Problems

P18.1 **Assume the binary prototype vectors**

$$\mathbf{p}_1 = \begin{bmatrix} 1 \\ 1 \\ -1 \\ -1 \end{bmatrix}, \qquad \mathbf{p}_2 = \begin{bmatrix} 1 \\ -1 \\ 1 \\ -1 \end{bmatrix}.$$

   i. **Design a continuous-time Hopfield network (specify connection weights) to recognize these patterns, using the Hebb rule.**

   ii. **Find the Hessian matrix of the high-gain Lyapunov function for this network. What are the eigenvalues and eigenvectors of the Hessian matrix?**

   iii. **Assuming large gain, what are the stable equilibrium points for this Hopfield network?**

i. First calculate the weight matrix from the reference vectors, using the supervised Hebb rule.

$$\mathbf{W} = \mathbf{p}_1(\mathbf{p}_1)^T + \mathbf{p}_2(\mathbf{p}_2)^T = \begin{bmatrix} 1 & 1 & -1 & -1 \\ 1 & 1 & -1 & -1 \\ -1 & -1 & 1 & 1 \\ -1 & -1 & 1 & 1 \end{bmatrix} + \begin{bmatrix} 1 & -1 & 1 & -1 \\ -1 & 1 & -1 & 1 \\ 1 & -1 & 1 & -1 \\ -1 & 1 & -1 & 1 \end{bmatrix},$$

which simplifies to

$$\mathbf{W} = \begin{bmatrix} 2 & 0 & 0 & 2 \\ 0 & 2 & -2 & 0 \\ 0 & -2 & 2 & 0 \\ -2 & 0 & 0 & 2 \end{bmatrix}.$$

ii. The Hessian of the high-gain Lyapunov function, from Eq. (18.54), is the negative of the weight matrix:

$$\nabla^2 V(\mathbf{a}) = \begin{bmatrix} -2 & 0 & 0 & -2 \\ 0 & -2 & 2 & 0 \\ 0 & 2 & -2 & 0 \\ 2 & 0 & 0 & -2 \end{bmatrix}.$$

The prototype patterns are orthogonal ($[\mathbf{p}_1]^T\mathbf{p}_2 = 0$). Thus, the eigenvalues are $\lambda_1 = -S = -4$ and $\lambda_2 = 0$. The eigenspace for $\lambda_1 = -4$ is

$$X = \text{span}\{\mathbf{p}_1, \mathbf{p}_2\}.$$

The eigenspace for $\lambda_2 = 0$ is the orthogonal complement of X:

$$X^\perp = \text{span}\left\{ \begin{bmatrix} 1 \\ 1 \\ 1 \\ 1 \end{bmatrix}, \begin{bmatrix} 1 \\ -1 \\ -1 \\ 1 \end{bmatrix} \right\},$$

where we have chosen two vectors that are orthogonal to both $\mathbf{p}_1$ and $\mathbf{p}_2$.

iii. The stable points will be $\mathbf{p}_1, \mathbf{p}_2, -\mathbf{p}_1, -\mathbf{p}_2$ since the negative of the prototype patterns will also be equilibrium points. There may be other equilibrium points, if other corners of the hypercube lie in the span $\{\mathbf{p}_1, \mathbf{p}_2\}$. There are a total of $2^4 = 16$ corners of the hypercube. Four will fall in X and four will fall in $X^\perp$. The other corners are partly in X and partly in X^T.

P18.2 **Consider a high-gain Hopfield network with a weight matrix and bias given by**

$$\mathbf{W} = \begin{bmatrix} -1 & -1 \\ -1 & -1 \end{bmatrix} \quad \text{and} \quad \mathbf{b} = \begin{bmatrix} 1 \\ -1 \end{bmatrix}.$$

18

    i. **Sketch a contour plot of the high-gain Lyapunov function for this network.**

    ii. **If the network is given the initial condition $\begin{bmatrix} 1 & 1 \end{bmatrix}^T$, where will the network converge?**

i.   First consider the high-gain Lyapunov function

$$V(\mathbf{a}) = -\frac{1}{2}\mathbf{a}^T\mathbf{W}\mathbf{a} - \mathbf{b}^T\mathbf{a}.$$

The Hessian matrix is

$$\nabla^2 V(\mathbf{a}) = -\mathbf{W} = \begin{bmatrix} 1 & 1 \\ 1 & 1 \end{bmatrix}.$$

Next, we need to compute the eigenvalues and eigenvectors:

$$|\nabla^2 V(\mathbf{a}) - \lambda \mathbf{I}| = \left| \begin{bmatrix} 1-\lambda & 1 \\ 1 & 1-\lambda \end{bmatrix} \right| = \lambda^2 - 2\lambda + 1 - 1 = \lambda(\lambda-2).$$

The eigenvalues are $\lambda_1 = 0$ and $\lambda_2 = 2$.

Now we can find the eigenvectors. For $\lambda_1 = 0$,

$$[\nabla^2 V(\mathbf{a}) - \lambda_1 \mathbf{I}] \mathbf{z}_1 = \mathbf{0},$$

and therefore

$$\begin{bmatrix} 1 & 1 \\ 1 & 1 \end{bmatrix} \mathbf{z}_1 = \mathbf{0} \text{ or } \mathbf{z}_1 = \begin{bmatrix} 1 \\ -1 \end{bmatrix}.$$

Similarly, for $\lambda_2 = 2$,

$$[\nabla^2 V(\mathbf{a}) - \lambda_2 \mathbf{I}] \mathbf{z}_2 = \mathbf{0}$$

and therefore

$$\begin{bmatrix} -1 & 1 \\ 1 & -1 \end{bmatrix} \mathbf{z}_2 = \mathbf{0} \text{ or } \mathbf{z}_2 = \begin{bmatrix} 1 \\ 1 \end{bmatrix}.$$

So the term

$$-\frac{1}{2}\mathbf{a}^T \mathbf{W} \mathbf{a}$$

has zero curvature in the direction $\mathbf{z}_1$ and positive curvature in the direction $\mathbf{z}_2$.

Now we have to account for the linear term. First plot the contour without the linear term, as in Figure P18.1.

The linear term will cause a negative slope in the direction of

$$\mathbf{b} = \begin{bmatrix} 1 \\ -1 \end{bmatrix}.$$

Therefore everything will curve down toward $\begin{bmatrix} 1 & -1 \end{bmatrix}^T$, as is shown in Figure P18.2.

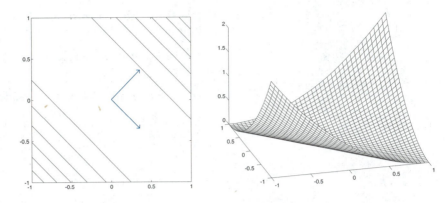

Figure P18.1 Contour Without Linear Term

ii. All trajectories will converge to $\begin{bmatrix} 1 & -1 \end{bmatrix}^T$, regardless of the initial conditions. As we can see in Figure P18.2, the energy function has only one minimum, which is located at $\begin{bmatrix} 1 & -1 \end{bmatrix}^T$. (Keep in mind that the output of the network is constrained to fall within the hypercube $\{ \mathbf{a} : -1 < a_i < 1 \}$.)

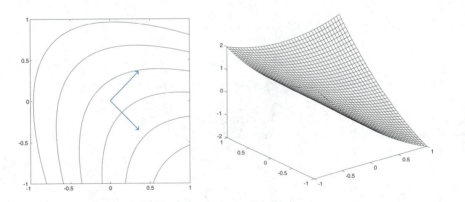

Figure P18.2 Contour Including Linear Term

P18.3 **Consider the following prototype vectors.**

$$\mathbf{p}_1 = \begin{bmatrix} 1 \\ 1 \end{bmatrix} \qquad \mathbf{p}_2 = \begin{bmatrix} -1 \\ 1 \end{bmatrix}$$

 i. **Design a Hopfield network to recognize these patterns.**

 ii. **Find the Hessian matrix of the high-gain Lyapunov function for this network. What are the eigenvalues and eigenvectors of the Hessian matrix?**

      iii. What are the stable points for this Hopfield network (assume large gain)? What are the basins of attraction?

      iv. How well does this network perform the pattern recognition problem?

i. We will use the Hebb rule to find the weight matrix.

$$\mathbf{W} = \mathbf{p}_1 (\mathbf{p}_1)^T + \mathbf{p}_2 (\mathbf{p}_2)^T = \begin{bmatrix} 1 & 1 \\ 1 & 1 \end{bmatrix} + \begin{bmatrix} 1 & -1 \\ -1 & 1 \end{bmatrix} = \begin{bmatrix} 2 & 0 \\ 0 & 2 \end{bmatrix}$$

The bias is set to zero.

$$\mathbf{b} = \begin{bmatrix} 0 \\ 0 \end{bmatrix}$$

ii. The Hessian matrix of the high-gain Lyapunov function is the negative of the weight matrix.

$$\nabla^2 V (\mathbf{a}) = -\mathbf{W} = \begin{bmatrix} -2 & 0 \\ 0 & -2 \end{bmatrix}$$

By inspection, we can see that there is a repeated eigenvalue.

$$\lambda_1 = \lambda_2 = -S = -2$$

The eigenvectors will then be

$$\mathbf{z}_1 = \begin{bmatrix} 1 \\ 0 \end{bmatrix} \text{ and } \mathbf{z}_2 = \begin{bmatrix} 0 \\ 1 \end{bmatrix},$$

or any linear combination. (The entire $\Re^2$ is the eigenspace for the eigenvalue $\lambda = -2$.)

iii. From Chapter 8 we know that when the eigenvalues of the Hessian are equal, the contours will be circular. Because the eigenvalues are negative, the function will have a single maximum at the origin. There will be four minima at the four corners of the hypercube $\{\mathbf{a}: -1 < a_i < 1\}$. There are also four saddle points. The high-gain Lyapunov function is displayed in Figure P18.3.

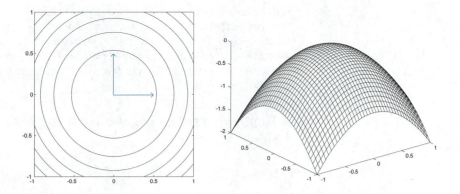

Figure P18.3 High-Gain Lyapunov Function for Problem P18.3

There are a total of nine stationary points. We could use the corollary to La-Salle's Invariance Theorem to show that the maximum point at the origin has a basin of attraction that only includes the origin itself. Therefore it is not a stable equilibrium point. The saddle points have regions of attraction that are lines. (For example, the saddle point at $\begin{bmatrix} -1 & 0 \end{bmatrix}^T$ has a region of attraction along the negative a_1 axis.) The four corners of the hypercube are the only attractors that have two-dimensional regions of attraction. The region of attraction for each corner is the corresponding quadrant of the hypercube. Figure P18.4 shows the low-gain Lyapunov function (with gain $\gamma = 1.4$) and illustrates convergence to a saddle point and to a minimum.

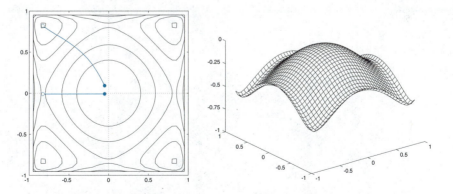

Figure P18.4 Lyapunov Function for Problem P18.3

iv. The network does not do a good job on the pattern recognition problem. Not only does it recognize the two prototype patterns, but it also "recognizes" the other two corners of the hypercube as well. The network will converge to whichever corner is closest to the input pattern, even though we only wanted it to store the two prototype patterns. Since every possible two-bit pattern has been stored, the network is not very useful. This is not unexpected, since the number of patterns that the Hebb rule is expected to store is only 15% of the number of neurons. Since we only have two neurons, we can't expect to successfully store many patterns. Try Exercise E18.2 for a better network.

P18.4 **A Hopfield network has the following high-gain Lyapunov function:**

$$V(\mathbf{a}) = -\frac{1}{2}(7(a_1)^2 + 12a_1a_2 - 2(a_2)^2).$$

   i. Find the weight matrix.

   ii. Find the gradient vector of the Lyapunov function.

   iii. Find the Hessian matrix of the Lyapunov function.

   iv. Sketch a contour plot of the Lyapunov function.

   v. Sketch the path that a steepest descent algorithm would follow for $V(\mathbf{a})$ with an initial condition of $\begin{bmatrix} 0.25 & 0.25 \end{bmatrix}^T$.

i. $V(\mathbf{a})$ is a quadratic function, which can be rewritten as

$$V(\mathbf{a}) = -\frac{1}{2}(7(a_1)^2 + 12a_1a_2 - 2(a_2)^2) = -\frac{1}{2}\mathbf{a}^T\begin{bmatrix} 7 & 6 \\ 6 & -2 \end{bmatrix}\mathbf{a}.$$

Therefore the weight matrix is

$$\mathbf{W} = \begin{bmatrix} 7 & 6 \\ 6 & -2 \end{bmatrix}.$$

ii. Since $V(\mathbf{a})$ is a quadratic function, we can use Eq. (8.38) to find the gradient.

$$\nabla V(\mathbf{a}) = -\frac{1}{2}\begin{bmatrix} 7 & 6 \\ 6 & -2 \end{bmatrix}\mathbf{a}$$

iii. From Eq. (8.39), the Hessian is

$$\nabla^2 V(\mathbf{a}) = -\begin{bmatrix} 7 & 6 \\ 6 & -2 \end{bmatrix} = \begin{bmatrix} -7 & -6 \\ -6 & 2 \end{bmatrix}.$$

iv. To compute the eigenvalues,

$$\left| \nabla^2 V(\mathbf{a}) - \lambda \mathbf{I} \right| = \left| \begin{bmatrix} -7-\lambda & -6 \\ -6 & 2-\lambda \end{bmatrix} \right| = \lambda^2 + 5\lambda - 50 = (\lambda + 10)(\lambda - 5).$$

The eigenvalues are $\lambda_1 = -10$ and $\lambda_2 = 5$.

Now we can find the eigenvectors. For $\lambda_1 = -10$,

$$[\nabla^2 V(\mathbf{a}) - \lambda_1 \mathbf{I}] \mathbf{z}_1 = \mathbf{0},$$

and therefore

$$\begin{bmatrix} 3 & -6 \\ -6 & 12 \end{bmatrix} \mathbf{z}_1 = \mathbf{0} \text{ or } \mathbf{z}_1 = \begin{bmatrix} 2 \\ 1 \end{bmatrix}.$$

Similarly, for $\lambda_2 = 5$,

$$[\nabla^2 V(\mathbf{a}) - \lambda_2 \mathbf{I}] \mathbf{z}_2 = \mathbf{0}$$

and therefore

$$\begin{bmatrix} -12 & -6 \\ -6 & -3 \end{bmatrix} \mathbf{z}_2 = \mathbf{0} \text{ or } \mathbf{z}_2 = \begin{bmatrix} 1 \\ -2 \end{bmatrix}.$$

Note that this is a saddle point case, since $\lambda_1 < 0 < \lambda_2$. There will be negative curvature along $\mathbf{z}_1$ and positive curvature along $\mathbf{z}_2$. The contour plot of the high-gain Lyapunov function is shown in Figure P18.5.

18

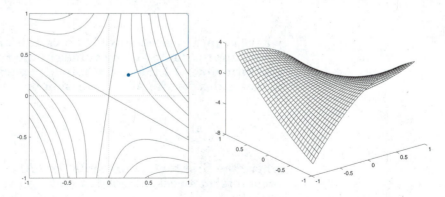

Figure P18.5 High-Gain Lyapunov Func. & Steepest Descent Trajectory

v. The steepest descent path will follow the negative of the gradient and will be perpendicular to the contour lines, as we saw in Chapter 9. When the trajectory hits the edge of the hypercube, it follows the edge down to the minimum point. The resulting trajectory is shown in Figure P18.5.

The high-gain Lyapunov function is only an approximation, since it assumes infinite gain. As a comparison, Figure P18.6 illustrates the Lyapunov function, and the Hopfield trajectory, for a gain of 0.5.

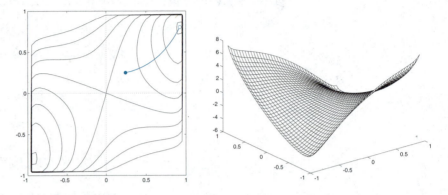

Figure P18.6 Lyapunov Function & Hopfield Trajectory

P18.5 **The Hopfield network has been used for applications other than content-addressable memory. One of these other applications is analog-to-digital (A/D) conversion [HoTa86]. The function of the A/D converter is to take an analog signal y, and convert it into a series of bits (zeros and ones). For example, a two-bit A/D converter would try to approximate the signal y as follows:**

$$y \cong \sum_{i=1}^{2} a_i 2^{(i-1)} = a_1 + a_2 2,$$

where a_1 and a_2 are allowed values of 0 or 1. (This A/D converter would approximate analog values in the range from 0 to 3, with a resolution of 1.) Tank and Hopfield suggest the following performance index for the A/D conversion process:

$$J(\mathbf{a}) = \frac{1}{2}\left(y - \sum_{i=1}^{2} a_i 2^{(i-1)}\right)^2 - \frac{1}{2}\left(\sum_{i=1}^{2} 2^{2(i-1)} a_i (a_i - 1)\right),$$

where the first term represents the A/D conversion error, and the second term forces a_1 and a_2 to take on values of 0 or 1.

Show that this performance index can be written as the Lyapunov function of a Hopfield network and define the appropriate weight matrix and bias vector.

The first step is to expand the terms of the performance index.

$$\left(y - \sum_{i=1}^{2} a_i 2^{(i-1)}\right)^2 = y^2 - 2y \sum_{i=1}^{2} a_i 2^{(i-1)} + \sum_{j=1}^{2}\sum_{i=1}^{2} a_i a_j 2^{(i-1)+(i-1)},$$

$$\left(\sum_{i=1}^{2} 2^{2(i-1)} a_i (a_i - 1)\right) = \sum_{i=1}^{2} (a_i)^2 2^{2(i-1)} - \sum_{i=1}^{2} a_i 2^{2(i-1)}$$

If we substitute these terms back into the performance index we find

$$J(\mathbf{a}) = \frac{1}{2}\left(y^2 + \sum_{\substack{j=1 \\ i \neq j}}^{2}\sum_{i=1}^{2} a_i a_j 2^{(i-1)+(i-1)} + \sum_{i=1}^{2} a_i (2^{2(i-1)} - 2^i y)\right).$$

The first term is not a function of $\mathbf{a}$. Therefore, it does not affect where the minima will occur, and we can ignore it.

We now want to show that this performance index takes the form of a high-gain Lyapunov function:

$$V(\mathbf{a}) = -\frac{1}{2}\mathbf{a}^T \mathbf{W}\mathbf{a} - \mathbf{b}^T \mathbf{a}.$$

This will be the case if

$$\mathbf{W} = \begin{bmatrix} 0 & -2 \\ -2 & 0 \end{bmatrix} \text{ and } \mathbf{b} = \begin{bmatrix} y - \frac{1}{2} \\ 2y - 2 \end{bmatrix}.$$

In this Hopfield network, unlike the content-addressable memory, the input to the network is the scalar y, which is then used to compute the bias vector. In the content-addressable memory, the inputs to the network were vector patterns, which became the initial conditions on the network outputs.

Note that in this network the transfer function must limit the output to the range $0 < a < 1$. One transfer function that could be used is

$$f(n) = \frac{1}{(1 - e^{-\gamma n})}.$$

18

Epilogue

In this chapter we have introduced the Hopfield model, one of the most influential neural network architectures. One of the reasons that Hopfield was so influential was that he emphasized the practical considerations of the network. He described how the network could be implemented as an electrical circuit, and VLSI implementations of Hopfield-type networks were built at an early stage.

Hopfield also explained how the network could be used to solve practical problems in pattern recognition and optimization. Some of the applications that Hopfield proposed for his networks were: content-addressable memory [Hopf82], A/D conversion [TaHo86] and linear programming and optimization tasks, such as the traveling salesman problem [HoTa85].

One of Hopfield's key contributions was the application of Lyapunov stability theory to the analysis of his recurrent networks. He also showed that, for high-gain amplifiers, the Lyapunov function for his network was a quadratic function, which was minimized by the network. This led to several design procedures. The idea behind the development of the design techniques was to convert a given task into a quadratic minimization problem, which the network could then solve.

The Hopfield network is the last topic we will cover in any detail in this text. However, we have certainly not exhausted all of the important neural network architectures. In the next chapter we will give you some ideas about where to go next to explore the subject further.

Further Reading

[Ande72]   J. Anderson, "A simple neural network generating an inter-active memory," *Mathematical Biosciences*, vol. 14, pp. 197–220, 1972.

Anderson proposed a "linear associator" model for associative memory. The model was trained, using a generalization of the Hebb postulate, to learn an association between input and output vectors. The physiological plausibility of the network was emphasized. Kohonen published a closely related paper at the same time [Koho72], although the two researchers were working independently.

[AnSi77]   J. A. Anderson, J. W. Silverstein, S. A. Ritz and R. S. Jones, "Distinctive features, categorical perception, and probability learning: Some applications of a neural model," *Psychological Review*, vol. 84, pp. 413–451, 1977.

This article describes the brain-state-in-a-box neural network model. It combines the linear associator network with recurrent connections to form a more powerful autoassociative system. It uses a nonlinear transfer function to contain the network output within a hypercube.

[CoGr83]   M. A. Cohen and S. Grossberg, "Absolute stability of global pattern formation and parallel memory storage by competitive neural networks," *IEEE Transactions on Systems, Man and Cybernetics*, vol. 13, no. 5, pp. 815–826, 1983.

Cohen and Grossberg apply LaSalle's Invariance Theorem to the analysis of the stability of competitive neural networks. The network description is very general, and the authors show how their analysis can be applied to many different types of recurrent neural networks.

[Gros67]   S. Grossberg, "Nonlinear difference-differential equations in prediction and learning theory," *Proceedings of the National Academy of Sciences*, vol. 58, pp. 1329–1334, 1967.

This early work of Grossberg's discusses the storage of information in dynamically stable configurations.

18

[Hopf82]   J. J. Hopfield, "Neural networks and physical systems with emergent collective computational properties," *Proceedings of the National Academy of Sciences*, vol. 79, pp. 2554–2558, 1982.

This is the original Hopfield neural network paper, which signaled the resurgence of the field of neural networks. It describes a discrete-time network that behaves as a content-addressable memory. Hopfield demonstrates that the network evolves so as to minimize a specific Lyapunov function.

[Hopf84]   J. J. Hopfield, "Neurons with graded response have collective computational properties like those of two-state neurons," *Proceedings of the National Academy of Sciences*, vol. 81, pp. 3088–3092, 1984.

Hopfield demonstrates how an analog electrical circuit can function as a model for a large network of neurons with a graded response. The Lyapunov function for this network is derived and is used to design a network for use as a content-addressable memory.

[HoTa85]   J. J. Hopfield and D. W. Tank, " 'Neural' computation of decisions in optimization problems," *Biological Cybernetics*, vol. 52, pp. 141–154, 1985.

This article describes the application of Hopfield networks to the solution of optimization problems. The traveling salesman problem, in which the length of a trip through a number of cities with only one visit to each city is minimized, is mapped onto a Hopfield network.

[Koho72]   T. Kohonen, "Correlation matrix memories," *IEEE Transactions on Computers*, vol. 21, pp. 353–359, 1972.

Kohonen proposed a correlation matrix model for associative memory. The model was trained, using the outer product rule (also known as the Hebb rule), to learn an association between input and output vectors. The mathematical structure of the network was emphasized. Anderson published a closely related paper at the same time [Ande72], although the two researchers were working independently.

[LiMi89]   J. Li, A. N. Michel and W. Porod, "Analysis and synthesis of a class of neural networks: Linear systems operating on a closed hypercube," *IEEE Transactions on Circuits and Systems*, vol. 36, no. 11, pp. 1405–1422, November 1989.

This article investigates a class of neural networks described by first-order linear differential equations defined on a closed hypercube (Hopfield-like networks). Wanted and unwanted equilibrium points fall at the corners of the cube. The authors discuss design procedures that minimize the number of spurious equilibrium points.

[McPi43]   W. McCulloch and W. Pitts, "A logical calculus of the ideas immanent in nervous activity," *Bulletin of Mathematical Biophysics.*, vol. 5, pp. 115–133, 1943.

This article introduces the first mathematical model of a neuron in which a weighted sum of input signals is compared to a threshold to determine whether or not the neuron fires.

[TaHo86]   D. W. Tank and J. J. Hopfield, "Simple 'neural' optimization networks: An A/D converter, signal decision circuit and a linear programming circuit," *IEEE Transactions on Circuits and Systems*, vol. 33, no. 5, pp. 533–541, 1986.

The authors describe how Hopfield neural networks can be designed to solve certain optimization problems. In one example the Hopfield network implements an analog-to-digital conversion.

18

Exercises

E18.1 In the Hopfield network example starting on page 18-7 we used a gain of $\gamma = 1.4$. Figure 18.3 displays the Lyapunov function for that example. The high-gain Lyapunov function for the example is shown in Figure 18.9.

    i. Show that the minima of the Lyapunov function for this example will be located at points where $n_1 = n_2 = f(n_1) = f(n_2)$. (Use Eq. (18.42) and set the gradient of $V(\mathbf{a})$ to zero.)

    ii. Investigate the change in location of the minima as the gain is varied from $\gamma = 0.1$ to $\gamma = 10$.

    iii. Sketch the contour plot for several different values of gain in this interval. You will probably need to use MATLAB for this.

E18.2 In Problem P18.3 we used the supervised Hebb rule to design a Hopfield network to recognize the following patterns:

$$\mathbf{p}_1 = \begin{bmatrix} 1 \\ 1 \end{bmatrix} \quad \mathbf{p}_2 = \begin{bmatrix} -1 \\ 1 \end{bmatrix}.$$

If we use another design rule [LiMi89], we find the following weight matrix and bias

$$\mathbf{W} = \begin{bmatrix} 1 & 0 \\ 0 & -10 \end{bmatrix} \quad \mathbf{b} = \begin{bmatrix} 0 \\ 11 \end{bmatrix}.$$

    i. Graph the contour plot for the high-gain Lyapunov function, if this weight matrix and bias are used.

    ii. Discuss the difference between the performance of this Hopfield network and the one designed in Problem P18.3.

    iii. Write a MATLAB M-file to simulate the Hopfield network. Use the **ode45** routine. Plot the responses of this network for several initial conditions.

E18.3 A Hopfield network has the following high-gain Lyapunov function:

$$V(\mathbf{a}) = -\frac{1}{2}((a_1)^2 + 2a_1 a_2 + 4(a_2)^2 + 6a_1 + 10a_2).$$

    i. Find the weight matrix and bias vector for this network.

    ii. Find the gradient and Hessian for $V(\mathbf{a})$.

    iii. Sketch a contour plot of $V(\mathbf{a})$.

    iv. Find the stationary point(s) for $V(\mathbf{a})$. Use the corollary to LaSalle's Invariance Theorem to find as much information as you can about basins of attraction for any stable equilibrium points.

E18.4 In Problem P18.5 we demonstrated how a Hopfield network could be designed to operate as an A/D converter.

    i. Sketch the contour plot of the high-gain Lyapunov function for the two-bit A/D converter network using an input value of $y = 0.5$. Locate the minimum points.

    ii. Repeat part (i) for an input value of $y = 2.5$.

    iii. Use the answers to parts (i) and (ii) to explain how the network will operate. Will the network perform the A/D conversion correctly?

E18.5 Assume the binary prototype vectors

$$\mathbf{p}_1 = \begin{bmatrix} -1 \\ 1 \\ 1 \\ -1 \end{bmatrix}, \qquad \mathbf{p}_2 = \begin{bmatrix} 1 \\ -1 \\ 1 \\ -1 \end{bmatrix}.$$

    i. Design a continuous-time Hopfield network (specify connection weights and biases only) to recognize these patterns, using the Hebb rule.

    ii. Find the Hessian matrix of the high-gain Lyapunov function for this network. What are the eigenvalues and eigenvectors of the Hessian matrix?

    iii. Assuming large gain, what are the stable equilibrium points for this Hopfield network?

18

E18.6 In Exercise E7.7 we asked the question: How many prototype patterns can be stored in one weight matrix? Repeat that problem using the Hopfield network. Begin with the digits "0" and "1". (The digits are shown at the end of this problem.) Add one digit at a time up to "6", and test how often the correct digit is reconstructed after randomly changing 2, 4 and 6 pixels.

    i. First use the Hebb rule to create the weight matrix for the digits "0" and "1". Then randomly change 2 pixels of each digit and apply the noisy digits to the network. Repeat this process 10 times, and record the percentage of times in which the correct pattern (without noise) is produced at the output of the network. Repeat as 4 and 6 pixels of each digit are modified. The entire process is then repeated when the digits "0", "1" and "2" are used. This continues, one digit at a time, until you test the network when all of the digits "0" through "6" are used. When you have completed all of the tests, you will be able to plot three curves showing percentage error versus number of digits stored, one curve each for 2, 4 and 6 pixel errors.

ii. Repeat part (i) using the pseudoinverse rule (see Chapter 7), and compare the results of the two rules.

iii. For extra credit, repeat part (i) using the method described in [LiMi89]. In that paper it is called Synthesis Procedure 5.1.

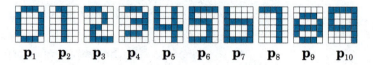

$\mathbf{p}_1$ $\quad$ $\mathbf{p}_2$ $\quad$ $\mathbf{p}_3$ $\quad$ $\mathbf{p}_4$ $\quad$ $\mathbf{p}_5$ $\quad$ $\mathbf{p}_6$ $\quad$ $\mathbf{p}_7$ $\quad$ $\mathbf{p}_8$ $\quad$ $\mathbf{p}_9$ $\quad$ $\mathbf{p}_{10}$

19 Epilogue

Objectives

We have discussed many of the key neural network architectures and learning rules and have explained how they can be used to design networks for applications in pattern recognition, function approximation, adaptive filtering, etc. Of course it is impossible for one text to provide in-depth coverage of all important neural networks. The field is extremely broad and is changing very rapidly.

In this chapter we want to give you a few ideas about where to go next. We will discuss some of the networks we were not able to cover in detail in this text, and will provide some references for further reading.

19

Theory and Examples

Chapter 3 provided a preview of the types of networks covered in this text. If you recall, Chapter 3 presents three neural networks and applies them to a simple pattern recognition problem. The three networks are the perceptron, the Hamming network and the Hopfield network. The perceptron is an example of a feedforward network, which we later generalized to multilayer perceptron networks. We discussed feedforward networks in Chapters 4, 7 and 10–12 (perceptron, linear associator, ADALINE, multilayer perceptron). The Hamming network is an example of a competitive network. We presented competitive networks in Chapters 14–16 (Kohonen layers, self-organizing feature map, learning vector quantizers, Grossberg network, ART network). The Hopfield network is an example of a dynamic associative memory network. The continuous-time Hopfield network was presented in Chapter 18.

In this chapter we will discuss some of the neural networks we did not have space to present in detail in previous chapters. These networks are related to the networks we have covered, and they fit into the three categories of network presented in Chapter 3 — feedforward networks, competitive networks and dynamic associative memory networks. We will present these other networks in the context of these three categories.

In addition to current neural network research, we will also discuss some of the classical foundations of neural networks. In previous chapters we described some principles in linear algebra, optimization and stability theory that have contributed to neural networks. In this chapter we will indicate some of the other disciplines that have supplied ideas and algorithms to the field.

The final section of this chapter lists some current neural network journals and textbooks that can assist you in your future studies.

The list of networks that we discuss in the remainder of this chapter is not comprehensive, and even if it were complete at the time of publication, it would be out of date within a few weeks. However, we hope this list will indicate the breadth of the field and will give you a place to start in your further study of neural networks.

Feedforward and Related Networks

Radial Basis Networks

First introduced in the solution of real multivariable interpolation problems, the radial basis function (RBF) network consists of two layers. The neurons in the first layer do not use the weighted sum of inputs and the sigmoid transfer function, which are typical of multilayer networks. Instead, the outputs of the first-layer neurons, each of which represents a *basis function*, are determined by the distance between the network input and the "center" of the basis function. As the input moves away from a given center, the neuron output drops off rapidly to zero. The second layer of the RBF network is linear and produces a weighted sum of the outputs of the first layer. The neurons in the RBF network have localized receptive fields because they only respond to inputs that are close to their centers. This is in contrast to the standard multilayer networks, where the sigmoid function creates a global response. The RBF network trains faster than multilayer perceptron networks, but requires many neurons for high-dimensional input spaces. [Powe87], [BrLo88], [MoDa89], [PoGi90]

CMAC (Cerebellar Model Articulation Controller)

Like the radial basis networks, the CMAC is a network that uses hidden units with localized receptive fields. This allows efficient learning. The CMAC was developed by Albus (1971) as a model of the cerebellum. He later applied the network to the control of robotic manipulators. In its initial form, the CMAC was implemented by a table look-up procedure. [Albu71], [Albu75]

Polynomial Networks

In Chapters 3, 4 and 10 we discussed the limitations of single-layer networks. They can only learn to classify patterns that are linearly separable. In Chapter 11 we illustrated that this limitation could be overcome by using multilayer networks, which could implement arbitrary decision regions. Another solution to this problem is to use a different type of neuron in a single layer. Instead of computing a linear combination of the inputs, the neurons can compute a more complex function, such as a polynomial. The following networks are examples of polynomial networks.

Functional Link Network

The neurons in the functional link network receive the standard linear combination of input elements plus higher-order terms. The higher-order terms include groups of products of different input elements. [Pao89]

Group Method of Data Handling (GMDH)

The group method of data handling (GMDH) was introduced by A.G. Ivakhnenko in 1968. Each neuron in this network has exactly two inputs. The output of each neuron is a general quadratic multinomial combination of the two inputs. Each layer of the network increases the degree of the polynomial created by the network. [Ivak71]

19

Sigma-Pi Network

This network is a generalization of multilayer perceptron networks that incorporates product terms into the net input of each neuron. The net input to each neuron is equal to a weighted sum of all signals impinging on that neuron, as well as a weighted sum of selected products of these signals. [RuMc86], [HeNo95]

Modular Network

This network is a compromise between the networks with localized receptive fields, like the radial basis function network and the CMAC, and global networks, like the multilayer perceptron. It consists of a number of expert networks, each of which can be a multilayer network, followed by a gating network that combines the outputs of the expert networks into one overall output. [JaJo91a], [JaJo91b]

Adaptive Critic

The basic adaptive critic system, which is normally used in control system applications, consists of two networks: the critic network and the action network. The purpose of the critic network is to evaluate the system performance in the absence of a true error measurement. The action network is then updated based on information from the critic network. The system is trained using reinforcement learning, which is somewhere between supervised and unsupervised learning. The system does not have access to a target output, but it does receive a reinforcement signal, such as "success" or "failure." [BaSu83], [Sutt84]

Variations of Backpropagation

Many variations on backpropagation, other than those of Chapter 12, have been proposed. This has probably been the most active area of neural network research since 1986. We discuss a few of the more successful backpropagation variations below.

Quickprop

Quickprop is a heuristic modification of backpropagation, in which the step size is determined by assuming that the error surface is quadratic and that the derivative with respect to one weight is independent of the other weights. [Fahl89]

Rprop

This procedure is designed to overcome the problem caused by the derivative of the sigmoid function being small when the magnitude of the net input is large. This may cause the gradient of the performance index to be small, even when far from a minimum point. Steepest descent would then produce very small steps. In Rprop the step size is not a function of the magnitude of the gradient. If the sign of the derivative for a given weight remains the same over several iterations, then the magnitude of the step size increases. If the sign of the derivative oscillates, then the magnitude of the step size decreases. [RiBr93]

Cascade-Correlation

The cascade-correlation learning architecture (Fahlman and Lebiere, 1990) is an example of a network growing procedure. It begins with no hidden nodes and can be trained with the LMS algorithm. Then hidden nodes are added to the network one at a time. Each new hidden node has a connection from each of the inputs and from each of the pre-existing hidden nodes. Each hidden node is connected to each output node. [FaLe90]

Network Pruning

One of the problems with training neural networks, as we discussed in Chapter 11, is a lack of generalization. If the network has too many parameters it can overfit the data. The error on the training set can become very small, but when data points outside the training set are presented, the error is large. One approach to improve network generalization is to reduce the number of parameters in the network. Network pruning eliminates certain weights after the network has been trained. Examples are Optimal Brain Damage [LeDe90] and Optimal Brain Surgeon [HaSt93].

Regularization

Another solution to network overfitting is to add a term to the performance index, a complexity penalty, which accounts for the size of the network. In other words, the modified performance index would consist of two parts, one a function of the squared error and the other a function of the number of network parameters (or their size). The training process attempts to minimize the squared error while using the least complex network. Two examples of regularization are the weight decay procedure [Hinto89], and the weight elimination method [WeRu91].

Stopped Training

This procedure, like regularization, is used to achieve better generalization in trained networks. The idea is to separate the data set into three parts: the training set, the validation set and the testing set. The training set is used to compute the gradient and to determine the weight update. The validation set is used to decide when to stop training. The test set is used to compare the performance of different networks. The training is stopped when the error on the validation set begins to increase. This keeps the network from overfitting on the training set. [Sarl95]

19

Probabilistic Neural Network

The probabilistic neural network is actually a parallel implementation of a standard Bayesian classifier. It is a three-layer network that can perform pattern classification. In its standard form, the probabilistic network is not trained. The training vectors simply become the weight vectors in the first layer of the network, in a manner similar to the Hamming network. The advantage of the PNN is that it does not require training. The disadvantage is that the weight matrix can be very large if there are many vectors in the training set. If the training set is too large, a clustering operation may have to be performed to reduce the size. [Spec90]

Generalized Regression Neural Network

Like the PNN, the generalized regression neural network does not require an iterative training procedure. While the PNN is used for classification problems, the GRNN is used for the estimation of continuous variables, as in standard regression techniques. It is related to the radial basis function network and the CMAC and is based on a standard statistical technique called kernel regression. [Spec91]

Multilayer Networks with Time Delays

Multilayer feedforward networks can approximate any Borel-integrable function, but they cannot incorporate any time dependency. For this reason, a number of researchers have proposed networks that combine multilayer perceptrons with time delays, some of which include feedback connections.

Time-Delay Neural Network

The time-delay neural network (TDNN) is a multilayer feedforward network in which the outputs of a layer are buffered several time steps and then fully connected to the next layer. It has been applied most often to speech recognition tasks. [LaHi88], [WaHa89].

Finite Impulse Response Multilayer Perceptron

The finite impulse response (FIR) multilayer perceptron network is a generalization of the TDNN. The FIR network is a multilayer network with each weight replaced by a finite impulse response filter. This network was first applied to time series prediction. [Wan90a], [Wan 90b], [Wan94]

Pipelined Recurrent Neural Network

The pipelined recurrent neural network (PPRN) consists of a number of modules, each of which receives an appropriately delayed version of the input signal. Each module is a fully connected recurrent network with a single output neuron. The modules operate sequentially, with the output of one module feeding into the succeeding module. It is more complex than the

TDNN and FIR networks because it has both feedforward and feedback (recurrent) connections and therefore has infinite memory. However, the modularity of the network allows efficient training. The PPRN was designed for adaptive prediction of nonstationary signals. [HaLi95]

Nonlinear Autoregressive Moving Average (NARMA) Network

The NARMA network is based on the linear ARMA model used in time series analysis and system identification. It consists of a single multilayer network that has two sets of inputs. The first set consists of the input signal and delayed values of the input signal. The second set of inputs consists of delayed values of the network output. The network is used for identification and control of dynamic systems and the prediction of time series. [NaPa90]

Elman Network

The Elman network is a two-layer network with feedback connections from the output of the hidden layer to its input. The feedback paths allow Elman networks to learn to recognize and generate temporal patterns as well as spatial patterns. [Elma90]

Real-Time Recurrent Network

The real-time recurrent network (RTRN) has a structure similar to the discrete-time Hopfield network, except that it contains hidden neurons. The RTRN has two layers: a hidden layer and an output layer. Both layers receive two sets of inputs. The first set consists of delayed values of all neuron outputs (both hidden and output neurons). The second set consists of external input signals. The RTRN, with its associated learning rule, is able to run continuously and to learn in real-time. It has the disadvantage that, because it is fully connected, it may require many neurons and excessive computation. [WiZi89]

Training Multilayer Networks with Delays

The multilayer networks described in the previous section, as well as other dynamic networks, cannot normally be trained with the standard backpropagation algorithm because of the time dependence. They require the use of dynamic backpropagation. There are two basic structures for dynamic backpropagation. One evolves forward through time, while the other evolves backward through time.

Backpropagation Through Time

The backpropagation through time (BTT) algorithm for dynamic networks is an extension of the backpropagation algorithm for static networks. It can be derived by unfolding the network forward through time to produce a multilayer feedforward network — a set of a layers for each time step. The backpropagation process effectively moves backward through time. The

19

BTT algorithm is characterized by relatively low computational cost and relatively high storage requirements. The standard BTT algorithm is not suitable for real-time operation because the output of the network for all time steps must be computed before the gradient is calculated (by back-propagating through the entire time sequence). (See Exercise E11.5 for an example of the BTT concept.) [RuMc86], [Werb90]

Forward Perturbation Algorithm

The forward perturbation algorithm (also referred to as the real-time re-current learning algorithm, the sensitivity method or the recursive back-propagation algorithm) is designed for real-time operation. The gradient is updated at each time step — forward through time. This algorithm is char-acterized by relatively high computational cost and relatively low storage requirements. (See Problems P11.4 and P11.9 for an example of the for-ward perturbation concept.) [WiZi89], [NaPa91]

Competitive Networks

Counterpropagation

The counterpropagation network (CPN) combines a competitive layer of in-stars with a layer of outstars. The CPN can be used for data compression, function approximation or pattern association. It combines supervised and unsupervised training. [Hech87], [Hech88]

Neocognitron

The neocognitron, a hierarchical network, is one of the most complex net-works yet developed. The neurons in each layer of the network receive con-nections from only a localized subset of the neurons in the previous layer. The neocognitron is designed for pattern recognition, in particular hand-written character recognition, and is relatively insensitive to distortion and scaling of patterns. [FuMi83], [Fuku88]

ART Networks

There are many variations of the ART network other than the ART1 net-work described in Chapter 16. The ART1 network was designed for unsu-pervised categorization of binary patterns. Later networks were modified to handle analog patterns, and some networks also include supervised learning. [CaGr87], [CaGr90], [CaGrMa92], [CaGrRo91], [CaGrRe91], [CaRo95]

Dynamic Associative Memory Networks

The Hopfield network is the only dynamic associative memory network presented in this text. A number of related networks have been suggested in the literature.

Li-Michel Networks

This class of network is described by a system of first-order linear differential equations defined on a closed hypercube. The design procedure for these networks guarantees that the number of spurious equilibrium points is as small as possible and that the basin of attraction for each prototype pattern is as large as possible. These networks are closely related to the Hopfield model, and the design procedures can be applied directly to the Hopfield model. [LiMi89], [MiFa90]

Boltzman Machine

A Hopfield network will converge to a local minimum of the Lyapunov function, but there is no guarantee that it will converge to a global minimum. In the Boltzman machine, noise is used in an attempt to reach the global minimum. The technique is called simulated annealing and is analogous to metallurgical annealing, in which a body of metal is heated to near melting and then slowly cooled according to a specified schedule. The high temperatures cause thermal agitation, which prevents the metal from becoming frozen in a high energy (brittle) state. In the Boltzman machine, noise is added to the network trajectory so that it will not be trapped in a local minimum. The magnitude of the noise is decreased over time, so that the network will eventually converge. [GeGe84], [AkHi85]

Bidirectional Associative Memory

The bidirectional associative memory (BAM) is related to the Hopfield network and also has some similarity to the ART architecture. It consists of two layers and uses the forward and backward information flow between the layers to perform a search for a stored stimulus-response association. The network evolves to a local minimum of the "energy" surface, which is a two-pattern resonance state, with each pattern at the output of one layer. [Kosk87], [Kosk88]

Brain-State-in-a-Box

The brain-state-in-a-box (BSB) is a dynamic associative memory model that preceded the Hopfield model. This discrete-time model was derived as an extension of the linear associator. Feedback was added, and a saturating linear transfer function was used to contain the network response within a hypercube. As with the high-gain Hopfield network, the stable points correspond to corners of the hypercube. [AnSi77]

19

Classical Foundations of Neural Networks

Many of the techniques used in neural networks are related to procedures that have been developed in other fields of study. This fact is often overlooked by newcomers to the field. In this section we want to review just a few of the ideas from other disciplines that are closely related to current neural network architectures or learning rules.

Statistics

Many classes of neural networks are functionally equivalent to standard procedures in mathematical statistics. For example, single-layer feedforward networks (including functional-link neural networks and polynomial neural networks) are basically generalized linear models. Two-layer feedforward networks are closely related to projection pursuit regression. Probabilistic neural networks are identical to kernel discriminant analysis. General regression neural networks are identical to Nadaraya-Watson kernel regression. Kohonen competitive networks are similar to k-means cluster analysis. Hebbian learning is closely related to principal component analysis. [Smit93], [Sarle94], [BaCo94], [Brid90], [MacK92], [Joll86], [HwLa94]

Physics/Statistical Mechanics

Several neural networks were inspired by work in physics, and in particular, by statistical mechanics. For instance, the Hopfield model was so influential because it was shown to be analogous to the Ising-spin model of magnetic materials that is used in statistical mechanics. The Boltzman machine is based on the principle of simulated annealing, which also comes out of the statistical physics literature. [ShKi72], [KiSh78], [Pere84], [Pere92]

Biology/Psychology

The connection between neural networks and ideas in biology and psychology is clear. However, even though the entire field of neural networks is inspired by these disciplines, we often fail to keep up with the current developments in these areas. [Thom75], [Gros82], [ChSe92], [Ande95]

Books and Journals

Neural Network Journals

The references we have provided in this chapter represent just the tip of the iceberg of neural network research and application. To keep up with the current neural network activity, you may wish to survey the following list of journals. Some of them are addressed solely to neural networks, others cover broader subject areas but devote significant space to neural network topics.

- *Applied Optics*
- *Biological Cybernetics*
- *Cognitive Science*
- *Connection Science*
- *IEEE Transactions on Circuits and Systems*
- *IEEE Transactions on Neural Networks*
- *IEEE Transactions on Systems, Man, and Cybernetics*
- *International Journal of Neural Systems*
- *Journal of Artificial Neural Networks*
- *Journal of Cognitive Neuroscience*
- *Journal of Neuroscience*
- *Machine Learning*
- *Network: Computation in Neural Systems*
- *Neural Computation*
- *Neural Networks*
- *Proceedings of the National Academy of Sciences*

Neural Network Textbooks

We have also included a list of neural network textbooks. We hope you have found our textbook to be satisfactory, but to obtain the deepest understanding of a subject, it is worthwhile to investigate it from several points of view. Each of these textbooks takes a slightly different approach to the subject.

- *Self-Organization and Associative Memory*, 3rd Edition, T. Kohonen, Springer-Verlag, 1989.
- *Adaptive Pattern Recognition and Neural Networks*, Y.-H. Pao, Addison-Wesley, 1989.
- *Neurocomputing*, R. Hecht-Nielsen, Addison-Wesley, 1990.
- *Introduction to the Theory of Neural Computation*, J. Hertz, A. Krogh and R. G. Palmer, Addison-Wesley, 1991.

19

- *Neural Networks: Algorithms, Applications, and Programming Techniques*, J. A. Freeman and D. M. Skapura, Addison-Wesley, 1991.

- *Neural Computing: An Introduction*, 2nd Edition, R. Beale and T. Jackson, Adam Hilger, 1991.

- *Introduction to Artificial Neural Systems*, J. Zurada, West Publishing, 1992.

- *An Introduction to the Modeling of Neural Networks*, P. Peretto, Cambridge University Press, 1992.

- *Neural Networks and Fuzzy Systems*, B. Kosko, Prentice-Hall, 1992.

- *Neural Networks for Pattern Recognition*, A. Nigrin, MIT Press, 1993.

- *Digital Neural Networks*, S. Y. Kung, Prentice-Hall, 1993.

- *Neural Networks for Statistical Modeling*, M. Smith, Van Nostrand Reinhold, 1993.

- *Advanced Methods in Neural Computing*, P. D. Wasserman, Van Nostrand Reinhold, 1993.

- *Neural Networks: A Tutorial*, M. Chester, Prentice-Hall, 1993.

- Neural Networks for Optimization and Signal Processing, A. Cichocki and R. Unbehauen, John Wiley & Sons, 1993.

- *Neural Networks: A Comprehensive Foundation*, S. Haykin, Macmillan, 1994.

- *Neural Network Principles*, R. L. Harvey, Prentice-Hall, 1994.

- *Fundamentals of Neural Networks: Architectures, Algorithms, and Applications*, L. Fausett, Prentice-Hall, 1994.

- *Fundamentals of Artificial Neural Networks*, M. H. Hassoun, MIT Press, 1995.

- *An Introduction to Neural Networks*, J. A. Anderson, MIT Press, 1995.

- *Self-Organizing Maps*, T. Kohonen, Springer-Verlag, 1995.

Epilogue

We hope that this text has helped shed some light on the field of neural networks and that it will encourage you to explore the subject further. The field is broad and is expanding rapidly. There will certainly be many new developments in neural networks in the coming years. The concepts discussed in this text will provide you with a good foundation to pursue further studies in this area. In this chapter we have suggested some places where you can go to continue your neural network exploration.

19

Further Reading

Radial Basis Networks

[BrLo88]   D. S. Broomhead and D. Lowe, "Multivariable functional interpolation and adaptive networks," *Complex Systems*, vol. 2, pp. 321–355, 1988.

[MoDa89]   J. E. Moody and C. J. Darken, "Fast learning in networks of locally-tuned processing units," *Neural Computation*, vol. 1, pp. 281–294, 1989.

[PoGi90]   T. Poggio and F. Girosi, "Networks for approximation and learning," *Proceedings of the IEEE*, vol. 78, pp. 1481–1497, 1990.

[Powe87]   M. J. D. Powell, "Radial basis functions for multivariable interpolation: A review," in *Algorithms for the Approximation of Functions and Data*, J. C. Mason and M. G. Cox, eds., Oxford, England: Clarendon Press, pp. 143–167, 1987.

CMAC

[Albu71]   J. S. Albus, "A theory of cerebellar function," *Mathematical Biosciences*, vol. 10, pp. 25–61, 1971.

[Albu75]   J. S. Albus, "A new approach to manipulator control: The cerebellar model articulation controller (CMAC)," *Journal of Dynamic Systems, Measurement and Control, Transactions of the ASME*, vol. 97, pp. 220–227, 1975.

Polynomial Networks

Functional Link

[Pao89]   Y.-H. Pao, *Adaptive Pattern Recognition and Neural Networks*, Reading, MA: Addison-Wesley, 1989.

Group Method of Data Handling (GMDH)

[Ivak71]   A. G. Ivakhnenko, "Polynomial theory of complex systems," *IEEE Transactions on Systems, Man, and Cybernetics*, vol. 12, pp. 364–378, 1971.

Sigma-Pi Networks

[HeNo95]   M. Heywood and P. Noakes, "A framework for improved training of sigma-pi networks," *IEEE Transactions on Neural Networks*, vol. 6, no. 4, pp. 893–903, 1995.

[RuMc86]   D. E. Rumelhart and J. L. McClelland, *Parallel Distributed Processing, Explorations in the Macrostructure of Cognition*, vol. 1, Cambridge, MA: MIT Press, 1986.

Modular Network

[JaJo91a]   R. A. Jacobs and M. I. Jordan, "A competitive modular connectionist architecture," in *Advances in Neural Information Processing Systems 3*, R. P. Lippman, J. E. Moody and D. J. Touretzky, eds., pp. 767–773, San Mateo, CA: Morgan Kaufmann, 1991.

[JaJo91b]   R. A. Jacobs, M. I. Jordan, S. J. Nowlan and G. E. Hinton, "Adaptive mixtures of local experts," *Neural Computation*, vol. 3, pp. 79–87, 1991.

Adaptive Critic

[BaSu83]   A. R. Barto, R. S. Sutton and C. W. Anderson, "Neuronlike adaptive elements that can solve difficult learning control problems," *IEEE Transactions on Systems, Man, and Cybernetics*, vol. 13, pp. 834–846, 1983.

[Sutt84]   R. S. Sutton, "Temporal credit assignment in reinforcement learning," Ph.D. Dissertation, University of Massachusetts, Amherst, MA, 1984.

Variations of Backpropagation Learning

Quickprop

[Fahl89]   S. E. Fahlman, "Fast learning variations on back-propagation: An empirical study," in *Proceedings of the 1988 Connectionist Models Summer School* (Pittsburgh 1988), D. Touretzky, G. Hinton and T. Sejnowski, eds., pp. 38–51, San Mateo, CA: Morgan Kaufmann, 1989.

Rprop

[RiBr93]   M. Riedmiller and H. Braun, "A direct adaptive method for faster backpropagation learning: The RPROP algorithm", *Proceedings of the IEEE International Conference on Neural Networks*, San Francisco: IEEE, 1993.

Cascade Correlation

[FaLe90]   A. E. Fahlman and C. Lebiere, "The cascade-correlation learning architecture," in *Advances in Neural Information Processing Systems 2*, D. Touretzky, ed., San Mateo, CA: Morgan Kaufmann, pp. 524–532, 1990.

19

Pruning

[HaSt93]   B. Hassibi, D. G. Stork and G. J. Wolff, "Optimal brain surgeon and general network pruning," *Proceedings of the IEEE International Joint Conference on Neural Networks*, vol. 2, pp. 441–444, 1992.

[LeDe90]   Y. Le Cun, J. S. Denker and S. A. Solla, "Optimal Brain Damage," in *Advances in Neural Information Processing Systems 2*, D. Touretzky, ed., San Mateo, CA: Morgan Kaufmann, pp. 598–604, 1990.

Regularization

Weight Decay

[Hinto89]   G. E. Hinton, "Connectionist learning procedures," *Artificial Intelligence*, vol. 40, pp. 185–234, 1989.

Weight Elimination

[WeRu91]   A. S. Weigand, D. E. Rumelhart and B. A. Huberman, "Generalization by weight elimination with application to forecasting," in *Advances in Neural Information Processing Systems 3*, R. Lippman, J. Moody and D. Touretzky, eds., San Mateo, CA: Morgan Kaufmann, pp. 575–582, 1991.

Stopped Training

[Sarle95]   W. S. Sarle, "Stopped training and other remedies for overfitting," to appear in *Proceedings of the 27th Symposium on the Interface*, 1995.

Probabilistic Neural Network

[Spec90]   D. F. Specht, "Probabilistic neural networks," *Neural Networks*, vol. 3, no. 1, pp. 109–118, 1990.

Generalized Regression Neural Network

[Spec91]   D. F. Specht, "A general regression neural network," *IEEE Transactions on Neural Networks*, vol. 2, no. 6, pp. 568–576, 1991.

Multilayer Networks with Time Delays

Time-Delay Neural Network

[LaHi88]   K. J. Lang and G. E. Hinton, "The development of the time-delay neural network architecture for speech recognition," Technical Report CMU-CS-88-152, Carnegie-Mellon University, Pittsburgh, PA, 1988.

[WaHa89]   A. Waibel, T. Hanazawa, G. Hinton, K. Shikano and K. J. Lang, "Phoneme recognition using time-delay neural networks," *IEEE Transactions on Acoustics, Speech and Signal Processing*, vol. 37, pp. 328–339, 1989.

Finite Impulse Response (FIR) Network

[Wan90a]   E. A. Wan, "Temporal backpropagation for FIR neural networks," *IEEE International Joint Conference on Neural Networks*, vol. 1, San Diego, CA, pp. 575–580, 1990.

[Wan90b]   E. A. Wan, "Temporal backpropagation: An efficient algorithm for finite impulse response neural networks," in *Proceedings of the 1990 Connectionist Models Summer School*, D. S. Touretzky, J. L. Elman, T. J. Sejnowski and G. E. Hinton, eds., San Mateo, CA: Morgan Kaufmann, pp. 131–140, 1990.

[Wan94]   E. A. Wan, "Time series prediction by using a connectionist network with internal delay lines," in *Time Series Prediction: Forecasting the Future and Understanding the Past*, A. S. Weigend and N. A. Gershenfeld, eds., Reading, MA: Addison Wesley, pp. 195–217, 1994.

Pipelined Recurrent Neural Network

[HaLi95]   S. Haykin and L. Li, "Nonlinear adaptive prediction of nonstationary signals," *IEEE Transactions on Signal Processing*, vol. 43, no. 2, pp. 526–535, 1995.

Nonlinear Autoregressive Moving Average (NARMA) Network

[NaPa90]   K. S. Narendra and K. Parthasarathy, "Identification and control of dynamical systems using neural networks," *IEEE Transactions on Neural Networks*, vol. 1, no. 1, pp. 4–27, 1990.

Elman Network

[Elma90]   J. L. Elman, "Finding structure in time," *Cognitive Science*, vol. 14, pp. 179–211, 1990.

19

Real-Time Recurrent Network

[WiZi89] R. J. Williams and D. Zipser, "A learning algorithm for continually running fully recurrent neural networks," *Neural Computation*, vol. 1, pp. 270–280, 1989.

Training Multilayer Networks with Time Delays

Backpropagation Through Time

[RuMc86] D. E. Rumelhart and J. L. McClelland, *Parallel Distributed Processing, Explorations in the Macrostructure of Cognition*, vol. 1, Cambridge, MA: MIT Press, 1986.

[Werb90] P. J. Werbos, "Backpropagation through time: What it is and how to do it," *Proceedings of the IEEE*, vol. 78, pp. 1550–1560, October 1990.

Forward Perturbation Algorithm

[NaPa91] K. S. Narendra and K. Parthasarathy, "Gradient methods for the optimization of dynamical systems containing neural networks," *IEEE Transactions on Neural Networks*, vol. 2, pp. 252–262, 1991.

[WiZi89] R. J. Williams and D. Zipser, "A learning algorithm for continually running fully recurrent neural networks," *Neural Computation*, vol. 1, pp. 270–280, 1989.

Competitive Networks

Counterpropagation

[Hech87] R. Hecht-Nielsen, "Counterpropagation Networks," *Applied Optics*, vol. 26, pp. 4979–4984, December 1987.

[Hech88] R. Hecht-Nielsen, "Applications of Counterpropagation Networks," *Neural Networks*, vol. 1, no. 2, pp. 131–139, 1988.

Neocognitron

[FuMi83] K. Fukushima, S. Miyake and T. Ito, "Neocognitron: A neural network model for a mechanism of visual pattern recognition," *IEEE Transactions on Systems, Man, and Cybernetics*, vol. 13, no. 5, pp. 826–834, 1983.

[Fuku88] K. Fukushima, "Neocognitron: A hierarchical neural network capable of visual pattern recognition," *Neural Networks*, vol. 1, pp. 119–130, 1988.

ART

[CaGr87b]   G. A. Carpenter and S. Grossberg, "ART2: Self-organization of stable category recognition codes for analog input patterns," *Applied Optics*, vol. 26, no. 23, pp. 4919–4930, 1987.

[CaGr90]   G. A. Carpenter and S. Grossberg, "ART3: Hierarchical search using chemical transmitters in self-organizing pattern recognition architectures," *Neural Networks*, vol. 3, no. 23, pp. 129–152, 1990.

[CaGrMa92]   G. A. Carpenter, S. Grossberg, N. Markuzon, J. H. Reynolds and D. B. Rosen, "Fuzzy ARTMAP: A neural network architecture for incremental learning of analog multidimensional maps," *IEEE Transactions on Neural Networks*, vol. 3, pp. 698–713, 1992.

[CaGrRo91]   G. A. Carpenter, S. Grossberg and D. B. Rosen, "Fuzzy ART: Fast stable learning and categorization of analog patterns by an adaptive resonance system," *Neural Networks*, vol. 4, pp. 759–771, 1991.

[CaGrRe91]   G. A. Carpenter, S. Grossberg and J. Reynolds, "ARTMAP: Supervised real-time learning and classification of nonstationary data by a self-organizing neural network," *Neural Networks*, vol. 4, pp. 565–588, 1991.

[CaRo95]   G. A. Carpenter and W. D. Ross, "ART-EMAP: A neural network architecture for object recognition by evidence accumulation," *IEEE Transactions on Neural Networks*, vol. 6, no. 4, pp. 805–818, July 1995.

Associative Memory Recurrent Networks

19

Li-Michel Networks

[LiMi89]   J. Li, A. N. Michel and W. Porod, "Analysis and synthesis of a class of neural networks: Linear systems operating on a closed hypercube," *IEEE Transactions on Circuits and Systems*, vol. 36, no. 11, pp. 1405–1422, November 1989.

[MiFa90]   A. N. Michel and J. A. Farrell, "Associative memories via artificial neural networks," *IEEE Control Systems Magazine*, April, pp. 6–17, 1990.

Boltzman Machine

[AcHi85]   D. H. Ackley, G. F. Hinton and T. J. Sejnowski, "A learning algorithm for Boltzman machines," *Cognitive Science*, vol. 9, pp. 147–169, 1985.

[GeGe84]   S. Geman and D. Geman, "Stochastic relaxation, Gibbs distributions, and the Bayesian restoration of images," *IEEE Transactions on Pattern Analysis and Machine Intelligence*, vol. 6, pp. 721–741, 1984.

Bidirectional Associative Memory

[Kosk87]   B. Kosko, "Adaptive bidirectional associative memories," *Applied Optics*, vol. 26, pp. 4910–4918, 1987.

[Kosk88]   B. Kosko, "Bidirectional associative memories," *IEEE Transactions on Systems, Man, and Cybernetics*, vol. 18, no. 1, pp. 49–60, 1988.

Brain-State-in-a-Box

[AnSi77]   J. A. Anderson, J. W. Silverstein, S. A. Ritz and R. S. Jones, "Distinctive features, categorical perception, and probability learning: some applications of a neural model," *Psychological Review*, vol. 84, pp. 413–351, 1977.

Classical Techniques

Statistics

[BaCo94]   P. V. Balakrishnan, M. C. Cooper, V. S. Jacob, and P. A. Lewis, "A study of the classification capabilities of neural networks using unsupervised learning: A comparison with k-means clustering," *Psychometrika*, vol. 59, pp. 509–525, 1994.

[Brid90]   J. S. Bridle, "Probabilistic interpretation of feedforward classification network outputs, with relationships to statistical pattern recognition," in *Neurocomputing: Algorithms, Architectures and Applications*, F. Fogleman-Soulie and J. Herault, eds., Berlin: Springer-Verlag, pp. 227–236, 1990.

[HwLa94]   J.-N. Hwang, S.-R. Lay, M. Maechler, R. D. Martin and J. Schimert, "Regression modeling in back-propagation and projection pursuit learning," *IEEE Transactions on Neural Networks*, vol. 5, no. 3, pp. 342–353, 1994.

[Joll86]   I. T. Jolliffe, *Principal Component Analysis*, New York: Springer-Verlag, 1986.

[MacK92]   D. J. C. MacKay, "A practical Bayesian framework for backpropagation networks," *Neural Computation*, vol. 4, pp. 448–472, 1992.

[Sarle94]   W. S. Sarle, "Neural networks and statistical models," *Proceedings of the Nineteenth Annual SAS Users Group International Conference*, Cary, NC: SAS Institute, pp. 1538–1550, 1994.

[Smit93]   M. Smith, *Neural Networks for Statistical Modeling*, New York: Van Nostrand Reinhold, 1993.

Physics/Statistical Mechanics

[KiSh78]   S. Kirkpatrick and D. Sherrington, "Infinite-range models of spin-glasses," *Physical Review, Series B*, vol. 17, pp. 4384–4403, 1978.

[Pere84]   P. Peretto, "Collective properties of neural networks: A statistical physics approach," *Biological Cybernetics*, vol. 50, pp. 51–62, 1984.

[Pere92]   P. Peretto, *An Introduction to the Modeling of Neural Networks*, Cambridge, England: Cambridge University Press, 1992.

[ShKi72]   D. Sherrington and S. Kirkpatrick, "Spin-glasses," *Physical Review Letters*, vol. 35, 1972.

Biology/Psychology

[Ande95]   J. A. Anderson, *An Introduction to Neural Networks*, Cambridge, MA: MIT Press, 1995.

[ChSe92]   P. S. Churchland and T. J. Sejnowski, *The Computational Brain*, Cambridge, MA: MIT Press, 1992.

[Gros82]   S. Grossberg, *Studies of Mind and Brain*, Boston: D. Reidel Publishing Co., 1982.

[Thom75]   R. F. Thompson, *Introduction to Physiological Psychology*, New York: Harper and Row, 1975.

19

A Bibliography

[AcHi85]   D. H. Ackley, G. F. Hinton and T. J. Sejnowski, "A learning algorithm for Boltzman machines," *Cognitive Science*, vol. 9, pp. 147–169, 1985. (Chapter 19)

[Albe72]   A. Albert, *Regression and the Moore-Penrose Pseudoinverse*, New York: Academic Press, 1972. (Chapter 7)

[Albu71]   J. S. Albus, "A theory of cerebellar function," *Mathematical Biosciences*, vol. 10, pp. 25–61, 1971. (Chapter 19)

[Albu75]   J. S. Albus, "A new approach to manipulator control: The cerebellar model articulation controller (CMAC)," *Journal of Dynamic Systems, Measurement and Control, Transactions of the ASME*, vol. 97, pp. 220–227, 1975. (Chapter 19)

[Ande72]   J. A. Anderson, "A simple neural network generating an interactive memory," *Mathematical Biosciences*, vol. 14, pp. 197–220, 1972. (Chapter 1, 13, 18)

[Ande95]   J. A. Anderson, *An Introduction to Neural Networks*, Cambridge, MA: MIT Press, 1995. (Chapter 19)

[AnRo88]   J. A. Anderson and E. Rosenfeld, *Neurocomputing: Foundations of Research*, Cambridge, MA: MIT Press, 1989. (Chapters 1, 10)

[AnSi77]   J. A. Anderson, J. W. Silverstein, S. A. Ritz and R. S. Jones, "Distinctive features, categorical perception, and probability learning: Some applications of a neural model," *Psychological Review*, vol. 84, pp. 413–451, 1977. (Chapters 18, 19)

[BaCo94]   P. V. Balakrishnan, M. C. Cooper, V. S. Jacob, and P. A. Lewis, "A study of the classification capabilities of neural networks using unsupervised learning: A comparison with k-means clustering," *Psychometrika*, vol. 59, pp. 509–525, 1994. (Chapter 19)

[Barn92]   E. Barnard, "Optimization for training neural nets," *IEEE Transactions on Neural Networks*, vol. 3, no. 2, pp. 232–240, 1992. (Chapter 12)

A

[BaSu83] A. R. Barto, R. S. Sutton and C. W. Anderson, "Neuronlike adaptive elements that can solve difficult learning control problems," *IEEE Transactions on Systems, Man, and Cybernetics*, vol. 13, pp. 834–846, 1983. (Chapters 4, 19)

[Batt92] R. Battiti, "First and second order methods for learning: Between steepest descent and Newton's method," *Neural Computation*, vol. 4, no. 2, pp. 141–166, 1992. (Chapters 9, 12)

[Brid90] J. S. Bridle, "Probabilistic interpretation of feedforward classification network outputs, with relationships to statistical pattern recognition," in *Neurocomputing: Algorithms, Architectures and Applications*, F.Fogleman-Soulie and J. Herault, eds., Berlin: Springer-Verlag, pp. 227–236, 1990. (Chapter 19)

[Brog91] W. L. Brogan, *Modern Control Theory*, 3rd Ed., Englewood Cliffs, NJ: Prentice-Hall, 1991. (Chapters 4, 5, 6, 8, 9, 17)

[BrLo88] D. S. Broomhead and D. Lowe, "Multivariable functional interpolation and adaptive networks," *Complex Systems*, vol. 2, pp. 321–355, 1988. (Chapter 19)

[CaGr87a] G. A. Carpenter and S. Grossberg, "A massively parallel architecture for a self-organizing neural pattern recognition machine," *Computer Vision, Graphics, and Image Processing*, vol. 37, pp. 54–115, 1987. (Chapter 16)

[CaGr87b] G. A. Carpenter and S. Grossberg, "ART2: Self-organization of stable category recognition codes for analog input patterns," *Applied Optics*, vol. 26, no. 23, pp. 4919–4930, 1987. (Chapters 16, 19)

[CaGr90] G. A. Carpenter and S. Grossberg, "ART3: Hierarchical search using chemical transmitters in self-organizing pattern recognition architectures," *Neural Networks*, vol. 3, no. 23, pp. 129–152, 1990. (Chapters 16, 19)

[CaGrMa92] G. A. Carpenter, S. Grossberg, N. Markuzon, J. H. Reynolds and D. B. Rosen, "Fuzzy ARTMAP: A neural network architecture for incremental learning of analog multidimensional maps," *IEEE Transactions on Neural Networks*, vol. 3, pp. 698–713, 1992. (Chapters 16, 19)

[CaGrRe91] G.A. Carpenter, S. Grossberg and J. Reynolds, "ARTMAP: Supervised real-time learning and classification of nonstationary data by a self-organizing neural network," *Neural Networks*, vol. 4, pp. 565–588, 1991. (Chapters 16, 19)

[CaGrRo91] G. A. Carpenter, S. Grossberg and D. B. Rosen, "Fuzzy ART: Fast stable learning and categorization of analog patterns by an adaptive resonance system," *Neural Networks*, vol. 4, pp. 759–771, 1991. (Chapter 19)

[CaRo95] G. A. Carpenter and W. D. Ross, "ART-EMAP: A neural network architecture for object recognition by evidence accumulation," *IEEE Transactions on Neural Networks*, vol. 6, no. 4, pp. 805–818, July 1995. (Chapter 19)

[Char92] C. Charalambous, "Conjugate gradient algorithm for efficient training of artificial neural networks," *IEEE Proceedings*, vol. 139, no. 3, pp. 301–310, 1992. (Chapter 12)

[ChSe92] P. S. Churchland and T. J. Sejnowski, *The Computational Brain*, Cambridge, MA: MIT Press, 1992. (Chapter 19)

[CoGr83] M. A. Cohen and S. Grossberg, "Absolute stability of global pattern formation and parallel memory storage by competitive neural networks," *IEEE Transactions on Systems, Man, and Cybernetics*, vol. 13, no. 5, pp. 815–826, 1983. (Chapters 17, 18)

[DARP88] *DARPA Neural Network Study*, Lexington, MA: MIT Lincoln Laboratory, 1988. (Chapter 1)

[Elma90] J. L. Elman, "Finding structure in time," *Cognitive Science*, vol. 14, pp. 179–211, 1990. (Chapter 19)

[Fahl89] S. E. Fahlman, "Fast learning variations on back-propagation: An empirical study," in *Proceedings of the 1988 Connectionist Models Summer School*, D. Touretzky, G. Hinton and T. Sejnowski, eds., San Mateo, CA: Morgan Kaufmann, pp. 38–51, 1989. (Chapters 12–19)

[FaLe90] A. E. Fahlman and C. Lebiere, "The cascade-correlation learning architecture," in *Advances in Neural Information Processing Systems 2*, D. Touretzky, ed., San Mateo, CA: Morgan Kaufmann, pp. 524–532, 1990. (Chapter 19)

[FrSk91] J. Freeman and D. Skapura, *Neural Networks: Algorithms, Applications, and Programming Techniques*, Reading, MA: Addison-Wesley, 1991. (Chapter 14)

[FuMi83] K. Fukushima, S. Miyake and T. Ito, "Neocognitron: A neural network model for a mechanism of visual pattern recognition," *IEEE Transactions on Systems, Man, and Cybernetics*, vol. 13, no. 5, pp. 826–834, 1983. (Chapter 19)

A

[Fuku88]   K. Fukushima, "Neocognitron: A hierarchical neural network capable of visual pattern recognition," *Neural Networks*, vol. 1, pp. 119–130, 1988. (Chapter 19)

[GeGe84]   S. Geman and D. Geman, "Stochastic relaxation, Gibbs distributions, and the Bayesian restoration of images," *IEEE Transactions on Pattern Analysis and Machine Intelligence*, vol. 6, pp. 721–741, 1984. (Chapter 19)

[Gill81]   P. E. Gill, W. Murray and M. H. Wright, *Practical Optimization*, New York: Academic Press, 1981. (Chapters 8, 9)

[GrMi89]   S. Grossberg, E. Mingolla and D. Todorovic, "A neural network architecture for preattentive vision," *IEEE Transactions on Biomedical Engineering*, vol. 36, no. 1, pp. 65–84, Jan. 1989. (Chapter 15)

[Gros67]   S. Grossberg, "Nonlinear difference-differential equations in prediction and learning theory," *Proceedings of the National Academy of Sciences*, vol. 58, pp. 1329–1334, 1967. (Chapter 18)

[Gros68]   S. Grossberg, "Some physiological and biochemical consequences of psychological postulates," *Proceedings of the National Academy of Sciences*, vol. 60, pp. 758–765, 1968. (Chapter 13)

[Gros76]   S. Grossberg, "Adaptive pattern classification and universal recoding: I. Parallel development and coding of neural feature detectors," *Biological Cybernetics*, vol. 23, pp. 121–134, 1976. (Chapters 1, 15, 16)

[Gros80]   S. Grossberg, "How does the brain build a cognitive code?" *Psychological Review*, vol. 88, pp. 375–407, 1980. (Chapter 1)

[Gros82]   S. Grossberg, *Studies of Mind and Brain*, Boston: D. Reidel Publishing Co., 1982. (Chapters 13, 15, 16, 19)

[Gros90]   S. Grossberg, "Neural networks: From foundations to applications," Short-Course Notes, Boston University, Boston, MA, May 6–11, 1990. (Chapter 15)

[HaMe94]   M. T. Hagan and M. Menhaj, "Training feedforward networks with the Marquardt algorithm," *IEEE Transactions on Neural Networks*, vol. 5, no. 6, pp. 989–993, 1994. (Chapter 12)

[HaLi95]   S. Haykin and L. Li, "Nonlinear adaptive prediction of nonstationary signals," *IEEE Transactions on Signal Processing*, vol. 43, no. 2, pp. 526–535. (Chapter 19)

[HaSt93]   B. Hassibi, D. G. Stork and G. J. Wolff, "Optimal brain sur-geon and general network pruning," *Proceedings of the IEEE International Joint Conference on Neural Networks*, vol. 2, pp. 441–444, 1992. (Chapter 19)

[Hebb 49]   D. O. Hebb, *The Organization of Behavior*, New York: Wiley, 1949. (Chapters 1, 7, 13)

[Hech87]   R. Hecht-Nielsen, "Counterpropagation networks," *Applied Optics*, vol. 26, pp. 4979–4984, December 1987. (Chapter 19)

[Hech88]   R. Hecht-Nielsen, "Applications of counterpropagation net-works," *Neural Networks*, vol. 1, no. 2, pp. 131–139, 1988. (Chapter 19)

[Hech90]   R. Hecht-Nielsen, *Neurocomputing*, Reading, MA: Addi-son-Wesley, 1990. (Chapter 14)

[HeNo95]   M. Heywood and P. Noakes, "A framework for improved training of sigma-pi networks," *IEEE Transactions on Neu-ral Networks*, vol. 6, no. 4, pp. 893–903, 1995. (Chapter 19)

[Himm72]   D. M. Himmelblau, *Applied Nonlinear Programming*, New York: McGraw-Hill, 1972. (Chapters 8, 9)

[Hinto89]   G. E. Hinton, "Connectionist learning procedures," *Artifi-cial Intelligence*, vol. 40, pp. 185–234, 1989. (Chapter 19)

[Hopf82]   J. J. Hopfield, "Neural networks and physical systems with emergent collective computational properties," *Proceedings of the National Academy of Sciences*, vol. 79, pp. 2554–2558, 1982. (Chapters 1, 18)

[Hopf84]   J. J. Hopfield, "Neurons with graded response have collec-tive computational properties like those of two-state neu-rons," *Proceedings of the National Academy of Sciences*, vol. 81, pp. 3088–3092, 1984. (Chapter 18)

[HoTa85]   J. J. Hopfield and D. W. Tank, " 'Neural' computation of de-cisions in optimization problems," *Biological Cybernetics*, vol. 52, pp. 141–154, 1985. (Chapter 18)

[HoSt89]   K. M. Hornik, M. Stinchcombe and H. White, "Multilayer feedforward networks are universal approximators," *Neu-ral Networks*, vol. 2, no. 5, pp. 359–366, 1989. (Chapter 11)

[Hube88]   D. H. Hubel, *Eye, Brain, and Vision*, New York: Scientific American Library, 1988. (Chapter 15)

A

[HwLa94]   J.-N. Hwang, S.-R. Lay, M. Maechler, R. D. Martin and J. Schimert, "Regression modeling in back-propagation and projection pursuit learning," *IEEE Transactions on Neural Networks*, vol. 5, no. 3, pp. 342–353, 1994. (Chapter 19)

[Ivak71]   A. G. Ivakhnenko, "Polynomial theory of complex systems," *IEEE Transactions on Systems, Man, and Cybernetics*, vol. 12, pp. 364–378, 1971. (Chapter 19)

[Jaco88]   R. A. Jacobs, "Increased rates of convergence through learning rate adaptation," *Neural Networks*, vol. 1, no. 4, pp 295–308, 1988. (Chapter 12)

[JaJo91a]   R. A. Jacobs and M. I. Jordan, "A competitive modular connectionist architecture," in *Advances in Neural Information Processing Systems 3*, R. P. Lippman, J. E. Moody and D. J. Touretzky, eds., pp. 767–773, San Mateo, CA: Morgan Kaufmann, 1991. (Chapter 19)

[JaJo91b]   R. A. Jacobs, M. I. Jordan, S. J. Nowlan and G. E. Hinton, "Adaptive mixtures of local experts," *Neural Computation*, vol. 3, pp. 79–87, 1991. (Chapter 19)

[John01]   G. L. Johnson, "Contributions to the comparative anatomy of the mammalian eye, chiefly based on ophthalmoscopic examination," *Philosophical Transactions of the Royal Society of London*, Series B., vol. 194, pp. 1–82, Plate 1, 1901. (Chapter 15)

[Joll86]   I. T. Jolliffe, *Principal Component Analysis*, New York: Springer Verlag, 1986. (Chapter 19)

[KiSh78]   S. Kirkpatrick and D. Sherrington, "Infinite-range models of spin-glasses," *Physical Review, Series B*, vol. 17, pp. 4384–4403, 1978. (Chapter 19)

[Koho72]   T. Kohonen, "Correlation matrix memories," *IEEE Transactions on Computers*, vol. 21, pp. 353–359, 1972. (Chapters 1, 13, 18)

[Koho87]   T. Kohonen, *Self-Organization and Associative Memory*, 2nd Ed., Berlin: Springer-Verlag, 1987. (Chapters 13, 14)

[Kosk87]   B. Kosko, "Adaptive bidirectional associative memories," *Applied Optics*, vol. 26, pp. 4910–4918, 1987. (Chapter 19)

[Kosk88]   B. Kosko, "Bidirectional associative memories," *IEEE Transactions on Systems, Man, and Cybernetics*, vol. 18, no. 1, pp. 49–60, 1988. (Chapter 19)

[LaHi88]   K. J. Lang and G. E. Hinton, "The development of the time-delay neural network architecture for speech recognition," Technical Report CMU-CS-88-152, Carnegie-Mellon University, Pittsburgh, PA, 1988. (Chapter 19)

[LaSa67]   J. P. LaSalle, "An invariance principle in the theory of stability," in *Differential Equations and Dynamic Systems*, J. K. Hale and J. P. Lasalle, eds., New York: Academic Press, pp. 277–286, 1967. (Chapter 17)

[LeCu85]   Y. Le Cun, "Une procedure d'apprentissage pour reseau a seuil assymetrique," *Cognitiva*, vol. 85, pp. 599–604, 1985. (Chapter 11)

[LeDe90]   Y. Le Cun, J. S. Denker and S. A. Solla, "Optimal brain damage," in *Advances in Neural Information Processing Systems 2*, D. Touretzky, ed., San Mateo, CA: Morgan Kaufmann, pp. 598–604, 1990. (Chapter 19)

[Leib90]   D. Lieberman, *Learning, Behavior and Cognition*, Belmont, CA: Wadsworth, 1990. (Chapter 13)

[LiMi89]   J. Li, A. N. Michel and W. Porod, "Analysis and synthesis of a class of neural networks: Linear systems operating on a closed hypercube," *IEEE Transactions on Circuits and Systems*, vol. 36, no. 11, pp. 1405–1422, November 1989. (Chapter 18, 19)

[MacK92]   D. J. C. MacKay, "A practical bayesian framework for back-propagation networks," *Neural Computation*, vol. 4, pp. 448–472, 1992. (Chapter 19)

[McPi43]   W. McCulloch and W. Pitts, "A logical calculus of the ideas immanent in nervous activity," *Bulletin of Mathematical Biophysics*, vol. 5, pp. 115–133, 1943. (Chapters 1, 4, 18)

[MiFa90]   A. N. Michel and J. A. Farrell, "Associative memories via artificial neural networks," *IEEE Control Systems Magazine*, April, pp. 6–17, 1990. (Chapter 19)

[MiPa69]   M. Minsky and S. Papert, *Perceptrons*, Cambridge, MA: MIT Press, 1969. (Chapters 1, 4)

[MoDa89]   J. E. Moody and C. J. Darken, "Fast learning in networks of locally-tuned processing units," *Neural Computation*, vol. 1, pp. 281–294, 1989. (Chapter 19)

[NaPa90]   K. S. Narendra and K. Parthasarathy, "Identification and control of dynamical systems using neural networks," *IEEE Transactions on Neural Networks*, vol. 1, no. 1, pp. 4–27, 1990. (Chapter 19)

A

[NaPa91]   K. S. Narendra and K. Parthasarathy, "Gradient methods for the optimization of dynamical systems containing neural networks," *IEEE Transactions on Neural Networks*, vol. 2, pp. 252–262, 1991. (Chapter 19)

[NgWi90]   D. Nguyen and B. Widrow, "Improving the learning speed of 2-layer neural networks by choosing initial values of the adaptive weights," *Proceedings of the IJCNN*, vol. 3, pp. 21–26, July 1990. (Chapter 12)

[Pao89]   Y.-H. Pao, *Adaptive Pattern Recognition and Neural Networks*, Reading, MA: Addison-Wesley, 1989. (Chapter 19)

[Park85]   D. B. Parker, "Learning-logic: Casting the cortex of the human brain in silicon," Technical Report TR-47, Center for Computational Research in Economics and Management Science, MIT, Cambridge, MA, 1985. (Chapter 11)

[Pere84]   P. Peretto, "Collective properties of neural networks: A statistical physics approach," *Biological Cybernetics*, vol. 50, pp. 51–62, 1984. (Chapter 19)

[Pere92]   P. Peretto, *An Introduction to the Modeling of Neural Networks*, Cambridge, England: Cambridge University Press, 1992. (Chapter 19)

[PoGi90]   T. Poggio and F. Girosi, "Networks for approximation and learning," *Proceedings of the IEEE*, vol. 78, pp. 1481–1497, 1990. (Chapter 19)

[Powe87]   M. J. D. Powell, "Radial basis functions for multivariable interpolation: A review," in *Algorithms for the Approximation of Functions and Data*, J. C. Mason and M. G. Cox, eds., Oxford, England: Clarendon Press, pp. 143–167, 1987. (Chapter 19)

[RiBr93]   M. Riedmiller and H. Braun, "A direct adaptive method for faster backpropagation learning: The RPROP algorithm," *Proceedings of the IEEE International Conference on Neural Networks*, San Francisco: IEEE, 1993. (Chapter 19)

[RiIr90]   A. K. Rigler, J. M. Irvine and T. P. Vogl, "Rescaling of variables in back propagation learning," *Neural Networks*, vol. 3, no. 5, pp 561–573, 1990. (Chapter 12)

[Rose58]   F. Rosenblatt, "The perceptron: A probabilistic model for information storage and organization in the brain," *Psychological Review*, vol. 65, pp. 386–408, 1958. (Chapters 1, 4)

[Rose61]   F. Rosenblatt, *Principles of Neurodynamics*, Washington DC: Spartan Press, 1961. (Chapter 4)

[RuHi86]   D. E. Rumelhart, G. E. Hinton and R. J. Williams, "Learning representations by back-propagating errors," *Nature*, vol. 323, pp. 533–536, 1986. (Chapter 11)

[RuMc86]   D. E. Rumelhart and J. L. McClelland, eds., *Parallel Distributed Processing: Explorations in the Microstructure of Cognition*, vol. 1, Cambridge, MA: MIT Press, 1986. (Chapters 1, 11, 14, 19)

[Sarle94]   W. S. Sarle, "Neural networks and statistical models," *Proceedings of the Nineteenth Annual SAS Users Group International Conference*, Cary, NC: SAS Institute, pp. 1538–1550, 1994. (Chapter 19)

[Sarle95]   W. S. Sarle, "Stopped training and other remedies for overfitting," to appear in *Proceedings of the 27th Symposium on the Interface*, 1995. (Chapter 19)

[Scal85]   L. E. Scales, *Introduction to Non-Linear Optimization*, New York: Springer-Verlag, 1985. (Chapters 8, 9, 12)

[Shan90]   D. F. Shanno, "Recent advances in numerical techniques for large-scale optimization," in *Neural Networks for Control*, Miller, Sutton and Werbos, eds., Cambridge, MA: MIT Press, 1990. (Chapter 12)

[ShKi72]   D. Sherrington and S. Kirkpatrick, "Spin-glasses," *Physical Review Letters*, vol. 35, 1972. (Chapter 19)

[SlLi91]   J.-J. E. Slotine and W. Li, *Applied Nonlinear Control*, Englewood Cliffs, NJ: Prentice-Hall, 1991. (Chapter 17)

[Smit93]   M. Smith, *Neural Networks for Statistical Modeling*, New York: Van Nostrand Reinhold, 1993. (Chapter 19)

[Spec90]   D. F. Specht, "Probabilistic neural networks," *Neural Networks*, vol. 3, no. 1, pp. 109–118, 1990. (Chapter 19)

[Spec91]   D. F. Specht, "A general regression neural network," *IEEE Transactions on Neural Networks*, vol. 2, no. 6, pp. 568–576, 1991. (Chapter 19)

[StDo84]   W. D. Stanley, G. R. Dougherty and R. Dougherty, *Digital Signal Processing*, Reston VA: Reston Publishing Co., 1984. (Chapter 10)

[Stra76]   G. Strang, *Linear Algebra and Its Applications*, New York: Academic Press, 1980. (Chapters 5, 6)

A

[Sutt84]   R. S. Sutton, "Temporal credit assignment in reinforcement learning," Ph.D. Dissertation, University of Massachusetts, Amherst, MA, 1984. (Chapter 19)

[TaHo86]   D. W. Tank and J. J. Hopfield, "Simple 'neural' optimization networks: An A/D converter, signal decision circuit and a linear programming circuit," *IEEE Transactions on Circuits and Systems*, vol. 33, no. 5, pp. 533–541, 1986. (Chapter 18)

[Thom75]   R. F. Thompson, *Introduction to Physiological Psychology*, New York: Harper and Row, 1975. (Chapter 19)

[Toll90]   T. Tollenaere, "SuperSAB: Fast adaptive back propagation with good scaling properties," *Neural Networks*, vol. 3, no. 5, pp. 561–573, 1990. (Chapter 12)

[vanT75]   H. F. J. M. van Tuijl, "A new visual illusion: Neonlike color spreading and complementary color induction between subjective contours," *Acta Psychologica*, vol. 39, pp. 441–445, 1975. (Chapter 15)

[VoMa88]   T. P. Vogl, J. K. Mangis, A. K. Zigler, W. T. Zink and D. L. Alkon, "Accelerating the convergence of the backpropagation method," *Biological Cybernetics*, vol. 59, pp. 256–264, Sept. 1988. (Chapter 12)

[vond73]   C. von der Malsburg, "Self-organization of orientation sensitive cells in the striate cortex," *Kybernetic*, vol. 14, pp. 85–100, 1973. (Chapter 15)

[WaHa89]   A. Waibel, T. Hanazawa, G. Hinton, K. Shikano and K. J. Lang, "Phoneme recognition using time-delay neural networks," *IEEE Transactions on Acoustics, Speech and Signal Processing*, vol. 37, pp. 328–339, 1989. (Chapter 19)

[Wan90a]   E. A. Wan, "Temporal backpropagation for FIR neural networks," *IEEE International Joint Conference on Neural Networks*, vol. 1, pp. 575–580, San Diego, CA, 1990. (Chapter 19)

[Wan90b]   E. A. Wan, "Temporal backpropagation: An efficient algorithm for finite impulse response neural networks," in *Proceedings of the 1990 Connectionist Models Summer School*, D. S. Touretzky, J. L. Elman, T. J. Sejnowski and G. E. Hinton, eds., San Mateo, CA: Morgan Kaufmann, pp. 131–140, 1990. (Chapter 19)

[Wan94]   E. A. Wan, "Time series prediction by using a connectionist network with internal delay lines," in *Time Series Prediction: Forecasting the Future and Understanding the Past*, A. S. Weigend and N. A. Gershenfeld, eds., Reading, MA: Addison-Wesley, pp. 195–217, 1994. (Chapter 19)

[WeRu91]   A. S. Weigand, D. E. Rumelhart and B. A. Huberman, "Generalization by weight elimination with application to forecasting," in *Advances in Neural Information Processing Systems 3*, R. P. Lippman, J. E. Moody and D. J. Touretzky, eds., San Mateo, CA: Morgan Kaufmann, pp. 575–582, 1991. (Chapter 19)

[Werbo74]   P. J. Werbos, "Beyond regression: New tools for prediction and analysis in the behavioral sciences," Ph.D. Thesis, Harvard University, Cambridge, MA, 1974. Also published as *The Roots of Backpropagation*, New York: John Wiley & Sons, 1994. (Chapter 11)

[Werb90]   P. J. Werbos, "Backpropagation through time: What it is and how to do it," *Proceedings of the IEEE*, vol. 78, pp. 1550–1560, October 1990. (Chapter 19)

[WhSo92]   D. White and D. Sofge, eds., *Handbook of Intelligent Control*, New York:Van Nostrand Reinhold, 1992. (Chapter 4)

[WiHo60]   B. Widrow, M. E. Hoff, "Adaptive switching circuits,"*1960 IRE WESCON Convention Record*, New York: IRE Part 4, pp. 96–104, 1960. (Chapters 1, 10)

[WiSt 85]   B. Widrow and S. D. Stearns, *Adaptive Signal Processing*, Englewood Cliffs, NJ: Prentice-Hall, 1985. (Chapter 10)

[WiWi 88]   B. Widrow and R. Winter, "Neural nets for adaptive filtering and adaptive pattern recognition," *IEEE Computer Magazine*, March 1988, pp. 25–39. (Chapter 10)

[WiZi89]   R. J. Williams and D. Zipser, "A learning algorithm for continually running fully recurrent neural networks," *Neural Computation*, vol. 1, pp. 270–280, 1989. (Chapter 19)

A

B Notation

Basic Concepts

Scalars: small *italic* letters.....*a,b,c*

Vectors: small **bold** nonitalic letters.....**a,b,c**

Matrices: capital **BOLD** nonitalic letters.....**A,B,C**

Language

Vector means a column of numbers.

Row vector means a row of a matrix used as a vector (column).

General Vectors and Transformations (Chapters 5 and 6)

$$\chi = \mathcal{A}(y)$$

Weight Matrices

Scalar Element

$$w_{i,j}^{k}(t)$$

i - row, j - column, k - layer, t - time or iteration

Matrix

$$\mathbf{W}^{k}(t)$$

Column Vector

$$\mathbf{w}_{j}^{k}(t)$$

Row Vector

$$_{i}\mathbf{w}^{k}(t)$$

Bias Vector

Scalar Element

$$b_{i}^{k}(t)$$

Vector

$$\mathbf{b}^{k}(t)$$

Input Vector

Scalar Element

$$p_i(t)$$

As One of a Sequence of Input Vectors

$$\mathbf{p}(t)$$

As One of a Set of Input Vectors

$$\mathbf{p}_q$$

Net Input Vector

Scalar Element

$$n_i^k(t) \ \ \text{or} \ \ n_{i,q}^k$$

Vector

$$\mathbf{n}^k(t) \ \ \text{or} \ \ \mathbf{n}_q^k$$

Output Vector

Scalar Element

$$a_i^k(t) \ \ \text{or} \ \ a_{i,q}^k$$

Vector

$$\mathbf{a}^k(t) \ \ \text{or} \ \ \mathbf{a}_q^k$$

Transfer Function

Scalar Element

$$a_i^k = f^k(n_i^k)$$

Vector

$$\mathbf{a}^k = \mathbf{f}^k(\mathbf{n}^k)$$

Target Vector

Scalar Element

$$t_i(t) \ \ \text{or} \ \ t_{i,q}$$

Vector

$$\mathbf{t}\,(t) \ \text{ or } \ \mathbf{t}_q$$

Set of Prototype Input/Target Vectors

$$\{\mathbf{p}_1, \mathbf{t}_1\}, \{\mathbf{p}_2, \mathbf{t}_2\}, \dots, \{\mathbf{p}_Q, \mathbf{t}_Q\}$$

Error Vector

Scalar Element

$$e_i\,(t) \ = \ t_i\,(t) - a_i\,(t) \ \text{ or } \ e_{i,\,q} \ = \ t_{i,\,q} - a_{i,\,q}$$

Vector

$$\mathbf{e}\,(t) \ \text{ or } \ \mathbf{e}_q$$

Sizes and Dimensions

Number of Layers, Number of Neurons per Layer

$$M, S^k$$

Number of Input Vectors (and Targets), Dimension of Input Vector

$$Q, R$$

Parameter Vector (includes all weights and biases)

Vector

$$\mathbf{x}$$

At Iteration k

$$\mathbf{x}\,(k) \ \text{ or } \ \mathbf{x}_k$$

Norm

$$\|\mathbf{x}\|$$

Performance Index

$$F\,(\mathbf{x})$$

Gradient and Hessian

$$\nabla F\,(\mathbf{x}_k) \ = \ \mathbf{g}_k \ \text{ and } \ \nabla^2 F\,(\mathbf{x}_k) \ = \ \mathbf{A}_k$$

B

Parameter Vector Change

$$\Delta \mathbf{x}_k = \mathbf{x}_{k+1} - \mathbf{x}_k$$

Eigenvalue and Eigenvector

$$\lambda_i \text{ and } \mathbf{z}_i$$

Approximate Performance Index (single time step)

$$\hat{F}(\mathbf{x})$$

Transfer Function Derivative

Scalar

$$\dot{f}(n) = \frac{d}{dn}f(n)$$

Matrix

$$\dot{\mathbf{F}}^m(\mathbf{n}^m) = \begin{bmatrix} \dot{f}^m(n_1^m) & 0 & \dots & 0 \\ 0 & \dot{f}^m(n_2^m) & \dots & 0 \\ \vdots & \vdots & & \vdots \\ 0 & 0 & \dots & \dot{f}^m(n_{S^m}^m) \end{bmatrix}$$

Jacobian Matrix

$$\mathbf{J}(\mathbf{x})$$

Approximate Hessian Matrix

$$\mathbf{H} = \mathbf{J}^T\mathbf{J}$$

Sensitivity Vector

Scalar Element

$$s_i^m \equiv \frac{\partial \hat{F}}{\partial n_i^m}$$

Vector

$$\mathbf{s}^m \equiv \frac{\partial \hat{F}}{\partial \mathbf{n}^m}$$

Marquardt Sensitivity Matrix

Scalar Element

$$\tilde{s}_{i,h}^{m} \equiv \frac{\partial v_h}{\partial n_{i,q}^{m}} = \frac{\partial e_{k,q}}{\partial n_{i,q}^{m}}$$

Partial Matrix (single input vector $\mathbf{p}_q$) and Full Matrix (all inputs)

$$\tilde{\mathbf{S}}_{q}^{m} \text{ and } \tilde{\mathbf{S}}^{m} = \left[\tilde{\mathbf{S}}_{1}^{m} \ \tilde{\mathbf{S}}_{2}^{m} \ ... \ \tilde{\mathbf{S}}_{Q}^{m} \right]$$

Parameters for Backpropagation and Variations

Learning Rate and Momentum
α and γ

Learning Rate Increase, Decrease and Percentage Change
η , ρ and ζ

Conjugate Gradient Direction Adjustment Parameter
β_k

Marquardt Parameters
μ and ϑ

Feature Map Terms

Distance Between Neurons
d_{ij} - distance between neuron i and neuron j

Neighborhood
$N_i(d) = \{j, d_{ij} \leq d\}$

Grossberg and ART Networks

On-Center and Off-Surround Connection Matrices

$$^{+}\mathbf{W}^{1} = \begin{bmatrix} 1 & 0 & \cdots & 0 \\ 0 & 1 & \cdots & 0 \\ \vdots & \vdots & & \vdots \\ 0 & 0 & \cdots & 1 \end{bmatrix} \text{ and } ^{-}\mathbf{W}^{1} = \begin{bmatrix} 0 & 1 & \cdots & 1 \\ 1 & 0 & \cdots & 1 \\ \vdots & \vdots & & \vdots \\ 1 & 1 & \cdots & 0 \end{bmatrix}$$

B

Excitatory and Inhibitory Biases

$${}^{+}\mathbf{b} \text{ and } {}^{-}\mathbf{b}$$

Time Constant

$$\varepsilon$$

Relative Intensity

$$\bar{p}_i = \frac{p_i}{P} \text{ where } P = \sum_{j=1}^{S^1} p_j$$

Instar and Outstar Weight Matrices

$$\mathbf{W}^{1:2} \text{ and } \mathbf{W}^{2:1}$$

Orienting Subsystem Parameters

$$\alpha, \beta \text{ and } \rho = \frac{\alpha}{\beta} \text{ (vigilance)}$$

ART1 Learning Law Parameter

$$\zeta$$

Lyapunov Stability

Lyapunov Function

$$V(\mathbf{a})$$

Zero Derivative Set, Largest Invariant Set and Closure

$$Z, L \text{ and } L^\circ$$

Bounded Lyapunov Function Set

$$\Omega_\eta = \{\mathbf{a} : V(\mathbf{a}) < \eta\}$$

Hopfield Network Parameters

Circuit Parameters

$$T_{i,j}, C, R_i, I_i, \rho$$

Amplifier Gain

$$\gamma$$

C 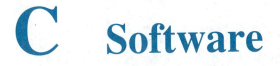 Software

Introduction

We have used MATLAB, a numeric computation and visualization software package, in this text. However, MATLAB is not essential for using this book. The computer exercises can performed with any available programming language, and the *Neural Network Design Demonstrations*, while helpful, are not critical to understanding the material covered in this book.

MATLAB is widely available and, because of its matrix/vector notation and graphics, is a convenient environment in which to experiment with neural networks. We use MATLAB in two different ways. First, we have included a number of exercises for the reader to perform in MATLAB. Many of the important features of neural networks become apparent only for large scale problems, which are computationally intensive and not feasible for hand calculations. With MATLAB, neural network algorithms can be quickly implemented, and large scale problems can be tested conveniently. If MATLAB is not available, any other programming language can be used to perform the exercises.

The second way in which we use MATLAB is through the *Neural Network Design Demonstrations*, which are on a disk included with this book. These interactive demonstrations illustrate important concepts in each chapter. The icon to the left identifies references to these demonstrations in the text.

MATLAB version 4.0 or later, or the student edition of MATLAB version 4.0, should be installed on your hard drive in a directory (for a DOS machine) or a folder (for a Macintosh) named MATLAB. To create this directory or folder and complete the installation process, follow the instructions given in the MATLAB documentation. Take care to follow the guidelines given for setting the path. A few of the demonstrations require the MathWorks' *Neural Network Toolbox* 1.0 or later.

After the software has been loaded into the MATLAB directory on your computer, it can be invoked by typing **nnd** at the MATLAB prompt. All demonstrations are easily accessible from a master menu.

This book is accompanied by 58 demonstrations that can be run from within MATLAB.

Overview of Demonstration Files

The demonstration files consist of two directories, NNDESIGN and MININNET. The first directory NNDESIGN contains all the demonstrations and functions that the demonstrations use.

The second directory MININNET contains a few key functions borrowed from the *Neural Network Toolbox* (NNT). These functions allow many of the demonstrations to run without the Toolbox. However, you should only install this directory if you do not have the NNT. Having both the Toolbox and the MININNET directory installed may result in unpredictable results due to multiple versions of the borrowed functions.

Demo Requirements

Many of the demonstrations do not require either the MININNET directory or the *Neural Network Toolbox*. Some functions require either the MININNET directory or the Toolbox, and a few require the Toolbox.

The last section of this appendix lists all the demonstrations and indicates the requirements for each. You can see the same list from within MATLAB by typing `help nndesign` after installing the NNDESIGN directory.

Running the Demonstrations

You can run the demonstrations directly by typing their names at the MATLAB prompt. Typing `help nndesign` brings up a list of all the demos you can choose from.

Alternatively, you can run the Neural Network Design splash window (`nnd`) and then click the Contents button. This will take you to a graphical Table of Contents. From there you can select chapters with buttons at the bottom of the window and individual demonstrations with popup menus.

Sound

Many of the demonstrations use sound. In many cases the sound adds to the understanding of a demonstration. In other cases it is there simply for fun. If you need to turn the sound off you can give MATLAB the following command and all demonstrations will run quietly:

`nnsound off`

To turn sound back on:

`nnsound on`

You may note that demonstrations that utilize sound often run faster when sound is off. In addtion, on some machines which do not support sound errors can occur unless the sound is turned off.

List of Demonstrations

Many of the demonstrations are followed by one of two symbols to indicate the resources required to run them:

+ Requires either MININNET functions or the *Neural Network Toolbox*.

* Requires the *Neural Network Toolbox*.

General

> nnd - Splash screen.
> nndtoc - Table of contents.
> nnsound - Turn Neural Network Design sounds on and off.

Chapter 2, Neuron Model and Network Architectures

> nnd2n1 - One-input neuron demonstration.+
> nnd2n2 - Two-input neuron demonstration.+

Chapter 3, An Illustrative Example

> nnd3pc - Perceptron classification demonstration.+
> nnd3hamc - Hamming classification demonstration.+
> nnd3hopc - Hopfield classification demonstration.+

Chapter 4, Perceptron Learning Rule

> nnd4db - Decision boundaries demonstration.+
> nnd4pr - Perceptron rule demonstration.+

Chapter 5, Signal and Weight Vector Spaces

> nnd5gs - Gram-Schmidt demonstration.
> nnd5rb - Reciprocal basis demonstration.

Chapter 6, Linear Transformations for Neural Networks

> nnd6lt - Linear transformations demonstration.
> nnd6eg - Eigenvector game.

Chapter 7, Supervised Hebbian Learning

> nnd7sh - Supervised Hebb demonstration.

Chapter 8, Performance Surfaces and Optimum Points

> nnd8ts1 - Taylor series demonstration #1.
> nnd8ts2 - Taylor series demonstration #2.
> nnd8dd - Directional derivatives demonstration.
> nnd8qf - Quadratic function demonstration.

C

Chapter 9, Performance Optimization

nnd9sdq - Steepest descent for quadratic function demonstration.
nnd9mc - Method comparison demonstration.
nnd9nm - Newton's method demonstration.
nnd9sd - Steepest descent demonstration.

Chapter 10, Widrow-Hoff Learning

nnd10nc - Adaptive noise cancellation demonstration.
nnd10eeg - Electroencephalogram noise cancellation demonstration.
nnd10lc - Linear pattern classification demonstration.

Chapter 11, Backpropagation

nnd11nf - Network function demonstration.+
nnd11bc - Backpropagation calculation demonstration.*
nnd11fa - Function approximation demonstration.*
nnd11gn - Generalization demonstration.*

Chapter 12, Variations on Backpropagation

nnd12sd1- Steepest descent backpropagation demonstration #1.*
nnd12sd2 - Steepest descent backpropagation demonstration #2.*
nnd12mo - Momentum backpropagation demonstration.*
nnd12vl - Variable learning rate backpropagation demonstration.*
nnd12ls - Conjugate gradient line search demonstration.*
nnd12cg - Conjugate gradient backpropagation demonstration.*
nnd12ms - Maquardt step demonstration.*
nnd12m - Marquardt backpropagation demonstration.*

Chapter 13, Associative Learning

nnd13uh - Unsupervised Hebb demonstration.+
nnd13hd - Hebb with decay demonstration.+
nnd13edr - Effect of decay rate demonstration.+
nnd13gis - Graphical instar demonstration.+
nnd13is - Instar demonstration.+
nnd13os - Outstar demonstration.+

Chapter 14, Competitive Networks

nnd14cc - Competitive classification demonstration.+
nnd14cl - Competitive learning demonstration.+
nnd14fm1 - 1-D feature map demonstration.*
nnd14fm2 - 2-D feature map demonstration.*
nnd14lv1 - LVQ1 demonstration.*
nnd14lv2 - LVQ2 demonstration.*

Chapter 15, Grossberg Network

nnd15li - Leaky integrator demonstration.
nnd15sn - Shunting network demonstration.
nnd15gl1 - Grossberg layer 1 demonstration.
nnd15gl2 - Grossberg layer 2 demonstration.
nnd15aw - Adaptive weights demonstration.

Chapter 16, Adaptive Resonance Theory

nnd16al1 - ART1 layer 1 demonstration.
nnd16al2 - ART1 layer 2 demonstration.
nnd16os - Orienting subsystem demonstration.
nnd16a1 - ART1 algorithm.

Chapter 17, Stability

nnd17ds - Dynamical system demonstration.

Chapter 18, Hopfield Network

nnd18hn - Hopfield network demonstration.

Index